To the children I work with
who make my job really a joy.

FIFTH EDITION

Articulation and Phonology in Speech Sound Disorders

A Clinical Focus

Jacqueline Bauman-Waengler

Speech-Language Specialist, Pleasant Valley School District

Camarillo, California

PEARSON

Boston   Columbus   Indianapolis   New York   San Francisco   Hoboken
Amsterdam   Cape Town   Dubai   London   Madrid   Milan   Munich   Paris   Montréal   Toronto
Delhi   Mexico City   São Paulo   Sydney   Hong Kong   Seoul   Singapore   Taipei   Tokyo

Vice President and Editorial Director: Jeffery W. Johnston
Executive Editor: Ann Castel Davis
Editorial Assistant: Janelle Criner
Executive Field Marketing Manager: Krista Clark
Senior Product Marketing Manager: Christopher Barry
Project Manager: Kerry Rubadue
Program Program Manager: Joe Sweeney
Operations Specialist: Deidra Skahill
Text Designer: Jouve

Cover Design Director: Diane Ernsberger
Media Producer: Autumn Benson
Media Project Manager: Tammy Walters
Full-Service Project Management: Jouve
Composition: Jouve
Printer/Binder: Edwards Brothers Malloy Jackson Road
Cover Printer: Edwards Brothers Malloy Jackson Road
Text Font: 10/12 Charis SIL Regular

Library of Congress Cataloging-in-Publication Data
Bauman-Wängler, Jacqueline Ann, author.
  [Articulatory and phonological impairments]
  Articulation and phonology in speech sound disorders : a clinical focus / Jacqueline Bauman-Waengler. – Fifth edition.
    p. ; cm.
  Preceded by Articulatory and phonological impairments / Jacqueline Bauman-Waengler. 4th ed. c2012.
  Includes bibliographical references and indexes.
  ISBN 978-0-13-381037-0—ISBN 0-13-381037-2
    I. Title.
  [DNLM: 1. Articulation Disorders.   2. Phonetics. WL 340.2]
  RC424.7
  616.85'5—dc23

                                                                              2014043309

10 9 8 7 6 5 4 3 2 1

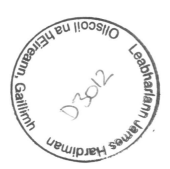

Loose Leaf Version ISBN 10: 0-13- 394891-9
ISBN 13: 978-0-13-394891-2

E-text ISBN 10: 0-13-404192-5
ISBN 13: 978-0-13-404192-6

Package ISBN 10: 0-13-409262-7
ISBN 13: 978-0-13-409262-1

Traditional Book ISBN 10: 0-13-381037-2
ISBN 13: 978-0-13-381037-0

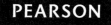

About the Author

JACQUELINE BAUMAN-WAENGLER has been a professor for more than 25 years. Her main teaching and clinical emphases are phonetics and phonology, including disorders of articulation and phonology in children and child language disorders. She has published and presented widely in these areas both nationally and internationally. In addition to the fifth edition of *Articulation and Phonology in Speech Sound Disorders: A Clinical Focus*, Bauman-Waengler has also published *Introduction to Phonetics and Phonology: From Concepts to Transcription* (2009) with Pearson. She is currently working as a speech/language specialist for Pleasant Valley School District (Camarillo, California).

Preface

The concept for this book grew out of a perceived need to create a bridge between theoretical issues in speech-language pathology and their clinical application. The goal for the fifth edition has remained the same: to tie strong academic foundations directly to clinical applications. To this end, every chapter contains suggestions for clinical practice as well as clinical examples and clinical applications. These features will assist the reader in developing an understanding of how basic concepts and theoretical knowledge form the core for clinical decision making in the assessment and remediation of speech disorders. Learning aids located at the end of every chapter include case studies, further readings, critical thinking, and multiple-choice questions.

New to This Edition

The fifth edition of *Articulation and Phonology in Speech Sound Disorders: A Clinical Focus* has several significant changes.

- *A modified title.* The title has changed somewhat to reflect the current use of "speech sound disorders," which is a new umbrella term that is critical to the field of articulation- and phonemic-based speech disorders.

- *Expanded topics of study.* In our constantly changing population, far more clinicians are dealing directly with individuals with varying dialects and children/adults who speak English as a second language. This edition includes updated research that reflects the changing landscape of the field, including expanded coverage on phoneme information in dialects in the United States as well as the needs of learners of English as a second language.

- *New clinical exercises.* This text includes a number of new, revised, or expanded clinical exercises to allow the student to master theoretical concepts by applying them to real-life situations. The eText edition of this text also contains embedded videos that can be used in conjunction with these clinical exercises, allowing for additional analysis or transcription opportunities.

- *Refined chapter organization.* A new chapter order has been developed so that Chapter 7 on Diagnosis now follows Chapter 6 on Assessment: Appraisal—Collection of Data. This change has been made to aid in the flow of concepts.

- *Categorical learning objectives.* These have been fine-tuned in each chapter so that the reader begins each chapter with a set of easily identifiable goals for his or learning. Each set of learning objectives provide the scaffolding to prepare readers for tests and quizzes and compartmentalize key concepts.

- *Chapter 1.* This has been revised to include a section on phonotactics of General American English. In addition, Chapter 1 reviews the most recent guidelines and definitions of the American Speech-Language-Hearing Association (ASHA) for establishing communication, language, articulation, and what is now considered to be "speech sound disorders." These definitions provide a more basic foundation for understanding later concepts, and the guidelines will be helpful in later clinical practice.

- *Chapter 8.* This chapter outlines several new features pertaining to dialects and English as a second language. First, Appalachian and Ozark English are detailed and contrasted. Second, the statistics on limited English proficient students have been updated, and new content on the Filipino/Tagalog phonemic system has been added. It is one of the five most frequently spoken languages by limited English proficient students.
- *Chapter 10.* The treatment of phonemic-based speech sound disorders has been expanded to include the concepts of the matrix for predicting phonological generalization. This concept is a radical departure from the traditional, phonetic-based treatment approaches and has much to offer children with a severe speech sound disorder.
- *Chapter 11.* This chapter is devoted to disorders that are traditionally considered speech sound disorders. Although a summary of assessment and remediation procedures appears in the text, each section contains updated references to lead the reader to additional possibilities.
- *Updated references.* References in each chapter have been updated to reflect the most recent research in the field.
- *The new DSM-5.* The nomenclature in this book reflects DSM-5 updates.

The eText edition of this text offers interactive digital features, including

- *Digital functionality.* The digital eText version of this title provides interactive tools to enhance students' experience with the material, including tools that allow students to search the text, make notes online, print important activities, and bookmark passages for later review.
- *Video links in each chapter.* Videos have been added to the eText edition. They give students an inside look at the world of communication disorders. These videos, chosen specifically for this text, illustrate critical concepts in easily digestible 2- to 3-minute clips.

  Videos in each chapter offer opportunities for students to transcribe words and sounds in children and adults that demonstrate multiple dialects and disorders. Additionally, students are exposed to real-life speech therapy lessons and dynamic interviews with professionals who specialize in articulation and phonology.

- *Linked glossary.* Key terms throughout the text are linked, giving students one-click access to crucial definitions.

Instructor's Resource Manual

To help instructors in preparing their courses, we have provided an Instructor's Resource Manual. This supplement is available online or can be obtained by contacting a Pearson sales representative. To download and print the Instructor's Resource Manual, go to www.pearsonhighered.com and then click on "Educators."

Acknowledgments

Preparing the fifth edition—as with previous editions—might appear at first to be a simple process but actually was a large time investment supported by many people. First, I would like to acknowledge Ann Davis who is the editor of this fifth edition; Joe Sweeney, program manager; John Shannon, project manager; and Jon Theiss, digital development editor. They have all been supportive and helpful as I have proceeded through this, at times, daunting task. A special thank you to Jon Theiss, digital development editor, who has really been patient with my struggles to prepare this edition for an enhanced eText version. Also thanks to Sharynne McLeod, PhD, Professor in Speech and Language Acquisition, Charles Sturt University, Australia, for responding to many questions and being a true colleague.

For this edition, I would like to say a special thanks to my reviewers: Stephen N. Calculator; University of New Hampshire; Toni B. Morehouse, University of Nebraska; and Steven Long, Marquette University. I hope that you can recognize many of the wonderful suggestions that guided me through these revisions.

Brief Contents

Contents

CHAPTER **6** Assessment and Appraisal: Collection of Data   143

CHAPTER **7** Diagnosis: Articulation- versus Phonemic-Based Speech Sound Disorders   177

Clinical Framework

Basic Terms and Concepts

LEARNING OBJECTIVES

When you have finished this chapter, you should be able to:

- Define communication, language, and speech.
- Define phonology, morphology, syntax, semantics, and pragmatics.
- Define communication disorder, speech disorder, and language disorder.
- Distinguish between articulation—articulation disorder, speech sound—speech sound disorder, phoneme—phonological disorders.

- Delineate phoneme and allophone.
- Compare and contrast terms that are used clinically and in research such as phonological disorder, speech sound disorder, speech delay, speech impairment, and residual speech sound disorder, for example.

Communication, Speech, and Language

Communication is central to our lives. We communicate in a number of ways—from text messaging to facial expressions. Simply defined, communication is the process of sharing information between individuals (Pence & Justice, 2008). When we think about the diversified population that we encounter within the discipline of communication disorders, a broader definition might be helpful. **Communication** is a process that consists of two or more people sharing information including facts, thoughts, ideas, and feelings. Early communication includes how to interact with other people and things, how to understand spoken language, and how to exchange information with others using gestures or symbols. Communication does not have to involve language and does not have to be vocalized (Justice & Redle, 2014; National Joint Committee for the Communicative Needs of Persons with Severe Disabilities, 2010). Deaf people communicate through gestures; babies communicate basic wants through crying. Communication refers to any way that we convey information from one person to another. For example, we use e-mail, text messaging, or phone calls as ways to communicate. In addition, smiling, waving, or raising your eyebrows at a comment are all examples of nonverbal communication. Sign languages, such as American Sign Language or Seeing Essential English, are nonverbal conventional linguistic systems used to communicate.

The most widely used means of communication is speech. **Speech** is the communication or expression of thoughts in spoken words, that is, in oral, verbal communication. Speech can be further divided into *articulation*, the motor production of speech sounds, *fluency*, the flow of speaking including rate and rhythm, and *voice* including vocal quality, pitch, loudness, and resonance (American Speech-Language-Hearing Association, 1993). The term *speech* is employed in various ways. Speech can be a more formal, spoken communication to an audience. For example: *Having to give a speech to her class was always frightening for Andrea.* Speech can indicate a manner of speaking: *Her speech was marked by a distinct Australian accent.* Speech is also used together with the term *language* to indicate the mental faculty of verbal communication: *The child's speech and language skills were tested as a portion of the diagnostic.* Based on this last example, it seems important to differentiate between speech and language. What are the distinctions between these two terms: *speech* versus *language*?

According to the American Speech-Language Hearing Association, **language** can be defined as a complex and dynamic system of conventional symbols that is used in various modes for thought and communication (American Speech-Language-Hearing Association Committee on Language, 1983). Among other variables, this definition further states that language is rule governed and is described by at least five linguistic parameters: phonological, morphological, syntactic, semantic, and pragmatic. Language is intricate and includes variability and change. In addition, all members of a language agree on the symbolic system that is used, and language is used to communicate in a variety of ways.

Within our definition of language are the terms *phonology*, *morphology*, *syntax*, *semantics*, and *pragmatics*. A brief definition of these words should be helpful in our understanding of language. One of these parameters, phonology, is of major importance in this text.

Subdivisions of Language

Phonology is the study of the sound system of language and includes the rules that govern its spoken form (Parker & Riley, 2010). Therefore, phonology analyzes which sound units are within a language. The sound system of English contains different vowels and consonants than that of Spanish, for example. Phonology also examines how these sounds are arranged, their systematic organization, and rule system. According to the English phonological rule system, no more than three consonants can be at the beginning of a syllable or word, such as in "street." In addition, certain consonant sounds cannot be arranged together. For example, an "sp" combination is acceptable in English ("spot" or "wasp"), whereas a "pf" cluster is not.

Another area of language is morphology. **Morphology** studies the structure of words; it analyzes how words can be divided into parts labeled *morphemes* (Crystal, 2010), each of which has an independent meaning. A **morpheme** is the smallest meaningful unit of a language. The word "cycle" is one morpheme meaning circular or wheel; however, the word "bicycle" contains two morphemes, "bi-" and "cycle," "bi" indicating two. In American English, plurality is often noted with the addition of an "s," such as "book" – "books," and "ed" can demonstrate past tense as in "cooked" or "talked." All of these units, "cycle," "bi-," "book" "-s," "cook," "talk," and "-ed" are morphemes of American English.

The third area of language is syntax. **Syntax** consists of organizational rules denoting word, phrase, and clause order; sentence organization and the relationship between words; word classes; and other sentence elements (Owens, 2008). We know that certain sentences, for example, are syntactically appropriate, such as "I really like to eat chocolate." or even "Chocolate, I really like to eat." However, a sentence such as "I eat like to really chocolate." would not be an acceptable sentence of American English. Within communication disorders, we examine the development of syntactical structures in children as well as the problems that certain populations, such as students learning English as a second language, might have when expressing themselves in complex syntactical sentences.

Semantics is the study of linguistic meaning and includes the meaning of words, phrases, and sentences (Parker & Riley, 2010). Semantics includes the fact that certain words have more than one meaning, such as "bat," and that words can have similar meanings, for example, "dog" and "canine." Also certain words share more or less common characteristics. "Cat," "dog," and "hamster" have certain commonalities, whereas "dog" and "boy" have properties that could be compared but seem not as related as the first three words. Semantics also includes phrase meanings as in the multiple interpretations of "a hot dog" and sentence meaning as in "She dressed and washed the baby."

The last term, **pragmatics**, refers to the study of language used to communicate within various situational contexts. Pragmatics includes, among other things, the reasons for talking, conversational skills, and the flexibility to modify speech for different listeners and social situations (Paul, 2007). Included in pragmatics would be the understanding that we talk differently to small children versus older adults; that certain situations typically dictate how and what we say (such as the communication in an interview will be quite different from a night out with your friends); and that we use certain facial expressions, body gestures, and word emphases to communicate very different meanings. For example, think of the sentence "Last night was really something" said with a smile and positive head nods versus the same sentence said with a scowl, negative head movements, and a different emphasis on "really." Within communication disorders, pragmatics may become a central issue when working with autistic children, for example. See Figure 1.1 for an overview of the divisions of communication.

To summarize, communication is the process of sharing information between/among individuals. Communication can be broadly divided into speech and language. Speech is the expression of thoughts in spoken words; it is oral, verbal communication. On the other hand, language is a complex, dynamic, and

> ## CLINICAL EXERCISES
>
> List two types of morphological endings that a child who deletes "s" at the end of a word might have difficulties with.
>
> The teacher refers a child to you from first grade. Based on an informal language sample, what could you analyze to examine each of the areas of language: phonology, morphology, syntax, semantics, and pragmatics?

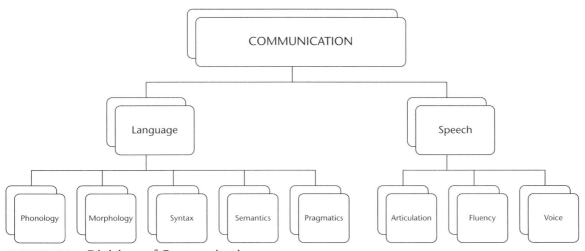

FIGURE 1.1 Divisions of Communication

Watch the following video of 4-year-old Ben and try to make comments about each of the following areas: phonology, morphology, syntax, semantics, and pragmatics.

rule-based system of conventional symbols that is used in diverse modalities for thought and communication. However, as practitioners, we deal with communication, speech, and language *disorders*. What characteristics would a disordered system demonstrate?

According to the 1993 guidelines of the American Speech-Language-Hearing Association (ASHA), a **communication disorder** is the impairment in the ability to receive, send, process, and comprehend concepts including verbal, nonverbal, and graphic symbol systems. In addition to hearing disorders, communication disorders are categorized into speech and language disorders. A **speech disorder** is used to indicate oral, verbal communication that is so deviant from the norm that it is noticeable or interferes with communication. Speech disorders are divided into articulation, fluency, and voice disorders. On the other hand, a **language disorder** is impaired comprehension and/or use of spoken, written, and/or other symbol systems. A language disorder may involve one or more of the following areas: phonology, morphology, syntax, semantics, and pragmatics. See Figure 1.2 for the subdivisions of communication disorders.

According to this classification, an impairment of the articulation of speech sounds is one example of a speech disorder. To understand this definition, it would be important to examine the terms *articulation* and *speech sounds*. In clinical practice, important distinctions are made between articulation and speech sounds versus phonology and phonemes. The following section defines and gives examples of how these words are used in our clinical practice within communication disorders.

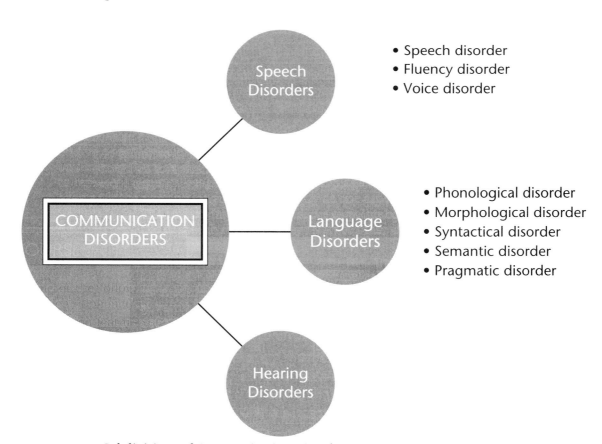

FIGURE 1.2 Subdivisions of Communication Disorders

Articulation and Speech Sounds: Phonology and Phonemes

The term *articulation* and its derivations are often used to describe an individual's speech. They might appear in a referral statement or within a diagnostic report; for example:

> Sandy was referred to the clinic because her parents were concerned about her *articulation* skills.
>
> Bob could *articulate* the sound correctly in isolation but not in word contexts.
>
> Joe's *articulation* disorder affected his speech intelligibility.

For the purpose at hand, **articulation** refers to the totality of motor movements involved in production of the actual sounds that comprise speech (Bauman-Waengler, 2009). The learning of articulatory skills is a developmental process involving the gradual acquisition of the ability to move the *articulators* (those structures that are important in forming the individual sounds) in a precise and rapid manner. Thus, *learning to articulate is a specific kind of motor learning.* Just as children become more adept at certain motor skills as they grow older, their articulation skills develop as well. For example, we do not expect the same level of articulatory abilities from a 2-year-old child as from a 6-year-old. Second, the definition suggests that errors in articulation result from relatively peripheral disturbances of these articulatory processes. Thus, the peripheral motor processes involved in the planning and execution of articulation are impaired; the central language capabilities of the individual remain intact. In summary, articulation is a specific, gradually developing motor skill that involves mainly peripheral motor processes.

Speech sounds are central units in any discussion of disordered speech. Although the human vocal tract is capable of producing a wide array of sounds, including coughing and burping, speech sounds are special sounds because they are associated with speech. **Speech sounds** represent physical sound realities; they are end products of articulatory motor processes. When talking about a child's s-production in the context of an articulation test, for example, we refer to the *speech sound* production of [s].

Speech sounds then are real, physical sound entities used in speech. But in addition to their *articulatory form*, they also have a linguistic function. *Linguistic function* includes, for example, the rules that address how specific sound units can be arranged to produce appropriate words and the phoneme concept. A **phoneme** is the smallest linguistic unit that is able, when combined with other such units, to distinguish meaning between words (Small, 2012). For example, "tick" has three phonemes /t/, /ɪ/, and /k/. We know that these are phonemes of American English because the word they form is meaningful. In contrast, /s/ is also a phoneme of American English as can be seen in "sick," /s/, /ɪ/, /k/, which differs from "tick" in one phoneme: /t/ versus /s/. As far as notation is concerned, speech sound productions are usually placed within brackets in phonetic transcription, whereas phoneme values are symbolized by slanted lines, or virgules. For example, [s] indicates that it was a sound someone actually pronounced in a specific manner. On the other hand, /s/ signifies the phoneme "s."

The idea of the phoneme is considered to be an abstraction. A phoneme is not a single, concrete, unchanging entity. A phoneme is an abstraction that is based on the many variations that occur for a particular sound because it is heard in differing contexts of conversational speech. This does not necessarily make the phoneme concept complex or difficult to understand. We constantly deal with abstractions. Take, for example, the concept "cat." A cat is not a single, unchanging entity. There are big cats and small cats, cats that are striped or solid colored of various shades. However, there are certain characteristics that we accept as being typical to the concept of "cat." We could say that the *cat concept* embraces a whole family of units that are related yet somehow are distinct.

Even two cats of the same size, color, and build will have slight variations that could be detected most certainly by the owners. If we apply this to the phoneme concept, we find a similar abstraction. So when we speak of a particular phoneme, /t/ for example, we are referring to the typical "t" but we also take into consideration the varieties of "t" that are used in various contexts and by different speakers. The term *allophone* is used to refer to the changes that occur in a phoneme when produced by speakers in differing contexts. **Allophones** are variations in phoneme realizations that do not change the meaning of a word when they are produced in differing contexts. Allophones are phonetic variations of a phoneme (Crystal, 2010). Within the phonological system of American English, there are many examples of allophones.

Several allophonic variations can occur with the /p/ phoneme, for example. At the beginning of a word as a single sound unit, /p/ is typically aspirated. Aspiration is that slight puff of air that you hear if you pronounce the word "pie" or "pot." This is transcribed as [pʰ], the small raised ʰ representing the puff of air or aspiration in phonetic transcription. However, /p/ is typically unaspirated following "s" as in "spy" or "spot," for example. If you pronounce these words, you will find that the puff of air, the aspiration that you noticed in "pie," is not present. However, these allophonic variations exemplified by aspiration or lack of aspiration do not have phonemic value within the phonological system of American English. In other words, we can hear these differences, but both aspirated and unaspirated p-sounds are considered one phoneme, /p/.

Phonology is the study of how phonemes are organized and function in a language. Phonology includes the inventory of phonemes of the language in question, thus a list of all the vowels and consonants that function in American English to differentiate meaning. However, phonology also focuses on how these phonemes are *organized* to convey meaning within a language system. Such a description would include how the phonemes can and cannot be arranged to form meaningful words. **Phonotactics** refers to the description of the allowed combinations of phonemes in a particular language. A more complete discussion of the phonotactics of American English will be presented in Chapter 2.

If one wants to refer to the physical reality, to the actual production, the term *speech sound* is used. From early to contemporary publications, such phoneme realizations have also been labeled **phonetic variations**. Speech sounds or phonetic variations can be

---

CLINICAL EXERCISES

Examples are given of allophonic variations with /p/. Can you think of similar allophonic variations with /t/ and /k/?

Say the word "leap" and then the word "cool" slowly. Concentrate on the production of [l]. Do you notice any differences between the first and the second [l] production? These two different productions are termed light "l" (leap) and dark "l" (cool) to denote the different types of productions. Discuss why this would be an allophonic variation in American English. In Russian, these two types of [l] productions have phonemic value.

Phonotactics of General American English include the fact that some phoneme combinations do not occur in American English words. An example would be /ʃ/ + /v/. General American English does have other /ʃ/ combinations, such as /ʃ/ + /r/ (e.g., shrink) or /ʃ/ + /t/ (e.g., wished). The /ʃ/ + /v/ combination does, however, occur in the phonological system of German. Words such as *Schwester* (/ʃvɛstəR/ "sister") document this as a *phonotactic* possibility in German.

Phonotactics also restricts some consonant clusters occurring in General American English to their use in certain word positions, for example, the clusters /sk/ and /ks/. Words or syllables can begin or end with /sk/ (e.g., *skate, risk*), however, this is not the case with /ks/. This cluster can occur only at the end of a syllable or word (e.g., *kicks*). This is a *phonotactic* characteristic of the phonological system of General American English.

TABLE I.I   Phoneme versus Speech Sound

Phoneme	Speech Sound
The smallest unit within a language that is able, when combined with other units, to establish word meanings and distinguish between them	Actual realizations of phonemes; referred to as *allophonic variations* or *phonetic variations*
Linguistic unit, an abstraction	Concrete, produced, transmitted, and perceived
Used in reference to a particular language system	Can be examined without referring to a specific language system
Basic unit within phonology	Basic unit within phonetics
Notation is within virgules / / (e.g., "the /s/ phoneme")	Notation is within brackets (e.g., "the [f] speech sound")

examined without reference to a given language system. This is not the case with phonemes. When using the term *phoneme,* we refer exclusively to the function of the sound in question: to its ability to signify differences in word meaning within a *specific* language (see Table 1.1). Two words that differ in only one phoneme value are called **minimal pairs**. Examples of minimal pairs are *dog* versus *log* and *dog* versus *dot.*

How do these terms relate to our clinical decision making? Speech sounds as end products of articulatory motor processes are the units we are describing when we use phonetic transcription to capture an individual's actual productions on an articulation test or spontaneous speech sample. Speech sounds and speech sound errors relate to articulatory deviations. However, what if we notice that a child's productions of *swing, sing, ring,* and *wing* all sound the same, for example, that they all sound like *wing*? The child is not using the necessary phonemic contrasts to signal differences between these words. Both listener and speaker will probably not be able to differentiate between these words because they sound identical. Now we are analyzing the child's phoneme system, the child's ability to use phonemes to establish and distinguish between word meanings. If this occurs consistently throughout the child's speech, we could conclude that the child's phoneme system is limited—that is, restricted when compared to the norm. Difficulties in using phonemes contrastively to distinguish meanings relate to *linguistic* abilities, to the individual's phonological system as one subcategory of language.

Speech sounds, then, are related to our motor, articulatory skills. On the other hand, phonemes represent our understanding of the phonological system of our particular language. Table 1.1 summarizes the differences between the phoneme and speech sound. Moving a step further, what would constitute an articulation disorder versus a phonological disorder? The next section defines each of these terms and provides clinical examples.

Speech Sound Disorders: Articulation and Phonological Disorders

Depending on the age of the child, most make some sound errors as they learn to say new words. A **speech sound disorder** occurs when difficulties making certain sounds continue past a certain age. Every sound has a different range of ages when a child should produce the sound accurately. If an individual's articulation deviates significantly from the norm, it may be diagnosed as an **articulation disorder**. An *articulation disorder*, as a subcategory of a speech disorder, is the atypical production of speech sounds characterized by substitutions, omissions, additions, or distortions that may interfere with intelligibility (American Speech-Language-Hearing Association, 2014). Articulation errors are typically

According to ASHA (2008), the term *phonological disorder* is a subset of a language disorder. In a different document, which is information for the public, ASHA states that a speech sound disorder includes problems with articulation (making sounds) **and** phonological processes (sound patterns) (2014). It appears that the present nomenclature has shifted slightly to include phonological difficulties under the category of speech sound disorders. This can be aptly summarized by Strand & McCauley (2008), who state that the term *phonological disorder* is used to refer to the entire range of developmental communication disorders in which sound production is primarily affected. In addition they add that more recently this broad range of disorders is referred to as *speech sound disorders*. However, this usage reserves the term *phonological disorders* to refer to a linguistic level of impairment. For the purpose at hand, these terms will be separated with the understanding that both terms could be under a broad terminological umbrella of speech sound disorder.

classified relative to a child's age, which translates into stages within this developmental process. Younger children are at an earlier stage in this development, whereas older children are at a later stage or may have completed the process. Depending on the age of the child, certain articulation errors may be considered to be typical (age-appropriate errors) or atypical (non–age-appropriate errors). When assessing an individual, we often gather information on the inventory of speech sounds used. The phonetic inventory is a list of all the speech sounds including their variations.

On the other hand, the term *phonology* is basic to the understanding of phonological disorders. When an individual's phonology deviates enough from the norm, this could lead to a phonological disorder. A **phonological disorder** refers to impaired comprehension of the sound system of a language and the rules that govern the sound combinations (ASHA, 2008; ASHA Ad Hoc Committee on Service Delivery in the Schools, 1993).

Phonology is closely related to other constituents of the language system, such as morphology, syntax, semantics, and pragmatics. A child's phonological system, therefore, can never be regarded as functionally separate from other aspects of the child's language growth. Several studies (e.g., Cummings, 2009; Edwards, Beckman, & Munson, 2004; Edwards, Fox, & Rogers, 2002; Morrisette & Gierut, 2002; Mortimer, 2007; Munson, Edwards, & Beckman, 2005a; Roberts, 2005; Storkel, 2001, 2003, 2004; Storkel & Rogers, 2000) have documented that delayed phonological development occurs concurrently with delayed lexical and grammatical development. Although the direct relationship between phonological and grammatical acquisition remains unclear, interdependencies certainly exist between these areas.

Assessment of a child with a phonological disorder would include gathering information about all phonemes that the child uses to distinguish meaning—the phonemic inventory. The **phonemic inventory** is the repertoire of phonemes used contrastively by an individual. When compared to the phonemic inventory of General American English, we might find that certain phonemes are not present in the child's speech—that is, the child's phonemic inventory is restricted.

In addition, we might analyze the child's phonotactics by examining the position in the word in which these phonemes occur—at the beginning, middle, or end of the word. Children who have

CLINICAL EXERCISES

Assume that a child produces the following variations: An s-sound produced with the tongue tip too far forward, transcribed as [s], an s-production with the tongue too far back, a so-called palatalized [s], [sʲ], and a lateral production of [s], [ɬ]. These three variations would be a portion of the phonetic inventory. What would be in the phonemic inventory?

Be careful to examine whether something is a variation of the same speech sound or a different phoneme when you construct the phonemic inventory.

difficulties with the organization of their phoneme system might not realize the phonotactics that are typical for American English. Their speech may demonstrate *phonotactic constraints;* in other words, the phoneme use is restricted, so the phonemes are not used in all possible word positions. The distinction between a speech sound/articulation disorder versus a phonological disorder remains decisively important. It keeps definitions clear and is applicable to diagnostic and intervention procedures. Therefore, for the purpose at hand, a distinction is made between articulation disorders, those in which the peripheral motor processes are disturbed, and phonological disorders, those in which the organization and function of the phonological system is impaired. This delineation is not without problems; delineating articulation from phonological difficulties is clinically not an either/or proposition. Often, a child will seem to display characteristics of both disorders. Although this division between articulation and phonological disorder may remain at times unclear, a systematic attempt to distinguish between them is one important aspect of clinical decision making. This dichotomy is used throughout this text and more fully developed in later chapters. Table 1.2 outlines several different terms that are used clinically and in the research in reference to speech sounds and speech sound disorders.

As you view this video of 5-year-old Tessa, make notes on which sounds the child can produce and which ones are still difficult for her to produce. Do you think her articulation is within normal limits for her age, or would you suggest one of the terms from Table 1.2 to describe her speech?

Now view this video of 5-year-old Caitlin. Do you notice any differences between Tessa and Caitlin in relationship to their speech and intelligibility?

TABLE 1.2 Speech Sounds and Speech Sound Disorders: Terminology

Term	Definition	Examples
Articulation	The totality of motor processes involved in the planning and execution of speech.	Describes the speech sound production of individuals (e.g., "The *articulation* of [s] was incorrect."). Describes tests that examine the production of speech sounds (e.g., "The clinician administered an *articulation* test.").
Articulation disorder	Difficulty with the motor production aspects of speech or an inability to produce certain speech sounds.	A diagnostic category that indicates that an individual's speech sound productions vary widely from the norm (e.g., "Tony was diagnosed as having an *articulation* disorder.").
Phonology	The study of the sound system of a language, examines the sound units of that particular language, how these sounds are arranged, their systematic organization, and rule system.	Describing the inventory and arrangement of sound units (e.g., the Spanish *phonological system* has fewer vowels than American English. The phoneme /s/ is present in Spanish, but not /z/.).
Phonological disorder	Impaired comprehension and/or use of the sound system of a language and the rules that govern the sound combinations.	The inventory of phonemes may be restricted (e.g., "Jonathan used the phoneme /t/ for /d, k, g, s, z, ʃ, ʒ, tʃ, dʒ/. He was diagnosed as having a phonological disorder.").
Persistent speech sound disorders	Errors that persist past the typical age of acquisition (i.e., 8 or 9 years old).	Children with this disorder show little spontaneous improvement, and their response to intervention is poor. There is commonly no known cause (Wren, Roulstone, & Miller, 2012).

(Continued)

TABLE 1.2 (Continued)

Term	Definition	Examples
Speech sound delay	Speech sound errors that are often noted as "normal" errors found in young children as they acquire specific sounds. A "delay" usually has the premise that the child will catch up and achieve normal development.	A category that is typically used in young children to denote a mismatch between the child's speech sound acquisition and what is considered to be a norm reference.
Deviant speech sound development	Speech sound errors that are not typically observed in the development of most young children.	A term that typically indicates a process that is not delayed but different. For example, Lindsey demonstrated substitutions, such as [s] for [p, b, t, d]. Her speech sound development appeared deviant.
Speech or phonological or disability	*Disability* is a complex phenomenon, reflecting the interaction between features of a person's body and features of the society in which he or she lives (World Health Organization, 2014). *Disability* is an umbrella term including impairments.	In reference to speech phonology, this would indicate a serious speech sound/ phonological difficulty that impacts the child's or person's functioning in society.
Speech or phonological impairment	An *impairment* is any loss or abnormality of physiological or anatomical structure or function (WHO, 2014).	In reference to speech or phonology, impairment is typically used synonymously with disorder. The anatomical/ physiological basis for the term is typically not a primary consideration.

CLINICAL APPLICATION

Inventory and Phonotactics

Jeff was referred to the school speech-language pathologist by his kindergarten teacher, who was worried about the lack of intelligibility of his speech. The clinician noted that Jeff's phonemic inventory was very restricted. The following phonemes were present in Jeff's speech: /p, b, t, d, k, g, m, n, ŋ, f, v, h, w/. Jeff's phonemic inventory did not include the following phonemes: /s, z, ʃ, ʒ, θ, ð, j, l, r, tʃ, dʒ/. In addition, certain phonotactic constraints were noted. At the beginning of a word, Jeff realized the above noted speech sounds. However, at the end of a word or syllable, he used only voiced sounds. Jeff's phonotactics did not employ voiceless sounds to terminate a word or syllable. Not only was Jeff's phonemic inventory limited but phonotactic constraints were also discovered.

SUMMARY

This chapter introduced the reader to several terms that are fundamental to the assessment and treatment of articulatory and phonological disorders. As an introduction, the terms *communication*, *speech*, and *language* were provided as well as the five subcategories of language: *phonology, morphology, syntax, semantics,* and *pragmatics*. Definitions and clinical applications were noted for *articulation, phonology,* *speech sound,* and the *phoneme* as a foundation for this understanding. Speech sound forms versus linguistic function were used to distinguish between the speech sound and the phoneme. Based on these definitions, differentiations between speech sound, articulation, and phonological disorders were presented as well as nomenclature that is widely used in clinic and research relative to these terms.

Speech Sound Disorder: Articulation

Sandy is a 6-year-old child who was seen in a diagnostic session at the speech and hearing clinic. Her parents were concerned about her inability to produce [s]. Based on an analysis of a spontaneous speech sample and an articulation test, it was found that Sandy misarticulated [s] and [z] in all transcribed situations because her tongue placement was too far forward during the productions. The child was able to differentiate her mispronunciations from norm productions of [s] and [z]. No other speech sounds were in error, and language skills were found to be within normal limits. Sandy used her distorted realizations in every position in which [s] and [z] should occur. Thus, she seemed to understand the organization of /s/ and /z/ within the language system. The clinician hypothesized that this child was having difficulties with the actual production level only, with the speech sounds [s] and [z], whereas the understanding of their phoneme function was intact.

Phonology: Phonological Disorder

Travis, a 6-year-old first-grader, was referred by his classroom teacher to the speech-language pathologist. The teacher said that although Travis's speech was fairly intelligible, she was concerned about speech and language problems she had noticed in class. Her second concern was that these difficulties might be impacting Travis's emerging literacy skills. According to the teacher, Travis was having difficulty distinguishing between certain sounds and words as the class progressed with elementary reading tasks.

An articulation test and a spontaneous speech sample were analyzed with the following results: Travis had difficulties with s-productions. At the end of a word or syllable, [s] was always deleted. At the beginning of a word or syllable, [s] was produced as [ʃ]. Interestingly enough, when the clinician analyzed other words, she found that Travis could produce [s], but not in its proper context. Thus, several words that contained [f] were articulated with normal sounding [s] realizations. Testing of minimal pairs containing /s/ and /ʃ/ revealed that Travis was having difficulty distinguishing between the phonemic values of the two sounds.

On language tests and in spontaneous conversation, Travis deleted the plural -s in the third person singular -s (e.g., "He, she, it walk"). Comprehension of these grammatical forms was often in error.

The clinician hypothesized that Travis had a phonological disorder—that he had difficulties with the phoneme function and the phonotactics of /s/. This problem was impacting his morphological development. Because of the noted problems in discrimination, this could also have an effect on his beginning reading skills.

The following small speech sample is from Tara, age 7;7.

rabbit	[wæbət]	ready	[wɛdi]
feather	[fɛdɚ]	arrow	[ɛwoʊ]
green	[gwin]	toothbrush	[tutbwəʃ]
this	[ðɪs]	thinking	[θɪŋkɪŋ]

(Continued)

(Continued)

that	[ðæt]	round	[waᵘnd]
rope	[woᵘp]	bridge	[bwɪdʒ]
rooster	[wustɚ]	street	[stwit]
bathing	[beˈdɪŋ]	thin	[θɪn]
nothing	[nʌtɪŋ]	them	[ðɛm]
bath	[bæt]	breathe	[bwid]

Which speech sound errors are noted in this sample?

Which sounds are substituted for the sounds in error?

Can any phonotactic restraints be noted in the correct productions of "th" and "r"?

Based on this limited information, do you think the child has an articulation disorder or a phonological disorder? Why?

TEST YOURSELF

1. The definition of *articulation* includes which one of the following?
   a. describes the systems and patterns of phonemes in a particular language
   b. includes phonotactics
   c. refers to the totality of motor processes involved in speech
   d. all of the above

2. The definition of *articulation disorder* reflects
   a. peripheral motor processes
   b. gradually developing motor skills
   c. the totality of motor processes involved in the planning and execution of speech
   d. all of the above

3. Which one of the following could be considered a portion of morphology?
   a. the multiple meanings of the word "trunk"
   b. that "un" could be added to "happy" to change its meaning
   c. that children know from a fairly early age that we talk to babies somehow differently
   d. that sentences can be combined with the word "and"

4. Which one of the following could be considered a portion of semantics?
   a. the multiple meanings of the word "trunk"
   b. that "un" could be added to "happy" to change its meaning
   c. that children know from a fairly early age that we talk to babies somehow differently

   d. that sentences can be combined with the word "and"

5. Which one of the following would *not* be considered a portion of phonology?
   a. linguistic function of phonemes
   b. addition of -s can indicate plurality
   c. phonotactics
   d. knowledge of the sound system of a language

6. Oral, verbal expression of language into words is
   a. phonology
   b. articulation
   c. speech
   d. pragmatics

7. The definition of phonology includes
   a. the description of the system and patterns of phonemes within a language
   b. the classification and description of how speech sounds are produced
   c. the oral, verbal expression of language
   d. the relatively peripheral motor processes involved in speech

8. The allowed combinations of phonemes in a particular language refer to the
   a. phonetic inventory
   b. phonemic inventory
   c. phonotactic constraints
   d. minimal pairs

9. Which one of the following is *not* included in the definition of phonological disorder?

a. problems in the language-specific function of phonemes

b. disturbances in the relatively peripheral motor processes that result in speech

c. disturbances represent an impairment of the understanding and organization of phonemes

d. phonemic errors

10. What is the smallest linguistic unit that can be combined with other such units to establish word meanings?

a. allophonic variation

b. speech sound

c. phoneme

d. phonotactic constraint

FURTHER READINGS

Bleile, K. (2013). *The manual of speech sound disorders: A book for students and clinicians* (3rd ed.). Stamford, CT: Cengage Learning.

Catford, J. (2002). *A practical introduction to phonetics* (2nd ed.). Oxford: Oxford University Press.

Handke, J. (2000). *The Mouton interactive introduction to phonetics and phonology.* Berlin, NY: Mouton de Gruyter.

Howard, S. (2010). Children with speech sound disorders. In J.S. Damico, N. Mueller, & M. Ball (Eds.), *The handbook of language and speech disorders* (pp. 339–361). West Sussex, UK: Wiley-Blackwell.

Waring, R., & Knight, R. (2013). How should children with speech sound disorders be classified? A review and critical evaluation of current classification systems. *International Journal of Language and Communication Disorders, 48,* 25–40.

Phonetics—Articulatory Phonetics

Speech Sound Form

LEARNING OBJECTIVES

When you have finished this chapter, you should be able to:

- Define phonetics and the branches of phonetics.
- List the differences in production and function of vowels versus consonants.
- Identify the three descriptive parameters that are used for vowel articulations, and classify the vowels of General American English using those three parameters.
- Differentiate between the various types of vowels.

- Identify and define the four parameters that are used to describe the articulation of consonants.
- Classify the consonants of American English according to their active and passive articulators, manner, and voicing characteristics.
- Define coarticulation and assimilation, and describe the different types of assimilatory processes.
- Identify the various types of syllable structures including the phonotactic restraints of General American English.

Phonetics: Definitions and Classification

The description and classification of speech sounds is the main aim of phonetics. Sounds may be identified with reference to their production (or "articulation"), their acoustic transmission, or their auditory reception. The most widely used description is articulatory, which is the main emphasis of this chapter.

Generally stated, phonetics is the science of speech. However, it might be useful to delineate speech in its entirety while also indicating the various divisions of phonetics. Thus defined, **phonetics** is the study of speech emphasizing the description and classification of speech sounds according to their production, transmission, and perceptual features. These three branches of phonetics are labeled *articulatory phonetics*, exemplifying speech production; *acoustic phonetics*, the study of speech transmission; and *auditory phonetics*, which examines speech perception.

Articulatory phonetics deals with the production features of speech sounds, their categorization, and classification according to specific details of their production. Central aspects include the way speech sounds are actually articulated, their objective similarities, and their differences. *Articulation* is typically used as a more general term to describe the overall speech production of individuals. Articulatory phonetics as a field of study attempts to document these processes according to specific parameters, such as the manner or voicing of the speech sound. Articulatory phonetics is closely aligned with speech sounds and speech sound disorders and is the main emphasis of this text.

Acoustic phonetics deals with the transmission properties of speech. Here, the frequency, intensity, and duration of speech sounds, for example, are described and categorized. If you have ever analyzed speech sounds according to their frequencies, this would be classified as one aspect of acoustic phonetics.

Within **auditory phonetics,** investigators focus on how we perceive sounds. Our ears are not objective receivers of acoustic data. Rather, many factors, including our individual experiences, influence our perception. Such factors are examined in the area of auditory phonetics.

In the context of this book, we are primarily interested in articulatory phonetics. This specialty area deals with the actualities of how speech sounds are formed. Directly related to this area of phonetics is, of course, articulation. An integral portion of articulatory phonetics is the description and classification of speech sounds. This knowledge is important for both the assessment and the treatment of speech sound/articulation disorders. Knowledge of the production features of speech sounds guides clinicians when they are evaluating the various misarticulations noted in a clinical evaluation. Thus, one important step in our diagnostic process involves gathering phonetic information on the exact way an individual misarticulates sounds.

Thus, articulatory phonetics *categorizes* and *classifies* the production features of speech sounds. A thorough knowledge of how vowels and consonants are generated remains essential for successful assessment and remediation of speech sound disorders. Although contemporary phonological theories have provided new ways of viewing the diagnosis and intervention of these disorders, knowledge of the speech sounds' production features secures a firm basis for using such procedures. Without this knowledge, phonological process analysis, for example, is impossible.

This chapter discusses articulatory-phonetic aspects of the speech sounds of General American English. The specific goals are to:

1. Provide a review of the production features of vowels and consonants
2. Introduce the concepts of coarticulation and assimilation as a means of describing how sounds change within a given articulatory context
3. Examine the structure of syllables including the phonotactics of General American English

The production of vowels and consonants as well as their subsequent language-specific arrangements into syllables and words depends on articulatory motor processes. If these processes are impaired, speech sound production will be disordered. Articulatory motor processes depend in turn on many anatomical-physiological prerequisites, which include respiratory, phonatory, or resonatory processes. For example, the speech problems of children with cerebral palsy often originate in abnormal respiratory, resonatory, and/or phonatory prerequisites for articulation. Therefore, the proper function of these basic systems must first be secured before any articulatory improvement can be expected. Articulatory motor ability is embedded in many different anatomical-physiological requisites, which are of fundamental importance to speech-language pathologists.

Basic knowledge in these areas is typically gained from courses and textbooks covering anatomy and physiology of the speech and hearing mechanisms rather than those directly related to impaired articulation and phonology. The anatomical-physiological aspects of such disorders are not

Watch the first 2 minutes of the following video with Alan Shain, who has cerebral palsy. Try to see if you can comment on his respiration, voice quality, and articulation. youtube.com/watch?v=JCrh2AMcO M4&list=PL637D650093F7D7A0

For more information about the respiratory, phonatory, resonatory, and articulatory characteristics of cerebral palsy, see Chapter 11.

BOX 2.1	Selected Readings in Anatomy and Physiology of the Speech and Hearing Mechanisms

Culbertson, W. R., Cotton, S. S., & Tanner, D. C. (2006). *Anatomy and physiology study guide for speech and hearing.* San Diego, CA: Plural.

Fuller, D. R., Pemental, J. T., & Peregoy, B. M. (2012). *Applied anatomy and physiology for speech-language pathology and audiology.* Baltimore: Lippincott Williams & Wilkins.

Netter, F. H. (2014). *Atlas of human anatomy* (6th ed.). Philadelphia: Saunders-Elsevier Health Sciences.

Seikel, J. A., King, D. W., & Drumwright, D. G. (2005). *Anatomy and physiology for speech and language* (3rd ed.). Clifton Park, NY: Delmar.

Zemlin, W. R. (1998). *Speech and hearing science: Anatomy and physiology* (4th ed.). Boston: Allyn & Bacon.

within the scope of this chapter. Box 2.1 offers references as an incentive for the reader to rediscover the wealth of information essential to the clinical assessment and remediation of articulatory and phonological impairments.

Vowels versus Consonants

Speech sounds are commonly divided into two groups: vowels and consonants. **Vowels** are produced with a relatively open vocal tract; *no significant constriction* of the oral (and pharyngeal) cavities is required. The airstream from the vocal folds to the lips is relatively unimpeded. Therefore, vowels are considered to be *open sounds*. In contrast, **consonants** have *significant constriction* in the oral and/or pharyngeal cavities during their production. For consonants, the airstream from the vocal folds to the lips and nostrils encounters some type of articulatory obstacle along the way. Therefore, consonants are considered to be *constricted sounds*. For most consonants, this constriction occurs along the sagittal midline of the vocal tract.

The *sagittal midline of the vocal tract* refers to the median plane that divides the vocal tract into right and left halves.

This constriction for consonants can be exemplified by the first sound in *top*, [t], or *soap*, [s]. For [t], the contact of the front of the tongue with the alveolar ridge occurs along the sagittal midline, whereas the characteristic s-quality is made by air flowing along this median plane as the tongue approximates the alveolar ridge. By contrast, during all vowel productions, the sagittal midline remains free. In addition, under normal speech conditions, General American English vowels are always produced with vocal fold vibration; they are voiced speech sounds. Only during whispered speech are vowels unvoiced. Consonants, on the other hand, may be generated with or without simultaneous vocal fold vibration; they can be voiced or voiceless. Pairs of sounds such as [t] and [d] exemplify this relevant feature. Pairs of similar sounds, in this case differing only in their voicing feature, are referred to as **cognates.** Voicing features constitute the main linguistically relevant differences that separate the consonant cognates such as [s] from [z] and [f] from [v]. The transcription of various vowels and consonants with examples of words in which these sounds could be used are in Table 2.1. Please note that various phonetic texts might transcribe sounds in somewhat different ways. Examples are provided to guide you with the transcription that is used in this textbook. See Appendix 2.1 for a list of how several textbooks vary in the transcription of vowels.

Vowels can also be distinguished from consonants according to the patterns of acoustic energy they display. Vowels are highly resonant, demonstrating at least two formant areas. Thus, vowels are more intense than consonants; in other words, they are typically louder than consonants. In this respect, we can say that vowels have greater sonority than consonants. **Sonority** of a sound is its loudness relative to that of other sounds with the same length, stress, and pitch (Ladefoged & Johnson, 2010). Because of the greater sonority of vowels over consonants, vowels are also referred to as **sonorants.** In English, the sonority scale from highest to lowest is the following: vowels → glides [w, j] → liquids [r] → [l] → nasals [m, n, ŋ] → voiced fricatives [z, v, ð] → voiceless fricatives [s, f, θ] → voiced stop-plosives [b, d, g] → voiceless stop-plosives [p, t, k] (O'Grady & Archibald, 2012). Because of the production features of a special group of consonants and their resulting sonority, certain consonants are also labeled sonorants. **Sonorant consonants** are produced with a relatively open expiratory passageway. When contrasted to other consonants, sonorant consonants demonstrate less obstruction of the airstream during their production. The sonorant consonants include the nasals ([m, n, ŋ]), the liquids ([l, r]), and the glides ([w, j]). The sonorants are distinguished from the **obstruents**, which are characterized by a complete or narrow constriction between the articulators hindering the expiratory airstream. The obstruents include the stop-plosives ([p, b, t, d, k, g]), the fricatives ([f, v, s, z, θ, ð, ʃ, ʒ, h), and the affricates ([ʧ, ʤ]).

There are also functional distinctions between vowels and consonants. In other words, vowels and consonants have different linguistic functions. This has often been referred to as the *phonological difference* between vowels and consonants (Crystal, 2010). The term *consonant* indicates this relationship: *con* meaning "together with" and *sonant* reflecting the tonal qualities that characterize vowels. Thus, consonants are those speech sounds that function linguistically *together with* vowels. As such, vowels serve as the center of syllables, as syllable nuclei. Vowels can constitute syllables by themselves as, for example, in the first syllable of *a-go* or *e-lope.* Vowels can also appear with one or more consonants, exemplified by *blue, bloom,* or *blooms.* Although there are many types of syllables, the vowel is always the center of the syllable, its nucleus. A small group of consonants can serve as the nuclei of syllables. A consonant that functions as a syllable nucleus is referred to as a **syllabic.** These form and functional differences are summarized in Table 2.2.

TABLE 2.1 IPA Symbols

Consonants		Vowels	
Symbol	Commonly Realized In	Symbol	Commonly Realized In
[p]	pay	[i]	eat
[b]	boy	[ɪ]	in
[t]	toy	[eɪ]	ape
[d]	doll	[ɛ]	egg
[k]	coat	[æ]	at
[g]	goat	[a]	father[1]
[m]	moon	[u]	moon
[n]	not	[ʊ]	wood
[ŋ]	sing	[oʊ]	boat
[θ]	think	[ɔ]	father[1]
[ð]	those	[ɑ]	hop
[f]	far	[aɪ]	tie
[v]	vase	[aʊ]	mouse
[s]	sun	[ɔɪ]	boy
[z]	zoo	[ɜ]	girl[1]
[ʃ]	shop	[ɝ]	bird
[ʒ]	beige	[ɚ]	winner
[ʧ]	chop	[ʌ]	cut
[ʤ]	job	[ə]	above
[j]	yes		
[w]	win		
[ʍ]	when[2]		
[l]	leap		
[r]	red		
[h]	hop		

[1]May be regional or individual pronunciation.

[2]Historically, the /ʍ/ was used in "wh" words such as "where" and "when" and was a voiceless sound. It has now merged with /w/ throughout much of the United States (Wolfram & Schilling-Estes, 2006).

When transcribing, syllabic consonants need a special notation. This is discussed in Chapter 3.

TABLE 2.2 Features Differentiating Vowels and Consonants

Vowels	Consonants
No significant constriction of the vocal tract	Significant constriction of the vocal tract
Open sounds	Constricted sounds
Sagittal midline of vocal tract remains open	Constriction occurs along sagittal midline of the vocal tract
Voiced	Voiced or unvoiced
Acoustically more intense	Acoustically less intense
Demonstrate more sonority	Demonstrate less sonority
Function as syllable nuclei	Only specific consonants can function as syllable nuclei

American English Vowels

Vowels are commonly described according to certain parameters (Abercrombie, 1967; Crystal, 2010; Heffner, 1975; Kantner & West, 1960; Shriberg & Kent, 2013):

1. The portion of the tongue that is involved in the articulation. Example: front versus back vowels.
2. The tongue's position relative to the palate. Example: high versus low vowels.
3. The degree of lip rounding or unrounding.

The vowel quadrilateral is a rough sketch of the inside of the oral cavity. As can be noted, the right axis is at a 90-degree angle, whereas the left axis is at a much wider angle. Think about this in relationship to the mouth and tongue. What implications do these differences have in relationship to vowel production and the movement capabilities of the front versus the back of the tongue? If you work with a child who has vowel difficulties, how could you use this information clinically?

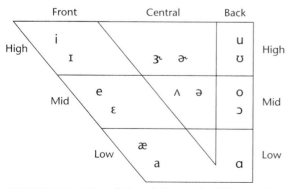

FIGURE 2.1 Vowel Quadrilateral of General American English Vowels

The four-sided form called a *vowel quadrilateral* is often used to demonstrate schematically the front–back and high–low positions. The form roughly represents the tongue position in the oral cavity (Figure 2.1).

The terms *tense/lax* and *open/close* are also used to describe vowels. *Tense* and *lax* refer to the degree of muscular activity involved in the articulation and to the length of the vowels in question (Shriberg & Kent, 2013). Therefore, tense vowels are produced with relatively more muscular activity and are longer in duration than lax vowels. The vowel [i] is considered to be a tense vowel, whereas [ɪ] is lax. When contrasting tense versus lax, one has to keep in mind that these oppositions refer to pairs of vowels that are productionally similar, i.e, to vowel cognates. For example, [i] and [ɪ] are considered to be "ee" type vowels, and [u] and [ʊ] are "oo" type vowels.

The terms *close* and *open* refer to the relative closeness of the tongue to the roof of the mouth. Again, only vowel cognates are usually characterized with these terms. Using the previous examples, [i] is more close - [ɪ] more open, [u] close - [ʊ] open.

There are two types of vowels: monophthongs and diphthongs. The quality of **monophthongs** remains the same throughout their entire production. They are pure vowels (Abercrombie, 1967). **Diphthongs** are vowels in which there is a change in quality during their production (Ladefoged & Johnson, 2010). The initial segment, the beginning portion of such a diphthong, is phonetically referred to as the **onglide** and its end portion as the **offglide.** Using this notation system, the following descriptions for the most common vowels of General American English are offered.

> "It should be noted that although monophthongs are often referred to as 'pure' vowels, no special virtue attaches to them" (Abercrombie, 1967, p. 60).

Front Vowels

[i]	A high-front vowel, unrounded, close, and tense.
[ɪ]	A high-front vowel, unrounded, open, and lax.
[e]	A mid-front vowel, unrounded, close, and tense. In General American English, this vowel is typically produced as a diphthong, especially in stressed syllables or when articulated slowly.
[ɛ]	A mid-front vowel, unrounded, open, and lax.
[æ]	A low-front vowel, unrounded, open, and lax.
[a]	A low-front vowel, unrounded, close, and tense. In General American English, the use of this vowel depends on the particular regional dialect of the speaker. In the New England dialect of the Northeast, one might often hear it.

All front vowels show various degrees of unrounding (lip spreading) with the high-front vowels showing the most. The lip spreading becomes less as one moves from the high-front vowels to the mid-front vowels, finally becoming practically nonexistent in the low-front vowel.

Back Vowels

[u]	A high-back vowel, rounded, close, and tense.
[ʊ]	A high-back vowel, rounded, open, and lax.
[o]	A mid-back vowel, rounded, close, and tense. This vowel is typically produced as a diphthong, especially in stressed syllables or when articulated slowly.
[ɔ]	A low mid-back vowel, rounded, open, and lax (Heffner, 1975). The use of this vowel depends on regional pronunciation.
[ɑ]	A low-back vowel, unrounded, open, and lax (Kantner & West, 1960). There seems to be some confusion in transcribing [ɔ] and [ɑ], although acoustic differences certainly exist. One distinguishing feature: The [ɔ] shows some degree of lip rounding, whereas [ɑ] does not.

Back vowels display different degrees of lip rounding in General American English. The high-back vowels [u] and [ʊ] often show a fairly high degree of lip rounding, whereas the low-back vowel [ɑ] is commonly articulated as an unrounded vowel.

Central Vowels

[ɝ]	A central vowel, rounded, tense with r-coloring. Rounding may vary, however, from speaker to speaker. [ɝ] is a stressed vowel. It is typically acoustically more intense, has a higher fundamental frequency, and has a longer duration when it is compared to a similar unstressed vowel such as [ɚ].

(Continued)

(Continued)

[ɚ]	A central vowel, rounded, lax with r-coloring. Again, lip rounding may vary from speaker to speaker. This lax vowel is an unstressed vowel.
[ɜ]	A central vowel, rounded, tense. [ɜ] is very similar in pronunciation to [ɝ], but it lacks any r-coloring. This vowel is heard in certain dialects. For example, [ɜ] might be found in a Southern dialect pronunciation of *bird* or *worth*. Also, it could be heard in the speech of children having difficulties producing the "r" sound.
[ʌ]	A lax, unrounded central vowel. It is a stressed vowel.
[ə]	A lax, unrounded central vowel. It is an unstressed vowel.

CLINICAL APPLICATION

Do Children Have Difficulties Producing Vowels?

Vowel errors in children developing phonological skills in a normal manner are relatively uncommon. However, children with phonological disorders may show deviant vowel patterns. Several studies (e.g., Davis, Jacks, & Marquardt, 2005; Pollock, 2013; Pollock & Berni, 2003; Reynolds, 2013; Stoel-Gammon & Herrington, 1990) have documented the presence of specific vowel problems in phonologically disordered children. Although certain vowel substitutions seem to be articulatory simplifications that could also occur in normal development, other errors appear to be idiosyncratic. Assessment of vowel qualities should be a portion of every diagnostic protocol. This can easily be achieved with any formal articulation test by transcribing the entire word rather than just the sound being tested.

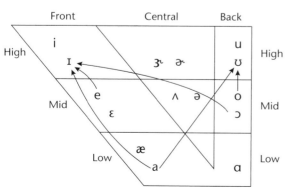

Watch, listen, and transcribe the short segment from 6-year-old Sandy. She says each word three times.

FIGURE 2.2 Vowel Quadrilateral with Rising Diphthongs

Diphthongs. As previously defined, a diphthong is a vowel sound that demonstrates articulatory movement resulting in a qualitative change during its production. Its initial portion, the onglide is acoustically more prominent and usually longer than the offglide. Common diphthongs in General American English are **rising diphthongs**. This means that when producing these diphthongs, essential portions of the tongue move from a lower onglide to a higher offglide position; thus, relative to the palate, the tongue moves in a rising motion. This can be demonstrated on the vowel quadrilateral as well (Figure 2.2).

Certain diphthongs are referred to as **centering diphthongs**. In this case, the offglide, or less prominent element of the diphthong, is a central vowel. Common in General American English is the use of the central vowel with r-coloring [ɚ] as an offglide. Thus, *fear* is often pronounced as [fɪɚ], *far* as [faɚ], and *bear* as [bɛɚ] (Ball & Rahilly, 1999). Theoretically, any vowel may be combined with [ə] or [ɚ] to form a centering diphthong; however, in General American English, certain centering diphthongs are more common than others. Thus, [ɪɚ], [ɛɚ], and [aɚ], which can be heard in *dear* [dɪɚ], *bear* [bɛɚ], or *farm* [faɚm], are far more prevalent than [iɚ] or [uɚ]. Lowe (1994) refers to the diphthongs that are paired with [ɚ] as **rhotic diphthongs**. Centering diphthongs are also seen transcribed with [r]. Thus, *dear* is transcribed as [dɪr], *bear* as [bɛr], or *farm* as [farm].

There are several ways to characterize diphthongs as single phonemic units in contrast to two separate vowels. Some transcribers use a bar or bow either above or below the two vowel symbols—[e͞ɪ], [e͜ɪ], or [e͡ɪ], for example. The author has chosen to use the transcription that elevates the offglide portion of the diphthong to indicate less intensity and length associated with it.

Discrepancies may be noted between the transcriptions of diphthongs offered in this text and the ones in other books. Because phonetic transcription is purely *descriptive*, never *prescriptive*, any transcription will, of course, vary according to the actual pronunciation. See Shriberg and Kent (2013) for a thorough discussion of the various ways diphthongs have been transcribed.

[eᶦ]	A **nonphonemic diphthong**.
	Nonphonemic diphthongs are those that the meaning of the word would *not* change if the vowel were to be pronounced as a monophthong [e] versus a diphthong [eᶦ]. Therefore, no change in meaning would result if just the onglide were realized. Words pronounced [beᶦk] or [bek], for example, would be recognized as the same word.
[oᵘ]	A nonphonemic diphthong.
[aᶦ]	A **phonemic diphthong**.
	Phonemic diphthongs are those in which the meaning *would* change in a particular word if only the vowel onglide were produced; in other words, if the vowel was realized as a monophthong. A realization of [a] instead of [aᶦ] will change the meaning in General American English as the words *sod* [sad] versus *sighed* [saᶦd] demonstrate.
[ɔᶦ]	A phonemic diphthong.
	The opposition [ʤɔ], *jaw*, versus [ʤɔᶦ], *joy*, exemplifies its phonemic value as a meaning-differentiating sound feature of English.
[aᵘ]	A phonemic diphthong.
	Oppositions such as [mas], *moss*, versus [maᵘs], *mouse*, exemplify its phonemic value.

See Appendix 2.1 for various ways the diphthongs and the rhotic diphthongs are transcribed in various current phonetic textbooks.

CLINICAL APPLICATION

Analyzing the Vowel System of a Child

Occasionally, the vowel system of a client may be restricted or show deviant patterns. In this case, a more in-depth analysis of the vowel productions may be necessary. Vowel systems can be analyzed using the vowel quadrilateral and knowledge of the diphthongs as guiding principles. Front, back, and central vowels as well as diphthongs can be checked in relationship to their accuracy and their occurrence in the appropriate contexts.

George, age 5;3, is a child with a deviant vowel system. George was being seen in the clinic for his phonological disorder. He was a gregarious child who loved to talk and would try to engage anyone who would listen in conversation. The only problem was that George was almost unintelligible. This made dialogue difficult, possibly more so for those who would patiently and diligently try to understand his continuing attempts to interact.

In addition to his many consonant problems, the following vowel deviations were noted:

Vowels Errors

Norm Production	→	Actual Production	Word Examples	Transcriptions		
[eᶦ]	→	[ɛ]	grapes	[greᶦps]	→	[dɛ]
			table	[teᶦbl̩]	→	[tɛboᵘ]
[i]	→	[ɪ]	feet	[fit]	→	[fɪ]
			teeth	[tiθ]	→	[tɪ]
			three	[θri]	→	[dɪ]
[ɛ]	→	[æ]	bed	[bɛd]	→	[bæt]
			feather	[fɛðɚ]	→	[fævə]

(Continued)

Norm Production	→	Actual Production	Word Examples	Transcriptions		
[u]	correct	[u]	shoe	[ʃu]	→	[tu]
			spoon	[spun]	→	[mun]
[ʊ]	correct	[ʊ]	book	[bʊk]	→	[bʊ]
[oʊ]	correct	[oʊ]	stove	[stoʊv]	→	[doʊ]
			nose	[noʊz]	→	[noʊ]
[ɑ]	correct	[ɑ]	mop	[mɑp]	→	[mɑ]
			blocks	[blɑks]	→	[bɑ]

George's productions of the back vowels [u], [ʊ], [oʊ], and [ɑ] are on target. The front vowels do show a deviant pattern, however. Not only is the diphthong [eɪ] produced as a monophthong but also the articulatory position of the vowel substitution for [e] is realized lower as [ɛ]. This tendency to lower vowels is also noted in the other productions with front vowels in which [i] becomes [ɪ] and [ɛ] becomes [æ].

American English Consonants

Four phonetic categories are used to transcribe consonants: (1) active articulator (organ of articulation), (2) passive articulator (place of articulation), (3) manner of articulation, and (4) voicing features. Most textbooks state that only place, manner, and voicing are used to characterize individual consonants (Edwards, 2003; Shriberg & Kent, 2013). However, they nevertheless often include the active articulator. For example, the term *lingual* as in *lingua-dental* or *lingua-palatal* designates the active articulator. However, when contrasting the lingua-dental sounds [θ] and [ð] to the lingua-palatal sounds [ʃ] and [ʒ], it becomes clear that different portions of the tongue are actively involved in the articulation. The term *lingual* alone does not specify these differences. This text emphasizes the detailed knowledge of production features for specific therapy goals. By adding a category specifically designating the active articulator, valuable clarification of consonant articulation is achieved.

Active Articulator/Organ of Articulation. Consonants are sounds characterized by the articulators creating a partial or total obstruction of the expiratory airstream. There are active and passive articulators. **Active articulators**, or what has been termed **organs of articulation**, are the parts within the vocal tract that actually move to achieve the articulatory result (Crystal, 2010). In describing the consonants of General American English, we are referring specifically to the movements of the lower lip and portions of the tongue. The structures actively involved in the articulation of the consonants of General American English and the resulting phonetic descriptors can be found in Table 2.3. Figure 2.3 is a display of the divisions of the tongue.

Passive Articulator/Place of Articulation. The **passive articulator** or the **place of articulation** denotes the area within the vocal tract that remains motionless during consonant articulation. It is the part that the active articulator approaches or contacts directly (Crystal, 2010). The upper lip and teeth, the palate, and the velum are the main places of articulation when describing the consonants of General American English. See Table 2.4 for the passive structures of articulation and their resulting phonetic descriptors. Figure 2.4 is a display of the structures of the oral cavity as active (organ of articulation) and passive articulators (places of articulation).

Manner of Articulation. The **manner of articulation** refers to the type of constriction that the active and passive articulators produce for the realization of a particular consonant. There are various manners of articulation, ranging from complete closure for the production of stop-plosives to a very limited constriction of the vocal tract for the

TABLE 2.3 Phonetic Description: Active Articulator/Organ of Articulation

Active Articulator	Phonetic Descriptor	Examples
Lower lip	Labial	[p], [b], [m], [f], [v], [w], [ʍ]
Tip of tongue	Apical	[s], [z], [θ], [ð], [r],[1] [l]
Lateral rims of tongue[2]	Coronal	[t], [d], [n], [ʃ], [ʒ], [tʃ], [dʒ]
Surface of tongue	Dorsum	
Anterior portion	Predorsal	[s], [z]
Central portion	Mediodorsal	[j], [r]
Posterior portion	Postdorsal	[k], [g], [ŋ]

[1]The transcription used officially by the International Phonetic Association for the General American English "r" is [ɹ]. See an explanation under the section "Rhotics."

[2]The term *coronal* designates the apex and the lateral rims of the tongue. Whereas the term *blade* of the tongue also includes its apex, it characterizes an extension into predorsal areas as well. In order to delineate the action of the active articulator as closely as possible, the terms *coronal* and *predorsal* will be used instead of *blade*.

production of glides. The following manners of articulation are used to account phonetically for the consonants of General American English.

Stop-Plosives During the production of stop-plosives, complete occlusion is secured at specific points in the vocal tract. Simultaneously, the velum is raised so that no air can escape through the nose. The expiratory air pressure builds up naturally behind this closure (stop); compression results, which is then suddenly released (plosive). Examples of stop-plosives are [p] and [b].

Fricatives Fricatives result when active and passive articulators approximate each other so closely that the escaping expiratory airstream causes an audible friction. As with the stops, the velum is raised for all fricative sounds. Two examples of fricatives are [f] and [v]. Some fricatives, referred to as **sibilants**, have a sharper sound than others because of the presence of high-frequency components. In General American English [s], [z], [ʃ], and [ʒ] belong to the sibilants.

Nasals These consonants are produced with the velum lowered so that the air can pass freely through the nasal cavity. However, there is complete occlusion within the oral cavity between the active and passive articulators. These sounds have been called *nasal stops* because of the occlusion of the active and passive articulators and the ensuing free air passage through the nasal cavity (Ball & Rahilly, 1999). The nasals of General American English are [m], [n], and [ŋ].

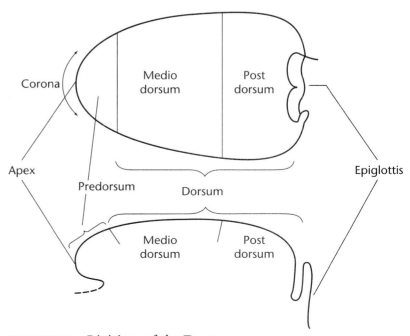

FIGURE 2.3 Divisions of the Tongue

TABLE 2.4 Phonetic Description: Passive Articulators/Place of Articulation

Passive Articulators	Phonetic Descriptor	Examples
Upper lip	Labial	[p], [b], [m], [w], [ʍ]
Upper teeth	Dental	[f], [v], [θ], [ð]
Alveolar ridge	Alveolar	[t], [d], [n], [s], [z], [l]
Surface of hard palate	Palatal	
Anterior portion	Prepalatal	[ʃ], [ʒ],[1] [r]
Central portion	Mediopalatal	[j], [r]
Posterior portion	Postpalatal	(does not normally occur in General American English)
Soft palate	Velar	[k], [g], [ŋ]

[1][ʃ] and [ʒ] are also referred to as *postalveolar sounds,* indicating a place of articulation just posterior to the highest point of the alveolar ridge. This text includes both of these places of articulation to describe [ʃ] and [ʒ].

Affricates. For affricate sounds, two phases can be noted. First, a complete closure is formed between the active and passive articulators, and the velum is raised. As a consequence of these articulatory conditions, expiratory air pressure builds up behind the blockage formed by the articulators—the stop phase, which is considered the first portion of the affricate. Second, the stop is then slowly (in comparison to the plosives)

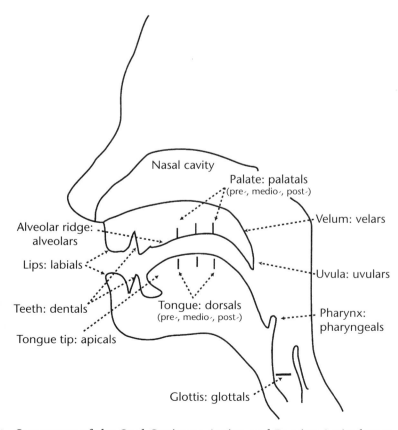

FIGURE 2.4 Structures of the Oral Cavity as Active and Passive Articulators

The rhotic "r" is officially transcribed by the International Phonetic Association as [ɹ], an upside down "r" to indicate, as mentioned above, an "r" production where the tongue tip is raised toward the alveolar ridge, The retroflexed is characterized by [ɻ], an upside-down *r* with a retroflexed diacritic. According to the International Phonetic Alphabet the [r] symbol is officially reserved for the alveolar trilled "r" sound, which can be heard in Spanish, for example. Because trilled "r" sounds do not exist in General American English and to prevent complicating matters unnecessarily, it is customary to use the [r] symbol for both the bunched and the retroflexed "r" sounds. However, you will see in some textbooks that the General American English rhotic is transcribed as [ɹ]. In reference to General American English, [r] and [ɹ] typically indicate the same sound, the "r" as in "rabbit."

released orally, resulting in the friction portion of the speech sound. Affricates should *not* be viewed as a stop plus fricative combination similar to consonant blends or clusters, such as [ks], in which the stop portion is formed by active and passive articulators, which differ in their placement. Rather, affricates are single uniform speech sounds characterized by a slow release of a stopping phase into a homorganic (*hom* = same) friction element. The two most prominent affricates of General American English are [tʃ] and [dʒ].

Glides. For the realization of glides, the constriction between active and passive articulators is not as narrow as for fricatives. In addition to this relatively wide articulatory posture, glides are also characterized by a gliding movement of the articulators from a relatively constricted into a more open position. The sounds [w] and [j] are considered glides. According to the classification of the International Phonetic Alphabet, [w] and [j] are considered approximants. **Approximants** are consonants in which there is a much wider passage of air, resulting in a smooth (as opposed to turbulent) airflow for these voiced sounds.

Laterals. These sounds are established by a midline closure but lateral openings within the oral cavity. Consequently, the expiratory airstream can pass around one or both sides of the tongue. [l] is the only lateral consonant of General American English. The laterals together with the rhotics are collectively referred to as **liquids**. According to the classification system of the International Phonetic Alphabet [l] is considered a lateral approximant.

Rhotics. The phonetic characteristics of the rhotics are especially difficult to describe. First, there are at least two types of rhotic productions: *retroflexed* and *bunched*. Second, the actual forming of rhotics is highly context dependent. Thus, the production easily changes, depending on the features of the surrounding sounds. In addition, the positioning of the tongue for individual speakers is highly variable. Generally, the *retroflexed* rhotics are produced with the

CLINICAL APPLICATION

When Active/Passive Articulators, Manner, and Voicing Are Not Enough

In analyzing the articulatory requisites for the realization of [ʃ], we find that it can be described—according to voicing, active and passive articulators, and manner—as a voiceless coronal-prepalatal fricative. This is a general phonetic description; however, another production characteristic of [ʃ] is lip rounding. Describing such an additional feature becomes necessary because some children with "sh" problems do not realize the rounding. In fact, the resulting aberrant production may result entirely from the absence of this lip-rounding feature.

TABLE 2.5 Phonetic Description: Manner of Articulation

Manner of Articulation	Phonetic Descriptor	Examples
Complete blockage	Stop-plosive	[p], [b], [t], [d], [k], [g]
Partial blockage	Fricative	[f], [v], [s], [z], [ʃ], [ʒ], [θ], [ð]
Nasal emission	Nasal	[m], [n], [ŋ]
Release of stop portion to a homorganic fricative portion	Affricate	[tʃ], [dʒ]
Gliding motion from a more closed to a more open position	Glide	[w], [ʍ], [j]
Lateral airflow	Lateral	[l]
Retroflex blade or bunched dorsum	Rhotic	[r]

CLINICAL EXERCISES

The child you are working with has a [w] for [r] substitution. At first, why might you avoid words with [r] + high-back vowels, such as "root" or "roof"? Reflect on the production of [w] with its high-back tongue placement.

Manner of articulation: If a child produces [t] for [s], what does the child need to understand to achieve [s]? Can you think of any ways to demonstrate this to the child?

TABLE 2.6 Phonetic Description: Voicing

Voicing	Phonetic Descriptor	Examples
With vocal fold vibration	Voiced	[b], [d], [g], [m], [n], [ŋ], [v], [z], [ʒ], [ð], [w], [j], [l], [r]
Without vocal fold vibration	Voiceless	[p], [t], [k], [f], [s], [ʃ], [θ], [ʍ], [h]

[1]The active and passive articulators, manner, and voicing features are based on the phonetic descriptions provided by Bronstein (1960) and Kantner and West (1960). These features are seen as descriptive and may, therefore, vary somewhat from speaker to speaker.

tongue tip in a retroflexed position (*retro* = back, *flex* = turn). The bunched rhotics, on the other hand, show an elevation of the whole corpus of the tongue toward the palate. Perhaps a better classification for [r] is the term *approximant*, which is used within the International Phonetic Alphabet. In this case, [r] is a central approximant. According to the International Phonetic Alphabet, there are two symbols used for the central rhotic approximants. The [ɹ] is a postalveolar approximant in which the tongue tip is raised and points directly upward toward the rear of the alveolar ridge. The [ɻ] is a retroflex production characterized by the tongue tip elevated and bent backward in a more retroflexed position. Officially, there is no International Phonetic Alphabet symbol for the bunched r-production (Ball & Rahilly, 1999). Refer to Table 2.5 for the various manners of articulation with examples of the consonants of General American English.

Voicing. **Voicing** is the term used to denote the presence or absence of simultaneous vibration of the vocal cords, resulting in voiced or voiceless consonants. The voiced and voiceless consonants of General American English are summarized in Table 2.6.

Far more precision may often be necessary to describe how specific consonants are produced. However, this framework of active articulator (organ of articulation), passive articulator (place of articulation), manner of articulation, and voicing provides a fairly accurate description of General American English consonants.

The following phonetic descriptions classify the consonants of General American English according to the parameters of voicing, active and passive articulators, and manner of production.[1]

[p]	Voiceless bilabial stop-plosive
	Because active and passive articulators are the lower and upper lips, one should actually say labio-labial. However, the term *bilabial* is usually preferred.
[b]	Voiced bilabial stop-plosive
[t]	Voiceless coronal-alveolar stop-plosive
[d]	Voiced coronal-alveolar stop-plosive
[k]	Voiceless postdorsal-velar stop-plosive
[g]	Voiced postdorsal-velar stop-plosive
[f]	Voiceless labio-dental fricative
[v]	Voiced labio-dental fricative
[s]	Voiceless apico-alveolar or predorsal-alveolar fricative
	The [s] (and [z]) can be produced in one of two ways: with the tongue tip up (i.e., an apico-alveolar fricative [sibilant]) or with the tongue tip resting behind the lower incisors (i.e., predorsal-alveolar fricative [sibilant]).
[z]	Voiced apico-alveolar or predorsal-alveolar fricative
[ʃ]	Voiceless coronal-prepalatal or coronal-postalveolar fricative with lip rounding
[ʒ]	Voiced coronal-prepalatal or coronal-postalveolar fricative with lip rounding.
[θ]	Voiceless apico-dental or interdental fricative
	The [θ] and [ð] are typically produced with either the tongue tip resting behind the upper incisors (i.e., apico-dental) or with the tongue tip slightly between the upper and lower incisors (i.e., interdental).
[ð]	Voiced apico-dental or interdental fricative
[m]	Voiced bilabial nasal
[n]	Voiced coronal-alveolar nasal
[ŋ]	Voiced postdorsal-velar nasal
[w]	Voiced labial-velar glide or approximant with lip rounding. The velar passive articulator refers to the body of the tongue being raised toward the velum.
[ʍ]	Voiceless labial-velar fricative (International Phonetic Alphabet, 2005) with lip rounding. The velar passive articulator refers to the body of the tongue being raised toward the velum.
[j]	Voiced mediodorsal-mediopalatal glide or approximant
[l]	Voiced apico-alveolar lateral or lateral approximant
[r]	Voiced mediodorsal-mediopalatal rhotic approximant (bunched) or voiced apico-prepalatal rhotic approximant (retroflexed)
	Here, the term *apico* refers to the underside of the apex of the tongue.
[h]	Voiceless unlocalized open consonant (an aspirate) or glottal fricative
	Although this sound is sometimes classified as a laryngeal or glottal fricative, in General American English, there is normally no constriction at the laryngeal, pharyngeal, or oral levels. See Heffner (1975) for a discussion of the [h] production in General American English.
[tʃ]	Voiceless coronal-alveolar stop portion followed by a voiceless coronal-postalveolar fricative portion
[dʒ]	Voiced coronal-alveolar stop portion followed by a voiced coronal-postalveolar fricative portion

CLINICAL EXERCISES

Which type of [s] do you use, the tongue tip up (coronal-alveolar) or the tip down (predorsal-alveolar)? Say a few words with [s] and note the position of your tongue. Try producing both types of [s] productions.

Some clinicians use only the tongue tip down version of [s] to remediate [s] difficulties. Why might this be the [s] production of choice if the child produces [θ] as a substitution and always goes back to this sound if you try to achieve a coronal-alveolar [s] production?

CLINICAL APPLICATION

Rhotic Errors versus Central Vowels with R-Coloring

Children with "r" problems, thus, rhotic consonant difficulties, often produce the central vowels with r-coloring ([ɝ] and [ɚ]) in error. However, that is not always the case. Note the following patterns seen in Latoria's speech.

Norm Production	→	Actual Production	Word Example	Transcriptions		
Rhotics						
[tr]	→	[tw]	tree	[tri]	→	[twi]
[br]	→	[bw]	bridge	[brɪʤ]	→	[bwɪʒ]
[r]	→	[w]	ring	[rɪŋ]	→	[wɪŋ]
[br]	→	[bw]	zebra	[zibrə]	→	[zibwə]
[r]	→	[w]	garage	[gərɑʒ]	→	[ʤəwɑ]
[θr]	→	[θw]	thread	[θrɛd]	→	[θwɛd]
[tr]	→	[tw]	treasure	[trɛʒɚ]	→	[twɛʒɚ]
Central Vowels with R-Coloring						
[ɚ]	correct	[ɚ]	feather	[fɛðɚ]	→	[fɛdɚ]
[ɚ]	correct	[ɚ]	soldier	[soʊldʒɚ]	→	[soʊʒɚ]
[ɚz]	correct	[ɚz]	scissors	[sɪzɚz]	→	[sɪzɚz]
[ɝ]	correct	[ɝ]	birthday	[bɝθdeɪ]	→	[bɝdeɪ]

On the one hand, Latoria has a [w] for [r] substitution ([r] → [w]) for the rhotic consonant [r]. On the other, she can produce the central vowels with r-coloring accurately.

Sounds in Context: Coarticulation and Assimilation

Until now, this textbook has discussed articulatory characteristics of speech sounds as discrete units. However, the articulators do not move from sound to sound in a series of separate steps. Speech consists of highly variable and overlapping motor movements. Sounds within a given phonetic context influence one another. For example, if the [s] production in *see* is contrasted to the one in *Sue*, it can be seen that [s] in *see* is produced with some spreading of the lips, whereas there is lip rounding in *Sue*. This difference results from the influence of the following vowel articulations: [i], a vowel with lip spreading, facilitates this feature in the [s] production in *see*, whereas the lip rounding of [u] influences the production of [s] in *Sue*. These types of modifications are grouped together under the term *coarticulation*. **Coarticulation** describes the concept that the articulators are continually moving into position for other segments over a stretch of speech. The result of coarticulation is referred to as *assimilation*. The term **assimilation** refers to adaptive articulatory changes by which one speech sound becomes similar, sometimes identical, to a neighboring sound segment. Such a change may affect one, several, or all of a sound's phonetic constituents; that is, a sound may change its active and passive articulators, manner, and/or voicing properties under the articulatory influence of another sound. Assimilation processes are perfectly natural consequences of normal speech production and are by no means restricted to developing speech in young children. Because the two segments become more alike, assimilatory processes are also referred to as *harmony processes.*

Watch, listen, and transcribe the video segment of Hope, who is 5 years old. She says each word three times.

There are different *types* and *degrees* of assimilatory processes. In regard to the different types of assimilatory processes, the following should be noted:

1. Assimilatory processes modifying directly adjacent sounds are called *contact* (or *contiguous*) *assimilations*. If at least one other segment separates the sounds in question, especially when the two sounds are in two different syllables, one speaks of *remote* (or *noncontiguous*) *assimilation*.

CLINICAL EXERCISES

If the child says [lɛloᵘ] for "yellow," how could you determine whether this is an [l] for [j] substitution or an assimilation process?

If a child said [tɛdəpoᵘn] for "telephone," could this be an assimilation process? Explain.

The following assimilation processes were noted in the results of children's articulation tests:

Contact

"jumping" [ʤʌmpɪŋ], typical transcription → [ʤʌmbɪŋ] with assimilation

If the two segments are contrasted, the [mp] in [ʤʌmpɪŋ] becomes [mb] in the assimilated production [ʤʌmbɪŋ]. In this case, the voiced [m], a *voiced* nasal, impacts the normally *voiceless* [p], the result is a voiced [b].

"skunk" [skʌŋk], typical transcription → [stʌŋk] with assimilation

If the two segments are contrasted, the [sk] in [skʌŋk] becomes [st] in the assimilated production [stʌŋk]. The articulatory placements of the active and passive articulators for [s], a *coronal-alveolar*, influence the stop-plosive [k], a *postdorsal-velar*, moving the production forward to a *coronal-alveolar* [t].

Remote

"yellow" [jɛloᵘ], typical transcription → [lɛloᵘ] with assimilation

The position of the active and passive articulators are impacted when the [j] at the beginning of the word (a mediodorsal-mediopalatal) becomes identical to the following [l]. This is a very common assimilation process in children. In this context, the influence of the [l] impacts the [j]. They are both glides, and only the active and passive articulators differentiate the two.

"telephone" [tɛləfoᵘn], typical transcription → [tɛdəfoᵘn] with assimilation

The [t] at the beginning of the word is the driving force for this assimilation. If the two words are compared, the [l] has changed to a [d] from a lateral to a stop-plosive, similar to the [t] at the beginning of the word. However, the voicing of the [l] has been maintained so that the resulting sound is a voiced stop-plosive, a [d].

2. Assimilations can be either *progressive* or *regressive*. In progressive assimilation, a segment influences a following sound in a linear manner. This is also referred to as *perseverative assimilation* (Crystal, 2010; Ladefoged & Johnson, 2010). The previously noted contact assimilations for *jumping* and *skunk* and the remote assimilation for *telephone* are examples of progressive assimilation. A previously articulated sound influenced a following sound.

[ʤʌmpɪn] becomes [ʤʌm$\overrightarrow{b}$ɪn]

[skʌŋk] becomes [$\overrightarrow{st}$ʌŋk]

[tɛləfoᵘn] becomes [$\overrightarrow{tɛd}$əfoᵘn]

In regressive assimilation, a sound segment influences a preceding sound. If "is she" [ɪz ʃi] is pronounced [ɪʒ ʃi], changing [s] into [ʒ], regressive assimilation is noted. The [ʃ] has impacted the articulation of the [z] so that it is changed to a fricative similar to [ʃ] but with voicing [ʒ]. Regressive assimilations are also known as *anticipatory* assimilations (Crystal, 2010; Ladefoged & Johnson, 2010).

The following are examples of progressive and regressive assimilation processes:

Progressive

"ice cream" [aˈskrim], typical pronunciation ⟶ [aˈstrim] with assimilation

The [sk] is assimilated to [st]. In the typical pronunciation, there is articulatory movement from [s] to [k]. The tongue moves, first towards the front of the mouth (apico-alveolar for [s]), and then the back of the tongue becomes active for the postdorsal-velar [k]. The second production [aˈstrim] is much simpler in movement. The forward placement of the [s] articulation moves the stop-plosive from a back production to a more fronted one. This is progressive contact assimilation.

"television" [tɛləvɪʒən] ⟶ [tɛdəvɪʒən]

In this example, [l] is assimilated to [d] because of the influence of the beginning [t] in "television." The lateral [l] is now articulated very similarly to the beginning [t]; however, the voicing of the [l] is maintained, thus [d]. This is progressive remote assimilation.

Regressive

"pumpkin" [pʌmkɪn] ⟶ [pʌŋkɪn]

Here the [m] is assimilated to a [ŋ] because of the impact of the [k]. Again, ease of production has changed the nasal [m], a front sound, to a nasal that is very close in production to the [k]. Both the [k] and [ŋ] are back sounds (postdorsal-velar). This is regressive contact assimilation.

"bathtub" [bæθtʌb] ⟶ [θæθtʌb]

Active, passive articulators and manner are impacted as [θ] influences the previous segment [b]. The result is that [b] is replaced by [θ]: This is regressive remote assimilation.

In regard to the different degrees of assimilatory influence, one distinguishes between phonemic assimilation and phonetic similitude (Ball & Rahilly, 1999). An altered segment that is perceived to be a different phoneme altogether is termed *phonemic assimilation*. *Phonetic similitude* occurs when the change in the segment is such that it is still perceived by speakers of a language as nothing more than a variation of the original segment. A phonemic assimilation could be exemplified by the change in *ten girls* [tɛn gɝlz] to [tɛŋ gɝlz]; the [n] completely changes to [ŋ] because of the influence of the following postdorsal-velar stop-plosive [g]. An example of a phonetic similitude would be the lip rounding of [s] in *soup* [sʷup] (the ʷ denotes lip rounding) as the [s] is influenced by the lip rounding of the following [u]. This would still be perceived as [s], not another sound value; the [sʷ] is an allophone of /s/.

Assimilation processes can also be total or partial. Total assimilation occurs when the changed segment and the source of the influence become identical. Partial assimilation exists when the changed segment is close to, but not identical to, the source segment.

The following are examples of total and partial assimilation processes:

Total   "window"   [wɪndoᵛ] → [wɪnoᵛ]

"Pontiac"   [pɑntiæk] → [pɑniæk]

In these two examples, the [d] and [t] are gone, the only remaining sound is the [n], and, thus, there is total assimilation.

Partial "handkerchief"

[hæŋkətʃɪf] → [hæŋkətʃɪf]

In this example, the nasality of the sound is present, but the placement of the active and passive articulators has changed from a coronal-alveolar [n] to a postdorsal-velar [ŋ].

The term *coalescence* is used when two neighboring segments are merged into a new and different segment. An example of coalescence would be the realization of *sandwich* [sænwɪtʃ] as [sæmɪtʃ]. The [n] and [w] have fused into the resulting [m]. This assimilation demonstrates the bilabial features for the articulation of [w] with the nasality of the [n]. The result is a bilabial nasal [m].

Children at different stages of their speech-language development tend to use assimilation processes in systematic ways. This is of obvious interest to clinicians whose task is to separate normal from impaired phonological development. In normally developing children and those with disordered phonology, syllable structure can also impact their production possibilities. This is discussed in the next section.

> Typical assimilation processes and the ages at which these processes occur in children are discussed in Chapter 5.

CLINICAL APPLICATION

Assimilation Processes and Articulation Testing

Assimilatory or harmony processes often occur during an articulation test. It is important to recognize these processes so that the test scoring will not be negatively impacted. The author has frequently observed the following assimilation processes:

Word	Expected Response	Child's Response	Impact on Scoring
Santa	[sæntə]	[sænə] total assimilation	Could be scored as an omission of [t]
sandwich	[sænwɪtʃ]	[sæmɪtʃ] total assimilation (coalescence)	Could be scored as an omission of [w] and an [m]/[n] substitution
presents	[prɛzənts]	[prɛzəns] total assimilation	Could be scored as an omission of [t]

A less common example was observed for Danny, age 4;3:

bath	[bæθ]	[θæθ]	[θ]/[b] substitution
bathtub	[bæθtʌb]	[θæθʌb]	[θ]/[b] substitution

However, Danny could produce [b] correctly in all other contexts. Note the correct production of [b] at the end of *bathtub*. This was an example of a regressive remote assimilation.

Syllable Structure

If we are asked to break words down into component parts, syllables seem to be more natural than sounds. For example, speakers of unwritten languages characteristically use syllable, not sound, divisions. They may even resist the notion that any further breakdown is possible (Ladefoged & Johnson, 2010). Also, preschool children use syllabification if they try to analyze a word. It is only after children are exposed to writing that they begin to understand the possibility of dividing words into sounds. Thus, syllables appear to be easily recognizable units.

Counting the number of syllables in a word is a relatively simple task. Probably all will agree on the number of syllables in the word *away* or *articulation*, for example. What we might disagree on are the beginning and end points of the syllables in question. To arrive at a consensus, it is first necessary to differentiate between written and spoken syllables.

A dictionary has written syllabification rules. We learn that the word *cutting* is to be divided cut-ting. However, differences may, and often do, exist between written and spoken syllables. The written syllabification rules for *cutting* do not reflect the way we would syllabify the word when speaking. The divisions [kʌ tɪŋ] would be more probable during normal speech. An awareness of existing differences between spoken and written syllable boundaries is important for speech-language specialists.

Determining spoken syllables can be especially problematic because a dictionary of rules for the boundaries of *spoken* syllables does not exist. Thus, two competent speakers of a given language may syllabify the same word in different ways. Words such as *hammer* and *window* would probably not cause problems. However, how should one syllabify *telephone*, as [tɛ lə foᵘn] or as [tɛl ə foᵘn]? That is, does [l] belong to the second or to the first syllable? Variations in the syllabification of spoken words do indeed exist between speakers. To understand this, a look at the syllable structure might be a good way to begin.

Structurally, the syllable can be divided into three parts: *peak, onset,* and *coda.* The **peak** is the most prominent, acoustically most intense part of the syllable. Although vowels are clearly more prevalent as syllable peaks, consonants are not strictly excluded. Consonants that serve as the syllable peak are referred to as *syllabics.* A peak may stand alone, as in the first syllable of the word *a-way*, or it can be surrounded by other sounds, as in *tan* or *bring.*

The **onset** of a syllable consists of all the segments prior to the peak, whereas the **coda** is made up of all the sound segments of a syllable following its peak. The segments that compose the onset are also termed *syllable releasing* sounds, and those of the coda are termed *syllable arresting* sounds. Thus, the onset of *meet* [mit] is [m]; that is, [m] is the syllable releasing sound. The coda, or syllable arresting sound, of *meet* is [t]. This applies also to consonant blends within one syllable. The onset of *scratched* is [skr], its peak is [æ], and the coda is [tʃt]. Not all syllables have onsets or codas. Both syllables of *today* [tudeᴵ] lack a coda, whereas *off* [ɑf] does not have an onset. The number of segments that an onset or a coda may contain is regulated by the phonotactic rules of the language in question. General American English syllables can have one to three segments in an onset (ray, stay, stray) and one to four segments in a coda (sit, sits, sixth [sɪksθ], sixths [sɪksθs]).

The peak and coda together are referred to as the **rhyme**. Therefore, in the word *sun*, the onset is "s" and the rhyme is "un." Syllables that do not contain codas are called **open** or **unchecked syllables**. Examples of open, unchecked syllables are *do* [du], *glee* [gli], or the first syllable of *rebound* [ri baᵘnd]. Syllables that do have codas are called **closed** or **checked syllables**, such as in *stop* [stɑp] or the first syllable in *window* [wɪn].

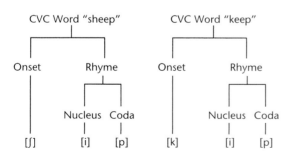

The words "sheep" and "keep" have the same rhyme. Therefore, these words "rhyme."

Every language has its own syllable structure rules, its own set of phonotactic restraints. The sonority scale highly influences the syllable structure rules. The general rule is that more sonorous elements are closer to the syllable nucleus, whereas less sonorant elements are farther away. The rules of phonotactics in General American English operate around this sonority hierarchy. The nucleus or peak of the syllable has maximal sonority, the sonority decreasing as you move away from the nucleus. Recall the sonority hierarchy from most sonorous (vowels) to the least [p, t, k]:

vowels → [w, j] → [r] → [l] → [m, n, ŋ] →[h] → [v, z, ʒ, ð] → [f, s, ʃ, θ] → [b, d, g] → [p, t, k]

This sonority hierarchy explains why the combination [sl] occurs only at the onset, whereas [ls] is only at the coda of a syllable. The [l] has more sonority than the [s]; therefore, it needs to be closer to the nucleus, which results in words such as [slip] and [pʌls] but not [lsip] or [pʌsl]. It should be noted that the [s] violates this principle often in General American English and in other languages (O'Grady & Archibald, 2012). Therefore, the combination [st] does occur as an onset in the word "stop," for example. The following represents a list of the phonotactic constraints of General American English

1. All syllables have a nucleus.
2. No /h/ is in the syllable coda. Although a word ends in the letter "h" such as "sigh" there is no /h/.
3. Complex onsets (those containing more than one element) cannot contain affricates /tʃ/ or /dʒ/.
4. The first consonant in a complex onset must be an obstruent (stop-plosive or fricative).
5. The second consonant in a complex onset cannot be a voiced obstruent (no voiced stop-plosives or fricatives).
6. If the first consonant in a complex onset is not an /s/, the second must be a liquid (/l, r/) or glide (/w, j/), for example, "flower" or "twin."
7. No glides are in codas of syllables. Words may end with the letter "w" for example, "cow" but that is spelling, not pronunciation.
8. If there is a complex coda, the second consonant cannot be /ŋ/, /ʒ/, or /ð/.
9. If the second consonant in a complex coda is voiced, so is the first.
10. Non-alveolar nasals /m, ŋ/ must be homorganic with the next segment (e.g., in "singer" /sɪŋgɚ/, the /ŋ/ and /g/ are homorganic).
11. Two obstruents in the same coda must share voicing (e.g., "bets" /ts/ and "beds" /dz/) (Haspelmath & Sims, 2010).

These phonotactic rules vary in every language. It is important to remember when working with individuals who are learning English as a second language. The phonotactics of their native language may influence their pronunciation patterns in English. For example, Cantonese has no consonant combinations (if the labialized /k/, /kʷ/ is counted as a consonant); therefore, no complex onsets or codas exist (except for colloquial Cantonese). This may impact the speaker's production capabilities in General American English.

The use of specific syllable structures is often neglected when analyzing the speech characteris-tics of children. However, they do seem to play an important developmental role. A child's first words consist typically of open or unchecked syllables, such as [bɑ] for *ball* or [mɪ] for *milk*. If children start to produce closed syllables, they usually contain only single-segment

CLINICAL EXERCISES

Johnny has an [s] problem and is beginning to work on two-syllable words (see page 34). Can you make up a list of 10 words that order the principles from easy to hard for type of syllables (5 words) and the degree of syllable stress (5 words)?

Now Johnny is working on consonant clusters with [s] at the beginning of a word. According to the principle of the number of consonants in a cluster, order the following words from easy to hard: spot, street, scratch, slide, stop, skunk, swim, spring. Based on production features of [s] and the other consonants in the cluster, try to state a rationale for further ordering the words.

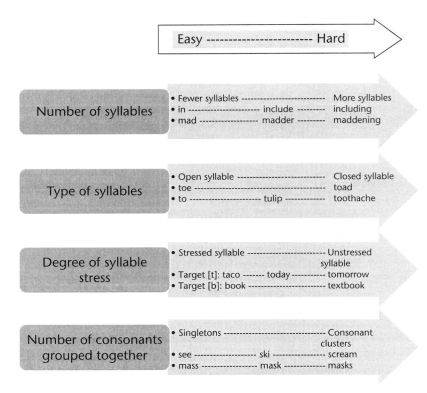

codas. Similarly, two-syllable words at this stage of development consist usually of open syllables (e.g., Ingram, 1976; Menn, 1971; Velten, 1943). Productions such as [be^{I} bi] for *baby* or [ti pɑ] for *teapot* are examples.

The ease of syllable production can be affected by at least three circumstances: (1) the *number of syllables* in an utterance, (2) the *type of syllable* (open versus closed), and (3) the *degree of syllable stress* (stressed or unstressed). Generally, fewer syllables, open syllables, and stressed syllables facilitate accurate productions of specific target sounds. Another concept that could be included is (4) the *number of consonants that are grouped together*. Single consonants (singletons) are easier to produce than consonant clusters. Therefore, a word with just a single consonant is easier to produce than a similarly structured word with consonant clusters. The diagram above represents these four factors based on ease of production.

SUMMARY

This chapter presented a broad definition of phonetics and three subdivisions: articulatory, acoustic, and auditory phonetics. Within articulatory phonetics, an overview of vowels and consonants was given, and the form and function of vowels and consonants of General American English were discussed. Both vowels and consonants were classified according to their articulatory production features and their linguistic functions. Phonetic descriptors were given to provide the clinician with a detailed account of articulatory action during normal production of vowels and

consonants. These features can later be contrasted to those noted in the impaired sound realizations of children and adults with speech sound disorders.

In the second portion of this chapter, coarticulation, assimilation processes, and syllable structure were defined and examined. Coarticulation and resulting assimilatory processes were described as normal articulatory consequences that regularly occur in the speech of individuals. Assimilatory processes were defined according to the type and degree of sound modification. Examples were given of assimilatory processes in children and of the possible impact these processes could have on articulation test results. The last section, on syllable structure, defined the parts of the syllable and examined the phonotactic rules for syllable structure in General American English. It was suggested that an analysis of syllable structures could provide the clinician with additional knowledge when evaluating individuals with speech sound disorders.

CASE STUDY

The following sample is from Tina, age 3;8.

dig	[dɛg]	cat	[tæt]
house	[haʊθ]	bath	[bæt]
knife	[naf]	red	[led]
duck	[dʊt]	ship	[sɪp]
fan	[vɛn]	ring	[wɪŋ]
yes	[wɛt]	thumb	[dʌm]
boat	[bot]	that	[zæt]
cup	[tʊp]	zip	[wɪp]
lamp	[wæmp]	key	[di]
goat	[dot]	win	[jɪn]

Compare the typical vowel productions to those noted in the sample according to

1. The portion of the tongue that is involved in the articulation (front, central, back).
2. The tongue's position relative to the palate (high, mid, low). For example:

    dig   [dɛg]   a high-front vowel changed to a mid-front vowel

Compare the typical consonant productions to those noted in the sample according to voicing, active/passive articulators, and manner characteristics.

     house   [haʊθ]   a voiceless apico-alveolar (predorsal-alveolar) fricative [s] is changed to a voiceless interdental (apico-dental) fricative [θ]

Continue to analyze the vowel and consonant changes for the other words contained in this sample.

THINK CRITICALLY

1. Some young children have trouble producing [s] and [z]; they substitute [θ] and [ð] for these sounds. Thus, the word *Sue* would be pronounced [θu] and *zoo* as [ðu]. Compare the two articulations and see whether you might be able to describe to a child of age 6 what he or she would have to do to change the articulation from [θ] and [ð] to [s] to [z].

2. Children often have trouble with the lip rounding associated with the sh-sounds ([ʃ] and [ʒ]). Which type of vowel contexts would promote lip rounding? Can you find five words that you could use to assist in the lip rounding of [ʃ]?

3. Identify the following assimilation processes according to the parameters: contact versus remote, progressive versus regressive, phonemic assimilation, phonetic similitude, or coalescence.

news	[nuẓ]	however	news-paper	[nuspeˈpɚ]
panty	[pænti]	→	[pæni]	
did you	[dɪd ju]	→	[dɪd ʒu]	
incubate	[ɪnkjubeˈt]	→	[ɪŋkjubeˈt]	
misuse	[mɪsjuz]	→	[mɪʃuz]	

4. Identify the following syllable structures according to (a) onset, peak, and coda and (b) closed or open syllables. For example:

   win.dow → [wɪn.doʊ]
   1st syllable: onset-peak-coda, closed syllable
   2nd syllable: onset-peak, open syllable
   telephone
   wagon
   shovel
   banana
   pajamas

5. You are testing [k] sounds in the initial, medial, and final positions with a child who is 4 years old with a [t] for [k] substitution. You would like to keep the syllable structure and the stress consistent for all the words used. Therefore, all words should be two syllables in length, stress should be on the same syllable, and syllable structures should be comparable. Find six words that could be used for a 4-year-old child which would test [k] under these conditions.

TEST YOURSELF

1. Which one of the following is *not* included in the definition of phonetics?
   a. the production features of speech sounds
   b. the organizational system of speech sounds
   c. the transmission properties of speech sounds
   d. the perceptual bases of speech sounds

2. Which one of the subdivisions of phonetics would examine the frequency, intensity, and duration of speech sounds?
   a. articulatory phonetics
   b. acoustic phonetics
   c. auditory phonetics

3. If you were studying how foreign students perceive various speech sounds of General American English, which branch of phonetics would you be studying?
   a. articulatory phonetics
   b. acoustic phonetics
   c. auditory phonetics

4. If you were studying how the production of [s] varies in General American English versus Spanish, which branch of phonetics would you be studying?
   a. articulatory phonetics
   b. acoustic phonetics
   c. auditory phonetics

5. Vowels are defined as having
   a. no simultaneous vocal fold vibration under normal conditions
   b. articulatory constriction along the sagittal midline of the vocal tract
   c. relatively unimpeded airstream from the vocal folds to the lips
   d. relatively less acoustic intensity than consonants

6. Which consonants are considered to be sonorant consonants?
   a. fricatives and affricates
   b. stop-plosives
   c. all voiced consonants
   d. nasals, liquids, and glides

7. The vowel [i] is described phonetically as a
   a. high-front vowel that is unrounded and lax
   b. mid-front vowel that is unrounded and tense
   c. high-front vowel that is unrounded and tense
   d. high-back vowel that is unrounded and tense

8. The consonant [l] is described phonetically as a
   a. voiced apico-alveolar lateral approximant
   b. voiced coronal-alveolar glide
   c. voiced predorsal-alveolar lateral-approximant
   d. voiced postdorsal-velar lateral-approximant

9. A very young child says [ɡɑɡ] for *dog*. This is which type of assimilation process?
   a. regressive phonemic assimilation
   b. progressive phonemic assimilation
   c. regressive phonetic similitude
   d. coalescence

10. A young child says [nɔˈni] for *noisy*. This is which type of assimilation process?
    a. progressive contact phonemic assimilation
    b. regressive contact phonemic assimilation
    c. progressive remote phonemic assimilation
    d. progressive remote phonetic similitude

11. Which one of the following words has an unchecked syllable structure?
    a. cupcake   c. jumping
    b. tomato   d. bathtub

12. What is the rhyme of "reached"?
    a. [i]   c. [itʃt]
    b. [itʃ]   d. [it]

FURTHER READINGS

Ashby, P. (2005). *Speech sounds.* London: Routledge.

Bauman-Waengler, J. (2009). *Introduction to phonetics and phonology: From concepts to transcription.* Boston: Pearson/Allyn & Bacon.

Davenport, M., & Hannahs, J. (2006). *Introducing phonetics and phonology.* London: Arnold.

Garn-Nunn, P., & Lynn, J. (2004). *Calvert's descriptive phonetics* (3rd ed.). New York: Thieme.

Ladefoged, P. (2005). *Vowels and consonants* (2nd ed.). Malden, MA: Blackwell.

Yavaş, M. (2005). *Applied English phonology.* Malden, MA: Blackwell.

APPENDIX 2.1 Phonetic Symbols Used in Current Phonetic Transcription Textbooks

Word Example: Diphthongs	Bauman-Waengler (2009)	Edwards (2003)	Garn-Nunn & Lynn (Calvert's, 2004)	Shriberg and Kent (2013)	Small (2012)
buy, my	[aɪ] or [ɑɪ] depending on pronunciation	[aɪ]	[aɪ]	[a͞ɪ]	[aɪ]
bay, may	[e] monophthong, [eɪ] diphthong	[e]	[e] monophthong, [eɪ], diphthong	[e] monophthong, [e͞ɪ] diphthong	[e] monophthong, [eɪ], diphthong
boat, home	[o] monophthong, [oʊ] diphthong	[o]	[o] monophthong, [oʊ], diphthong	[o] monophthong, [o͞ʊ] diphthong	[o] monophthong, [oʊ], diphthong
cow, loud	[aʊ]	[aʊ]	[aʊ]	[a͞ʊ]	[aʊ]
boy, hoist	[ɔɪ]	[ɔɪ]	[ɔɪ]	[ɔ͞ɪ]	[ɔɪ]
Word Examples: Rhotic Diphthongs					
fear, beer	[ɪɚ]	[ɪr]	[ɪr]	[ɪr]	[ɪr]
bear, mare	[ɛɚ]	[ɛr]	[ɛr]	[ɛr]	[ɛr]
more, floor	[oɚ] or [ɔɚ] depending upon pronunciation	[ɔr]	[ɔr]	[ɔr]	[ɔr]
bar, far	[ɑɚ]	[ɑr]	[ɑr]	[ɑr]	[ɑr]

Phonetic Transcription and Diacritics

LEARNING OBJECTIVES

When you have finished this chapter, you should be able to:

- Define phonetic transcription and explain why it is a notational system.
- Describe how the International Phonetic Alphabet is used.
- Explain the value of transcription for speech-language therapists.
- Define diacritics.
- Identify the diacritics used to delineate consonant and vowel sounds.
- Identify the diacritics used to mark stress, duration, and syllable boundaries.

VIRTUALLY every book on speech sound disorders contains a brief discussion of phonetic transcription. In such a section, the symbols and diacritics of the International Phonetic Alphabet are listed with a comment on the importance of accurate transcription for the assessment procedure. This underplays its importance, however; accurate transcription forms *the* basis for the diagnosis of articulatory-phonological impairments. If clinicians cannot correctly identify and transcribe the productions of their clients, their therapy will not be as goal directed as it should be. Transcribing words phonetically is also an invaluable aid in documenting change as therapy progresses. It is a vital skill in assessing and treating speech sound disorders.

Nevertheless, in training and in clinical practice, phonetic transcription seems to be one of the most neglected areas of study. Although transcription skills are as indispensable as they are difficult to master, the chance to learn them is often limited to one undergraduate course. This meager knowledge base is seldom systematically expanded or revisited in other courses or in most clinical experiences. Many practicing clinicians simply do not feel comfortable with phonetic transcription and, therefore, unfortunately use it as infrequently as possible.

Phonetic transcription is more than just transposing perceived sounds into "strange" symbols; it is above all a process of fine-tuning one's auditory perception for the purpose of successful clinical intervention. Perceptual skills improve with systematic efforts to listen carefully to, and differentiate accurately among, subtle changes in sound quality. Although this is not a workbook on phonetic transcription (this section does not offer nearly enough information for such a course), it does emphasize and treat phonetic transcription in considerably more detail than textbooks on speech sound disorders usually do.

The first goal of this chapter is to introduce the International Phonetic Alphabet as a notational system used to document norm productions of vowels and consonants of General American English. However, the transcription of disordered speech requires more than that. It needs additional signs, diacritical marks that can be added to basic transcription symbols to indicate additional sound values. They provide a means of documenting irregular articulatory events. Therefore, this chapter's second goal is to present and discuss some of the more common diacritical marks. Clinical comments are included to exemplify the use of these diacritics. The third goal of this chapter is to examine the clinical implications of phonetic transcription, including the use of diacritics. Examples are provided to demonstrate how phonetic transcription can be used in the assessment and treatment process.

Phonetic Transcription as a Notational System

Speech is a fleeting event, existing for only the shortest time period—so short, in fact, that if artificial means are not used, its existence could not be documented even immediately after the event. Historically, all writing systems were invented to make speech events last longer, to preserve them.

Traditional writing systems do a great job in preserving *what* has been said, but they fall grossly short in indicating *how* it has been said, even though this can be just as important. For example, a speech-language specialist needs to document the details of a child's aberrant sound realizations. There are no letters in our alphabet for laterally produced s-sounds, for instance. Professionals clearly need more information about *how* a specific speech event has been executed than about *what* has been said. For these special purposes, traditional writing systems are useless. Special ones had to be invented to serve these needs. *Phonetic transcription* systems were devised to document real actualizations of speech events.

Today, the frequently revised International Phonetic Alphabet is probably the most widely accepted transcription system in the world (Figure 3.1). The International Phonetic Association, founded in 1886, published the first International Phonetic Alphabet in 1888. It offers a one-to-one correspondence between phoneme realizations and sound symbols. However, at the same time, many additional signs can be used to identify modifications in the original production. Generally, the International Phonetic Alphabet serves the professional interests of speech-language pathologists well. Its symbols capture much of what we are interested in. Occasionally, one may be forced to add to the inventory of available symbols to characterize an irregular production. That, though, is to be expected because phonetic transcription systems are typically designed to transfer standard (but highly impermanent) speech events adequately into (more durable) readable signs. In *aberrant* speech, just about anything can happen, and this may well necessitate additional characters to indicate unusual articulatory events. If such an additional characterization becomes necessary, the specific phonetic value of any added sign must, of course, be described precisely and in detail. If other professionals cannot reliably "read" the transcribed materials, they cannot accurately retransform the symbols into the original phonetic events; that is, they still will not know how the sound was actualized. Under such circumstances, any phonetic transcription becomes pointless.

Transcription is separated into two types: Broad and narrow. The more general type of transcription is referred to as **broad transcription**, which is based on the phoneme system of the particular language; each symbol represents a phoneme. Because of the fact that phonemes within a language system are noted, this type of transcription is also referred to as **phonemic transcription**. For broad transcription, the symbols are placed within slashes / /, which are termed *virgules*. Thus, /p/ would indicate phonemic transcription.

A second type of transcription is **narrow transcription**. This type records the sound units with as much production detail as possible. This notation encompasses both the use of the broad classification system noted in the International Phonetic Alphabet as well as extra symbols, which can be added to give a particular phonetic value; in other words,

THE INTERNATIONAL PHONETIC ALPHABET (revised to 2005)

CONSONANTS (PULMONIC)

© 2005 IPA

	Bilabial	Labiodental	Dental	Alveolar	Postalveolar	Retroflex	Palatal	Velar	Uvular	Pharyngeal	Glottal
Plosive	p b			t d		ʈ ɖ	c ɟ	k g	q ɢ		ʔ
Nasal	m	ɱ		n		ɳ	ɲ	ŋ	N		
Trill	B			r					R		
Tap or Flap		ⱱ		ɾ		ɽ					
Fricative	ɸ β	f v	θ ð	s z	ʃ ʒ	ʂ ʐ	ç ʝ	x ɣ	χ ʁ	ħ ʕ	h ɦ
Lateral fricative				ɬ ɮ							
Approximant		ʋ		ɹ		ɻ	j	ɰ			
Lateral approximant				l		ɭ	ʎ	L			

Where symbols appear in pairs, the one to the right represents a voiced consonant. Shaded areas denote articulations judged impossible.

CONSONANTS (NON-PULMONIC)

Clicks		Voiced implosives		Ejectives	
ʘ	Bilabial	ɓ	Bilabial	ʼ	Examples:
ǀ	Dental	ɗ	Dental/alveolar	pʼ	Bilabial
ǃ	(Post)alveolar	ʄ	Palatal	tʼ	Dental/alveolar
ǂ	Palatoalveolar	ɠ	Velar	kʼ	Velar
ǁ	Alveolar lateral	ʛ	Uvular	sʼ	Alveolar fricative

OTHER SYMBOLS

ʍ	Voiceless labial-velar fricative	ɕ ʑ	Alveolo-palatal fricatives
w	Voiced labial-velar approximant	ɺ	Voiced alveolar lateral flap
ɥ	Voiced labial-palatal approximant	ɧ	Simultaneous ʃ and x
ʜ	Voiceless epiglottal fricative		
ʢ	Voiced epiglottal fricative		Affricates and double articulations can be represented by two symbols joined by a tie bar if necessary. k͡p t͡s
ʡ	Epiglottal plosive		

VOWELS

	Front	Central	Back
Close	i • y	ɨ • ʉ	ɯ • u
	ɪ ʏ	ʊ	
Close-mid	e • ø	ɘ • ɵ	ɤ • o
Open-mid	ɛ • œ	ɜ • ɞ	ʌ • ɔ
	æ	ɐ	
Open	a • ɶ		ɑ • ɒ

Where symbols appear in pairs, the one to the right represents a rounded vowel.

SUPRASEGMENTALS

ˈ	Primary stress	ˌfoʊnəˈtɪʃən
ˌ	Secondary stress	
ː	Long	eː
ˑ	Half-long	eˑ
˘	Extra-short	ĕ
|	Minor (foot) group	
‖	Major (intonation) group	
.	Syllable break	ɹi.ækt
‿	Linking (absence of a break)	

DIACRITICS

Diacritics may be placed above a symbol with a descender, e.g. ŋ̊

̥	Voiceless	n̥ d̥	̤	Breathy voiced	b̤ a̤	̪	Dental	t̪ d̪
̬	Voiced	s̬ t̬	̰	Creaky voiced	b̰ a̰	̺	Apical	t̺ d̺
ʰ	Aspirated	tʰ dʰ	̼	Linguolabial	t̼ d̼	̻	Laminal	t̻ d̻
̹	More rounded	ɔ̹	ʷ	Labialized	tʷ dʷ	̃	Nasalized	ẽ
̜	Less rounded	ɔ̜	ʲ	Palatalized	tʲ dʲ	ⁿ	Nasal release	dⁿ
̟	Advanced	u̟	ˠ	Velarized	tˠ dˠ	ˡ	Lateral release	dˡ
̠	Retracted	e̠	ˤ	Pharyngealized	tˤ dˤ	̚	No audible release	d̚
̈	Centralized	ë	̴	Velarized or pharyngealized	ɫ			
̽	Mid-centralized	̽e	̝	Raised	e̝	(ɹ̝ = voiced alveolar fricative)		
̩	Syllabic	n̩	̞	Lowered	e̞	(β̞ = voiced bilabial approximant)		
̯	Non-syllabic	e̯	̘	Advanced Tongue Root	e̘			
˞	Rhoticity	ɚ a˞	̙	Retracted Tongue Root	e̙			

TONES AND WORD ACCENTS

LEVEL			CONTOUR		
e̋ or ˥	Extra high		ě or ˇ	Rising	
é ˦	High		ê ˆ	Falling	
ē ˧	Mid		e᷄ ˊ	High rising	
è ˨	Low		e᷅ ˏ	Low rising	
ȅ ˩	Extra low		e᷈ ˜	Rising-falling	
↓	Downstep		↗	Global rise	
↑	Upstep		↘	Global fall	

FIGURE 3.1 The International Phonetic Alphabet (revised to 2005)

Source: Copyright 2005 International Phonetic Association. Reproduced by permission. Available http://www.langsci.ucl.ac.uk/ipa/ipachart.html

to characterize specific production features. This type of transcription is also denoted as **phonetic transcription** because it includes phonetic, production feature details. For narrow transcription, the symbols are placed within brackets [ ]. For example, [tʰ] would be narrow transcription exemplifying a sound unit [t] with aspiration [ʰ]. Another way to look at broad and narrow transcription would be to refer back to the definitions of *phoneme* and *allophone* (see pages 5–6). Broad transcription notes the differences in *phonemes*, whereas narrow transcription exemplifies *allophones*. As clinicians, we are often analyzing disordered speech; therefore, additional symbols may be added to the basic sound unit to characterize allophonic variation. These notations are termed *diacritics* and are discussed in the next section. At other times, the actual production may be so different that another phoneme symbol will be needed. For example, a child may produce "th" for "s" in all words. We could summarize this as a difference in a child's phonemic system; broad transcription exemplified by /θ/ for /s/ could be used. On the other hand, narrow transcription is employed if a child's tongue placement of "s" is just a bit too far forward, and the result does not sound like "th" but rather a distorted "s." A marker, a diacritic, is added to "s." This narrow transcription is [s̪], the small symbol under the "s" indicating a dentalized production, one in which the tongue is approaching the front teeth; that is, the tongue is slightly forward, giving the "s" a distorted quality.

CLINICAL COMMENTS

This dichotomy between broad and narrow transcription, or phonemic versus phonetic transcription, relates directly to the difference between a phonemic and a phonetic inventory. A *phonemic inventory* contains all the phonemes that a child uses contrastively. Because /θ/ and /s/ are two different phonemes, if a child uses both contrastively, for example contrasts "sink" and "think," both would be included in the phonemic inventory. However, if he or she uses /θ/ for all /s/ phonemes, then only /θ/ would be included in the phonemic inventory, not /s/. On the other hand, the phonetic inventory includes, but is not limited to, the phonetic details that are categorized by the use of diacritics. Therefore, if a child says [sʷ] (lip rounded [s]), [s̪] (dentalized [s]), and [sʲ] (palatalized [s]) for /s/, then /s/ is part of the phonemic inventory, but all three variants [sʷ], [s̪], and [sʲ] would be contained in the phonetic inventory. Related to [s] productions, the lateral "s" [ɬ] is considered to be so different in its production from /s/ that it is considered to be a separate phoneme. This is due to the fact that lateralization is considered to be a *primary* articulation. Therefore, if a child says [ɬ] for *all* /s/ phonemes, then /ɬ/ is in the phonemic and phonetic inventory, but /s/ would not be included in either.

The dichotomy between phonetic and phonemic transcription often leads to transcribers using brackets, [ ], and slashes, / /, interchangeably. However, as noted in the previous chapter, brackets, [ ], should be used when listening to and transcribing actual productions. This notation indicates actual realizations, the concrete productions of a speech sound. Therefore, if we are transcribing a child's speech, the brackets, [ ], should be used. If we are summarizing a phonemic inventory, then phonemic or broad transcription might be sufficient. As speech-language clinicians, however, we often assess disordered speech. In this case, narrow transcription will probably be used to note as much detail as possible. Narrow transcription is a necessity when the individual's speech patterns demonstrate errors that cannot be perceptually classified as phonemes of that given language.

Phonetic transcription is a purely *descriptive* enterprise. Occasionally, beginning transcription materials consist of lists of orthographically presented words (*book, table, snail,* and so on) that students then have to transfer into phonetic symbols. Such a practice can be misleading. It supports the mistaken notion that there is a *prescriptive* part to phonetic transcription that provides some guiding principle about how words are supposed to be pronounced. This is also suggested by dictionaries: Each entry tells the reader how to spell a word correctly, and the following symbols indicate how the word "should be" pronounced. There is, of course, nothing wrong with spelling out how words are commonly pronounced, but any jump from how they *are* pronounced to how they *should be* pronounced has nothing to do with the idea behind or practice of phonetic transcription.

Why Use Phonetic Transcription?

Accurate phonetic transcription is an indispensable clinical tool for speech-language pathologists. That is why it has to be taken so seriously, especially when it is used to assess and remediate impaired articulation and phonology. Without a reliable record of how a child or adult realized a particular speech sound, we simply do not have enough information for goal-directed intervention, nor can we document changes in production that might occur during therapy. Phonetic transcription provides a reasonably accurate written record of what was said and what it sounded like.

Admittedly, phonetic transcription is somewhat troublesome and time consuming. In addition, it certainly has its own problems. Some rules have to be strictly observed to overcome these problems. The first thing any aspiring transcriber has to understand is that the human ear is not a microphone. We are unable to *receive* only; we must always *perceive*; that is, people automatically judge and interpret incoming acoustic signals based on their experience with those signals. In respect to spoken language, this means that when listening to the incoming acoustic signal, the listener unwillingly "distorts" it in the direction of former experiences, including how the listener would have produced it. This "built-in" tendency is the greatest danger to any serious transcription effort. Any higher degree of accuracy is very difficult to attain if perceptual biases rule transcription efforts. To overcome the tendency to "interpret" what was heard requires considerable goodwill, patience, and special training.

Several other problems must be considered when using phonetic transcription. For example, many circumstances can affect our transcription, such as the age of the client or an unusual vocal quality. Other factors may produce large variations in the inter- and intrajudge reliability of transcriptions, including the intelligibility of the client, the position of the sound in the word, and whether narrow or broad transcription is used (Shriberg & Lof, 1991). Shriberg and Kent (2013) provide an excellent overview of the sources of variation and the factors that affect the reliability of phonetic transcription. These problems are very real, and caution must be exercised when using phonetic transcription. On the other hand, we cannot simply disregard transcription because of its inherent problems or use a private system of noting sound realizations. Instead, the importance of developing good, reliable transcription skills should be stressed. These skills will prove to be an invaluable resource in the assessment and treatment of speech sound disorders.

Diacritics

Diacritics are marks added to sound transcription symbols to give them a particular phonetic value. The set of basic phonetic transcription symbols represents language-specific typical productions. Because speech-language pathologists deal mostly with aberrant articulatory events, it follows that diacritical marks are of special importance when characterizing the speech of their clients. Diacritics are needed to note the clients' deviant sound qualities.

Numerous diacritics are noted in Figure 3.1. Although these diacritics have functioned fairly effectively, extensions to the International Phonetic Alphabet (extIPA) were developed specifically to address the transcription of disordered speech. The extIPA symbols, first published in 1990, were revised in 2002 and 2008. See Figure 3.2 for a list of the extIPA symbols. The following discussion on diacritics includes only those frequently used by clinicians. Readers should refer to Figures 3.1 and 3.2 for special transcription needs as they develop.

extIPA SYMBOLS FOR DISORDERED SPEECH
(Revised to 2008)

CONSONANTS (other than on the IPA Chart)

	bilabial	labiodental	dentolabial	labioalv.	linguolabial	interdental	bidental	alveolar	velar	velophar.
Plosive		p̪ b̪	p̠̃ b̠̃	p̪ b̪	t̼ d̼	ẗ̪ d̪̈				
Nasal			m̠̃	m̪	n̼	n̪̈				
Trill					r̼	r̪̈				
Fricative median			f̠̃ ṽ̠	f̪ v̪	θ̼ ð̼	θ̪̈ ð̪̈	ḧ̪ ḧ̪			ʩ
Fricative lateral+median								ʪ ʫ		
Fricative nareal	m̃							ñ̥	ŋ̃	
Percussive	w̃w						ʭ			
Approximant lateral					l̼	l̪̈				

Where symbols appear in pairs, the one to the right represents a voiced consonant. Shaded areas denote articulations judged impossible.

DIACRITICS

↔	labial spreading	s̪	⁀	strong articulation	f͈	˵	denasal	m̃
ꟹ	dentolabial	v̺		weak articulation	v̜	˶	nasal escape	v̂
	interdental/bidental	n̪̈	\	reiterated articulation	p\p\p	˷	velopharyngeal friction	s̴
=	alveolar	t̠	,	whistled articulation	s̩	↓	ingressive airflow	p↓
~	linguolabial	d̼	→	sliding articulation	θs	↑	egressive airflow	!↑

CONNECTED SPEECH

(.)	short pause
(..)	medium pause
(...)	long pause
f	loud speech [{f laʊd f}]
ff	louder speech [{ff laʊdə ff}]
p	quiet speech [{p kwaɪət p}]
pp	quieter speech [{pp kwaɪətə pp}]
allegro	fast speech [{allegro fɑst allegro}]
lento	slow speech [{lento sloʊ lento}]
crescendo, ralentando, etc. may also be used	

VOICING

	pre-voicing	˳z
	post-voicing	z˳
	partial devoicing	z̬
	initial partial devoicing	ˌz
	final partial devoicing	z̧
	partial voicing	ˌs
	initial partial voicing	ˌs
	final partial voicing	ş
=	unaspirated	p꞊
ʰ	pre-aspiration	ʰp

OTHERS

(C̄), (C̄), (V̄)	indeterminate sound, consonant, vowel	ⱡ	Velodorsal articulation
(P̄l.v̄l̄s̄), (N̄)	indeterminate voiceless plosive, nasal, etc	¡	sublaminal lower alveolar percussive click
( )	silent articulation (ʃ), (m)	!¡	alveolar and sublaminal clicks (cluck-click)
(( ))	extraneous noise, e.g. ((2 sylls))	*	sound with no available symbol

© ICPLA 2008

FIGURE 3.2 ExtIPA Symbols for Disordered Speech (revised to 2008)

Source: Reprinted by permission of the International Clinical Phonetics and Linguistics Association.

Diacritics Used with Consonants

These symbols describe deviations from normal tongue placement for consonants.

Dentalization.   This term refers to an articulatory variation in which the tongue approaches the upper incisors. It is marked by [ˌ] placed under the IPA symbol. For example, the symbol [d] stands for a coronal-alveolar voiced stop. A dentalized realization results when a child places the tip of the tongue not against the alveolar ridge, as the

IPA symbol indicates, but against the inside of the upper incisors. A *dentalized realization* is transcribed as

[d̪] = dentalized [d]

[d̪] occurs quite often as the result of coarticulation. Compare [d]-productions in the words *widow* and *width*. The articulatory influence of the following [θ], an addental or even interdental sound, will probably "dentalize" normally alveolar [d] realizations. Dentalized s-sounds, [s̪], and [z̪] frequently occur in the speech of children (Smit, 1993b).

Palatalization. Another modification of consonant articulation is *palatalization*. Only sounds for which the palate is *not* the place of articulation can be palatalized. If the place of articulation is the alveolar ridge or the upper incisors, palatalization occurs if the anterior portions of the tongue approach prepalatal or mediopalatal portions of the palate; that is, when the active and passive articulators are positioned somewhat posteriorly. For velar consonants, palatalization indicates the movement of the articulators in the direction of the palate to a more anterior articulation. Palatalization causes a typical change in the quality of the sound(s) in question. The diacritical mark for palatalization is a superscript j added to the right of the basic IPA symbol:

[sʲ] = palatalized [s]

[tʲ] = palatalized [t]

Velarization. This term refers to a more posterior tongue placement (in the direction of the velum) for palatal sounds. The diacritical mark for velarization is a superscript ɣ placed to the right of the IPA symbol. Thus [tˠ] is a velarized [t]. An exception is the so-called dark [l], which may be transcribed in two different ways. In General American English, this dark [l] is usually heard in word-final positions, for example, in *pull* or *shawl*; as a syllabic, such as in *little* or *bottle*; preceding a consonant exemplified by *salt* or *build*; and preceding high-back vowels [u] (*loop*) or [ʊ] (*look*) (Small, 2012). The velarization in these cases is often so prominent that even main phonetic characteristics of [l], the articulation of the tongue tip against the alveolar ridge, are sometimes no longer present. In such a case, the velarization actually replaces the typical apico-alveolar l-articulation. The velarized production is an allophonic variation of [l], it does not change the meaning of the word in question. Velarized [l]-productions are transcribed [ɫ] or [lˠ]:

[fuɫ] = velarized [l]-sound

[kulˠ] = velarized [l]-sound

The so-called dark and light l-sounds are discussed in more detail in Chapter 9.

Lateralization. [l] is the only lateral in General American English. It cannot be lateralized because it is a lateral already. If during any consonant production other than [l] air is released laterally, we speak of *lateralization*. For example, [s] can and often becomes lateralized. Articulations of [s] and [z] require a highly accurate placement of frontal parts of the tongue *approximating* the alveolar ridge, not touching the alveolar ridge. This precarious position must be maintained throughout the entire sound duration, a motorically difficult task, especially for young children. To make things easier, children sometimes establish direct contact between the active and passive articulators. Under these circumstances, the airstream cannot, of course, escape centrally any longer. In an attempt to maintain the fricative effect of [s], children then release the air laterally into the cheeks. The result is a conspicuous [s] variation, a lateral lisp. Lateralization is considered a primary articulation; therefore, the production features are changed so much that a different phoneme results. For example,

Problems with s-Sounds

Dentalized, palatalized, and lateralized [s] realizations are frequent distortions noted in children. In some children, the dentalized [s] may co-occur with a "th" for "s" substitutions ([s] → [θ] or [s] → [s̪]), as in the following productions:

"Santa Claus" [θæn tə klɑs̪] for [sæn tə klɑz]

The tongue position that is too far forward for children's [s]-productions may fluctuate slightly, so that the production is perceived at times as [s̪] and at other times as [θ]. When it is perceived as [s̪], it is an allophonic variation of [s]. However, if it is heard as [θ], the production has crossed phonemic boundaries; it is now perceived as a different phoneme. It is interesting to note that certain children may also use this dichotomy systematically: [θ] may be realized at the beginning of a word or syllable, whereas [s̪] is produced at the end of a word or syllable, for example. Such a possibility should be considered in our assessment.

Differentiating among dentalized, palatalized, and lateralized [s]-productions may seem difficult at first. However, clear perceptual qualities distinguish the three forms. Dentalized [s]-sounds, [s̪], have a "dull" quality; they lack the sharp, high-frequency characteristic of typical [s]-productions. On the other hand, lateralized [s]-sounds, [ɬ], have a distinct noise component to them that is typically rather conspicuous. If the airflow is just on one side (either right or left), a speech-language specialist typically observes a distortion of the lips and even jaw to the side of the air escape. Palatalized [s] variations, [sʲ], perceptually approach a [ʃ] quality. Palatalization of [s] is marked by the anterior portions of the tongue approaching parts of the palate, resulting in a slightly posterior placement of the articulators. If [s] is compared to [ʃ], one notes that [ʃ] realizations also require a more posteriorly placed articulation (apico-alveolar [s] versus coronal-prepalatal [ʃ]).

the voiceless lateral "s" is a phoneme of the Navajo language, whereas the voiced lateral has phonemic value in Mongolian (Ladefoged & Maddieson, 1996). The lateral "s" production is categorized as an apico-alveolar lateral fricative. According to the International Phonetic Alphabet, [ɬ] is the voiceless apico-alveolar fricative, and [ɮ] is its voiced counterpart.

[sɪp] → [ɬɪp] = a lateralized [s]

[zɪp] → [ɮɪp] = a lateralized [z]

The extIPA also provides symbols to distinguish among productions that demonstrate *both* lateral and central airflow (as opposed to just lateral). The symbols for those are

[su] → [ꞎsu] = a voiceless alveolar fricative with lateral and central airflow

[zu] → [ɭzu] = a voiced alveolar fricative with lateral and central airflow

Voice Symbols

Devoicing of Voiced Consonants   Under normal circumstances, vowels and more than half of our consonants are voiced. If these sounds become completely devoiced in a speech sample, the speech needs to be marked. In cases of total devoicing, the International Phonetic Alphabet symbol for the voiceless counterpart of the voiced sound, its unvoiced cognate, is usually indicated.

[ʃus] for "sho<u>es</u>"

[tip] for "<u>d</u>eep"

In this case, the phonemic value has changed from /z/ to /s/ in "shoes" and from /d/ to /t/ in "deep."

Partial Devoicing   Often, however, the sound in question is only partially devoiced. This is considered an allophonic variation of the voiced consonant. The diacritic for partial devoicing is a small circle in parentheses placed under the sound symbol:

[ʃuz̥]

[brɛd̥]

These examples are transcribed according to the extIPA, which differentiates initial devoicing [◌̥] and final devoicing [◌̥].

Voicing Voiceless Consonants   Voiceless consonants may also be voiced, especially if they occur between two vowels. A casual pronunciation of *eighteen* might serve as an example.

If voiceless consonants become totally voiced, the phoneme value has changed and the segment is transcribed with the respective symbol:

[eˈtin] → [eˈdin]

Partial Voicing If voiceless consonants become partially voiced, that is, are allophonic variations of the consonant, the diacritical mark is a lowercase *v* in parentheses under the respective sound symbol:

[eˈt̬in] for "eighteen"

Initial and final partial voicing are [̬] and [̬], respectively.

Aspiration and Nonaspiration of Stop-Plosives
Stop-plosives (as well as other consonants) are often described according to two parameters: fortis and lenis. *Fortis* refers to relatively more articulatory effort, whereas *lenis* refers to comparatively less effort. Most voiceless stop-plosives are realized as fortis consonants, whereas voiced stop-plosives are usually articulated as lenis productions. (One can note the increased articulatory effort on the level of air pressure by contrasting [t] and [d] with a hand in front of the mouth.) The sudden release of the articulatory effort in fortis stop-plosives leads typically to aspiration. This aspiration is noted by using a small superscript h following the voiceless stop-plosive sound:

"table" [tʰeˈbəl]

Stop-plosives, which are normally aspirated, are not marked unless the aspiration is excessive.

Voiceless stop-plosives that are normally aspirated may be produced without this fortis aspiration. In this case, the diacritic for unaspirated stops, [⁼], could be added.

"pie" [p⁼aɪ]

This example indicates that a normally aspirated [p] has occurred without aspiration. This may not appear significant; however, if you have ever tried to learn French with its unaspirated voiceless stop-plosives (such as in "Paris"), you might understand the difficulty. Children may also not aspirate stop-plosives when they are usually aspirated. This can lead to the clinical impression of a voiced stop-plosive.

Unreleased Stop-Plosives
Stop-plosives can be modified in another manner. Unreleased stop-plosives result when the articulatory closure is maintained and not—as usual—released. Although voiceless unreleased stops are more obvious because of their loss of aspiration, voiced stops can be unreleased as well. Unreleased stops typically occur at the end of an utterance or at the end of one-word responses. To indicate an unreleased articulation, the diacritical mark [̚] is added:

Boy, was it hot.

[bɔˈ wʌz ɪt hɑt ̚]

CLINICAL COMMENTS

Partial Voicing and Devoicing
Partial voicing and devoicing are difficult to discern and to transcribe correctly. The first impression of transcribers is often some minor qualitative variance—the sound is somehow "off." Such a first impression is usually a good reason to focus subsequently on the voicing–devoicing opposition. This two-step procedure makes it easier to arrive at the difficult judgment: partially voiced or partially devoiced.

Also, General American English has a tendency to devoice (or partially devoice) final consonants. The following are examples from Daniel, age 4;7.

"stove"	[stoᵘv]	→	[stoᵘf]	total devoicing
"slide"	[slaˈd]	→	[slaˈd̥]	partial devoicing
"flag"	[flæg]	→	[flæg̥]	partial devoicing
"nose"	[noᵘz]	→	[noᵘs]	total devoicing

The general devoicing tendency in final positions suggests that realizations like these should probably not be considered aberrant productions.

Watch and listen to and then transcribe the following video of Marissa and Gail, both 6 years old, saying the following words: dog, tick, coop, good, keg, deed, and dig. Each child says each word three times. Note the partial and total devoicing as well as the interdental articulations.

Voiceless stop-plosives are usually aspirated at the beginning of words; however, they are not aspirated in consonant clusters. Word-final aspiration is variable (Edwards, 2003).

CLINICAL COMMENTS

Transcribing Unreleased Consonants

Unreleased stop-plosives should be noted *during* the simultaneous transcription of a client's speech. Just listening to and transcribing from recordings can be misleading because, when recorded, unreleased stop-plosives can sound similar to consonant omissions. During live transcriptions, we can hear and at least partially see the actual articulation. This provides a much better basis for our judgment regarding an unreleased stop-plosive production or a consonant deletion.

The following transcriptions come from an articulation test of Billy, age 4;3:

"cup"	[kʌp]	→	[tʌp˺]
"music"	[mjuzɪk]	→	[mudɪk˺]
"book"	[bʊk]	→	[bʊk˺]
"feet"	[fit]	→	[fit˺]
"watch"	[wɑtʃ]	→	[wɑt˺]
"sandwich"	[sænwɪtʃ]	→	[gæmɪt˺]

Unreleased stop-plosives seldom warrant therapeutic intervention. Billy's case was different. In addition to his many articulation errors, unreleased consonants contributed substantially to a decrease in his intelligibility.

CLINICAL COMMENTS

Syllabics

In spontaneous speech, adults often reduce the unstressed final syllable, as in the following example:

He broke the bottle.

[hi broᵘk ðə bɑtl̩]

Children can also demonstrate the use of syllabics. For example:

"little" [lɪtl̩]

"scratching" [skræ tʃn̩]

The boy is fishing; he has a fishing pole.

[ðə bɔɪ ɪz'fɪʃn̩ hi hæz ə'fɪʃn̩ poᵘl]

Although such syllabics obviously need to be noted and transcribed, they are considered norm realizations.

Syllabic Consonants Unstressed syllables easily become *reduced syllables*. This means that their vowel nucleus practically disappears. If the vowel nucleus is reduced, the following consonant becomes a syllabic; that is, it becomes the peak of that syllable. This is especially the case in unstressed final syllables when a nasal or the lateral follows the preceding vowel. The proper diacritic mark for such an occurrence is a straight line directly under the syllabic consonant.

fɪʃɪŋ → fɪʃən → fɪʃn̩

Labialization/Nonlabialization of Consonants Consonants, with the exception of [ʃ] and [w], are typically produced without lip rounding. Lip rounding is a production feature of both of these consonants. If a normally unrounded consonant is produced with lip rounding, for example, a normally unrounded [s], this is referred to as *labializing the sound in question.* The diacritic for labialized consonants is a superscript w placed to the right of the symbol in question. When consonants that are normally rounded (such as [ʃ] and [w]) are produced without lip rounding, this is considered nonlabialization. The diacritic for labial spreading [↔] is placed under the symbol in question [ʃ̵] to indicate nonlabialization. Labialized consonants can be the result of assimilation processes, as in the following example:

"soup" [sʷup] = labialized [s] due to the influence of the rounded [u] vowel

Labialization of normally unrounded consonants from assimilation is noted, but it is not considered a speech sound problem. On the other hand, [ʃ] is usually produced with at least some degree of lip rounding. The following example indicates [ʃ] without lip rounding:

"ship" [ʃ̵ɪp] = nonlabialized [ʃ]

Unrounded [ʃ] realizations can also result from assimilation; however, some children unround [ʃ] in all contexts. This is considered an aberrant production and should be noted. It usually affects the quality of the [ʃ], making it sound somewhat "off," qualitatively different from a typical production.

Derhotacization Derhotacization is the loss of r-coloring for the consonant [r] and the central vowels with r-coloring, [ɝ] and [ɚ], respectively. Derhotacized central vowels are transcribed as [ɝ] and [ə]. However, [r], as in *rabbit*, can lose its characteristic r-coloring as well. Children often substitute a [w] for this sound. Another possibility is the substitution of [ʋ], which is a voiced labiodental approximant. For [ʋ], the lower lip approximates the upper teeth. It is very similar to the voiced [w] but with the teeth and lips held in the position used to articulate the letter "vee." The [ʋ] sound, in contrast, also lacks the high-back tongue position of [w], which is considered a labio-*velar* approximant.

Watch, listen to, and transcribe the following video of Summer who is 6 years old. Note the lack of lip rounding on the "sh" words and transcribe them accordingly. What other speech sound difficulties do you note with Summer?

Diacritics Used with Vowels

Rounding/Unrounding of Vowels   There are vowels that have lip rounding as one of their production features and others that are typically produced with no lip rounding—[u] versus [i], for example. The rounding or unrounding of the lips is an important feature of vowel realizations. However, for several reasons, some clients may delete or inappropriately add these characteristics. This results in a distortion of the respective sound quality. The International Phonetic Alphabet offers one symbol to indicate lip rounding (in normally unrounded vowels) and one for unrounding of vowels when they are typically produced with lip rounding. The signs are placed directly under the vowel symbol in question and consist of a small *c*-type notation, which indicates unrounding (or less rounding than is considered normal) when open to the right. When this *c* is reversed, creating an opening to the left, it denotes rounding (or more rounding than is normally the case):

[ṷ] = unrounded [u]

[ɛ̹] = rounded [ɛ]

Changes in Tongue Placement for Vowels   Deviations in tongue positioning affect vowel as well as consonant articulations. Different vowel qualities are established essentially by different sizes and forms of the vocal tract. Two main factors determining these sizes and forms pertain to the location of the raised portion of the tongue (front and back dimensions) and to the extent to which the tongue is raised in the direction of the hard or soft palate (high and low dimensions).

Raised/Lowered Tongue Position   The International Phonetic Alphabet offers a set of

---

CLINICAL COMMENTS

Rounding and Unrounding of [ʃ]

Rounded [s]- and unrounded [ʃ]-sounds are frequent sibilant realizations of children. These may be aberrant productions or context-based assimilation processes. The following is an excerpt from a transcription of Matt, age 4;6:

The boy is swinging really high.
[ðə bɔˈ ɪz sʷwɪŋən rili haˈ]

My mommy made vegetable soup.
[maˈ mɑmi meˈd vɛdʒəbəl sʷup]

In addition to Matt's unorthodox pronunciation of *vegetable*, we note that his [s]-sounds are rounded. In the given context, they may be regressive assimilation processes influenced by the rounding of the following [w] or [u].

This does not seem to be the case in Chris's transcription, which is based on an articulation test and a spontaneous speech sample.

"fish"	[fɪʃ]	→	[fɪ ʃ̮]
"watch"	[wɑtʃ]	→	[wɑ ʃ̮]
"chicken"	[tʃɪkən]	→	[ʃ̮ɪkən]
"shovel"	[ʃʌvəl]	→	[ʃ̮ʌvəl]

At lunch I ate a peanut butter sandwich.
[æt lʌn ʃ̮ aˈ eˈt ə pinət bʌtɚ ʃ̮ænɪʃ̮]

I wish I had some new tennis shoes, like Michael Jordan.
[aˈ wɪʃ̮ aˈ hæd sʌm nu tɛnə ʃ̮uz laˈk maˈkəl ʃordən]

Chris, in contrast to Matt, unrounds his "sh"-sounds even when they precede a rounded vowel, as in the word shoes. He also occasionally uses [ʃ] for [s]-, [tʃ]-, and [dʒ]-sounds.

diacritics that signals the direction of tongue heights on the vertical plane, leading to deviations from norm vowel productions. The diacritic [ᴛ] under the vowel symbol marks a lower elevation, whereas the diacritic [⊥] under the character marks a higher elevation of the tongue than is normally the case for the production of the vowel in question. For example,

$$[s\underset{\tau}{\mathrm{I}}t]$$

would state that the high-front elevation of the tongue for standard [ɪ] articulation has not been reached in this realization; that is, the tongue articulation was lower than normal, resulting in a perceptible distortion for [ɪ]. Trying to describe our auditory impression of this sound, we would say that it shifted in the direction of (but not reaching) the sound quality of [e].

Similarly, the transcription

$$[b\underset{\perp}{\mathrm{I}}t]$$

would indicate a higher-than-normal elevation of the tongue for [ɪ], resulting in a quality that approaches [i] characteristics.

The same principle applies to all vowels. A question that logically follows is whether it makes a difference which symbol we use if the vowel is somewhere between two qualities. In other words, do a raised [e] ([e̝]) and a lowered [ɪ] ([ɪ̞]) signify the same vowel quality? The answer is no. In our previous example, the speech-language specialist must decide whether this vowel realization sounded more like an [e]- or an [ɪ]-type vowel. Based on the transcriber's auditory perception, the basic vowel quality must first be chosen, and then the modifying diacritic mark should be added to it. This is easier to understand if you refer again to the definitions of *phoneme* and *allophone*. These symbols are indicating allophonic variations in a vowel phoneme. Therefore, the phoneme that you understood must first be selected and then the diacritic added to indicate an allophone.

> Think of the symbol as a pointer with its base the top of the T-type notation. If the pointer projects down [ᴛ], the tongue has been lowered; if it points up [⊥], the tongue has been raised.

Advanced/Retracted Tongue Position There are also diacritics signaling tongue variations on the horizontal plane that lead to deviations from norm productions. They indicate a tongue position that is too far forward or too far back for a normal production of the vowel in question. The diacritic for vowels produced with a tongue more advanced than usual is [+]. More retracted protrusions are marked by the diacritic [−]. Both are placed under the vowel symbol.

> [ɛ̟] is an [ɛ] vowel with an advanced tongue articulation; the tongue placement is more forward than is typically the case.
>
> [ʊ̠] is an [ʊ] vowel with a retracted tongue articulation; the tongue placement is too far back.

CLINICAL COMMENTS

Noting Changes in Tongue Positions for Vowels

Changes in the position of the tongue for vowel realizations are often perceptually difficult to target. Although transcribers are aware that the vowel quality is slightly distorted, they may not be sure what has caused this deviation. If the tongue has been lowered or raised, the vowel quality will sound somehow similar to the neighboring vowel on the vertical plane of the vowel quadrilateral. Thus, a lowered [ɛ] will have a certain [æ] quality, or a raised [ʊ] will approach [u]. The best reference source in these cases is the vowel quadrilateral. However, this is not so simple if the tongue movements pertain to the horizontal plane—that is, to a tongue position too advanced or retracted. One point of reference is that front vowels that demonstrate a retracted tongue position and back vowels that demonstrate a tongue position that is too far forward sound somewhat "centralized"—that is, their distinct qualities appear reduced. Therefore, although the vowel can still be identified as the respective front or back vowel, it approaches a [ʌ]-type quality.

Nasality Symbols During the production of most General American English speech sounds, the velum is tensed to block the escape of the expiratory air through the nasal cavity. The only exception to this rule is for the nasals. This is what—quite correctly—the textbooks tell us. However, in reality, the conditions are not always so clear-cut. If a nasal follows a vowel, for example, nasality often seeps into the vowel segment; the preceding vowel becomes nasalized:

$$[tæn] \rightarrow [t\tilde{æ}n]$$

As long as the nasality does not overstep the boundary line of natural assimilatory processes, this nasality remains unmarked. Speakers and listeners perceive these variations as normal. However, if the nasality is perceived as being excessive, or hypernasal, we need to place the "tilde" [~] (which you may have encountered in Spanish language classes) over the respective sound(s). As speech-language specialists, we encounter hypernasality prominently in the speech of clients with dysarthrias and cleft palates.

Denasality is also encountered in the speech of our clients. The symbol for denasality is the tilde with a slash through it, placed above the nasal consonant:

$$ni \rightarrow \tilde{n}i$$

This symbol refers to a reduction of nasal quality. Only nasal consonants can be denasalized. If nasal consonants are perceived as having a total lack of nasal quality (having a completely oral quality), then the symbol for the resulting homorganic voiced stop is used:

$$ni \rightarrow di$$

Assimilation and Dialect

One of the characteristics of African-American dialect is the total regressive assimilation of postvocalic nasals (e.g., Moran, 1993; Wolfram, 1989). The assimilation process is regressive in that the nasal following the vowel changes the characteristic of the preceding vowel into a nasalized vowel. It is considered a *total* assimilation process because the postvocalic nasal consonant is totally gone. The following examples demonstrate this process:

"pen"	[pɛn]	→	[pɛ̃n]	→	[pɛ̃]
"thumb"	[θʌm]	→	[θʌ̃m]	→	[θʌ̃]

These pronunciations were noted on an articulation test from a child, age 4;3, speaking African-American dialect:

"broom"	[brum]	→	[brũ]
"gum"	[gʌm]	→	[gʌ̃]
"sandwich"	[sæn wɪtʃ]	→	[sæ̃ wɪtʃ]
"ice cream"	[aˈs krim]	→	[aˈs krĩ]

The total regressive assimilation process are dialectal in nature. In the African-American dialect, they represent a pronunciation possibility.

Diacritics for Stress, Duration, and Syllable Boundaries

Stress Markers Every multisyllabic word has its own stress pattern, which our clients may or may not realize in a regular manner. The main purpose for all stress realizations is to emphasize certain syllables over others, thus creating a hierarchy of prominence among them.

Primary Stress The order of prominence is actualized by differences in loudness, pitch, and duration, the loudness differences being the most striking of the three. Generally, two different loudness levels are observed. The loudest syllable is said to have the *primary stress*. It is marked by a superscript short straight line in front of the respective syllable.

"syllable" [ˈsɪ lə bəl]

"railway" [ˈreˈl weˈ]

"superior" [sə ˈpɪr i ɚ]

Secondary Stress The next loudest syllable bears the *secondary stress*. It is indicated by a subscript short straight line in front of the syllable in question.

"supermarket" [ˈsu pɚ ˌmɑr kət]

"signify" [ˈsɪg nə ˌfaˈ]

"phonetic" [ˌfə ˈnɛ tɪk]

CLINICAL COMMENTS

Displacement of Stress

Clients with dysarthrias have typical difficulties with stressing. The following transcription exemplifies such a possible displacement of stress.

"birthday"	
Norm speaker:	[ˈbɝθ ˌdeɪ]
Dysarthric speaker:	[ˌbɝθ ˈdeɪ]
"umbrella"	
Norm speaker:	[ˌəm ˈbrɛ lə]
Dysarthric speaker:	[ˈʌm ˌbrə lə]

Some people find it difficult to distinguish among specific stressed versus unstressed syllables in words. For them, it may be of help to know that in General American English, different loudness levels characterizing stress go usually (but not always) hand in hand with changes in pitch; thus, the louder the syllable, the higher the pitch. To pay attention to pitch differences first then may aid in discriminating among differing levels of loudness in stressing. It is also helpful to know that many (but again, not all) words in General American English have their primary (or secondary) stress emphasis on the first syllable. A third possibility for those with difficulty in distinguishing stress differences is to vary systematically the loudness in each of the syllables of the word in question, [ˈdʒɛˌloʊ] versus [ˌdʒɛˈloʊ], for example. Typically, one version of that particular word will sound clearly more acceptable than the other. By a process of elimination, one can often determine the appropriate stress pattern.

Duration Symbols Sounds take up different amounts of time in continuous speech. We are so used to these measurable differences in sound duration that we register changes in these typical lengths automatically as "too short" or "too long." If that is our perceptual impression, we have to indicate it by means of diacritic markers. Normal (i.e., inconspicuous) sound duration remains unmarked.

Lengthening Longer than normal duration is signaled by either one or two dots following the sound symbol in question. The more dots, the longer the sound.

[fɪt]	standard vowel duration
[fɪ·t]	slightly longer than normal vowel duration
[fɪːt]	clearly longer than normal vowel duration

Shortening Shorter than normal speech sound productions also occur. Different degrees of shortening are, as a rule, not indicated. The diacritic mark for any shortened sounds is [̆] placed above the respective sound symbol.

Shortening sounds can lead to cutting off a portion of their phonetic properties. Young children with unstable [s]-sounds sometimes shorten the normally fairly long s-segments to something that may sound like the release portion of [t]. If onset and holding portions of [t] are also identifiable, the obvious transcription would be [t]. However, if that is not the case—that is, if we indeed have an [s]-impression—we would transcribe this as [š].

Syllable Boundaries Syllable boundaries are indicated by a period placed between the syllables.

"reliable"	[ri.laɪ.ə.bəl]
"attention"	[ə.tɛn.ʃən]

Additional Symbols The following symbols are not diacritics but are often used when transcribing aberrant speech.

Glottal Stop The glottal stop ([ʔ]) is produced when a closed glottis is suddenly released after a buildup of subglottal air pressure. The release of air pressure creates a popping noise. The glottal stop is considered an allophonic variation of some stop-plosive productions and can serve to release vowels in stressed syllables or separate successive vowels between words:

"oh"	[ʔoᵁ]	releasing a vowel
"Anna asks"	[ænə ʔæsks]	separating successive vowels

Some children with articulatory or phonological impairments use the glottal stop as a sound substitution.

Bilabial Fricatives The voiceless ([ɸ]) and voiced ([β]) bilabial fricatives are not phonemes of General American English but can also be used as sound substitutions in aberrant speech. For example, a child might substitute a bilabial fricative for the labiodentals [f] or [v] or possibly produce the [p] and/or [b] as a fricative, resulting in [ɸ] or [β]. Both sounds are produced by bringing the lips together so that a horizontally long but vertically narrow passageway is left between them for the voiceless or voiced breath stream to pass.

Palatal Fricatives The voiceless [ç] and voiced [ʝ] mediodorsal-mediopalatal fricatives may be heard as substitutions for [ʃ] and [ʒ]. These aberrant productions are characterized by a more posterior positioning of the articulators than for [ʃ] or [ʒ]. Thus, the place of constriction for both active and passive articulators shifts from coronal-postalveolar (or prepalatal) to this mediodorsal-mediopalatal position. The voiceless [ç] sounds similar to a voiceless [j].

> The bilabial fricatives are phonemes in several languages. For example, [ɸ] is a phoneme of Japanese, whereas [β] has phonemic value in Spanish.

Postdorsal-Velar Fricatives When attempting to produce the postdorsal-velar stops [k] and [g], some children may not raise the tongue sufficiently to create a complete closure. In this case, a fricative may result. The symbols for the postdorsal-velar fricatives are [x] for the voiceless sound and [ɣ] for its voiced cognate.

Postdorsal-Uvular Stops These sounds may again be heard by a child who is attempting to produce [k] or [g]. In this case, the client produces a stop-plosive, but the place of articulation is too far back in the mouth, resulting in a sound that might be perceived as having a "guttural" quality. The voiceless postdorsal-uvular stop is transcribed [q], and its voiced counterpart is noted as [G].

Flap, Tap, or One-Tap Trill The flap, tap, or what is also known as the *one-tap trill* [ɾ], is a frequent allophonic variation of [t] and [d]. This variation often occurs when stop-plosives are preceded and followed by vowels, as in *city* or *butter*. The flap, tap, one-tap trill is articulated with a single tap of the

CLINICAL APPLICATION

The ExtIPA and Multiple Interdentality

Multiple interdentality, a label dating back to at least the 1930s (Froeschels, 1931, 1937), may often be seen in our clinical population. It is used to describe an immature speech habit in which children produce [t], [d], [l], and [n] with their tongue tip too far forward. In other words, the tongue tip is between their teeth—that is, an interdental production. According to the ExtIPA chart (see Figure 3.2), we see that there is a way to transcribe these sounds in the following manner:

[t̪], [d̪], [n̪], [l̪]

Children with multiple interdentality often have difficulty with [s] and [z] as well. These sounds are also produced interdentally and end up sounding like "th" sounds, thus [θ] and [ð].

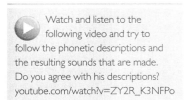

Watch and listen to the
following video and try to
follow the phonetic descriptions and
the resulting sounds that are made.
Do you agree with his descriptions?
youtube.com/watch?v=ZY2R_K3NFPo

tongue tip against the alveolar ridge or possibly just with a movement of the tongue tip in the direction of the alveolar ridge. This is considered a normal and acceptable allophonic variation of [t] and [d].

"butter"   [bʌɾɚ]

"ladder"   [læɾɚ]

Clinical Implications

Phonetic transcription and, especially, its diacritic marks appear at first glance to be complicated to handle and difficult to remember. The obvious question arises as to how these diacritics could be helpful in our assessment and therapeutic process.

First, accurate phonetic transcription involves ear training, a sharpening of our auditory discrimination abilities. These skills are indispensable for clinical expertise, something that can never be emphasized enough. Second, phonetic transcription and, especially, the use of diacritic marks provides a generally agreed-upon, professional way to note certain deviations from norm productions. This system allows clinicians to communicate freely with other professionals within the field of communication sciences and disorders. Transcription symbols can be translated back into actual speech events in the same way that musicians can read notes and translate them back into tunes. Third, by being aware of the many variations that can occur, accurate phonetic transcriptions allow for additional diagnostic complexity that would not be considered without this knowledge. If we do not know what to listen for—unreleased stops or partial devoicing, for example—we might not identify some of these variations. And fourth, diacritics can be used very effectively to document change over time during a remediation process. Often, therapy involves a systematic change of a child's articulation, which evolves slowly into a standard, norm production in more complex environments such as words or sentences, for example. Diacritics can be used to document this change. A child's articulation of [s] might evolve from [θ] to [s̪] and finally to a norm [s] production. Diacritics offer a way to document this change. By not using diacritics and just saying that the [s] is "distorted," we are not documenting the systematic nature of the change.

The realizations of [s] illustrate well how the use of diacritics can have valuable practical consequences for assessment and intervention. Knowing what to listen for, we find that what once sounded like simply a distorted [s] can now be specified as the actual aberrant form presented: a palatal versus a lateral versus a dentalized [s]-distortion, for example. All these variations can be noted using the respective diacritic marks. In addition, to the clarification that the notation system provides, detailed knowledge about actual realizations is indispensable for assessing and successfully remediating [s] errors. By establishing that the [s] appears distorted, we are saying only that its typical production is not a norm production. We have addressed the *acceptability* issue of the sound realization but not its aberrant *production* features, the most important information for clinical purposes. However, by comparing a child's actual articulatory features with the known features for typical [s]-productions, we will know precisely which placement characteristics need to be changed therapeutically.

Identifying an [s]-distortion as a palatal [s], for example, gives detailed information that can be used when planning therapy. A palatal [sʲ] is produced with the tongue tip too far back in the direction of the palatal area. Because of this tongue position, the palatal [s] has a [ʃ]-like quality. All other production features are usually in accordance with norm [s]-articulations; the lateral edges of the tongue are raised, and the sagittal grooving necessary for the [s] is present as well. It may be possible, therefore, that a child needs only to move the tongue tip to a more anterior position to produce a more normal sounding [s]. By applying this knowledge, therapy becomes not only more goal directed but also much simpler—with the consequence of saving time and possible frustration.

The advantage of knowing how children actually produce the distorted speech sound becomes even more obvious if we compare two distorted sound productions, one palatal [s] ([sʲ]) and one dentalized [s] ([s̪]), for example. The [s̪] is characterized by a tongue placement too far forward. In this case, children need to move the tongue posteriorly to obtain [s]. This would be in direct contrast to the procedure necessary for the [sʲ] in which a more frontal placement for active and passive articulators becomes necessary. Detailed knowledge of a client's production features then proves to be an important asset leading to expedient therapeutic intervention.

Theoretically and practically, the importance of the preceding discussion seems rather obvious. Its essential ingredient is our ability to note and differentiate among changes in sound quality as the basis for our remedial task. By fine-tuning transcription skills, not only are the listener's discrimination and transcription capabilities increased, but also the effectiveness of the whole intervention process improves.

Based on the author's clinical experience, Table 3.1 offers the most frequently used symbols.

TABLE 3.1 Commonly Used Transcription Symbols

Phonemic Symbol	Definition	Use
[ɬ]	Voiceless apico-alveolar lateral fricative	Indicates a lateral [s].
[ɮ]	Voiced apico-alveolar lateral fricative	Indicates a lateral [z].
[ʋ]	Voiced labiodental approximant	May be used as a substitution for [r].
[ɜ]	Central vowel without r-coloring heard in a stressed word position	Identification of problems with [r] that may be related to lack of r-coloring in the stressed central vowels.
[ə]	Central vowel without r-coloring heard in an unstressed word position	Identification of problems with [r] that may be related to lack of r-coloring in the unstressed central vowels.
[ʔ]	Glottal stop	May be used as a substitution for stop-plosives (or other consonants).

Diacritic	Definition	Use
̪	Dentalized, tongue approaches the upper incisors	[s̪], [z̪] An s-production in which the articulators are too far forward and the s-production approaches a [θ] or [ð] quality
j	Palatalized, articulators approach the palate	[sʲ], [zʲ] For [s] and [z], these productions sound more qualitatively like [ʃ].
[↔]	Unrounded production	[ʃ] No lip rounding on production and may occur with affricate productions.
̚	Unreleased stop-plosive	[t̚] May at first sound like a consonant deletion but movement of the articulators is noted.
[t̪], [d̪], [n̪], [l̪]	Interdentalized productions	Some young children may show interdental productions on any or all of these sounds that will also be evident in s-productions.

CLINICAL APPLICATION

Using Diacritics in the Assessment Process

Andy, age 6;2, was referred to the speech-language specialist by his classroom teacher. According to the teacher, his main problem seemed to be his "speech," which she described as being somewhat difficult to understand and containing many sound errors. After a thorough appraisal, the speech-language specialist was concerned that Andy might have a phonological disorder. When first listening to Andy's spontaneous speech, in addition to his w/r substitutions, she thought that he used [θ] realizations for th-, s-, and sh-sounds. The clinician was worried that Andy was not able to differentiate between these phonemes. She had to admit, though, that there were some qualitative differences among the productions that she could not quite describe. She decided to continue with her assessment, paying special attention to these sounds. She also used some pictures that pinpointed the th-, s-, and sh-sounds in an elicited speech sample. After carefully listening to Andy's actual productions and later to the video clip, the clinician arrived at the following results:

One-Word Articulation Test Results

Norm Production	→	Actual Production	Word Examples	Transcriptions
[s], [z]	→	[s̪], [z̪]	sun	[sʌn] → [s̪ʌn]
			bus	[bʌs] → [bʌs̪]
			zoo	[zu] → [z̪u]
			All consonant clusters with [s]	[s] + consonant → [s̪] + consonant
[ʃ]	→	[sʲ]	shoe	[ʃu] → [sʲu]
			fish	[fɪʃ] → [fɪsʲ]
			dishes	[dɪʃəz] → [dɪsʲəz]
[θ]	Correct	[θ]	thumb	[θʌm] → [θʌm]
[ð]	Correct	[ð]	feather	[fɛðɚ] → [fɛðə]

Selected Spontaneous Speech Sample

I have a red toothbrush. My mommy tells me every night to brush my teeth.
[aɪ hæv ə wɛd tuθbwəsʲ maɪ mɑmi tɛlz̪ mi ɛvri naɪt tu bwʌsʲ maɪ tiθ]

Today in school we made an art picture.
[tudeɪ ɪn s̪kul wi meɪd ən ɑt pɪksʲə]

We cut out all sorts of things with scissors and pasted them on this sheet of paper.
[wi kʌt aʊt ɑl s̪ɔəts̪ ʌv θɪŋkz̪ wɪθ s̪ɪz̪əz̪ ænd peɪstəd ðɛm ɑn ðɪs̪ sʲit ʌv peɪpə]

Andy did actually differentiate among the th-, s-, and sh-sounds with a dentalized production—[s̪, z̪] for /s/ and /z/, a palatalized [sʲ] for /ʃ/, and correct "th" realizations. In this case, careful transcription and the use of diacritics made a difference in the outcome of this assessment.

SUMMARY

Assessment procedures and results should be accurate, professional, and accomplished in a manner that is accountable. This chapter introduced the International Phonetic Alphabet as a widely used system that can provide these requisites for the assessment of speech sound disorders. The International Phonetic Alphabet was developed to document actual phonetic realizations of speech events. It is a means of transferring highly impermanent speech events into more durable graphic representations. Such a system offers the speech-language specialist a way to substantiate assessment results, document changes in therapy, and communicate effectively with other professionals. Transcription should never be considered just an option; accurate transcription is a necessity for professional evaluations.

To increase the effectiveness of the International Phonetic Alphabet, certain diacritic marks are used to add production details to the meaning of the basic symbol. These marks are indispensable to the documentation of many of the unusual realizations of our clients. In addition to those diacritics noted on the International Phonetic Alphabet chart, the extensions to this chart, the ExtIPA can be used for disordered speech. Such diacritics were itemized, explained, and exemplified in the second section of this chapter. This section also offered clinical comments on many of the diacritics as well as actual phonetic transcriptions utilizing these marks.

The last section of this chapter demonstrated how phonetic transcription and the detailed knowledge acquired through its use in assessment procedures benefit the intervention and remediation processes. First, the accuracy needed for the transcription task promotes the fine-tuning of perceptual skills, a clinical proficiency that will, by its very nature, enhance the likelihood of successful intervention. Second, the specificity gained through phonetic transcription, including diacritics, translates into a far more goal-directed treatment approach, which increases clinical efficacy. Third, phonetic transcription and diacritics can be used to document systematic changes in therapy which can evolve in children's speech.

CASE STUDY

The following transcription is from Jordan, age 5;6. The first transcription is broad transcription; the second one is narrow transcription.

Broad Transcription			
sit	[sɪt]	soap	[soᵘp]
sing	[sɪŋ]	soup	[sup]
sock	[sɑk]	summer	[sʌmɚ]
sun	[sʌn]	bus	[bʌθ]
miss	[mɪs]	toss	[tɑs]
goose	[gus]	race	[reᶦs]
house	[haᵘs]	pass	[pæs]
zoo	[zu]	zap	[zæp]
bees	[biz]	news	[nuz]
rose	[roᵘz]	trees	[triz]
Narrow Transcription			
sit	[s̪ɪt]	soap	[s̪ʲoᵘp]
sing	[s̪ɪŋ]	soup	[s̪ʲup]
sock	[s̪ʲɑk]	summer	[s̪ʲʌmɚ]

(Continued)

Narrow Transcription (*Continued*)			
sun	[s̠ʌn]	bus	[bʌθ]
miss	[mɪs̠]	toss	[tɑsʲ]
goose	[gusʲ]	race	[reˈs̠]
house	[haᵘsʲ]	pass	[pæs̠]
zoo	[zʲu]	zap	[z̠æp]
bees	[biz̠]	news	[nuzʲ]
rose	[roᵘzʲ]	trees	[triz̠]

Based on this small sample, make a list of the consonants contained in the phonetic versus the phonemic inventory. What additional information do the diacritics provide? Do you see a pattern for the palatalized versus dentalized [s] and [z]?

THINK CRITICALLY

1. What is the difference in production between [s̠], and [θ]? Which articulatory features would you need to change to produce a standard [s]? How would you explain this to a child?
2. What are the production features of [ʃ]? What would you do to change the production to a standard [ʃ]? Are there any v͞owel contexts you could use to assist in acquiring this standard production?
3. The following transcription is from a child, age 4;2. Label the diacritics and state which ones are context related and which ones would be considered aberrant productions.

   [aˈ wʌnt t̥u go t̥u s̠ʌ bitʃ↔]

   I want to go to the beach.

   [sʲæli ɬɛd wi kʊd˧ goᵘ]

   Sally said we could go.

   [dæɾɪ wʌnts̠ tu sʷwɪm]

   Daddy wants to swim.

   [ɪt wɪl bi f̬ʌn

   It will be fun.
4. Put in the syllable boundaries and the primary stress markers for the following words:

   outspoken

   inspiration

   national

   monumental

   October
5. Identify the following symbols. Which sound(s) might be the actual target(s) for a child who produces these sounds?

   [x]　　[ʔ]　　[ʧ]　　[ȷ̊]

TEST YOURSELF

1. Diacritics can be used for?
   a. Documenting results from an articulation test
   b. Demonstrating specific articulatory changes during the process of therapy
   c. both a and b
   d. none of the above

2. Which one of the following is *not* a diacritic used with vowels?
   a. [ₜ]
   b. [₊]
   c. [̞]
   d. [ˑ]

3. Which one of the following would indicate a nasalized [s]?
   a. [s:]
   b. [ṣ]
   c. [s̃]
   d. [sʲ]

4. Which one of the following would be a standard pronunciation?
   a. [ʒu] zoo
   b. [bɛɾi] Betty
   c. [sʲɪŋɚ] singer
   d. [kɪ̪pkeep

5. In the transcription [kætl̩], what does the diacritic under the [l] indicate?
   a. that the [l] is partially devoiced
   b. that the [l] is unreleased
   c. that the [l] is lateralized
   d. that the [l] is the syllable nucleus of the second syllable

6. The voiced labiodental approximant is transcribed as
   a. [β]
   b. [ɣ]
   c. [ʋ]
   d. [j̜]

7. The voiced labiodental approximant may be substituted for which sound?
   a. [s]
   b. [r]
   c. [l]
   d. [ʃ]

8. Which one of the transcriptions would indicate "bird" without the r-coloring on the vowel?
   a. [bɝd]
   b. [bɛd]
   c. [bɪ̩d]
   d. [bɔd]

9. Which one of the following transcriptions indicates excessive aspiration?
   a. [kʰip]
   b. [kɪ̩ p]
   c. [kɪ̩p]
   d. [kĩp]

10. The transcription [ʊ̞] would indicate which one of the following?
    a. a vowel position that is too far forward
    b. a vowel position that is too far back
    c. a vowel that is less rounded than usual
    d. a vowel that is more rounded than usual

FURTHER READINGS

Bauman-Waengler, J. (2009). *Introduction to phonetics and phonology: From concepts to transcription.* Boston: Pearson/Allyn & Bacon.

Garcia Lecumberri, M., & Maidment, J. (2000). *English transcription course.* London: Arnold.

Harbers, H. M. (2013). *A phonetics workbook for students: Building a foundation for transcription.* Boston: Pearson.

International Phonetic Association. (1999). *Handbook of the International Phonetic Association: A guide to the use of the International Phonetic Alphabet.* Cambridge: Cambridge University Press.

Shriberg, L., & Kent, R. (2013). *Clinical phonetics* (4th ed.). Boston: Allyn & Bacon.

Small, L. (2012). *Fundamentals of phonetics: A practical guide for students* (3rd ed.). Upper Saddle River, NJ: Pearson.

Theoretical Considerations and Practical Applications

CHAPTER

4

LEARNING OBJECTIVES

When you have finished this chapter, you should be able to:

- Trace how the term speech sound evolved into the phoneme concept.
- Describe the Chomsky and Halle (1968) distinctive feature classification.
- Identify markedness and how it is used to classify sound classes.
- Define natural phonology.
- List examples of the common phonological processes.

- Distinguish linear from the nonlinear (multilinear) phonologies.
- Describe autosegmental phonology and its use of a tiered representation.
- Explain the metrical trees in relationship to strong and weak stressing.
- Describe the characteristics of feature geometry.
- Understand the importance of optimality theory as a constraint-based approach.

THEORIES are very practical. They are based on confirmed observations or systematic experiments. As such, they try to abstract from many practical experiences, attempting to find order and rules amid seemingly entangled details. Theories can also serve as blueprints for practical tasks. For example, phonological theories attempt to explain the structure and function of phonemic systems that can then be applied to both normal and disordered phonological systems. Various theories, such as natural phonology, which generated phonological processes, have resulted in analysis procedures that are often used to evaluate the phonological systems of children.

Theories are relevant to the diagnosis and treatment of individual clients. Because theories guide and direct clinical work, they are fundamentally important to the diagnostic and therapeutic process. For example, as stated earlier, many students and clinicians are currently using phonological processes to describe patterns of errors and to determine therapeutic goals. The concept of phonological processes evolved from the theory of natural phonology (Donegan & Stampe, 1979; Stampe, 1969, 1972, 1973). The theory of natural phonology applied certain principles of generative grammar, itself another theory that has revolutionized the way professionals view language. Both of these theories have resulted in major changes in the way we view diagnostics and therapy within communication disorders. Different types of analyses are now employed diagnostically, and a major shift in therapy has occurred because of the impact of these theories.

Theories also offer a *variety* of clinical possibilities. Each theory provides a somewhat different perspective on the problem to be solved. Therefore, if one theory is used, assessment and treatment will vary from those suggested by a second theory. This gives clinicians several possible directions and approaches from which they can choose. Each theory and its application provide clinicians unique problem-solving advantages. Without such strategies, certain details would go unnoticed, and valuable diagnostic information would be lost. Thus, theories provide a means of maximizing diagnostic and therapeutic skills. They are significant to clinicians' professional work.

However, theories come and go. What was theoretically important in the 1960s and seemed to hold practical, clinical significance may be outdated and clinically irrelevant in these times. This is caused by a number of factors, probably the most important being the relative ease with which a theory can be applied to clinical practice. Even memorable theoretical constructs will fall by the wayside if they are cumbersome and difficult for clinicians to implement. Because the focus of this text is clinical application, theoretical models that have proven clinically irrelevant will be discussed but only briefly. References will be given to guide the reader to further information if more knowledge is desired.

Chapters 2 and 3 deal primarily with production features of articulation—with speech sound forms.The focus in this chapter shifts to phonology—to speech sound function. This shift is a consequence of the fact that contemporary theories in our field are phonological theories; they clearly emphasize the function of the phoneme as a meaning-differentiating unit.

The first goal of this chapter is to introduce the reader to some basic terminology and principles underlying many of the contemporary phonological theories. The second goal is to present several phonological theories that have been applied clinically within the discipline. Each phonological theory is discussed in relationship to its theoretical framework, how it developed, and how it functions. Finally, clinical implications are suggested for each of the presented theories.

Phonology

What Is Phonology?

Phonology can be defined as the description of the systems and patterns of phonemes that occur in a language. It involves determining the language-specific phonemes and the rules that describe the changes that take place when these phonemes occur in words (Ladefoged & Johnson, 2010). Within this system, the smallest entity that can be distinguished by its contrasting function within words is called the *phoneme*. The phoneme is, thus, the central unit of phonology.

Many different theoretical frameworks for phonological investigations exist. However, these various approaches all have one fundamentally important commonality, the differentiation between two levels of sound presentation:

1. The *phonetic level* with sounds (phones, allophones) as central units
2. The *phonemic level* represented by phonemes

How Does Phonology Work?

To understand the concept of phonology, it is important to differentiate clearly between speech sounds and phonemes. Speech sounds (phones, allophones) are physical *forms* that are the result of physiological processes and that have verifiable acoustic properties. Speech sounds are viewed from the end product of their production. When a child, for example, in spontaneous speech demonstrates a specific type of articulation resulting in an entity we can transcribe, we are examining speech sounds or what has been referred

Phonology as a concept and discipline has undergone considerable changes. The original French and German terms *phonologie* (Baudouin de Courtenay, 1895) and *Phonologie* (Trubetzkoy, 1931), respectively, were, under the influence of structuralism. These terms were replaced by *functional phonetics* (Jakobson, 1962; Martinet, 1960). The term *functional phonetics* emphasized the functional aspect of speech sounds. Phonology has also been called *phonemics* (Sapir, 1925), underlining the linguistic function of the phoneme. The term *phonology* is presently preferred and used by most professionals within the field of communication disorders.

to as *phones* or *allophones*. *Phonemes*, on the other hand, are defined in terms of their linguistic *function*—that is, in terms of their ability to establish meaningful units in a language. If we analyze a child's systematic use of units to establish meaning between words, such as "bat" versus "hat," we are examining the phonemes of that child's system.

How Did the Concept of the Phoneme Develop?

Phoneme as a term first appeared in publications toward the end of the nineteenth century when linguists and phoneticians found it necessary to expand the former single-sound concept into a two-dimensional concept:

1. speech sounds as production realities
2. speech sounds in their meaning-establishing and meaning-distinguishing function, as "phonemes"

In their works, the British phonetician Henry Sweet (1845–1912), the German Eduard Sievers (1850–1932), and the Swiss Jost Winteler (1846–1929) laid the foundation for the understanding of this duality. However, historically, Baudouin de Courtenay deserves the credit for introducing the *concept of the phoneme* in 1870. (The word *phoneme* existed prior to this time, but it was used as another label for speech sound.) N. H. Kruszewski (1881), a student of Baudouin de Courtenay, further popularized the term in his dissertation. Baudouin de Courtenay interpreted the proposed sound duality as differences between a physiologically concrete sound realization and its mental image. Influenced by the thinking of his time, Baudouin de Courtenay interpreted phonemes as primarily *psychological* sound units, as "psychic equivalents of the sound" (Lepschy, 1970, p. 60), as the sound "intended" by the speaker and "understood" by listeners. This was in contrast to the actually articulated sound, which was seen as a physiological fact. Similarly, the Russian linguist L.V. Ščerba, who succeeded Baudouin de Courtenay, defined the phoneme as "the shortest general sound image of a given language which can be associated with meaning images, and can differentiate words" (Lepschy, 1970, p. 62).

A definition of the phoneme and its relationship to phonology are found in Chapter 1.

The British phonetician Daniel Jones presented a more language-based phoneme concept in the first half of the twentieth century (Jones, 1938, 1950). He defined the phoneme as a "family of sounds in a given language which are related in character and are used in such a way that no one member ever occurs in a word in the same phonetic context as any other member" (Jones, 1950, p. 10). According to Jones's definition, as long as speech sounds are understood as belonging to the same category, they constitute a phoneme of that language. For example, as long as [s]-productions with all their verifiable phonetic differences (different speakers, various circumstances) are evaluated by listeners as being the same, as belonging to the s-category, these allophonic variations represent the single phoneme /s/ in that language.

Today's prevalent phoneme concept is still more functionally oriented. The specific *use* of the phoneme in a language is the primary emphasis. Nikolai S. Trubetzkoy and Roman Jakobson introduced this strictly functional phoneme concept (strongly influenced by Ferdinand de Saussure's [1916/1959] revolutionary new "structuralistic" way to look at language). Trubetzkoy, cofounder of the Prague School of Linguistics, wrote that "the phoneme can be defined satisfactorily neither on the basis of its psychological nature nor on the basis of its relation to the phonetic variants, but purely and solely on the basis of its function in the system of language" (Trubetzkoy, 1939/1969, p. 41).

One important aspect of a language's phonological system is its *phonemic inventory*. However, this is not the only variable used in characterizing different phonological systems. Edward Sapir (1921) pointed out that two languages having the same phoneme inventory can, nevertheless, have very different phonologies. Thus, although the inventories may be identical, the way these sound segments can and cannot be arranged to form words (phonotactics) may be quite different. Consequently, the *phonotactics*, or "permissible" sound arrangements within a language, is an important aspect of phonemes' "function" and is, therefore, an integral part of the phonology of a given language.

Speech Sound versus Phoneme: Clinical Application

Every utterance has two facets: an audible sequence of speech sounds and their specific meaning conveyed through this sequence. For example, if someone says, "Hey, Joe, over here," there is an audible sequence of sounds [heɪ dʒoʊ oʊvɚ hɪɚ] that conveys a specific meaning. Both the physical form of the speech sound and its language-specific function need to be realized for the utterance to be meaningful. If only one aspect, either speech sound form or function, is realized, a breakdown in the communicative process will occur. To apply this clinically, although a child may have the correct speech sound form, in other words, be able to produce [p]–[b], [t]–[d], and [k]–[g], this child might leave out these sounds at the end of a word. Thus, form is accurate, but the child's realization of the function is inadequate. In this case, "beet" sounds like "bee" and "keep" becomes "key." A breakdown in communication would probably occur.

Adequate form and function of all segments are basic requirements for meaningful utterances in any language. Form is established by the way the segment in question is produced by articulatory events. Segment function presupposes the observance of the language-specific rules regarding the arrangement of the speech sound segments. During an utterance, *form* and *function* become combined into meaning-conveying entities.

Segmental form and function also largely depend on one another. Without acceptable production features, sound segments cannot fulfill their functional task. If, for example, the word *key* is realized as *tea,* a frequent error made by children with t/k substitutions, elements of sound production have interfered with sound function. In this case, the phonological opposition between /t/ and /k/ has been destroyed. Segment function depends on normal segment form.

Also, segment form depends on proper segment function. Without observance of the phonotactic rules governing the language, an acceptable sound production will not relay the intended message. If, for example, a child produces a correct [s] but does not realize the phonotactic rules combining this [s] with other consonants in clusters, the meaning will be impaired. *Stop* might become *top*, or *hats* is realized as *hat*. For the purpose of effective verbal communication, regular segment form and function are indispensable.

CLINICAL EXERCISES

List three word examples in which lack of realization of the phonotactic rules for consonant clusters would change the meaning of the word.

Explain why speech sounds have been labeled as concrete entities and the phoneme as more of an abstraction.

Articulation and Phonological Theories and Therapies: Separation or Unity?

Historically, "correct" single-sound realizations were often the central focus of articulation work. Mastering how sound segments can and cannot be joined together to establish and convey meaning within the respective language was largely neglected. The underlying assumption was that speakers with defective articulation either "know" these rules already or will "learn" them through the various exercises that incorporated the sound in various contexts, for example. Articulation therapies focused on the realization of acceptable speech sound forms.

Today, it is often the other way around. The main orientation is the mastering of the phonological rules that govern the language-specific utilization of the sound segments. Children with phonemic-based disorders demonstrate difficulties with the function of the sound segment, with the rule-governed arrangement of these units. Thus, mastery of the phonological rules, not the speech sound realization, becomes the main goal. This can be exemplified by the multiple oppositions approach to therapy, which is based on the children's developing these functional contrasts that differentiate the meaning between words.

> The multiple oppositions approach is described in detail in Chapter 10.

Both intervention approaches have contributed substantially to the treatment of speech sound disorders. They represent outgrowths of different theoretical viewpoints. However, their high degree of mutual dependency implies that, for successful articulation work, these two approaches are not clinically a matter of "either or" but of "as well as." Of course, based on the specific clinical characteristics of an individual client, one approach may take precedence. If, for example, emphasis on speech sound form were the chosen approach, functional aspects would, nevertheless, also have to be considered. For example, a child who has just learned the speech sound [ʃ] (i.e., the form is learned) will practice this correct production in various syllable shapes according to phonotactic principles. In this example, function follows form. On the other hand, if speech sound function were the main goal, there might be a point in therapy when the clinician would need to consider aspects of speech sound form as well. For example, a child produces a speech sound that appears to be a correctly articulated [f]. However, the child uses this [f] as a substitution for [θ]. The word *bath* is articulated [bæf] and *thing* as [fɪŋ]. In words that normally are articulated with [f], the child uses a [p]; "fan" becomes "pan" and "fig" is articulated as "pig." The child is able to produce the form, but the function of the [f] would need to be taught. Contrasting the phonemes /f/ and /p/ in word pairs might help to establish the function of these two phonemes as meaning-differentiating units.

In summary, effective verbal communication always mirrors both aspects of speech sounds, acceptable form and function. Remediation must consider both sides of this duality; they represent two sides of the same coin.

CLINICAL APPLICATION

Phonological and Articulation Therapies Working Together

Toby was 5;2 when he was seen by the new speech/language specialist. Although he had previously received speech therapy, his speech was still considered very difficult to understand. A thorough assessment revealed that all fricative sounds were produced as stop-plosives. Thus, [f] and [v] were articulated as [p] and [b], and the voiceless and voiced [s] and [z], [ʃ] and [ʒ], as well as [θ] and [ð] were articulated as [t] and [d]. Toby often had difficulty discriminating words containing these phonemic oppositions. Thus, if the clinician asked him to point to the picture of a "pin" versus a "fin" or of a "vase" versus a "base," Toby would often be in error. After completing the evaluation, the clinician decided that Toby had a phonemic-based disorder: He did not understand the function of these phonemes in the language system.

The clinician began to work on differentiating and establishing these oppositions in meaningful contexts. Pictures and objects that contained these oppositions were used. The clinician noted that as Toby's discrimination abilities improved, he attempted to produce [f] and [v]; however, these realizations were consistently in error. As Toby struggled to correct the aberrant productions, the clinician realized that he was quickly becoming frustrated. The clinician used her knowledge of speech sound form to show Toby how to produce [f] and [v] in an acceptable manner. Toby was interested, responded quickly to this instruction, and soon could produce regular [f] and [v] sounds. He was very proud of his achievement and responded [naʊ aɪ kæn teɪ ɪt waɪt].

The next section of this chapter addresses specific phonological theories. Each section defines, exemplifies, and provides clinical examples when applicable to demonstrate the relevance of these theories to clinical assessment and treatment. This is a historical overview. If the application of the theoretical model is no longer used, its clinical application has been condensed.

Distinctive Feature Theories

Distinctive feature theories are attempts to determine the specific properties of a sound that serve to signal meaning differences in a language. The task is to determine which features are decisive for the identification of the various phonemes within a given language. Phonetic constituents that distinguish among phonemes are referred to as **distinctive features.**

What Are Distinctive Features?

How does one differentiate between apparent likenesses? For example, how do we distinguish among similar cars, houses, or streets? We look for discernible marks that might set the particular object apart from similar objects. A tree on the corner of a particular street, a brightly colored door on a house, for example, may serve as distinctive features that differentiate streets or houses. "A distinctive feature is any property that separates a subset of elements from a group" (Blache, 1978, p. 56).

A sound component is said to be distinctive if it serves to distinguish one phoneme from another. These units, which are smaller than sound segments, are considered to be "atomic" constituents of sound segments that cannot be broken down any further (Jakobson, 1949). Theoretically, an inventory of these properties would allow the analysis of phonemes not only of General American English but also of all languages. Thus, distinctive features are considered to be universal properties of speech segments.

How Do Distinctive Features Work?

Distinctive features are the smallest indivisible sound properties that establish phonemes. An inventory of distinctive sound features would demonstrate similarities and dissimilarities among phonemes. These similarities and differences are marked by the presence of certain properties in some phonemes and the absence of these properties in others. The term *binary* is used in most distinctive feature analyses to indicate these similarities and differences. A **binary system** uses a plus (+) and minus (−) system to signal the presence (+) or absence (−) of certain features.

Many different distinctive features must be considered to arrive at those that distinguish among phonemes. For example, consonants must be distinguished from vowels, voiced consonants from voiceless consonants, and nasals from nonnasals, to mention just a few. If /k/ and /g/ are considered, the following binary oppositions could be established:

/k/	/g/
is a consonant = + consonantal	is a consonant = + consonantal
is not a vowel = − vocalic	is not a vowel = − vocalic
is not voiced = − voice	is voiced = + voice

In this representation of similarities and dissimilarities, voicing is the only feature that distinguishes /k/ from /g/. Two sound segments are considered distinct and can, therefore, serve as phonemes *if at least one of their features is different.*

To expand slightly on this feature system, consider the phonemes /k/, /g/, and /ŋ/. As previously noted, /k/ and /g/ are distinguished from each other by the feature of voicing. How could this feature system be expanded to include the distinctive features that distinguish among /k/, /g/, and /ŋ/?

/k/	/g/	/ŋ/
+ consonantal	+ consonantal	+ consonantal
− vocalic	− vocalic	− vocalic
− voice	+ voice	+ voice
− nasal	− nasal	+ nasal

Although voice distinguishes /k/ from /g/ and /ŋ/, nasality is the feature that differentiates /g/ and /ŋ/, all of their other features being the same. In this example, nasality is the distinctive feature that creates an opposition between the phonemes /g/ and /ŋ/.

Presence or absence of the sound segments' distinctive features can be displayed in a matrix form. The Chomsky–Halle (1968) distinctive feature system is often noted in textbooks for speech-language pathologists. However, this is not the only distinctive feature system. Over the years, many distinctive feature systems have been developed (e.g., those by Jakobson, 1949; Jakobson, Fant, & Halle, 1952; Jakobson & Halle, 1956; Ladefoged, 1971; Singh and Polen, 1972). Each of these authors had a different idea about which distinctive features were important when distinguishing among phonemes. Most of the feature systems were binary; however, others (Ladefoged, 1971; Ladefoged & Johnson, 2010) used multivalued features. In addition, most distinctive feature systems used articulatory dimensions to classify the phonemes, although acoustic parameters have been used as well (Jakobson et al., 1952). One distinctive feature system is not necessarily superior to another. They were all developed to address somewhat different aspects of feature distinctions. In addition, many distinctive feature systems originated as a means of analyzing *universal* similarities and differences observed in phoneme systems of many different languages. This goal would of necessity incorporate feature modalities that are not required when analyzing General American English phonemes.

To summarize, the distinctive feature system is an attempt to document specific sound constituents that establish phonemes. Distinctive feature theories organize sound constituents according to some productional (or in some cases acoustic) properties that might be employed in languages to establish meaning differences. The result is a system of contrastive, linguistically relevant elements. Historically, many different feature systems exist, and many of the newer phonological theories, such as feature geometry, use their own somewhat different distinctive features. No one feature system has clear advantages over another. All distinctive feature systems reflect the authors' concept of those characteristics that most aptly define the phoneme.

How Did Distinctive Feature Theories Develop?

The original distinctive feature theory grew out of the phoneme concept and was further developed by the members of the Prague School in the 1930s. Very early in his work, Roman Jakobson, cofounder of the Prague School, hypothesized that the ultimate constituent of language was not the phoneme itself but its smaller components, its distinctive features. Jakobson stressed that these minimal differences serve the function of distinguishing among words that are different in meaning. It is these distinctive features that are functioning to distinguish between *bat* and *pat*, for example.

The Jakobson et al. (1952) system used 12 *acoustic* features based on the sound segments' spectrographic display. Such descriptions soon proved unsatisfactory for linguistic use because similar acoustic representations can be the result of a number of different articulatory gestures. This led to a revision of the original system. In 1956, Jakobson and Halle published a new distinctive feature system that included *articulatory* production features. Many of the later distinctive feature systems (Chomsky & Halle, 1968; Halle, 1962; Ladefoged & Johnson, 2010) were defined primarily according to articulatory features (or a combination of articulatory and acoustic parameters).

Distinctive Feature Theories: Clinical Application

Distinctive feature systems were developed as a means of analyzing phonemes and entire phoneme systems of languages. Each phoneme of the particular system was assessed to determine whether the distinctive feature was present (+) or absent (−). Although originally devised to analyze the regular realization of phonemes within and across languages, the use of distinctive features to analyze disordered speech could not be overlooked. When sound substitution features were compared to target sound features, similarities and differences could be noted.

Distinctive feature systems offered several advantages over the previous analysis systems of classifying errors according to substitutions, deletions, and distortions. First, they provided a more complete analysis. For example, sound substitutions can be broken down into several feature components, which can then be compared and analyzed. Second, and perhaps more important, distinctive feature systems concentrate on the features that distinguish phonemes within a language. Previous analysis procedures had at best focused on phonetic production aspects of speech sounds. With the impact of phonology on the field of communication disorders, this emphasis shifted to the phoneme and its function within the language system.

Distinctive feature analysis contrasted the features of the target sound to the substitution, resulting in a list of distinctive features that differentiated the two. This analysis could show whether (1) error sounds shared common features and (2) specific error patterns existed.

Therapeutic implications follow logically. If a child can be taught to discriminate between the presence and absence of these differentiating distinctive features, the aberrant sound productions should be easily remediated. However, can children really understand and differentiate between distinctive features? Jakobson's (1942/1968) hypothesis that children acquire features rather than sounds seems to support this assumption. If this is the case, therapy could facilitate this developmental process. In addition, if children acquire features rather than sounds, a certain amount of generalization should occur. Consequently, children should be able to generalize features from sounds that they can realize to others they cannot. This could be therapeutically useful. Children who can produce, for example, + voicing in one phonemic context should be able to generalize this + voicing to other phonemic contexts. Therefore, treatment of one phonemic opposition with specific distinctive features should lead to the norm production of other phonemic oppositions with the same distinctive feature oppositions. This would be a means of treating more than one phoneme in a time-efficient manner.

Over time, several distinctive feature therapy programs were developed (Blache, 1989; Compton, 1976; McReynolds & Engmann, 1975; Weiner & Bankson, 1978). However, for speech-disordered children, both the analysis procedures and the clinical applicability

Are distinctive features dated? Although distinctive feature therapy does seem to be "out," newer nonlinear (multilinear) phonological theories still rely heavily on distinctive features. Markedness, a concept developed in distinctive theory, is also an important aspect of one of the more contemporary phonological theories, "optimality theory". Markedness is also an important variable in the complexity approach (see Chapter 10).

of distinctive features have been difficult to use and questioned by several authors (Carney, 1979; Foster, Riley, & Parker, 1985). Some critical comments have focused on the fact that distinctive feature theory and distinctive features are abstract concepts: Distinctive features are theoretical concepts that were formulated to account for the sound patterns of languages. Carney further argued that a distinctive feature analysis based on the phoneme concept compels clinicians to ignore phonetic information. This phonetic information, exemplified by [s̪] or [ʃ], is not classifiable according to distinctive features and may lead to classifying errors inappropriately or not at all. For example, if a child produces a dentalized s-sound, [s̪], how is this classified? There is no distinctive feature for dentalized [s]. The clinician might ignore the distortion, declaring it a norm production, or could classify it as a [θ]. In both cases, valuable diagnostic and therapeutic information would be lost.

Generative Phonology

What Is Generative Phonology?

Generative phonology is an outgrowth of distinctive feature theory representing a substantial departure from previous phonological theories. Pregenerative theories of phonology—that is, those occurring prior to generative phonology (e.g., by Jakobson et al., 1952; Jakobson & Halle, 1956)—distinguished between two levels of realization: phonetic and phonemic. However, in pregenerative theories, both the phonetic and phonemic levels were analyzed by means of the actual productions, or the concrete realizations, of speech—for example, by using tape recordings of different language samples to assess the systems. Thus, pregenerative theories were developed around the *surface forms*. Surface forms, sometimes referred to as *surface-level representation,* are the actual end products of production. For example, if you transcribe a child's utterances, you are examining the surface form. The surface form is a phonetic sequence of units that have characteristic features. On the other hand, generative phonologies expanded this concept decisively to include what has been called the **underlying form or deep structure,** which is a purely theoretical concept that is thought to represent a mental reality at the core of language use (Crystal, 2010). Underlying forms exemplify the person's language competency as one aspect of his or her cognitive capacity.

The underlying forms also serve as points of orientation to describe regularities of speech reality as they relate to other areas of language, notably morphology and syntax.

Generative phonology then assumes two levels of sound representation, an abstract underlying form called *phonological representation* and its modified surface form, the *phonetic representation.* **Phonological rules** govern how this phonological representation (underlying representation or deep form) is transformed into the actual pronunciation (surface form).

Watch and listen to the first 2½ minutes of this lecture on surface and deep structure. Note the examples that are given to help you understand these concepts. youtube.com/watch?v=cnygrKrQvY0

How Does Generative Phonology Work?

This section introduces the distinctive features system that has been most widely used (Chomsky & Halle, 1968).

Generative Distinctive Features. The first accounts of a generative distinctive feature theory were presented by Noam Chomsky (1957). Chomsky and Morris Halle's (1968) *The Sound Pattern of English* is often cited as the major work in this area. They developed a new set of distinctive features that were different from those proposed by Jakobson and Halle (1956). In *The Sound Pattern of English*, the authors describe five features that establish and distinguish among phonemes: (1) major class features, (2) cavity features, (3) manner of articulation features, (4) source features, and (5) prosodic features.

The *major class features* characterize and distinguish among three sound production possibilities that result in different basic sound classes:

1. *Sonorant.* "Open" vocal tract configuration promoting voicing. General American English vowels, glides, nasals, and liquids belong to this category.
2. *Consonantal.* Sounds produced with a high degree of oral obstruction, such as stops, fricatives, affricates, liquids, and nasals.
3. *Vocalic.* Sounds produced with a low degree of oral obstruction (not higher than required for the high vowels [i] and [u]), such as vowels and liquids.

Cavity features refer to the active and/or passive place of articulation:

1. *Coronal.* Sounds produced with the apical/predorsal portion of the tongue ("the blade of the tongue raised from its neutral position," Chomsky & Halle [1968, page 304]). This cavity feature marks several consonants, for example, [t], [d], [s], [z], [n], and [l]. See Table 4.1 for additional consonants.
2. *Anterior.* Sounds produced in the frontal region of the oral cavity with the alveolar ridge being the posterior border, that is, labial, dental, and alveolar consonants. [m], [n], [b], [p], [f], [v], [d], and [t] are examples.
3. *Distributed.* Sounds with a relatively long oral-sagittal constriction, such as [ʃ], [s], and [z].

TABLE 4.1 General American English Consonant Matrix According to the Chomsky and Halle (1968) Distinctive Features

	p	b	t	d	k	g	θ	ð	f	v	s	z	ʃ	ʒ	tʃ	dʒ	m	n	ŋ	r	l	w	j	h
Sonorant	−	−	−	−	−	−	−	−	−	−	−	−	−	−	−	−	+	+	+	+	+	+	+	+
Consonantal	+	+	+	+	+	+	+	+	+	+	+	+	+	+	+	+	+	+	+	+	+	−	−	−
Vocalic	−	−	−	−	−	−	−	−	−	−	−	−	−	−	−	−	−	−	−	+	+	−	−	−
Coronal	−	−	+	+	−	−	+	+	−	−	+	+	+	+	+	+	−	+	−	+	+	−	−	−
Anterior	+	+	+	+	−	−	+	+	+	+	+	+	−	−	−	−	+	+	−	−	+	−	−	−
Nasal	−	−	−	−	−	−	−	−	−	−	−	−	−	−	−	−	+	+	+	−	−	−	−	−
Lateral	−	−	−	−	−	−	−	−	−	−	−	−	−	−	−	−	−	−	−	−	+	−	−	−
High	−	−	−	−	+	+	−	−	−	−	−	−	+	+	+	+	−	−	+	−	−	+	+	−
Low	−	−	−	−	−	−	−	−	−	−	−	−	−	−	−	−	−	−	−	−	−	−	−	+
Back	−	−	−	−	+	+	−	−	−	−	−	−	−	−	−	−	−	−	+	−	−	+	−	−
Round	−	−	−	−	−	−	−	−	−	−	−	−	−	−	−	−	−	−	−	−	−	+	−	−
Continuant	−	−	−	−	−	−	+	+	+	+	+	+	+	+	−	−	−	−	−	+	+	+	+	+
Delayed release	−	−	−	−	−	−	−	−	−	−	−	−	−	−	+	+	−	−	−	−	−	−	−	−
Voiced	−	+	−	+	−	+	−	+	−	+	−	+	−	+	−	+	+	+	+	+	+	+	+	−
Strident	−	−	−	−	−	−	−	−	−	−	−	−	−	−	−	−	−	−	−	−	−	−	−	−

4. *Nasal.* Sounds produced with an open nasal passageway—exemplified by the nasals [m], [n], and [ŋ].

5. *Lateral.* Sounds produced with lowered lateral rim portions of the tongue (uni- or bilateral). The only General American English example is [l].

6. *High.* Sounds produced with a high tongue position, vowels as well as consonants. Thus, [i], [u], [k], and [ŋ] would be [+ high].

7. *Low.* Vowels produced with a low tongue position—[ɑ], for example. The only consonants qualifying for this category are [h], [ʔ], and pharyngeal sounds. The latter are produced with the root of the tongue as an active articulator.

8. *Back.* Vowels and consonants produced with a retracted body of the tongue, for example, back vowels, velar and pharyngeal consonants.

9. *Round.* Production of vowels and consonants by rounding lips. [u] and [w] are [+ round].

Manner of articulation features specify the way that active and passive articulators work together to produce sound classes, signaling production differences between stops and fricatives, for example:

1. *Continuant.* "Incessant" sounds produced without hindering the airstream by any blockages within the oral cavity. Vowels, fricatives, glides, and liquids are [+ continuant]; stops, nasals, and affricates are [− continuant].

2. *Delayed release.* Sounds produced with a slow release of a total obstruction within the oral cavity. Affricates such as [tʃ] and [dʒ] are [+ delayed release].

3. *Tense.* Consonants and vowels produced with a relatively greater articulatory effort (muscle tension, expiratory air pressure). [p], [t], [k], [i], and [u], for example, are [+ tense]. [b], [d], [g], [ɪ], and [ʊ], by comparison, are [− tense].

Source features refer to subglottal air pressure, voicing, and stridency:

1. *Heightened subglottal pressure.* General American English voiceless aspirated stops ([p], [t], [k]) are [+ HSP] because their production requires an added amount of expiratory airflow that, after freely passing the glottis, accumulates behind the occlusion within the oral cavity.

2. *Voiced.* Produced with simultaneous vocal fold vibration. All General American English vowels, glides, liquids, nasals, voiced stops, fricatives, and affricates are [+ voiced]. [p], [t], [k], [f], [s], and [ʃ], by contrast, are [− voiced].

3. *Strident.* The term *strident* (making a loud or harsh sound) is a feature of General American English voiceless and voiced fricatives and affricates. However, the interdental fricatives [θ] and [ð] are [− strident].

Chomsky and Halle (1968) named *prosodic features* but did not discuss them. To see how several of these distinctive features apply to General American English consonants and vowels, see Tables 4.1 and 4.2.

Generative Naturalness and Markedness.

One aspect of distinctive feature theory that seems to have more direct clinical applicability and can be found in later theoretical constructs is the concept of *naturalness* and *markedness*. Naturalness and markedness can be seen as two ends of a continuum. The term **naturalness** designates two features: (1) the relative simplicity of a sound production and (2) its high frequency of occurrence in languages. In other words, more natural sounds are those that are considered easier to produce and occur in many languages of the world. **Markedness,** on the other hand,

TABLE 4.2 General American English Vowel Matrix According to the Chomsky and Halle (1968) Distinctive Features

	i	ɪ	e	ɛ	æ	ɑ	ɔ	o	ʊ	u	ʌ
Consonantal	−	−	−	−	−	−	−	−	−	−	−
Vocalic	+	+	+	+	+	+	+	+	+	+	+
Coronal	−	−	−	−	−	−	−	−	−	−	−
Anterior	−	−	−	−	−	−	−	−	−	−	−
High	+	+	−	−	−	−	−	−	+	+	−
Low	−	−	−	−	+	+	+	−	−	−	−
Back	−	−	−	−	−	+	+	+	+	+	+
Round	−	−	−	−	−	−	+	+	+	+	−
Tense	+	−	+	−	−	+	−	+	−	+	−

refers to sounds that are relatively more difficult to produce and are found less frequently in languages. For example, [p] is considered a natural sound (= unmarked). It is easy to produce and occurs in many languages around the world. On the other hand, the affricate [tʃ] is a marked sound: It is relatively more difficult to produce and is found infrequently in other languages.

Marked and unmarked features are typically used when referring to cognate pairs, such as /t/ and /d/, and sound classes, such as nasals. Sloat, Taylor, and Hoard (1978) describe the following sounds and sound classes according to markedness parameters:

Voiceless obstruents are more natural (unmarked) than voiced obstruents.

Obstruents are more natural (unmarked) than sonorants.

Obstruents include the stops, fricatives, and affricates. See Chapter 2 for a more complete definition.

Stops are more natural (unmarked) than fricatives.

Fricatives are more natural (unmarked) than affricates.

Low-front vowels appear to be the most natural (unmarked) vowels.

Close-tense vowels are more natural (unmarked) than open-lax vowels.

Anterior consonants are more natural (unmarked) than nonanterior consonants.

Consonants without secondary articulation are more natural (unmarked) than those with secondary articulation (such as simultaneous lip rounding).

The concept of naturalness versus markedness became a relevant clinical issue when it was observed that children with phonemic-based disorders have a tendency to substitute more unmarked, natural classes of segments for marked ones. For example, children substituted stops for fricatives and deleted the more marked member of a consonant cluster (Ingram, 1989b). Although the results of at least one investigation demonstrated contrary findings (McReynolds, Engmann, & Dimmitt, 1974), most investigations supported the notion that children and adults with speech disorders more frequently showed a change from marked segments to unmarked substitutions (Kirk, 2008; Menn & Velleman, 2010; Taps Richard & Barlow, 2011). Markedness is also an important variable in newer theoretical models such as optimality theory.

How Did Generative Phonology Develop?

Generative phonology represents the application of principles of generative (or transformational) grammar to phonology. Noam Chomsky first introduced the concept of generative grammar in 1957 in a book titled *Syntactic Structures*. Generative grammar departed radically from structuralistic and behavioristic approaches to grammar, which had dominated linguistic thought during the decades before Chomsky's work. Prior to the introduction of generative grammar, linguists had analyzed the surface forms of sentences into their constituent parts and looked at the parts of speech and the type of sentence structure. This type of analysis was found to be inadequate in various respects. An often-used example illustrates this point:

John is eager to please.

John is easy to please.

If the two sentences are analyzed according to a structuralistic point of view, the results will indicate that both sentences have exactly the same structure. However, this analysis does not reveal that the two sentences have drastically different meanings. In the first sentence, John wants to please— in the second sentence, the reference is to someone else pleasing John.

One aim of generative grammar was to provide a way to analyze sentences that would account for such differences. To do this, a concept that postulated not only a *surface*-level of realization but also a *deep*-level of representation was developed. *Competence* and *performance* were also terms that distinguished surface- from deep-levels of representation, competence representing the deep-level and performance relating to the surface-level. Language competence was viewed as the individual's knowledge of the rules of a language, whereas performance was actual language use in real situations. Structuralists and behaviorists had focused on an individual's performance; generative grammar shifted this focus to include the concept of an individual's language competence. The formulation of rules governing the events between the deep-level competence and surface-level performance was an important concept within generation grammar.

Distinctive Features and Generative Phonology: Clinical Application

Distinctive features and generative phonology are no longer used clinically. This is probably because of the difficulty of the analysis. Therefore, this explanation is offered as a brief overview of the principle behind using distinctive features to diagnose speech sound disorders.

Generative phonology was originally developed to analyze the phonological systems of languages. Its application to phonological development in children has its foundation in Smith's (1973) case study of his son Amahl. Other authors (e.g., Compton, 1976; Grunwell, 1975) extended these analysis principles to children with disordered phonemic systems. Generative phonology, applied in this manner, compares a child's phonological system to an adult's. Rules that described the differences between the deep- and surface-level representations were generated. To do this using distinctive feature system analysis, the target sound is compared to the child's substitution, noting the distinctive features that are different between the target and substitution.

Because the distinctive feature system is binary, (+) and (−), similarities and differences between target and substitution can be clearly ascertained. One of the advantages of this analysis is that it allows for a comparison of several sound substitutions to the target phoneme. For example, if a client substitutes [t] for [d], [z], and [ʃ], similarities and differences among all sound features can be compared. A second advantage of this analysis is that correctly and incorrectly realized features across several phonemes can be examined to see whether patterns exist. A pattern is characterized by frequent use of one or more identical distinctive features when the target sound and the sound substitution are compared.

Natural Phonology

What Is Natural Phonology?

"[Natural phonology] is a natural theory . . . in that it presents language as a natural reflection of the needs, capacities, and world of its users, rather than as a merely conventional institution" (Donegan & Stampe, 1979, p. 127). **Natural phonology** incorporates features of naturalness theories and was specifically designed to explain the normal development of children's phonological system. The theory of natural phonology postulates that patterns of speech are governed by an innate, universal set of phonological processes. **Phonological processes** are innate and universal; therefore, all children are born with the capacity to use the same system of processes. Phonological processes, as natural processes, are (1) easier for a child to produce and are substituted for sounds, sound classes, or sound sequences when children's motor capacities do not yet allow their norm realization, (2) operating as all children attempt to use and organize their phonological systems so that they can progress to the language-specific system that characterizes their native language, and (3) used to constantly revise existing differences among the innate patterns and the adult norm production. The theory points out prominent *developmental steps* children go through until the goal of adult phonology is reached in the children's early years. Disordered phonology is seen as an inability to realize this "natural" process of goal-oriented adaptive change.

How Does Natural Phonology Work?

The theory of natural phonology assumes that a child's innate phonological system is continuously revised in the direction of the adult phonological system. Stampe (1969) proposed three mechanisms to account for these changes: (1) limitation, (2) ordering, and (3) suppression. These mechanisms reflect properties of the innate phonological system as well as the universal difficulties children display in the acquisition of the adult sound system.

     Limitation occurs when differences between a child's and an adult's systems become *limited* to only specific sounds, sound classes, or sound sequences. Limitation can be exemplified by the following: A child might first use a more "natural" sound for a more marked one. For example, all fricatives might be replaced by homorganic stops (e.g., [f] → [p], [θ] → [t], [s] → [t]). Later, this global substitution of all fricatives by stops might become *limited* to only [s] and [z], so that "sun" becomes [tʌn] and "zoo" becomes [du], for example, but "fun" and "pig" are accurate.

     Ordering occurs when substitutions that appeared unordered and random become more organized. Ordering can be exemplified by the following: A child's first revisions may appear unordered. To stay with the stop for fricative example, a child might at first also devoice the voiced stops of the substitution; thus, ([s] → [t] and [z] → [t]). Thus, *Sue* is pronounced as [tu], but *zoo* is also articulated as [tu]. Later, the child might begin to "order" the revisions by voicing initial voiced stops but still retaining the stop substitution. Now *Sue* is [tu] and *zoo* is [du].

According to phonological processes, create your own example of "limitation" that could possibly occur in a child's speech.

A child produces the labiodentals [f] and [v] and the apico-dentals [θ] and [ð] as [p]. According to this phonological theory, give an example of how "ordering" might occur.

The term **suppression** refers to the abolishment of one or more phonological processes as children move from the innate speech patterns to the adult patterns. Suppression occurs when a previously used phonological process is not used any longer.

According to Stampe (1979), all children embark on the development of their phonological systems from the same beginnings. Stampe sees children as possessing a full understanding of the underlying representation of the adult phoneme system: That is, from the very beginning, children's perceptual understanding of the phonemic system mirrors that of adult's. Children just have difficulties with the peripheral, motor realization of the phonetic surface form. Many authors (e.g., Fey, 1992; Stoel-Gammon & Dunn, 1985) have questioned the validity of this idea. In addition, Stampe's account of phonological development presents children as passively suppressing these phonological processes. Other contemporary authors, notably Kiparsky and Menn (1977), see children as being far more actively involved in the development of their phonological systems.

In spite of such shortcomings, Edwards (1992) states that "it is not necessary to totally discard the notion of phonological processes just because we may not agree with all aspects of Stampe's theory of Natural Phonology, such as his view that phonological processes are 'innate' and his assumption that children's underlying representations are basically equivalent to the broad adult surface forms" (p. 234). Phonological process analysis has found widespread clinical application, although it is not used to *explain* developmental speech events, which was the original intent of natural phonologists, but to *describe* the deviations noted in the speech of children.

Because phonological processes are so central to the workings of natural phonology and to its clinical application, some of the more common processes are listed here with some explanatory remarks.

Phonological Processes

Although many different processes have been identified in the speech of normally developing children and those with phonemic-based disorders, only a few occur with any regularity. Those processes that are common in the speech development of children across languages are called **natural processes.**

Phonological processes are categorized as syllable structure processes, substitution processes, and assimilatory processes. **Syllable structure processes** describe those sound changes that affect the structure of the syllable. **Substitution processes** describe those sound changes in which one sound class is replaced by another. **Assimilatory processes** describe changes in which a sound becomes similar to, or is influenced by, a neighboring sound of an utterance.

Syllable Structure Processes

Cluster reduction. The articulatory simplification of consonant clusters into a single consonant, typically the more "natural" member of the cluster.

Example: [pun] for *spoon.*

Reduplication. This process is considered a syllable structure process because the syllable structure is "simplified"; that is, the second syllable becomes merely a repetition of the first. *Total reduplication* refers to the exact reduplication of the first syllable. In partial reduplication, the vowel in the second syllable is varied (Ingram, 1976).

Examples:

Total reduplication: [wɑwɑ] for *water.*

Partial reduplication: [babi] for *blanket.*

Weak syllable deletion. The omission of an unstressed syllable.

Example: [nænə] for *ba'nana.*

Final consonant deletion. The omission of a syllable-arresting consonant, a coda.

Example: [hɛ] for *head.*

Substitution Processes

Consonant cluster substitution. The replacement of one member of a cluster.

Example: [stwit] for *street.*

Note: This is additionally referred to as *gliding* to indicate the specific type of substitution.

Changes in the Active Articulator or Passive Articulator

Fronting. Sound substitutions in which the active and/or place of the passive is more anteriorly located than the intended sound. Prominent types include *velar fronting* (t/k substitution) and *palatal fronting* (s/ʃ substitution).

Examples: [ti] for *key*; [su] for *shoe.*

Labialization. The replacement of a nonlabial sound by a labial one.

Example: [fʌm] for *thumb.*

Alveolarization. The change of nonalveolar sounds, mostly interdental and labiodental sounds, into alveolar ones.

Example: [sʌm] for *thumb.*

Changes in Manner of Articulation

Stopping. The substitution of stops for fricatives or the omission of the fricative portion of affricates.

Examples: [tʌn] for *sun*; [dus] for *juice.*

Affrication. The replacement of fricatives by homorganic affricates.

Example: [tʃu] for *shoe.*

Deaffrication. The production of affricates as homorganic fricatives.

Example: [ʃiz] for *cheese.*

Denasalization. The replacement of nasals by homorganic stops.

Example: [dud] for *noon.*

Gliding of liquids/fricatives. The replacement of liquids or fricatives by glides.

Examples: [wɛd] for *red*; [ju] for *shoe.*

Vowelization (vocalization). The replacement of syllabic liquids and nasals, foremost [l], [ɚ], and [n], by vowels.

Examples: [teˈbo] for *table*; [lædʊ] for *ladder*.

Derhotacization. The loss of r-coloring in central vowels with r-coloring, [ɝ] and [ɚ].

Examples: [bɜd] for *bird*, [lædə] for *ladder*.

Changes in Voicing

Voicing. The replacement of a voiced for a voiceless sound.

Example: [du] for *two*.

Devoicing. The replacement of a voiceless for a voiced sound.

Example: [pit] for *beet*.

Assimilation processes can also be classified according to the type and degree of the assimilatory changes. For definitions and examples, see the section "Sounds in Context: Coarticulation and Assimilation" in Chapter 2.

Assimilatory Processes (Harmony Processes)

Labial assimilation. The change of a nonlabial into a labial sound under the influence of a neighboring labial sound.

Example: [fwɪŋ] for *swing*.

Velar assimilation. The change of a nonvelar into a velar sound under the influence of a neighboring velar sound.

Example: [gɑg] for *dog*.

Nasal assimilation. The influence of a nasal on a nonnasal sound.

Example: [mʌni] for *bunny*.

Note: The place of articulation is retained; only the manner is changed.

Liquid assimilation. The influence of a liquid on a nonliquid sound.

Example: [lɛloʊ] for *yellow*.

According to natural phonology, phonological processes are recognizable steps in the gradual articulatory adjustment of children's speech to the adult norm. This implies a chronology of phonological processes, specific ages at which the process could be operating and when the process should be suppressed. As useful as a chronology of normative data might seem for clinical purposes, tables of established age norms can easily be misleading. Individual variation and contextual conditions may play a large role in the use and suppression of phonological processes.

Ages of suppression of the various processes are discussed in Chapter 5.

To summarize, natural phonologists assume an innate phonological system that is progressively revised during childhood until it corresponds with the adult phonological output. Limitation, ordering, and suppression are the mechanisms for the revisions that manifest themselves in phonological processes. Phonological processes are developmentally conditioned simplifications in the realization of the phonological system in question. As these simplifications are gradually overcome, the phonological processes become suppressed.

How Did Natural Phonology Develop?

David Stampe introduced natural phonology in 1969. However, several of its basic concepts had been established considerably earlier, most prominent among them being the concepts of naturalness (markedness) and underlying versus surface forms, which are important aspects of generative phonology.

Jakobson (1942/1968) extended the concept of naturalness and markedness to *implied universals,* which could be found in different languages, children's acquisition of speech, and the deterioration of speech in aphasics. These universals were even used as a predictive device. Some examples include "fricatives imply stops" and "voiced stops imply voiceless stops." These examples would mean that if a language has fricatives, that language will have stops as well, and if a language has voiced stops in its inventory, the language will also have voiceless stops. Application of these two examples to children's acquisition of speech means that children will acquire stops before (homorganic) fricatives. Also, they acquire voiceless stops before voiced cognates. In an aphasic condition, the breakdown of speech would be characterized by the loss of the later-acquired sounds before the earlier-acquired ones. Thus, aphasics would lose fricatives before (homorganic) stops and voiced stops before voiceless ones. Whether these universal "laws" are generally valid under all of the previously mentioned conditions has been repeatedly questioned. However, these laws clearly exemplify the concepts of naturalness and markedness as universal phenomena.

Markedness theory also plays a central role in generative phonology and optimality theory (McCarthy & Prince, 1995; Prince & Smolensky, 1993). According to generative phonologists, markedness values are considered to be universal and innate. Thus, Jakobson with his concept of universal naturalness and Chomsky and Halle with their understanding of universal and innate naturalness set the stage for Stampe's natural phonology. Stampe incorporated the conceptual framework of naturalness into his theory of natural phonology.

At the same time, the meaning and use of the term *underlying form* changed drastically as it was incorporated into natural phonology. Within generative grammar, underlying forms—lexical as well as phonological—are highly abstract entities. They represent *assumed points of reference* that are necessary for the explanation of the many possible surface forms. In contrast, within the context of natural phonology, underlying forms as "models" for surface realizations suddenly gain some concrete reality. The underlying form is *the adult norm* that is the intended goal for children's production efforts.

Natural Phonology: Clinical Application. The concept of phonological processes within natural phonology has impacted both the assessment and the treatment of children with disordered phonological systems. Assessment procedures using phonological processes consist of contrasting the target word to a child's production. Aberrant productions are identified and labeled according to the phonological process that most closely matches the sound change. Typically, the processes are listed and the frequency of occurrence of individual processes is noted. Frequency of occurrence and the relative age of suppression play a role in targeting a process or processes for therapy. Depending on the age of the child, more frequent processes that should have been suppressed are commonly targeted for therapy.

Unlike other analysis procedures, phonological processes can account for changes in syllable or word structures and those that result from assimilations. Although phonological processes are not commonly used to identify sound distortions, they could be. For example, [s̱] could be labeled fronting and [sʲ] backing. Backing is considered an idiosyncratic process that can be found in the speech of children with phonemic-based disorders. **Backing** refers to a substitution in which the active and/or passive place of articulation is more posteriorly located than the intended sound.

Phonological Process Analysis.   A phonological process analysis is a means of identifying substitutions, syllable structure, and assimilatory changes that occur in clients' speech. Each error is identified and classified as one or more of the phonological processes. Patterns of errors are described according to the most frequent phonological processes present and/or to those that affect a class of sounds or sound sequences. Also, those phonological processes which affect a large number of sounds are noted due to their probable impact on intelligibility. The processes used to identify substitutions are again primarily based on production characteristics; however, they do account for sound and syllable deletions as well as several assimilation processes.

Several assessment protocols analyze phonological processes in articulation tests or in spontaneous speech (e.g., see Bankson & Bernthal, 1990; Hodson, 2004; Khan & Lewis, 2002; Lowe, 1996). All of them identify each aberrant production according to the phonological process or processes that best represent the changes that have occurred. Most protocols also summarize the phonological processes by counting the total number of specific processes. An example of transcribed articulation test results and language sample is provided in Appendix 4.1 for a child, H. H. (page 95). Appendix 4.1 (page 102) also provides a Phonological Process Analysis Summary Sheet filled out for H. H.

To analyze a speech sample according to phonological processes:

1. Identify the phonological process that best describes the change. More than one phonological process might apply to a given misarticulation. For example, if a child substitutes [d] for [s] ([s] → [d]), this needs to be identified as stopping and voicing.

2. Tally the number of times the child used each process. On the summary form, list the processes and their frequency of occurrence.

Phonological processes can be used to analyze substitutions and deletions, something that distinctive feature analysis was not able to do. In addition, phonological process analysis can generate patterns by noting the most frequent processes. It allows you to examine the sounds or sound classes that are most frequently included in the various phonological processes.

The next section introduces the more recent developments in phonological theories, the so-called nonlinear or multilinear phonological theories. They represent a radical departure from the conceptual framework that preceded them.

CLINICAL EXERCISES

A child demonstrates a high degree of fronting (velar only), cluster reduction, and final consonant deletion.

Can you give one example of each of these processes?

Which of these processes would probably affect intelligibility the most?

Watch and listen to this short video of 4-year-old Ben. See whether you can transcribe and note some of the phonological processes he uses. For example, listen to consonant clusters and his "th" sounds.

Linear versus Nonlinear Phonologies

What Are Linear and Nonlinear Phonologies?

Phonological theories, theories of generative phonology included, were based on the understanding that all speech segments are arranged in a sequential order. Consequently, underlying phonological representations and surface phonetic realizations, too, consisted of a string of discrete elements. For example:

Wow, what a test. [wa^ʊ wʌt ə tɛst]

The sequence of segments in this phrase begins with [w] and ends with [st]. All segments between follow each other in a specific order to convey a particular message. Such an assumption that all meaning-distinguishing sound segments are serially arranged characterizes all linear phonologies. Linear phonologies, exemplified by distinctive feature theories and early generative phonology, can be characterized as follows:

1. It emphasizes the linear, sequential arrangement of sound segments.
2. Each discrete segment of this string of sound elements consists of a bundle of distinctive features.
3. A common set of distinctive features is attributable to all sound segments according to a binary + and − system.
4. All sound segments have equal value, and all distinctive features are equal; thus, no one sound segment has control over other units.
5. The phonological rules generated apply only to the segmental level (as opposed to the suprasegmental level) and to those changes that occur in the distinctive features (Dinnsen, 1997).

Linear phonologies with sound segments (and their smaller distinguishing distinctive features) as central analytical units fail to recognize and describe larger linguistic units. Linear phonologies also do not account for the possibility that there could be a hierarchical interaction among segments and other linguistic units. Nonlinear or nonsegmental phonologies attempt to account for these factors.

Hierarchy refers to any system in which elements are ranked one above another.

Nonlinear (or what have been termed **multilinear**) **phonologies** are phonological theories in which segments are governed by more complex linguistic dimensions. The linear representation of phonemes plays a subordinate role. More complex linguistic dimensions—for example, stress, intonation, and metrical and rhythmical linguistic factors—may control segmental conditions. These theories explore the relationships among units of various sizes, specifically the influence of larger linguistic entities on sound segments. Therefore, rather than a linear view of equal-valued segments (in a left-to-right horizontal sequence), a hierarchy of factors is hypothesized to affect segmental units. Rather than a static sequence of segments of equal value (as in linear phonology), a dynamic system of features, ranked one above the other, is proposed. For example, syllable structure could affect the segmental level. A child may demonstrate the following pattern:

"man"	[mæn]	"window"	[wˡ doʊ]
"dog"	[dɑg]	"jumping"	[dʒʌ pɪ]
"ball"	[bɑl]	"Christmas tree"	[krɪ mə tri]

This child deletes the final consonant of each syllable in a multisyllabic word; however, no final consonant deletion occurs in one-syllable words. In this example, the number of syllables in a word interacts with and affects the segmental level. The number of syllables has priority over the segmental level: It determines segmental features. Nonlinear phonologies would rank syllable structure above the level of sound segments. Another factor that may affect the segmental level is stress. Children have a tendency to delete segments in unstressed syllables. The following transcriptions demonstrate this:

$$ba\text{'}nana \rightarrow [\text{'}næn\vartheta]$$

$$po\text{'}tato \rightarrow [\text{'}te^{\text{'}} to^{\upsilon}]$$

$$\text{'}telephone \rightarrow [\text{'}t\varepsilon fo^{\upsilon}n]$$

In these examples, the syllable stress clearly affects segmental realization; word stress has priority over the segmental level. "Instead of a single, linear representation (one unit followed by another with none having any superiority or control over other units), they [nonlinear phonologies] allow a description of underlying relationships that would permit one level of unit to be governed by another" (Schwartz, 1992, p. 271).

How Do Nonlinear Phonologies Work?

There are many different types of nonlinear/multilinear phonologies. Several new theories have been advanced and others have been modified. All nonlinear phonologies are based on a belief in the overriding importance of larger linguistic units influencing, even controlling, the realization of smaller ones. Nonlinear phonologies also attempt to incorporate this hierarchical order of linguistic elements into analytical procedures, using so-called *tiered representations* of features.

To describe the many different nonlinear phonologies is beyond the scope of this book. *The New Phonologies: Developments in Clinical Linguistics* (Ball & Kent, 1997) is an excellent source of more detailed information on autosegmental phonology, feature geometry, underspecification theory, dependency phonology, government phonology, grounded phonology, optimality theory, and gestural phonology.

This section is restricted to an introduction of nonlinear phonologies exemplified by autosegmental, metrical, feature geometry, and optimality theories. These theories are in no way superior to other nonlinear phonologies and have not gained widespread clinical applicability. However, they do seem valuable and offer the reader some newer insights into current phonological theories.

Autosegmental Phonology. John Goldsmith proposed **autosegmental phonology** in 1976. Originally, he presented this theory to account for tone phenomena in languages in which segmental features interact with varying tones. Although General American English is not a tone language, one application of autosegmental phonology is to the classification of affricates. Parker and Riley (2010) illustrate the essential problem in the following manner: According to the concept of linear (generative) phonology, features extend throughout a segment. Therefore, a segment such as /p/ is considered to be [− voice] throughout its entire segment, whereas /u/ is [+ voice] throughout its entirety. However, this is not the case with affricates. By definition, an affricate begins like a stop and ends like a fricative. The features that differentiate stops and fricatives are + *and* − continuant. This posed a problem for the linear phonologists because one segment cannot be designated as both a + and − distinctive feature. To get around this problem, the linear phonologists constructed the feature of "delayed release" to designate affricates. However, delayed release violates the construct of distinctive feature theory because this property does not extend throughout the entire segment.

Tone languages, which represent a large number of world languages, are distinguished by changes in the meaning of a word simply by changing the pitch level at which it is spoken. Thus, phonemic differences can be signaled by distinctive pitch levels known as *tones* or *tonemes* (Crystal, 2010). For example, in Mandarin Chinese, four different tones with the identical sound segments [ma] result in words that mean "mother," "hemp," "horse," and "scold." Autosegmental phonology placed these tones on a tier above the sound segments, demonstrating the overriding importance of these tones for the meaning of the word.

Autosegmental phonology proposed that changes within the boundary of a segment could be factored out and put onto another "tier." Thus a + and − continuant could be placed on another level to indicate the change within the segment boundary. A diagram of an affricate such as /tʃ/ would look accordingly:

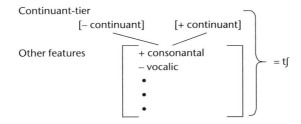

As can be seen, a single segment on one tier can be associated with more than one segment on another tier. Using the example of /tʃ/, the + consonantal segment can be associated with a + and − continuant on another tier. In fact, the term *autosegmental* refers to the concept that certain segments are autonomous—they do not have a one-to-one match on another level.

As mentioned earlier, Goldsmith's (1976) dissertation addressed tone phenomena in so-called tone languages. This concept was used to explain *one-to-many mappings* (one tone associated with more than one segment) and *many-to-one mappings* (more than one tone associated with one segment). However, this "tiered" organization can demonstrate many characteristics of children's speech as well—relationships between certain syllable types and production of sound segments, for example.

The following diagram depicts the skeletal tier of a Consonant-Vowel-Consonant (CVC) syllable:

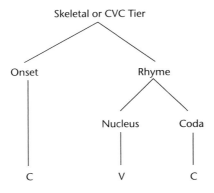

The feature spreading of autosegmental phonology supports the necessity of prioritizing words according to the surrounding vowels and consonants as therapy begins. For the child just learning a specific sound, it is important to think about how feature spreading may impact the sound acquisition. For example, if a child has trouble with the lip rounding of "sh" [ʃ], the child could use feature spreading as an aid. Words such as "shoe" or "bush" with the + lip rounding feature of the vowel would be helpful in promoting the lip rounding of [ʃ], whereas "ship" and "wish" with their – lip rounding feature would clearly not promote the necessary lip rounding.

Below is an example of a diagram in which a child deleted final consonants in two-syllable words. This diagram illustrates this relationship. C refers to consonant, V to vowel, and ∅ to a sound deletion:

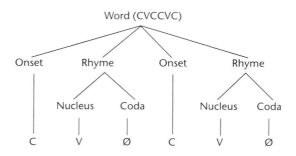

Autosegmental phonology also accounted for *feature spreading*. Certain features such as + and − rounding, for example, can spread to other vowels and consonants. There are two rules for spreading. First, + and − round spreads from a vowel to adjacent consonants within a syllable. Second, + and − round spreads from a consonant to an adjacent consonant up to a vowel. The following examples demonstrate the two types of feature spreading. The solid line is an inherent feature, whereas the dotted line represents a spread feature specification:

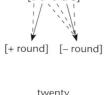

1. [+ and − round] spreads from a vowel to adjacent consonant. Note in the example that the rounding for the onglide portion of the diphthong in "soy", namely influences the beginning [s] in soy sauce whereas the unrounded offglide [ɪ] spreads to the second [s], the [s] in "sauce."

2. [+ and − round] spreads from a consonant to an adjacent consonant up to a vowel.

Feature spreading also occurs with such features as [+ voice] and [+ nasal].

To summarize, autosegmental phonology was originally conceived to account for cases in which a single segment is associated with two mutually exclusive features. It has since been expanded to demonstrate relationships between certain syllable types and consonant realizations. Feature spreading accounts for examples in which the feature or property of one segment spreads to adjacent segments.

Metrical Phonology. **Metrical phonology** (Liberman, 1975; Liberman & Prince, 1977) extended a hierarchical-based analysis to stress. In linear phonology, for example, stress was not handled in a binary + and − way; rather, stress could be assigned an infinite number of prominence values. The stress assignment rules of linear phonology produced a relative ordering within any given string of sound segments. This relative ordering can be used to analyze (1) the relative stressing of individual *words* within a sentence (sentence stress) as well as (2) the relative stressing of *syllables* within a word

(word stress). The following example demonstrates the linear phonology stress assignment of individual words (word stress) and when these words are placed within a sentence. The numeral 1 indicates the primary stress:

Word stress

a. customer
   1   3   2
b. services
   1   3   2

Sentence stress

c. customer services

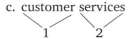

   1   2

d. He is the supervisor of customer services.
   4   6   5   1   7   2   3

This system of assigning stress to words within phrases appeared inadequate to Liberman and Prince. For example, the words *customer services* are assigned two different values in examples c and d even though the same words are used. Stress assignment rules in linear (generative) phonology were relational and changed depending on the prominence given to the words within a phrase.

Metrical phonologists proposed another concept for understanding and analyzing stress. "Metrical trees" are used to reflect the syntactic structure of an utterance. To show the relative prominence of each constituent in an utterance, a binary branching of these metrical trees represents stress patterns. One branch is labeled S for "stronger" stress and the other W for "weaker" stress. Applying this principle to an example, the following metrical tree can be drawn:

```
      /\
     W    S
     |    |
    big  brother
```

Thus, every tree in metrical phonology must have either a W S or an S W branching. This renders a binary stress representation. If the phrase is expanded, the following stress pattern emerges:

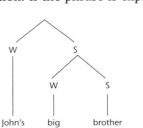

CLINICAL EXERCISES

According to autosegmental phonology, [+ and − round] spreads from a vowel to an adjacent consonant within a syllable. Show the + and − features on the words: "toothbrush, spoon," and "wood."

According to autosegmental phonology, [+ and − round] spreads from a consonant to an adjacent consonant up to a vowel. Show the + and − features for the words "swing, brushed," and "twist."

CLINICAL APPLICATION

Using Autosegmental Phonology to Analyze an Error Pattern

The following autosegmental chart is for a child who produces all initial consonant clusters (two- and three-sound clusters) as [d]:

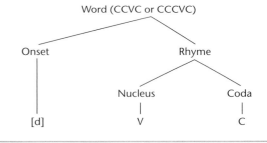

This pattern indicates that *brother* has more prominence than *big* and that the phrase *big brother* is more stressed than *John's*. The same relationship then is maintained between *big* and *brother* in both metrical representations.

CLINICAL APPLICATION

Using Metrical Phonology to Analyze an Error Pattern

The following metrical tree demonstrates a child's deletion of unstressed syllables in the two-syllable word *above* and the three-syllable word *umbrella*:

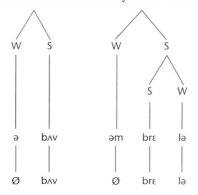

CLINICAL EXERCISES

Metrical phonology does provide an explanation as to why children maintain—and delete—certain syllables. Look at the following metrical trees for common words that children shorten.

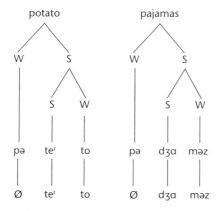

A child you are working with has difficulty with weak syllables. Draw the metrical tree for "elephant" and "telephone." Based on the metrical trees, what would you predict the child would say?

The second basic concept in metrical phonology pertains to the syllable. Although generative phonology indicates word boundaries, it does not consider the syllable structure. In metrical phonology the number of syllables within a word are considered as well as which consonants belong (or are hypothesized to belong) to each syllable. The notation uses the Greek letter sigma (σ) to indicate the individual syllables:

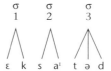

This hierarchical arrangement can also be used to include the *morphological* representation of the word with its syllabic divisions. The Greek symbol mu (μ) denotes the morphemes within this word:

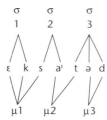

Such an analysis clearly indicates the difference between syllabic and morphological boundaries.

To summarize, metrical phonology is a theoretical construct that extends hierarchical analysis procedures to stress and syllable boundaries. Stress is analyzed according to a binary "strong" and "weak" system rather than to a relational numbering system that was used by earlier phonologies, including linear (generative) phonology. This hierarchical analysis has also been used when dividing words into syllables. Syllabic analyses allow for comparisons between syllable and morpheme boundaries.

Feature Geometry. **Feature geometry** represents a group of theories that have adopted the tiered representation of features used in autosegmental phonology. However, feature geometry theories have added a number of other hierarchically ordered feature tiers. Feature geometry attempts to explain why some features (but not others) are affected by assimilation processes (known as *spreading* or *linking* of features), whereas others are affected by neutralization or deletion processes (known as *delinking*) (Dinnsen, 1997). Feature geometry has several tier representations. Figure 4.1 is a feature geometry representation that is adapted from Bernhardt and Stemberger (1998). These features have been simplified to include only main areas that are pertinent for sounds of General American English.

In accordance with principles of nonlinear phonologies, feature geometry also uses hierarchically organized levels of representation, so-called tiers. These tiers interact with one another. Some features are designated as nodes, which means that these nodes may dominate more than one other feature and serve as a link between the dominated feature and higher levels of representation. For example, in Figure 4.1, the place node serves as a link among the labial, coronal, and dorsal nodes and the root node. Features at a higher level of representation are said to dominate other features. The place node, for example, dominates the different places of articulation (labial, coronal, and dorsal nodes). The place node must be activated, so to speak, before a specific place of articulation can be chosen. Or the laryngeal node as a higher level of representation must be functioning before [+ voice] can be designated. Features that are dominated are considered to be subordinate or at a lower level of representation.

The following is a brief explanation of the different nodes and features, summarized from Bernhardt and Stemberger (1998). Note, not all features mentioned by Bernhardt and Stemberger are present in the following list.

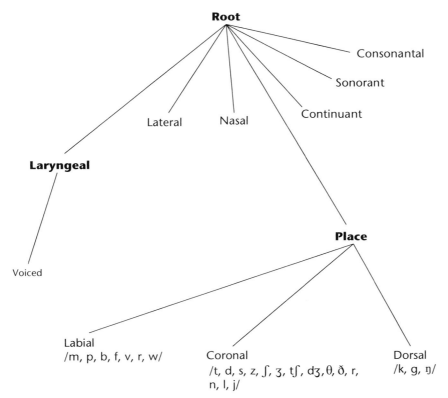

FIGURE 4.1 Feature Geometry of the English Consonant System
Adapted from Bernhardt and Stemberger (1998).

Note that distinctive features also play a central role in the newer nonlinear/multilinear phonologies. According to Bernhardt and Stemberger (1998), the distinctive elements for feature geometry are based on those of Chomsky and Halle (1968) except for the features for place of articulation, which follow Sagey (1986).

Laryngeal Features

1. [+ voiced] sounds produced with vocal fold vibration (e.g. [b, d, g, v, ð , z, ʒ])

Manner Features

1. [+ consonantal] sounds with a narrow constriction in the oral and/or pharyngeal cavities that significantly impede the flow of air (e.g., stops, affricates, nasals, fricatives, laterals are + consonantal).

2. [+ sonorant] sounds in which the pressure above the larynx allows the vocal cords to vibrate continuously without any rise in pressure above the larynx (e.g., voiced vowels, glides, liquids [r], and [l], [h])

3. [+ continuant] sounds in which air continues to move through the oral cavity (e.g., vowels, fricatives and affricates)

4. [+ nasal] sounds with the velum lowered so that air moves through the nasal cavity (e.g., nasals)

5. [+ lateral] sounds in which central airflow is blocked in the oral cavity but in which air is directed over at least one side of the tongue (e.g., laterals)

Place Features

Lips

[Labial] sounds made with more involvement of one or both lips (e.g., bilabials [p, b, m], labiodentals [f, v], [w], possibly [r] are + labial)

The tip of the tongue

[Coronal] sounds made with raising of the tip or blade of the tongue (e.g., [t, d, s, z, ʃ, ʒ, tʃ, dʒ, θ, ð , n, r, l, and j] plus high-front vowels are included)

The tongue body

[Dorsal] sounds made with the back of the tongue (e.g. [k, g, ŋ] (velars) and back vowels).

CLINICAL EXERCISES

Jake substitutes [t] and [d] for [k] and [g] in all word positions. The root node representing + consonantal (with stops) seems to be present.

At which level is the child having difficulty according to feature geometry? Examine the places of articulation under the place node.

Alexis produces a [w] for [r] and [j]. Which feature seems to dominate?

Another nonlinear theory, the *theory of radical underspecification* (Archangeli, 1988; Archangeli & Pulleyblank, 1994; Bernhardt, 1992b; Kiparsky, 1982; Pulleyblank, 1986), suggests that underlying representations contain only "unpredictable" features. A *predictable feature* is one that would be commonly associated with that particular segment or class of sounds. For example, nasals are typically voiced (although there are unvoiced nasals in some African languages). Voicing for nasals is then predictable and would not be contained in the underlying representation. Or because all sonorants are voiced, this is again a predictable feature and is not contained in the underlying representation. On the other hand, obstruents can be [+ voice] or [− voice]; therefore, the unpredictable nature of this feature is contained in the underlying representation.

Rules in nonlinear analysis are restricted to two basic operations: *spreading* (also known as *linking*) and *deletion* (also known as *delinking*) of phonological information from one tier to another. Spreading of features could be exemplified by the production of [gʌk] for *duck*. The coronal place node for /d/ is subject to the linking or assimilation from the dorsal place node feature of /k/. Thus, the dorsal place node of the final [k] in *duck* affects the initial [d]. The end result is that the initial [d] is produced as [g]. The place of articulation is moved from coronal [d] to dorsal [g]. Delinking could be exemplified by the production of [dʌ] for *duck*. Under the assumption that the underlying representation is intact, the final consonant slot for that production is delinked from the representation along with the actual features of /k/. Linking and delinking result from, and are constrained by, principles of association between tiers. These principles are outlined in Bernhardt and Stemberger (1998) and could be used as a reference for more detailed analysis procedures. For clinical application of these principles see Bernhardt, Bopp, Daudlin, Edwards, and Wastie (2010).

To summarize, one nonlinear phonology, feature geometry, theorizes that segments are composed of multitiered hierarchically organized features. Specific nodes that can dominate other features and link various levels of representation are designated. According to this theory, features can link (assimilate) or delink, causing neutralization or deletion. Principles of association are used to explain occurrences between tiers.

> **CLINICAL EXERCISES**
>
> The term underlying representation was discussed at the beginning of this chapter (page 68). The construct of radical underspecification is another theoretical idea about what the underlying representation actually is. In this case, it is thought that unpredictable features are contained in the underlying representation. What would be a predictable feature of [l] and [r] in General American English? What would be an unpredictable feature of the affricates? A predictable feature?

> **CLINICAL EXERCISES**
>
> According to nonlinear analysis, two basic operations may occur: *spreading* (also known as *linking*) and *deletion* (also known as *delinking*). Are the following transcriptions examples of spreading or delinking? Explain why for each: [lɛloᵘ] for "yellow," [kʌ] for "cup," [fɪndɚ] for "finger."

Optimality Theory. **Optimality theory,** first formalized by Prince and Smolensky (1993) and McCarthy and Prince (1995), is considered a constraint-based approach, not a rule-governed one as is feature geometry. Constraints are limits to what constitutes a possible pronunciation of a word. When constraints are applied linguistically, a set of grammatical universals is said to exist that includes the fact that all languages have syllables and that certain syllable patterns seem to be more (or less) common. For example, in General American English, there are words that begin with three consonants, such as *street*, but not any that begin with four consonants in a row. Therefore, we could say that General American English has a constraint on how many consonants can occur at the beginning of a word; three consonants are acceptable, but four are not. If compared to one another, languages demonstrate certain constraints. For example, Hawaiian allows no more than one consonant in a row, resulting in words such as *kanaka* for "man." When comparing this to English, which allows several consonants in a row, in such words as *street* and *sixths*, we could say that Hawaiian has a constraint against more than one consonant as an onset or as a syllable coda. Constraints characterize patterns that are and are not possible within or across languages. Applying this principle generally to children with speech sound disorders, we could state that child children who do not produce syllable codas thus evidencing final-consonant deletion, have a constraint against producing final codas.

Constraints are based on the principles of markedness. Thus, each constraint violation indicates markedness in that respect. Constraints are a means of (1) characterizing universal patterns that occur across languages, (2) demonstrating variations of patterns that occur between languages, and (3) determining markedness indicated by constraint violations (Archangeli & Langendoen, 1997).

> Markedness is discussed on pages 70–71 of this chap-ter.

Optimality theory, as a constraint-based approach, was originally developed to explain the differences that occur between and among languages. Optimality theory presupposes a universal grammar and states that constraints characterize universals; however, constraints can be violated. Some constraints are very important (within and across languages) and are rarely violated, whereas others are not as important and can be violated. If we examine constraints in this manner, we will find that the following universal trends are considered typical (unmarked) properties of syllables. To the right of the constraint is the name given to it by Archangeli and Langendoen (1997):

Syllables begin with a consonant.	ONSET
Syllables have one vowel	PEAK
Syllables end with a vowel.	NOCODA
Syllables have at most one consonant at an edge.	*COMPLEX

In examining this list, we can see whether there are constraint violations in General American English.

1. *Syllables begin with a consonant: ONSET.* Not all syllables begin with a consonant, as demonstrated by words such as *away* and *eat.* Probably in General American English most syllables do, however, begin with a consonant. This constraint can be violated (although it is maintained most of the time) in General American English.

2. *Syllables have one vowel: PEAK.* In General American English, this seems to be the case. Some syllables consist of syllabic consonants such as [bi.tl̩] or [fɪʃ.n̩]; however, no syllables contain two separate vowels. In General American English, the constraint of PEAK is *rarely,* if at all, violated.

3. *Syllables end with a vowel: NOCODA.* Not all syllables in General American English end with a vowel. Many syllables end with a consonant in words such as *hat, clock,* and *antique.* This constraint is violated in General American English.

4. *Syllables have at most one consonant at an edge: *COMPLEX.* This is also violated in General American English. Words such as *clocks* and *streets* demonstrate a violation of this constraint.

In summarizing, we could state that some of the previously mentioned constraints are violated, whereas others are not. This could lead to a rank ordering of constraints from those constraints that are never or rarely violated → to those that are sometimes violated → to those that are often violated. Those constraints that are *rarely* violated are considered higher-order constraints and are separated from others by a double arrow > >. Those constraints that are sometimes violated are separated from each other by a comma. Based on the previous discussion, the following rank ordering could be made:

PEAK > > ONSET, NOCODA, *COMPLEX

Thus, in General American English, the constraint PEAK (syllables have one vowel) is not violated. Therefore, it is separated from the others ONSET, NOCODA, and *COMPLEX. The other constraints, which can be violated, are separated by commas. Therefore, one important concept within optimality theory is the rank ordering of the constraints.

Optimality theory, like other linguistic theories, proposes an input (an underlying representation), an output (the surface representation), and a relation between the two. The only specification of the input is that it is linguistically well formed; it does not contain variables that are not grammatical. The output is the actual production. Optimality theory does not account for differences between the input and output in terms

CLINICAL EXERCISES

If you examine the four typical properties of syllables from Archangeli and Langendoen (1997) and think about the speech patterns noted in children with speech sound disorders, do they seem more to violate or adhere to these properties? Think about the high use of final consonant deletion or consonant cluster reduction.

of rules (as in generative grammar) or processes (as in natural phonology) but in terms of constraints. In optimality theory, the relation between the input and output is mediated by two formal mechanisms: the generator (GEN) and the evaluator (EVAL). The GEN links the input with potential outputs. It can add, delete, or rearrange, for example. The EVAL judges the outputs to determine which one is the *optimal* output. For any given input, such as [pɪg], which is the mental representation of the word *pig*, the GEN can generate an infinite number of possible phonetic outputs for that form. All these output forms compete with one another, but one output must be chosen as the optimal one. The EVAL evaluates all these different outputs and chooses the output that is the optimal response for that particular language. These output forms are evaluated through the constraints and their ranking within that language that thus restrict the possible output forms (Ball, 2002; Barlow, 2001).

Two types of constraints function within this mechanism: faithfulness and markedness. Faithfulness constraints require that input and output forms be identical to one another. If segments between the input and output are deleted, inserted, or rearranged, the faithfulness constraint is violated. If a child produces the word *skip* as [sɪp], then the faithfulness constraint has been violated. Markedness constraints require outputs to be unmarked or simplified in structure. *Unmarked features* are those that are easier to perceive or produce or those that occur frequently across languages. Consonant clusters are considered to be marked (see *COMPLEX mentioned previously). Thus, the child who produces *skip* as [skɪp] violates the markedness constraint. However, a child who says the word *skip* as [sɪp] has not violated this constraint; the output is unmarked or simplified.

As can be seen, faithfulness and markedness constraints are conflicting; there is an antagonistic relationship between the two. The conflict between faithfulness and markedness leads to violation of constraints. Every utterance violates some constraint; if faithfulness is maintained, then markedness is violated. (The most unmarked syllable would be something like [bɑ], so any more complex syllable structure would be in some violation of markedness.)

So how does the EVAL judge which one is the most optimal form? At this point, optimality theory postulates that the rank ordering of the constraints becomes the deciding factor. Lower-ranked constraints can be violated to satisfy higher-ranking constraints. In our previous example, ONSET, NOCODA, or *COMPLEX could be violated to satisfy PEAK.

If optimality theory is applied to phonological development, the hypothesis is that children acquire the correct ranking of the constraints as they develop. Immature patterns demonstrate that this ranking, according to the language in question, has not yet been mastered. Individual patterns of normal development are seen as products of the individual's idiosyncratic constraint rankings. Application of this to children with phonemic-based disorders indicates that these children also have their own unique constraint rankings. Our job is to find the rankings that would then account for the children's error patterns. The next step is to try to rerank the constraints so that they are

> Watch and listen to this video on optimality theory. youtube.com/watch?v=xsMea6QhLoA

CLINICAL EXERCISES

The following small sample is from Hector, age 4;6

Word Example	Transcription	Hector's Production
grapes	[greⁱps]	[deⁱ]
feet	[fit]	[fi]
teeth	[tiθ]	[ti]
stove	[stoᵘv]	[toᵘ]
spoon	[spun]	[un]
bed	[bɛd]	[ɛd]
book	[bʊk]	[ʊt]
nose	[noᵘz]	[noᵘ]
mop	[mɑp]	[mɑ]
pig	[pɪg]	[ɪd]

Consider the constraints ONSET, NOCODA, and *COMPLEX for Hector. Which constraints seem to be operating on a regular basis? Look at the four violations of his constraints. Do you see a pattern? Could this be used to reorganize his constraints?

TABLE 4.3 Summary of Terms and Examples for Optimality Theory

Constraint Based	Universal, languages differ in the ranking of constraints
Two Types of Constraints	Faithfulness and markedness
Markedness	Output is unmarked or simplified in structure
Faithfulness	Input and output forms are identical
	Conflict results in constraint violability: every output violates some constraint
Types of Markedness Constraints	Complex, Coda, Fricatives, Liquids (Liquid [l], Liquid [r])
Complex	Cluster reduction simplified "tree" ⇒ [ti], Violation = "tree" ⇒ [tri]
Coda	No syllable final consonants "team" ⇒ [ti], Violation "team" ⇒ [tim]
Fricatives	No fricatives "sip" ⇒ [tɪp], Violation = "sip" = [sɪp]
Liquids	No liquids "lip" ⇒ [wɪp], "rip" ⇒ [wɪp] Violation = "lip" ⇒ [lɪp], "rip" ⇒ [rɪp]
Liquid [l]	No liquid [l] "lose" ⇒ [wuz] Violation = "lose" ⇒ [luz]
Liquid [r]	No liquid [r] "rock" ⇒ [wɑk] Violation = "rock" ⇒[rɑk]
Types of Faithfulness Constraints	Max, Dep, Ident-Feature (Ident-[cons], Ident-[cont])
Max	Prohibits deletion "moon" ⇒ [mun] Violation = "moon" ⇒ [mu]
Dep	Prohibits insertion or addition of segments "sleep" ⇒ [slip] Violation = "sleep" ⇒ [sip]
Ident-feature	Prohibits changing any feature; input and output forms are the same "tree" ⇒ [tri] Violation = "tree" ⇒ [twi]
Ident-[cons]	Prohibits changing consonantal features, "bed" ⇒ [bɛd] Violation = "bed" ⇒ [bɛt]
Ident-[cont]	Prohibits changing continuant features, "sock" ⇒ [sɑk] Violation = "sock" ⇒ [tɑk]

more in line with the input. It is assumed that markedness constraints (thus, the typical simplification that occurs in relationship to the production features) must be demoted. *Demotion* is a process in which higher-ranking constraints that do not match the adult rankings become lower, thus the rankings will eventually match the adult ones. See Table 4.3 for a summary of terms and examples within optimality theory.

Optimality theory offers a new way to view both the acquisition of phonological patterns and the categorization of disordered phonological systems. The concept of constraints and demoting constraints reminds one of phonological process suppression. However, the theoretical optimality model and the information gained are far more detailed and give the clinician valuable information about what the child can do, not just what the child is incapable of doing.

How Did Nonlinear Phonology Develop?

John Firth, professor of general linguistics at the University of London, was a key figure in the development of modern linguistics in the United Kingdom. In a way, nonlinear phonology, too, can be traced back to Firth's (1948) so-called prosodic analysis. For the first time, Firth challenged the one-sided linguistic importance of the phonemic units in their consecutive linearity. He advocated the necessity for additional nonsegmental analyses, "prosodies," which represent larger linguistic entities, such as syllables, words, and phrases. He postulated that speech is a manifestation of consecutively ordered units *as well as* a manifestation of larger prosodic units that bind phonemes together into linguistically more comprehensive units. Firth theorized that different analytical systems may need to be set up to explain the range of contrasts involved. With this approach, known as *polysystemicism*, the concept of nonlinear phonology was born.

Contemporary nonlinear/multilinear phonologies are seen as an evolution process from generative phonology. Chomsky and Halle's (1968) major contribution, *The Sound Pattern of English*, was innovative in its description of two levels of representation, a surface phonetic representation and an underlying phonemic representation. Although the idea of distinctive features was taken from the Prague School of Linguistics, Chomsky and Halle understood the distinctive feature concept in a different way and modified it accordingly. Nonlinear phonologies adopt the generative concepts of distinctive features and surface-level and underlying representation. However, these new phonologies understand the surface-level representation in a very different way.

Chomsky and Halle's generative phonology described speech components in a linear manner: It was segment based. The components of any utterance were arranged in a sequence with one discrete segment following the next. A common set of distinctive features is attributed to all segments, and the assignment of a binary value specifies each feature. This limited the possibility of generating phonological rules in several respects. First, only whole segments could be deleted or added. The only other modifications that could occur in the segment were achieved by changing the + or − values of one or more distinctive features. (Thus, this system analyzes only additions, deletions, or substitutions; analysis of nonphonemic distortions is not possible.) Second, because all segments are equally complex and all distinctive features are equal within this system, there is no reason to expect that any one segment or any one distinctive feature might be affected by any given phonological rule. However, many observations and investigations have reported, for example, that certain sounds and sound classes appear to be especially vulnerable to assimilation, whereas others cause assimilation (Dinnsen, 1997). Third, early generative phonology adopted the division between the segmentals and the suprasegmentals that the structural linguists had used to describe and analyze speech events. However, such a division does not allow a vertical, hierarchical understanding of the interaction between segmental units and prosodic features. The nonlinear phonologies represent a challenge to the earlier segment-based approaches. "Nonlinear phonological theory is another step in the

CLINICAL APPLICATION

More Information—Feature Geometry versus Phonological Processes

Let's look at the difference between how feature geometry versus phonological processes would explain an example of a child who says [gʌ] for *duck* and [dʌ] for *dumb*. If phonological processes are assigned to these substitutions and deletions, the following results are noted:

"duck" [dʌk]	→	[gʌ] backing [d] → [g] final consonant deletion [k] → Ø
"dumb" [dʌm]	→	[dʌ] final consonant deletion [m] → Ø

Although these phonological processes are easily identifiable, they give no information about a child's underlying representation. Where to begin in therapy would be a relatively arbitrary choice that would be based on the number of times the processes were observed and the age at which they should be suppressed. Feature geometry demonstrates that the underlying representation for this child includes information about the dorsal place node, that is, about /k/ and /g/. This is evidenced by the dorsal production of [g] in [gʌ] for *duck*. Articulatory constraints, however, prevent realization of final consonants. If this was just a case of final consonant deletion, both *duck* and *dumb* should have been realized as [dʌ]. In the underlying representation, the child might be trying to differentiate between *duck* and *dumb*. This suggests that if the articulatory constraints could be eliminated, the child's g/d substitution (backing) might also be eliminated. The concept of feature geometry and underlying representation provides us with more insight into reasons for the child's output patterns.

evolution of our understanding of phonological systems" (Bernhardt & Stoel-Gammon, 1994, p. 126).

Although contemporary nonlinear phonologies began with Goldsmith's (1976) dissertation on autosegmental phonology, many different nonlinear phonological theories have since been proposed. This section has attempted to briefly introduce four nonlinear approaches: autosegmental phonology, metrical phonology, feature geometry, and optimality theory. However, the reader should keep in mind that many other nonlinear phonologies exist.

To summarize, many different nonlinear phonologies have been developed within the last decade or so. Some of them have been applied to case studies of children with disordered phonological systems. The results seem to indicate that these phonologies promise new insights into, and a deeper understanding of, the phonological system.

SUMMARY

This chapter first introduced some of the basic terminology and principles underlying contemporary phonological theories. The relationship between the sound form and the sound function (as phoneme) was established as a basis for understanding phonological theories. The development of the phoneme concept was traced historically to provide a foundation for the understanding of how phonological theories could evolve from this "new" concept. Clinical application of these basic principles stressed the interrelationship between sound–form and sound–function.

The remainder of this chapter summarized several phonological theories that impact the assessment and treatment of phonemic-based disorders. These theories were enumerated in a historical sequence. The linear phonologies were represented by distinctive feature theory, generative phonology, and natural phonology. The nonlinear phonologies included autosegmental, metrical, feature geometry, and optimality theory. Each phonological theory was discussed in regard to what the theoretical framework stands for, how it developed, how it functions, and its clinical implications.

The field of phonology is constantly evolving. Current phonological theories attempt to describe the phonological system with all its complexity in a different manner. Although some of the newer models have yet to stand the test of time and research, all offer new insights into the intricate nature of normal and impaired phonological systems.

CASE STUDY

The phonological process analysis procedure can be demonstrated using a slightly modified clinical example from Chapter 2, page 35. The following sample is from Tina, age 3;8.

dig	[dɛg]	boat	[bot]
house	[haʊθ]	cup	[tʌp]
knife	[nɑf]	lamp	[wæmp]
duck	[dʌt]	goat	[dot]
cat	[tæt]	ring	[wɪŋ]
bath	[bæt]	thumb	[tʌm]
red	[wed]	that	[dæt]
ship	[sɪp]	zip	[ðɪp]
fan	[fɛn]	key	[ti]
yes	[jɛθ]	win	[wɪn]

The following errors are noted:

[s] → [θ]	house, yes
[k] → [t]	duck, cat, cup, key
[θ] → [t]	bath, thumb
[r] → [w]	red, ring
[ʃ] → [s]	ship
[l] → [w]	lamp
[g] → [d]	goat
[ð] → [d]	that
[z] → [ð]	zip

Results are as follows:

	Target→Error	Phonological Process
[s] → [θ]	house, yes	fronting
[k] → [t]	duck, cat, cup, key	velar fronting
[θ] → [t]	bath, thumb	stopping + backing
[r] → [w]	red, ring	gliding
[ʃ] → [s]	ship	palatal fronting
[l] → [w]	lamp	gliding
[g] → [d]	goat	velar fronting
[ð] → [d]	that	stopping + backing
[z] → [ð]	zip	fronting

In summarizing the phonological processes, we see that fronting (including both velar and palatal fronting) affected five sounds (s → θ, k → t, ʃ → s, g → d, and z → ð). Both stopping + backing (θ → t and ð → d) and gliding (l, r → w) were noted on two different sounds.

If this sample is analyzed according to feature geometry, which two place features seem to be problematic for this child, one dominating on certain productions and one on others?

THINK CRITICALLY

The following are the results of an articulation test from Ryan, age 6;6:

horse	[hoᵘɚθ]	pig	[pɪk]	chair	[ʃɛɚ]
wagon	[wægən]	cup	[kʌp]	watch	[waʃ]
monkey	[mʌŋki]	swinging	[ʂwɪŋɪŋ]	thumb	[fʌm]
comb	[koᵘm]	table	[teˈbəl]	mouth	[maᵘf]
fork	[foɚk]	cat	[kæt]	shoe	[su]
knife	[nɑˈf]	ladder	[læɾɚ]	fish	[fɪs]
cow	[kaᵘ]	ball	[bɑl]	zipper	[ðɪpɚ]
cake	[keˈk]	plane	[pweˈn]	nose	[noᵘθ]

(*Continued*)

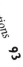
baby	[beˈbi]	cold	[koᵘd]	sun	[θʌn]
bathtub	[bæftəb]	jumping	[dʌmpən]	house	[haᵘθ]
nine	[naˈn]	TV	[tivi]	steps	[stɛp]
train	[tweˈn]	stove	[θtoᵘv]	nest	[nɛt]
gun	[gʌn]	ring	[wɪŋ]	books	[bʊkθ]
dog	[dɑg]	tree	[twi]	bird	[bɝd]
yellow	[wɛloᵘ]	green	[gwin]	whistle	[wɪθəl]
doll	[dɑl]	this	[dɪθ]	carrots	[kɛɚət]

Summarize the errors according to phonological processes. Which phonological processes occur most frequently?

TEST YOURSELF

1. Which one of the following does *not* belong to the phoneme/phonology concept?
   a. meaning-establishing and meaning-differentiating function of sound units
   b. underlying form or representation
   c. production realities
   d. sound unit function within a particular language system

2. Which one of the following is a major class feature that distinguishes sounds produced with a high degree of oral obstruction?
   a. sonorant
   b. consonantal
   c. vocalic
   d. coronal

3. Which one of the following statements concerning phonological processes is *not* true?
   a. they are innate
   b. they are universal
   c. children with different language backgrounds begin with different sets of phonological processes
   d. they are used to simplify productions for children in the developmental period

4. If a child says [wɑʃ] for *watch*, this is an example of which phonological process?
   a. stopping
   b. affrication
   c. deaffrication
   d. labialization

5. Which one of the following is true about non-linear/multilinear phonologies?
   a. segments are governed by more complex linguistic dimensions such as stress
   b. emphasis is on the sequential arrangement of sound segments
   c. all sound segments have equal value
   d. no one sound segment has control over the other units

6. Which one of the following terms is *not* representative of autosegmental phonology?
   a. tiers are separable and independent levels
   b. certain segments are autonomous and do not have a one-for-one match on another level
   c. strong and weak stresses are emphasized
   d. feature spreading is also a portion of this concept

7. According to metrical phonology, the word *potato* has which one of the following stress patterns?
   a. weak branching to "po," strong branching to "tato"; further divided into strong branching on "ta," weak branching on "to"
   b. strong branching on "po," weak branching to "tato"; further divided into strong branching on "ta," weak branching on "to"
   c. weak branching to "po," strong branching to "tato"; further divided into weak branching on "ta," strong branching on "to"

8. Which one of the following terms is *not* associated with feature geometry?
   a. spreading
   b. distinctive features
   c. faithfulness
   d. delinking

9. In optimality theory, the constraint "markedness" requires outputs to be
   a. the same as the input
   b. simplified in structure
   c. marked
   d. demoted

10. If a child produces [tɑ] for *stop*, then whi... the following constraints is violated?
   a. *COMPLEX
   b. *CODA
   c. *FRICATIVES
   d. MAX

FURTHER READINGS

Archangeli, D., & Langendoen, T. (1998). *Optimality theory: An overview*. Malden, MA: Blackwell.

Ball, M., & Kent, R. (1997). *The new phonologies: Developments in clinical linguistics*. San Diego, CA: Singular.

Ball, M., Mueller, N., & Rutter, B. (2011). *Phonology for Communication Disorders*. New York: Lawrence Erlbaum.

Bernhardt, B., & Stemberger, J. (2000). *Workbook in nonlinear phonology for clinical application*. Austin, TX: PRO-ED.

Lombardi, L. (2001). *Segmental phonology in optimality theory: Constraints and representations*. New York: Cambridge University Press.

APPENDIX 4.1

I. Single-Word Responses to Goldman-Fristoe Test of Articulation for Child H. H.

Target Word	Child's Production	Target Word	Child's Production
1. house	[hɑʊ]	17. rabbit	[wæbə]
2. telephone	[tɛfoʊ]	18. fishing	[bɪdɪn]
3. cup	[tʌp]	19. church	[tɜ]
4. gun	[dʌn]	20. feather	[bɛdə]
5. knife	[nɑˈ]	21. pencils	[pɛntə]
6. window	[wɪnoʊ]	22. carrot	[tɛwə]
7. wagon	[wædən]	orange	[oʊwɪn]
wheel	[wi]	23. bathtub	[bætə]
8. chicken	[tɪtə]	bath	[bæ]
9. zipper	[tɪpə]	24. thumb	[bʌm]
10. scissors	[tɪtə]	finger	[bɪnə]
11. duck	[dʌt]	ring	[wɪŋ]
yellow	[jɛwoʊ]	25. jump	[dʌmp]
12. vacuum	[ætu]	26. pajamas	[dæmi]
13. matches	[mætət]	27. plane	[beˈn]
14. lamp	[wæmp]	blue	[bu]
15. shovel	[dʌvə]	28. brush	[bʌs]
16. car	[tɑə]	29. drum	[dʌm]

	Child's Production
	[bæ]
	[tænə dɑ]
	[tɪtmə]
	[ti]
...rel	[twɜə]

Target Word	Child's Production
34. sleeping	[twipɪn]
bed	[bɛd]
35. stove	[doʊ]
this	child would not say

2. Transcription of H. H. According to Pre-, Inter-, and Postvocalic Positions

Target Word	Child's Production	Position	Description
1. house	[haʊ]	postvocalic	[s] deletion
2. telephone	[tɛfoʊ]	[unstressed syllable deletion—noted but not counted on matrices]	
		postvocalic	[n] deletion
3. cup	[tʌp]	prevocalic	[k]→[t]
4. gun	[dʌn]	prevocalic	[g]→[d]
5. knife	[naɪ]	postvocalic	[f] deletion
6. window	[wɪnoʊ]	intervocalic	[nd]→[n]
7. wagon	[wædən]	intervocalic	[g]→[d]
wheel	[wi]	postvocalic	[l] deletion
8. chicken	[tɪtə]	prevocalic	[tʃ]→[t]
		intervocalic	[k]→[t]
		postvocalic	[n] deletion
9. zipper	[tɪpə]	prevocalic	[z]→[t]
		vowel nucleus	[ɚ]→[ə]
10. scissors	[tɪtə]	prevocalic	[s]→[t]
		intervocalic	[z]→[t]
		nucleus + postvocalic	[ɚz]→[ə]
11. duck	[dʌt]	postvocalic	[k]→[t]
yellow	[jɛwoʊ]	intervocalic	[l]→[w]
12. vacuum	[ætu]	prevocalic	[v] deletion
		intervocalic	[kj]→[t]
		postvocalic	[m] deletion
13. matches	[mætət]	intervocalic	[tʃ]→[t]
		postvocalic	[z]→[t]
14. lamp	[wæmp]	prevocalic	[l]→[w]
15. shovel	[dʌvə]	prevocalic	[ʃ]→[d]
		postvocalic	[l] deletion
16. car	[tɑə]	prevocalic	[k]→[t]
		vowel nucleus	[ɚ]→[ə]*
17. rabbit	[wæbɪ]	prevocalic	[r]→[w]
		postvocalic	[t] deletion

Target Word	Child's Production	Position	Description
18. fishing	[bɪdɪn]	prevocalic	[f]→[b]
		intervocalic	[ʃ]→[d]
		postvocalic	[ŋ]→[n], this is considered a variation in regular pronunciation, not an error, so not counted
19. church	[tɜ]	prevocalic	[tʃ]→[t]
		vowel nucleus	[ɝ]→[ɜ]
		postvocalic	[tʃ] deletion
20. feather	[bɛdə]	prevocalic	[f]→[b]
		intervocalic	[ð]→[d]
		vowel nucleus	[ɚ]→[ə]
21. pencils	[pɛntə]	intervocalic	[ns]→[nt]
		postvocalic	[lz] deletion
this	child would not say		
22. carrot	[tɛwə]	prevocalic	[k]→[t]
		intervocalic	[r]→[w]
		postvocalic	[t] deletion
orange	[oᵘwɪn]	intervocalic	[r]→[w]
		postvocalic	[ndʒ]→[n]
23. bathtub	[bætə]	intervocalic	[θt]→[t]
		postvocalic	[b] deletion
bath	[bæ]	postvocalic	[θ] deletion
24. thumb	[bʌm]	prevocalic	[θ]→[b]
finger	[bɪnə]	prevocalic	[f]→[b]
		intervocalic	[ŋg]→[n]
		vowel nucleus	[ɚ]→[ə]
ring	[wɪŋ]	prevocalic	[r]→[w]
25. jump	[dʌmp]	prevocalic	[dʒ]→[d]
26. pajamas	[dæmi]	[unstressed syllable deletion—noted but not counted in matrices]	
		prevocalic	[dʒ]→[d]
		[i] at end noted as a diminutive, final consonant deletion not counted in matrices	
27. plane	[beˈn]	prevocalic	[pl]→[b]
blue	[bu]	prevocalic	[bl]→[b]
28. brush	[bʌs]	prevocalic	[br]→[b]
		postvocalic	[ʃ]→[s]
29. drum	[dʌm]	prevocalic	[dr]→[d]
30. flag	[bæ]	prevocalic	[fl]→[b]
		postvocalic	[g] deletion
31. Santa Claus	[tænə dɑ]	prevocalic	[s]→[t]

Target Word	Child's Production	Position	Description
		intervocalic	[nt]→[n], considered a normal assimilation, counted as correct
		intervocalic	[kl]→[d]
		postvocalic	[z] deletion
32. Christmas tree	[tɪtmə ti]	prevocalic	[kr]→[t]
		intervocalic	[sm]→[tm]
		intervocalic	[str]→[t]
33. squirrel	[twɜə]	prevocalic	[skw]→[tw]
		vowel nucleus	[ɝ]→[ɜ]
		postvocalic	[l] deletion
34. sleeping	[twipɪn]	prevocalic	[sl]→[tw]
		postvocalic	[ŋ]→[n] this is considered a variation in regular pronunciation, not an error, so not counted
bed	[bɛd]		
35. stove	[doʊ]	prevocalic	[st]→[d]
		postvocalic	[v] deletion

*[ɑɚ] is considered to be a centering diphthong; therefore, it is the nucleus of the syllable.

3. Phonological Processes for H. H.

Target Word	Child's Production	Position	Description
1. house	[haʊ]	postvocalic	final consonant deletion
2. telephone	[tɛfoʊ]		weak syllable deletion
		postvocalic	final consonant deletion
3. cup	[tʌp]	prevocalic	velar fronting
4. gun	[dʌn]	prevocalic	velar fronting
5. knife	[naˈ]	postvocalic	final consonant deletion
6. window	[wɪnoʊ]	intervocalic	[nd] → [n] cluster reduction
7. wagon	[wædən]	intervocalic	velar fronting
wheel	[wi]	postvocalic	final consonant deletion
8. chicken	[tɪtə]	prevocalic	stopping
		intervocalic	velar fronting
		postvocalic	final consonant deletion
9. zipper	[tɪpə]	prevocalic	stopping + devoicing
		vowel nucleus	derhotacization
10. scissors	[tɪtə]	prevocalic	stopping
		intervocalic	stopping + devoicing
		nucleus	derhotacization
		postvocalic	final consonant deletion

Target Word	Child's Production	Position	Description
11. duck	[dʌt]	postvocalic	velar fronting
yellow	[jɛwoᵘ]	intervocalic	gliding of liquids
12. vacuum	[ætu]	prevocalic	initial consonant deletion
		intervocalic	[kj] → [t] cluster reduction + cluster substitution (velar fronting)
		postvocalic	final consonant deletion
13. matches	[mætət]	intervocalic	stopping
		postvocalic	stopping + devoicing
14. lamp	[wæmp]	prevocalic	gliding of liquids
15. shovel	[dʌvə]	prevocalic	stopping + fronting + voicing
		postvocalic	final consonant deletion
16. car	[tɑə]	prevocalic	velar fronting
		nucleus	derhotacization
17. rabbit	[wæbɪ]	prevocalic	gliding of liquids
		postvocalic	final consonant deletion
18. fishing	[bɪdɪn]	prevocalic	stopping + labialization + voicing
		intervocalic	stopping + fronting + voicing
		postvocalic	not counted, normal variation
19. church	[tɜ]	prevocalic	stopping
		nucleus	derhotacization
		postvocalic	final consonant deletion
20. feather	[bɛdə]	prevocalic	stopping + labialization + voicing
		intervocalic	alveolarization + stopping
		nucleus	derhotacization
21. pencils	[pɛntə]	intervocalic	[ns] → [nt] cluster substitution (stopping)
		postvocalic	cluster deletion
22. carrot	[tɛwə]	prevocalic	velar fronting
		intervocalic	gliding of liquids
		postvocalic	final consonant deletion
orange	[oᵘwɪn]	intervocalic	gliding of liquids
		postvocalic	[ndʒ] → [n] cluster reduction
23. bathtub	[bætə]	intervocalic	[θt] → [t] cluster reduction
		postvocalic	final consonant deletion
bath	[bæ]	postvocalic	final consonant deletion
24. thumb	[bʌm]	prevocalic	stopping + labialization + voicing
finger	[bɪnə]	prevocalic	stopping + labialization + voicing
		intervocalic	[ŋg] → [n] cluster reduction + fronting
		nucleus	derhotacization
ring	[wɪŋ]	prevocalic	gliding of liquids

Target Word	Child's Production	Position	Description
25. jump	[dʌmp]	prevocalic	stopping
26. pajamas	[dæmi]		weak syllable deletion
		prevocalic	stopping
		postvocalic	diminutive—use of [i]
27. plane	[beˈn]	prevocalic	[pl] → [b] cluster reduction + voicing
blue	[bu]	prevocalic	[bl] → [b] cluster reduction
28. brush	[bʌs]	prevocalic	[br] → [b] cluster reduction
		postvocalic	palatal fronting
29. drum	[dʌm]	prevocalic	[dr] → [d] cluster reduction
30. flag	[bæ]	prevocalic	[fl] → [b] cluster reduction, cluster substitution (stopping + labialization + voicing)
		postvocalic	final consonant deletion
31. Santa Claus	[tænə dɑ]	prevocalic	stopping
		intervocalic	[nt] → [n] considered normal assimilation, not counted
		intervocalic	[kl] → [t] cluster reduction, cluster substitution (velar fronting + voicing)
		postvocalic	final consonant deletion
32. Christmas tree	[tɪtmə ti]	prevocalic	[kr] → [t] cluster reduction, cluster substitution (velar fronting)
		intervocalic	[sm] → [t] cluster reduction, cluster substitution (stopping)
		intervocalic	[str] → [t] cluster reduction
33. squirrel	[twɝə]	prevocalic	[skw] → [tw] cluster reduction, cluster substitution (velar fronting)
		nucleus	derhotacization
		postvocalic	final consonant deletion

4. Spontaneous Speech Sample for H. H.

Looking at Pictures

[dæ ə pɪtə əv ə tɑ]
That a picture of a dog.

[hi ə bɪ dɑ]
He a big dog.

[hi baʊ ən hæ ə tawə]
He brown and has a collar.

[oʊ dæ ɪt ə tɪti]
Oh, that is a kitty.

[wi hæf ə tɪti]
We have a kitty.

[wi dat aʊ tɪti ə wa:ŋ taˈm]
We got our kitty a long time.

Conversation with Mom

[tæn wi do tu mədanoᵘ]	[hi tʌm tu mədanə wɪt ʌt]
Can we go to McDonald?	He come to McDonald with us?
[aⁱ wʌ ə tibɜdə]	[xxxxx mɑⁱ haᵘ]
I want a cheeseburger.	xxxx My house.
[aⁱ wʌ fɛnfɑⁱθ]	[mɑmi lɛ do]
I want french fries.	Mommy let go.
[wɛ ɪt bɪwi]	[lɛ do naᵘ]
Where is Billy?	Let go now.

Talking about Summer Vacation

[wi doᵘf tu dæmɑt]	[si hæt wɑtə taᵘt]
We drove to Grandma's.	She has lot'a cows.
[si wɪf ɪn oᵘ +haⁱo]	[taᵘt ju noᵘ mu taᵘ]
She live in Ohio.	Cows, you know, moo cow.
[si hæt ə fɑm]	[deⁱ it ə ho wɑt]
She has a farm.	They eat a whole lot.

5. Phonological Process Analysis Summary Sheet

Processes	Number of Occurrences
Syllable Structure Changes	
Cluster reduction	_____
Cluster deletion	_____
Reduplication	_____
Weak syllable deletion	_____
Final consonant deletion	_____
Initial consonant deletion	_____
Other _____	_____
Substitution Processes	
Consonant cluster substitution	_____
Velar Fronting	_____
Palatal Fronting	_____
Fronting	_____
Labialization	_____
Alveolarization	_____
Stopping	_____
Affrication	_____
Deaffrication	_____
Denasalization	_____
Gliding of liquids	_____
Gliding of fricatives	_____

Vowelization   _____

Derhotacization   _____

Voicing   _____

Devoicing   _____

Other _____   _____

                               _____

                               _____

Assimilation Processes

Labial assimilation   _____

Velar assimilation   _____

Nasal assimilation   _____

Liquid assimilation   _____

Other _____   _____

                               _____

                               _____

6. SUMMARY of Phonological Processes for Child H. H.

Processes	Number of Occurrences
Syllable structure changes	
Cluster reduction	15
Cluster deletion	2
Reduplication	0
Weak syllable deletion	2
Final consonant deletion	16
Initial consonant deletion	1
Other _____	
Substitution processes	
Consonant cluster substitution	7
Velar Fronting	11
Palatal Fronting	1
Fronting	3
Labialization	5
Alveolarization	1
Stopping	20

Affrication	0
Deaffrication	0
Denasalization	0
Gliding of liquids	6
Gliding of fricatives	0
Vowelization	0
Derhotacization	7
Voicing	9
Devoicing	3
Other _____	_____
_____	_____
_____	

Assimilation processes

Labial assimilation	_____
Velar assimilation	_____
Nasal assimilation	_____
Liquid assimilation	_____
Other _____	_____
_____	_____
_____	

H. H. demonstrates only four different processes 10 or more times: fronting (= 15 times, velar fronting 11 times, palatal fronting 1 time, and fronting 3 times), cluster reduction (= 15 times), final consonant deletion (= 16 times), and stopping (= 20 times). If the articulation test results are examined, one can note that final consonant deletion impacts some of the fricatives, the stop-plosives, the nasals, one of the affricates, and the lateral [l], whereas stopping affects the fricatives and affricates. On the other hand, fronting is limited to [k], [g], and [ʃ].

Normal Phonological Development

LEARNING OBJECTIVES

When you have finished this chapter, you should be able to:

- Describe the primary function of the infant's respiratory, phonatory, resonatory, and articulatory systems at birth, and explain the general changes that occur before babbling begins.
- Identify the types of auditory perceptual skills that infants demonstrate prior to their first words.
- List characteristics of each of the prelinguistic stages.

- Explain the role of individual variability during the early period of speech sound development.
- Trace the consonant, vowel, and prosodic development in children from their first words to their early school years.
- Identify the factors that influence speech sound development in children learning English as a second language.
- Describe the relationship among phonological development, metaphonology, and learning to read.

THIS CHAPTER outlines the prelinguistic behavior and phonological development of children from birth to their school years. **Prelinguistic behavior** refers to all vocalizations prior to the first actual words. **Phonological development** refers to the acquisition of speech sound form and function within the language system. In accordance with current terminology, this sound acquisition process is now referred to as *phonological development* rather than as speech sound development as it was in the past. **Speech sound development** refers primarily to the gradual articulatory mastery of speech sound forms within a given language. Thus, a child's proficiency to produce standard speech sound patterns is measured. Phonological development, on the other hand, implies the acquisition of a functional sound system intricately connected to the child's overall growth in language. Learning to produce a variety of sounds is not the same as learning the contrasts among sounds that convey differences in meaning.

The first goal of this chapter is to explore briefly certain aspects of the structural and functional development that must occur prior to speech sound production in the infant. In addition, it discusses the development of specific perceptual skills.

The second goal is to examine some of the available information on speech sound development. Organized according to segmental form as well as prosodic development, this survey ranges from the prelinguistic stages to the near completion of the phonological system during the early school years. In reviewing the literature, an attempt will be made to discuss the various studies so that the reader will become aware of differences in design and purpose which have often resulted in contrasting outcomes. In addition, it should be noted that much of the literature focuses on children's acquisition of speech sounds. Little information is available on children's gradual development of the phonemic function and phonotactic constraints of these segments within a language. When possible, these studies are also included.

The third goal of this chapter is to highlight interdependencies among language acquisition, phonological development, and emerging literacy. Developing phonology cannot be meaningfully separated from other aspects of emerging language; it represents an integral part of a child's total language acquisition process. Although cognitive and motor abilities certainly play important roles in the unfolding of phonology, a child's acquisition of semantic, morphosyntactic, and pragmatic skills influences it as well.

Various studies have provided guidelines for determining whether a child demonstrates normal versus impaired phonological development. These "mastery" studies are typically based on the results of testing a large number of children, setting a percentage for each age group for normal articulation of the speech sound in question, and, finally, establishing age levels that are considered to be the time frame for acquisition of each sound. As important as these studies are, the role of individual variation, especially in a child's younger years, should not be underestimated. The development of speech sounds and the acquisition of a child's phonological system remains an individual process. Although certain trends can be noted when comparing these studies containing large numbers of children, each child's own differences continue to play a large role in the total acquisition process. Both factors—general trends noted in large-scale studies and a child's individual growth and development—are important factors to consider when evaluating whether a child has a speech sound disorder.

Aspects of Structural and Functional Development

As the infant begins its journey from primarily crying behavior to babbling and words, important anatomical structures that are prerequisites for sound production need to be taken into consideration. Both the structure and the function of respiratory, phonatory, resonatory, and articulatory mechanisms must change considerably before any regular articulatory processes can occur. These necessary changes, which continue through infancy and early childhood, are directly reflected in the transformation from prelinguistic to linguistic sound productions. The following summary presents a broad outline of the development of the respiratory, phonatory, resonatory, and articulatory systems during this time span.

The shape, size, and composition of the respiratory system are dramatically modified from infancy to adulthood. Newborns and infants are, of course, perfectly able to accumulate enough air pressure against a closed glottis to "phonate" quite impressively. Although small compared to those of adults, babies' lungs are, relative to their body size, proportionally large. Their subglottal pressure (the pressure that accumulates below the closed glottis) is considerable and continues to be so throughout childhood. For example, when comparable loudness levels are contrasted, children demonstrate higher subglottal pressure values than do adults (Stathopoulos & Sapienza, 1993). In addition, compared to the adult, only approximately one-third to one-half of the alveoli are present in the lungs of the newborn (Hislop, Wigglesworth, & Desai, 1986). It is not until a child is approximately 7 to 8 years old that the number of alveoli approaches the adult value (Hislop et al., 1986; Kent, 1997). It is also around this age that children's respiratory function demonstrates adult patterns. Developmental milestones in the respiratory system are summarized in Table 5.1.

TABLE 5.1   Milestones in the Development of the Respiratory System of the Child

Age	Typical Patterns
Birth	Rest breathing is approximately 30–80 breaths per minute. Frequent paradoxical breathing occurs, exemplified by the rib cage making an expiratory movement as the abdomen performs an inspiratory movement. Compared to the adult, only between one-third and one-half of the number of alveoli are present at birth.
1.5 to 3 years	Rest breathing rate decreases to approximately 20–30 breaths per minute at age 3. Respiratory control increasingly supports the production of longer utterances during this time frame. The number of alveoli increases rapidly, beginning to approximate adultlike values at the end of this period. Small conducting airways surrounding the alveoli increase their dimensions in a similar fashion.
7 to 8 years	Rest breathing is approximately 20 breaths per minute. Adultlike breathing patterns are now beginning to be achieved. The number of alveoli reaches adult values at age 8.

Source: Summarized from: Hislop, Wigglesworth, & Desai (1986), Kent (1997), Thurlbeck, (1982) and Zeltner, Caduff, Gehr, Pfenninger, & Burri, (1987).

The changes in the phonatory and resonatory systems from infancy to childhood are especially impressive. This anatomical-physiological development leads directly to their future possibilities to articulate specific speech sounds. However, in newborns, the larynx and vocal tract reflect exclusively **primary functions**, the life-supporting duties of the speech mechanism. The larynx and vocal tract are at this time unable to fulfill any **secondary functions**, those tasks, including articulation of speech sounds, that occur in addition to the life-supporting ones. For example, the oral cavity (with tongue and lips) and the pharyngeal cavity are used primarily for sucking and swallowing actions. The tongue, which in young infants fills out the oral cavity completely, leaves practically no space for the buccal area, the space between the outside of the gums and the inside of the cheeks. In addition, a prenatally acquired "sucking pad" (encapsulated structure of each cheek that supports the lateral rims of the tongue for more effective sucking action), helps to fill out this space entirely. The production of sounds under these conditions is severely restricted. The ability to produce speech sounds is a highly complex process that depends primarily on many anatomical-physiological changes that occur as a product of growth and maturation. See Figure 5.1 for the tongue displacement and the size of several anatomical structures of the newborn infant.

The larynx, too, has to develop structurally before it can effectively contribute to the speech process. In newborns, for example, the arytenoid cartilages and the large posterior portion of the cricoid cartilage are disproportionately large when compared to an adult larynx (Figure 5.2). The vocal processes, where the vocal folds attach, are also large in relationship to the other structures. This means that the vocal processes reach deeply into the vocal folds, thus stifling their vibratory action. In addition, the infant's larynx sits closely under the angle between neck and chin. This high, semifixated position of the larynx does not allow the vocal tract to be effectively elongated in a downward direction. This elongation is indispensable for some resonating effects during vowel articulation, for example.

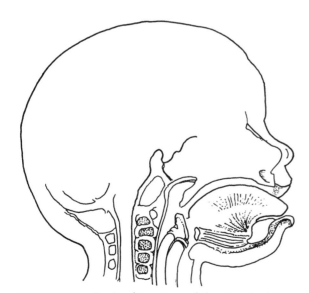

FIGURE 5.1   Sagittal Section of the Head of the Newborn Infant Demonstrating the Forward and Downward Placement of the Tongue

Source: Courtesy of Laura Gallardo.

POSTERIOR VIEW

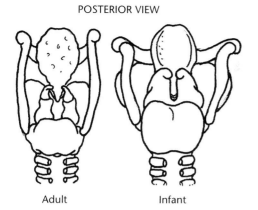

Adult   Infant

ANTERIOR VIEW

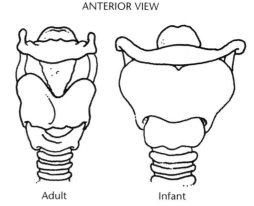

Adult   Infant

FIGURE 5.2 Posterior and Anterior Views of the Laryngeal Structures of an Adult and of an Infant
Source: Courtesy of Laura Gallardo.

Stabilization of the pharyngeal airway (necessary for an upright position) is another significant postnatal development. Anatomical changes include the downward displacement of the hyoid bone and larynx away from the base of the skull and the mandible and the loss of the aforementioned sucking pad. All of these changes must occur as prerequisites for the articulation of speech sounds.

After a child's first words, around the child's first birthday, the speech mechanism undergoes further enlargement and changes in form. Expansions of the laryngeal and pharyngeal cavities are prominent examples. These expansions co-occur with changes in the form and mobility of the arytenoid cartilages, soft palate, and tongue. The following changes characterize this development:

1. The thyroid cartilage enlarges more than the cricoid cartilage.
2. The epiglottis becomes larger and firmer.
3. The arytenoid cartilages, which were relatively large in the early stages of this development, now change little in size; they adapt structurally and functionally to the growth of the other laryngeal structures.
4. The vocal and ventricular folds—that is, the "true" and "false" vocal folds— lengthen. This has the effect that more of the vocal folds' muscular portion is now freed for normal vocal cord vibration.

Enlargement of the skull and laryngeal areas during childhood occurs mostly in posterior and vertical directions. This allows the velum more room and thus more mobility. However, the oral area is the site of the

To verify the decisive importance of movements of the larynx for normal vowel production, place your index finger lightly on the V-shaped notch of the thyroid cartilage of the larynx with the middle finger and thumb on either side of the lamina. In this position, articulate [i] versus [u]. The downward movement during [u] can easily be felt.

greatest changes in available space and resulting mobility of the anatomical structures. Because of these skeletal changes, the tongue no longer completely fills the mouth. In addition, the tongue and lips become elongated and acquire further mobility. The fine-tuning and coordination of the lip, mandible, tongue, and velar movements for regular voice and speech production are now increasingly acquired.

To summarize, during infancy, we see enormously complex developmental changes. The infant's larynx, mouth, and pharyngeal areas evolve from a mechanism able to serve only respiratory and feeding purposes to a vocal tract that is structurally and functionally ready to produce speech sounds.

Aspects of Perceptual Development

The last decade has produced a large amount of research examining young children's early processing of language. This is in part because of the rapid advances in noninvasive techniques to examine these processing abilities. These techniques include electroencephalography (EEG), event-related postentials (ERPs), magnetoencephalography (MEG), functional magnetic resonance imaging (fMRI), and near-infrared spectroscopy (NIRS). For a good review of these techniques, see Kuhl, 2010. Although it has often been documented that infants are able to discriminate minimal differences in speech sounds within the first months after their births (Best & McRoberts, 2003; Best, McRoberts, & Goodell, 2001; Houston & Jusczyk, 2000; Kuhl et al., 2006), their auditory experiences actually begin even before birth. Human fetuses are able to process auditory stimuli from the external world during the last trimester of pregnancy with a clear sensitivity to melody contours in language and music (Kisilevsky, Hains, Jacquet, Granier-Deferre, & Lecanuet, 2004; Mampe, Friederici, Christophe, & Wermke, 2009). Newborns prefer their mother's voice over other voices and will actively change their sucking rate to hear her voice more often than another female's voice (DeCasper & Fifer, 1980). And newborns' cry melody appears to be shaped by their native language (Mampe, Friederici, Christophe, & Wermke).

These results support the notion that infants start to pay attention and "learn" something about voice and speech prior to birth. However, what evidence do we have about the infant's and child's perception and discrimination of speech sounds and phonemic contrasts? The following is an overview of these perceptual skills.

- *Categorical perception.* **Categorical perception** refers to the tendency of listeners to perceive speech sounds (which are varied acoustically along a continuum) according to the phonemic categories of their native language. Thus, variations in voice onset time will produce a clear listener distinction between [ba] or [pa], as if an actual boundary divided the two. Based on changes in measured sucking rates, categorical perception for /b/ and /p/ in the syllables [ba] and [pa] has been demonstrated in infants as young as 1 month of age. Infants under 3 months of age can detect differences in place and manner of articulation for consonants. Studies related to the perception of phonemic contrasts in infants include those by Cohen and Cashon (2003), Houston and Jusczyk (2000), Jusczyk and Luce (2002), Mareschal and French (2000), Maye and Weiss (2003), and Maye, Werker, and Gerken (2002), for example.

- *Discrimination of nonnative sounds in infants.* If children demonstrate categorical perception between one and three months of age it was hypothesized that they might have an inborn ability to make these distinctions. To test this hypothesis, a task was devised in which the discrimination skills of infants were tested with unknown phonemes of nonnative languages—that is, languages to which they had not been exposed. Although adult nonnative speakers could not differentiate these pairs, results showed that infants up to approximately 6 to 8 months of age could indeed discriminate among nonnative sounds that were very similar in their production characteristics. During the second half of the first year of life, these discrimination abilities decrease, whereas discrimination of native speech sound perception increases (Best & McRoberts, 2003; Kuhl et al., 2006; Rivera-Gaxiola, Silva-Pereyra, & Kuhl, 2005). The conclusion drawn was that language experience may result in the loss of this ability. We do not distinguish between categories that are nonfunctional in our own native language.

- *Perceptual constancy.* The ability to identify the same sound across different speakers, pitches, and other changing environmental conditions is known as **perceptual constancy**. Perceptual constancy for vowels and consonants within different vowel contexts has been noted in children from 5½ to 10 months of age (Maye & Gerken, 2000; Werker & Fennell, 2004).

- *Perception of phonemic contrasts.* Shvachkin (1973) and Garnica (1973) examined the ability of toddlers from 10 to 22 months to associate minimally paired nonsense syllables to different objects. Could children learn to differentiate phonemes that signal word meaning differences? These studies found that all children had a developmental progression in the ability to make these distinctions; that is, some distinctions appear easier to detect than others. However, considerable variability was noted among the children as to which features were discriminated earlier and which later.

- *Early perceptual abilities related to language development and disorders.* Studies document that early perceptual abilities appear to be related to later language development in children; see, for example, those by Kuhl, Conboy, Padden, Nelson, and Pruitt (2005); Tsao, Liu, and Kuhl (2004) and Werker and Tees (2005). Tsao et al. (2004) measured speech discrimination in 6-month-old infants using a conditioned head-turn task. At 13, 16, and 24 months of age, language development was assessed in these same children using the MacArthur Communicative Development Inventory. Results demonstrated significant correlations between speech perception at 6 months of age and later language (word understanding, word production, and phrase understanding). The finding that speech perception performance at age 6 months predicts language at age 2 years supports the idea that phonetic perception may play an important role in language acquisition. Early perceptual studies may also show evidence of later difficulties, such as dyslexia (Bogliotti, 2003; Richardson, Leppaenen, Leiwo, & Lyytinen, 2003). For example, Lyytinen et al. (2001) investigated 107 children with a familial risk of dyslexia, comparing them to 93 children without familial risk. The earliest significant differences between groups were the categorical perception of speech sounds at a few days old (using brain potential responses to speech sounds) and head turning at 6 months old. No differences were found between the groups in other measures, such as parental reports of vocalization, motor behavior, or growth of vocabulary (using the MacArthur Communicative Development Scale) before age 2. Similarly, no group differences were found in cognitive and language development assessed by the Bayley Scales of Infant Development and the Reynell Developmental Language Scales before age 2.5.

An infant's early perceptual abilities include a wide range of competencies. Many of these abilities develop prior to the actual production of first words. It appears that the infant's early perceptual abilities may also impact later language development, whereas lack of specific skills may be a portion of the symptom complex of disordered language learning.

The next section examines another aspect of the infant's behavior: the prelinguistic stage, which describes vocalizations prior to the first real words. It also shows that specific competencies in this behavior will impact later language development.

Prelinguistic Stages: Before the First Words

Child language development is commonly divided into *prelinguistic behavior*, vocalizations prior to the first true words, and *linguistic development*, which starts with the appearance of these first words. This division is exemplified by the use of early nonmeaningful versus later meaningful sound productions. Jakobson's *discontinuity hypothesis* (1942/1968) clearly emphasized a sharp separation between these two phases. According to his theoretical notion, babbling is a random series of vocalizations in which many different sounds are produced with no apparent order or consistency. Such behavior is seen as clearly separated from the following systematic sound productions evidenced by the first words. The division between prelinguistic and linguistic phases of sound production, according to Jakobson, is often so complete that a child might actually undergo a period of silence between the end of the babbling period and the first real words.

Research since that time (e.g., Boysson-Bardies, 2001; Nathani, Ertmer, & Stark, 2006; Oller, 1980; Oller, Wieman, Doyle, & Ross, 1976; Stark, 1980, 1986) has repeatedly documented that (1) babbling behavior is not random but indicates that children's productions develop in a systematic manner, (2) the consonant-like sounds that are babbled are restricted to a small set of segments, and (3) the transition between babbling and first words is not abrupt but continuous; late babbling behavior and the first words are very similar in respect to the sounds used and the way they are combined. It also appears that children's perceptual abilities are quite developed before the first meaningful utterances. For example, some word comprehension is evident at approximately 7 to 9 months of age (Owens, 2008). The presence of phonemic contrasts in very young children has also been previously documented. Although this acquisition is gradual, more general contrasts begin at approximately 1 year of age. Findings such as these suggest that children's language systems starts to develop prior to the first spoken meaningful words during the prelinguistic period.

The following is an overview of the *prelinguistic stages* of production described by Stark (1986). Although these are referred to as *stages,* there is overlap from one period of development to the next. In addition, individual variations among children necessitate the use of approximate ages.

> *Stage 1: Reflexive crying and vegetative sounds (birth to 2 months).* This stage is characterized by a large proportion of reflexive vocalizations. *Reflexive vocalizations* include cries, coughs, grunts, and burps that seem to be automatic responses reflecting the physical state of the infant. *Vegetative sounds* may be divided into grunts and sighs associated with activity and clicks and other noises associated with feeding.

> *Stage 2: Cooing and laughter (2 to 4 months).* During this stage, *cooing* or *gooing* sounds are produced during comfortable states. Although these sounds are sometimes referred to as vowel-like, they also contain brief periods of consonantal elements that are produced at the back of the mouth. Early comfort sounds have quasi-resonant nuclei, in other words, they are produced as a syllabic nasal consonant or as a nasalized vowel (Nakazima, 1962; Oller, 1980). From 12 weeks on, a decrease in the frequency of crying is noted, and most infants' primitive vegetative sounds start to disappear. At 16 weeks, sustained laughter emerges (Gesell & Thompson, 1934).

Stage 3: Vocal play (4 to 6 months). Although there is some overlap between Stages 2 and 3, the distinguishing characteristics of Stage 3 include longer series of segments and the production of prolonged vowel- or consonant-like steady states. During this stage, the infant often produces extreme variations in loudness and pitch. When compared to those of older children, the transitions between segments in this stage are much slower and incomplete. In contrast to vowels in Stage 2, those in Stage 3 demonstrate more variation in tongue height and position.

Stage 4: Canonical babbling (6 months and older). Although **canonical babbling**, the collective term for the reduplicated and nonreduplicated babbling stages, usually begins around 6 months of age, most children continue to babble into the time when they say their first words. Stark (1986) describes reduplicated and nonreduplicated, or variegated, babbling as follows: **Reduplicated babbling** is marked by similar strings of consonant–vowel productions. There might be slight quality variations in the vowel sounds of these strings of babbles, but the consonants will stay the same from syllable to syllable. An example of this is [mama]. **Nonreduplicated** or **variegated babbling** demonstrates variation of *both* consonants and vowels from syllable to syllable. An example of this is [batə]. One major characteristic of this babbling stage is smooth transitions between vowel and consonant productions.

From the previous descriptions, one might conclude that these babbling stages are sequential in nature with a child first going through reduplicated babbling and later nonreduplicated babbling. This has indeed been documented by Elbers (1982), Oller (1980), and Stark (1986), to mention a few. However, more recent investigators have questioned this developmental pattern. For example, Mitchell and Kent (1990) assessed the phonetic variation of multisyllabic babbling in eight infants at 7, 9, and 11 months of age. Their findings showed that (1) nonreduplicated babbling was present from the time the infant began to produce multisyllabic babbling, it did not evolve from an earlier period of reduplicated babbling and (2) no significant difference existed between the amount of phonetic variation for the vocalizations when the infant was 7, 9, and 11 months old. These and other findings (Holmgren, Lindblom, Aurelius, Jalling, & Zetterstrom, 1986; Smith, Brown-Sweeney, & Stoel-Gammon, 1989) suggest that both reduplicated and variegated forms extend throughout the entire babbling period. At the beginning of Stage 4, babbling is used in a self-stimulatory manner; it is not used to communicate to adults. Toward the end of this stage, babbling may be used in ritual imitation games with adults (Stark, 1986). This is the beginning of imitative behavior and is an important milestone.

Stage 5: Jargon stage (10 months and older). This babbling stage overlaps with the first meaningful words. The **jargon stage** is characterized by strings of babbled utterances that are modulated primarily by intonation, rhythm, and pausing (Crystal, 1986). It sounds as if a child is actually attempting sentences but without actual words. Because many jargon vocalizations are delivered with eye contact, gestures, and intonation patterns that resemble statements or questions, parents are convinced that the child is indeed trying to communicate something to which they often feel compelled to respond (Stoel-Gammon & Menn, 1997).

> Watch and listen carefully to the video of 7½ month old Charlie. Which babbling stage does he seem to be in? youtube.com/watch?v=IyV2j4BsEM8.

The following section examines children's segmental productions toward the end of the canonical babbling stage. Because the productions cannot yet be said to be true vowels and consonants of a particular language system, they are referred to as **vocoids** and **contoids**, respectively. Pike (1943) introduced these terms to indicate *nonphonemic* speech sound productions.

Vocoids

Several early investigations with a large number of children were those carried out by Irwin and colleagues in the 1940s and 1950s (e.g., Chen & Irwin, 1946; Irwin, 1945, 1946, 1947a, 1947b, 1948, 1951; Irwin & Chen, 1946; Winitz & Irwin, 1958). According to the data on 57 children from 13 to 14 months of age, there was a continued predominance of the [ɛ], [ɪ], and [ʌ] vocoids. Thus, front and central vocoids were found to be favored over high and back vocoids. Later investigations (Davis & MacNeilage, 1990; Kent & Bauer, 1985) generated similar results.

Contoids

Several authors have investigated the contoids, which predominate in the late babbling stage. Locke (1983) provides an excellent overview of the results from three major investigations (Table 5.2). The agreement between these studies is far more striking than the differences. As the data in Table 5.2 indicate, the most frequent contoids were [h], [d], [b], [m], [t], [g], and [w]. The 12 most frequently produced contoids represent about 95% of all the segments transcribed in the three studies (Locke, 1983). These results stand in contrast to earlier statements that babbling consists of a great multitude of random vocalizations. On the contrary, these and other investigations (Locke, 1990; Ramsdell, Oller, Buder, Ethington, & Chorna, 2012; Vihman, Macken, Miller, Simmons, & Miller, 1985) suggest that only a rather limited set of phones is babbled.

Table 5.2 appears to indicate that the infants studied used no non-English sound segments. However, this is partially conditioned by the investigative methods employed and by the perceptual limitations inherent in phonetic transcription. As to the investigative

TABLE 5.2 Relative Frequency of English Consonantlike Sounds in the Babbling of 11- to 12-Month-Old American Infants[1]

Sound	More Frequent Consonants A[2]	B	C	Sound	Less Frequent Consonants A[2]	B	C
h	31.77	21.0	18.3	v	1.03	1.0	0
d	20.58	30.0	13.5	l	.96	1.0	1.6
b	9.79	5.0	10.0	θ	.85	0	0.4
m	6.69	1.0	7.2	z	.56	0	0
t	4.34	0	3.6	f	.37	0	0.4
g	4.15	12.0	8.4	ʃ	.37	0	0
s	3.45	0	0.4	ð	.34	0	0.8
w	3.39	17.0	8.4	ŋ	.33	1.0	3.2
n	2.65	1.0	4.4	ʒ	.10	0	0
k	2.12	1.0	6.3	r	.10	0	0
j	1.77	9.0	11.6	tʃ	0	0	0
p	1.63	0	1.6	dʒ	0	0	0
Totals	92.33	97.0	93.7		5.01	3.0	6.4

[1]The three investigations represented are *A:* Irwin, (1947a), *B:* Fisichelli (1950), *C:* Pierce and Hanna (1974).

[2]The *A* columns total less than 100% because the difference (2.66%) represents several sounds in Irwin's original tabulations that have no phonemic equivalent in General American English phonology (e.g., [ʔ ç χ]).

Source: Reprinted by permission from John L Locke, *Phonological Acquisition and Change.* Copyright © 1983 by Elsevier.

methodology, in the Irwin studies, only three non-English sounds were transcribed; the rest were ignored. The Fisichelli study considered exclusively English sounds. The Pierce and Hanna investigation, on the other hand, did document that the infants produced several non-English sounds with some frequency. Other investigations (e.g., Stockman, Woods, & Tishman, 1981) have confirmed the occurrence of non-English sounds in this late babbling period, although not to any high degree.

Syllable Shapes

During the later babbling periods, open syllables are still the most frequent type. In the Kent and Bauer (1985) study, for example, V, CV, VCV, and CVCV structures accounted for approximately 94% of all syllables produced. Although closed syllables were present, they were found to be very limited in the repertoires of these infants.

Babbling and Its Relationship to Later Language Development

Jakobson's (1968) discontinuity hypothesis denounced any link between babbling and later language development. However, babbling behavior is one aspect of early communication that is emerging as a predictor of later language ability. Several researchers have suggested that both the *quantity* and the *diversity* of vocalizations do indeed play a role in later language development.

Attempts have been made to correlate the quantity of vocalizations at a certain babbling age to later language performance (e.g., Brady, Marquis, Fleming, & McLean, 2004; Camp, Burgess, Morgan, & Zerbe, 1987; Kagan, 1971; McCune & Vihman, 2001; Paavola, Kunnari, & Moilanen, 2005; Rothgaenger, 2003). In these studies, *quantity* was defined as the number of vocalizations during a specific time. Although somewhat different criteria were used in the various studies, the results showed that the amount of prelinguistic vocalizations was positively related to later language measures.

Diversity of vocalizations was measured in infants by (1) the number of different consonant-like sounds heard in their babbling, (2) the number of structured CV

Based on the information from the prelinguistic stages, what stage should a child be in before you can hope to verbally stimulate him or her and possibly expect imitative behavior?

You are working in a birth to three-year program and have a child who you think is beginning to attempt to imitate simple babbling behavior. Based on the information on the most frequent babbled sounds, what type of syllables, vowels, and consonants might you want to attempt to use as stimulation?

CLINICAL APPLICATION

Knowledge of Babbling Stages and Diagnostics

Speech-language pathologists, especially those in early intervention services, are often confronted with children beyond 1 year of age who are still within the babbling stages of development. Knowledge of the babbling stages, which includes characteristics and approximate ages of occurrence, can be very helpful in our assessment process. Consider the following information from the parents of Megan, who is 16 months old.

The early intervention program was contacted by Megan's parents, who had been referred by the child's pediatrician. Megan was born 4 weeks premature and had been followed very closely by both the parents and the pediatrician. She had started to walk around 11 months of age, and the parents reported that all developmental milestones up to that point had been within normal limits. The parents were concerned because Megan did not have any real words. All their relatives' children had begun to talk when they were 10 to 12 months old.

The speech-language pathologist visited the family home and noted that Megan was a very active toddler who was busy with her toys and enjoyed attention. Occasionally, Megan produced utterances that consisted of single vowels, for example, [a], CV structures ([ba], [da], [ma]), and CVCV syllables ([mama], [babi], [dada], [dati]). According to the parents, repeated attempts at getting Megan to imitate these babbles had not met with success. It was observed (and the parents verified) that Megan did not use strings of babbles with any intonational patterns; that is, Megan did not produce jargon speech.

Based on these results, we could deduce that Megan is within the canonical babbling stage. However, she has not reached the point at which she is imitating these babbles in ritualized games with her parents, nor is she using jargon speech. According to the approximate ages presented, jargon speech begins around 10 months of age. Megan is now 16 months old. This information gives us a general idea of where Megan is within the period of prelinguistic development.

syllables, (3) the proportion of vocalizations containing a true consonant, and (4) the ratio of consonant-like sounds to vowel-like sounds (Bauer, 1988; Bauer & Robb, 1989; Boysson-Bardies, 2001; McCarthren, Warren, & Yoder, 1996; Munson, Edwards, & Beckman, 2005a; Nathani et al., 2006; Oller, Eilers, Neal, & Schwartz, 1999; Paul, 1991; Paul & Jennings, 1992; Reed, 2005; Rescorla & Ratner, 1996; Stoel-Gammon & Otomo, 1986; Whitehurst, Smith, Fischel, Arnold, & Lonigan, 1991). Summarizing the results of these methodologically varying studies, it appears that:

1. Less language growth is seen in children with more vocoid-babble compared to those with more contoid-babble.
2. Greater language growth is related to greater babble complexity.
3. Greater language growth is related to the increased diversity of contoid productions.

Prosodic Feature Development

Vowels and consonants are combined to produce syllables, words, and sentences. At the same time that we articulate these sound segments, pronunciation varies in other respects. For example, adults use a wide range of pitch and loudness variables that can change the meaning of what is said in a number of ways. Consider the sentence: "You want that.↘" said with a falling tone at the end compared to "You want that?↗" said with a rising tone at the end. (One can even imagine that if *that* is stressed and the vowel prolonged with an excessive rising tone in the second sentence, something incredible is being desired.) The sound segments in these two sentences [ju wʌnt ðæt] relate to *what* we say; *prosodic features* refer to *how* we say it. **Prosodic features** are larger linguistic units occurring across segments that are used to influence what we say. The linguistically most relevant prosodic features we realize in speech are pitch, loudness, and tempo variations (which include sound duration). They have specific functions and may be analyzed separately. If combined, they constitute the *rhythm* of a particular language or utterance.

The development of prosodic features in infants has gained considerable importance, and research supports the hypothesis positing a close interaction among prosodic features, early child-directed speech (motherese), and early language development (Bonvillian, Raeburn, & Horan, 1979; Delack & Fowlow, 1978; Fernald et al., 1989; Hallé, Boysson-Bardies, & Vihman, 1991; Hsu & Fogel, 2001; Jacobson, Boersma, Fields, & Olson, 1983; Kent & Murray, 1982; Robb & Saxman, 1990; Stern & Wasserman 1979; Turk, Jusczyk, & Gerken, 1995; Whalen, Levitt, & Wang, 1991). A better understanding of prosodic features and their development may offer us valuable insights into the transition from babbling to the first words and the close interconnection of segmental and prosodic feature acquisition.

Coinciding with the canonical babbling stage, or starting at approximately 6 months of age, the infant uses patterns of prosodic behavior. They then consistently employed certain features, primarily intonation, rhythm, and pausing (Crystal, 1986). Acoustic analysis shows that falling pitch is the most common intonation contour for the first year of life (Delack & Fowlow, 1978; Kent & Murray, 1982; Snow, 1998a, 1998b, 2000). Prosodic patterns continue to diversify toward the end of the babbling period to such a degree that names such as *expressive jargon* (Gesell & Thompson, 1934) and *prelinguistic jargon* (Dore, Franklin, Miller, & Ramer, 1976) have been applied to them. These strings of babbles typically sound like adult General American English intonation patterns, giving the impression of sentences without words.

Transition from Babbling to First Words

Several studies suggest that babbling and early words have much in common (e.g., Boysson-Bardies & Vihman, 1991; Davis & MacNeilage, 1990; Ferguson & Farwell, 1975; Kent & Bauer, 1985; Oller et al., 1976; Stark, 1980; Vihman, Ferguson, & Elbert, 1986). In fact, they are often so similar that difficulties arise in differentiating between the two. The main characteristics of the transition from babbling to first words include:

1. Primarily monosyllabic utterances
2. Frequent use of stop consonants followed by nasals and fricatives
3. Bilabial and apical productions
4. Rare use of consonant clusters
5. Frequent use of central, mid-front, and low-front vowels ([ʌ, ɛ, æ])

In spite of the similarities, data from Vihman and colleagues (1986) and Davis and MacNeilage (1990) revealed the following distinctions between babbling and first words:

1. A large diversity existed among the children's productions in each of the areas investigated (phonetic tendencies, consonant and vowel inventories, and word selection). The more words the children acquired, the more this diversity seemed to diminish (Vihman et al., 1986).
2. The majority of the children used voiced stops in babbling but not in words; [g] was the most prominent example of this (Vihman et al., 1986).
3. Vowels produced during babbling were used as substitutes for other vowel productions in words. The high-front vowel [i] was a frequent substitute (Davis & MacNeilage, 1990).
4. Productions were context dependent. For example, high-front vowels occurred more frequently following alveolars; high-back vowels following velars; and central vowels after labial consonants (Vihman, 1992). However, the Tyler and Langsdale (1996) study found little evidence of these context dependencies. The wide range of individual variability could in part explain the differences they encountered.

The First Fifty Words

Around a child's first birthday, a new developmental era begins: the *linguistic phase.* It starts the moment the first meaningful word is produced. That sounds plain enough, but there are some problems defining the first meaningful word. Must it be understood and produced by the child in all applicable situations and contexts? Must it have an adultlike meaning to the child? How do we categorize utterances that do not resemble our adult representation but are, nevertheless, used as words by the child in a consistent manner?

Most define the **first word** as an entity of relatively stable phonetic form that is produced consistently by a child in a particular context and is recognizably related to the adultlike word form of a particular language (Owens, 2008). Thus, if a child says [ba] consistently in the context of being shown a ball, this form would qualify as a word. If, however, the child says [dodo] when being shown the ball, this would not be accepted as a word because it does not approximate the adult form.

Children frequently use "invented words" (Locke, 1983) in a consistent manner, thereby demonstrating that they seem to have meaning for the children. These vocalizations—used consistently but without a recognizable adult model—have been called **proto-words** (Menn, 1978), **phonetically consistent forms** (Dore et al., 1976), **vocables** (Ferguson, 1976), and **quasi-words** (Stoel-Gammon & Cooper, 1984).

The time of the initial productions of words is usually called the *first-50-word stage*. This stage encompasses the time from the first meaningful utterance at approximately 1 year of age to the time when children begin to put two "words" together at approximately 18 to 24 months. Whether this stage is actually a separate developmental entity may be questioned. The first word may be a plausible starting point, but the strict 50-word cutoff point is, according to several studies, purely arbitrary (Ferguson & Farwell, 1975; Nelson, 1973). Nevertheless, it appears that children produce approximately 50 meaningful words before the next generally recognized stage of development, the *two-word stage*, begins.

During the first-50-word stage, there seems to be a large difference between the children's productional versus perceptual capabilities. For example, at the end of this stage, when children can produce approximately 50 words, they are typically capable of understanding around 200 words (Ingram, 1989a). This fact must have an effect on the development of semantic meaning as well as on the phonological system. It must be clearly understood that by analyzing children's verbal productions during this stage, we are looking at only one aspect of language development. Their perceptual, motor, and cognitive growth, as well as the influence of the environment, all play indispensable roles in this stage of language acquisition.

In examining the course of phonological development during this period, we see that it is heavily influenced by the individual words children are acquiring. Children are not just learning sounds, which they then use to make up words, but rather seem to learn word units that happen to contain particular sets of sounds. Ingram (2010) called this a *presystematic stage* in which contrastive words rather than contrastive phones (i.e., as phonemes) are acquired. The presystematic stage can be related to Cruttenden's (1981) *item learning* and *system learning* stages of early phonological development. In **item learning**, children first acquire word forms as unanalyzed units, productional wholes. Only later, characteristically after the first-50-word stage, does **system learning** occur, during which children acquire the phonemic principles of the phonological system in question.

The early portion of the item learning stage is known as the *holophrastic period*, the span of time during which children use one word to indicate a complete idea. In addition, the link between the object, its meaning, and the discrete sound segments used to represent the object is not yet firmly established. For example, a child might produce [da] to indicate a dog. The next day, the production might change somewhat, perhaps to [do]. This time, the production may not refer to a dog alone but also to a cow or horse. According to Piaget (1952), the child is still within the sensorimotor period of development and so has not yet achieved full imitative ability or object permanence. Sounds and meanings drift and change.

Segmental Form Development

Several authors (e.g., Ferguson & Farwell, 1975; Ingram, 1989b) have noted *phonetic variability* and a *limitation of syllable structures* and *sound segments* during the first-50-word stage. **Phonetic variability** refers to the unstable pronunciations of children's first 50 words. Although this has been well documented (Farwell, 1976; Kiparsky & Menn, 1977;

Stoel-Gammon & Cooper, 1984), it appears that some productions are more stable than others. Ferguson and Farwell call this category of words *stable forms.* However, the authors do not provide a measure for this stability, and from their examples, it is often unclear why certain words are considered more stable than others. To complicate matters, it seems that some children have a tendency to produce more stable articulations from the beginning of the first-50-word stage. Stoel-Gammon and Cooper (1984) and French (1989) provide data on children whose phonetic realizations were stable from the first real word.

The second characteristic of the first-50-word stage is the limitation of syllable structures and segmental productions used. From their relatively small repertoire of words, it would seem logical to conclude that children do not produce a large array of syllable structures and sound segments. However, what are the actual limitations during the first-50-word stage?

First, certain syllable types clearly predominate the first-50-word stage. These are CV, VC, and CVC syllables. When CVCV syllables are present, they are full or partial syllable reduplications. This, of course, does not mean that other syllable types do not occur. For example, the individual data from Ferguson and Farwell (1975), French (1989), Ingram (1974), Leopold (1947), Menn (1971), Stoel-Gammon and Cooper (1984), and Velten (1943) indicate that these syllables are indeed the most frequently occurring. However, the children produced other syllables as well. Menn's Daniel, for instance, produced CCVC [njaj], Leopold's Hildegard a CCVCV [priti], and Ferguson and Farwell's T a CVCVVC [wakuak]. If an individual child is examined to see whether patterns emerge, differences can be found. Certain children seem to favor specific types of syllables. For example, some children evidence CVC structures to a moderate degree from the very beginning of this stage. With others, CVC syllables appear only later and do not constitute any major part of the children's phonology until after the first-50-word stage (Ingram, 1976).

Second, what are the speech sound limitations that can be observed during the first-50-word stage? More specifically, which vowels and consonants are present, and which ones are not? Two studies by Jakobson (1942/1968) and Jakobson and Halle (1956) have had a large impact on this question. After studying several diary reports of children from various linguistic backgrounds, they concluded that the first consonants are labials, most commonly [p] or [m]; these first consonants are followed by [t] and later [k]; fricatives are present only after the respective homorganic stops have been acquired; and the first vowel is [a] or [ɑ], followed by [u] and/or [i].

Over the years, Jakobson's postulated universals have undergone a good deal of scrutiny. Although most of the investigators (e.g., Oller et al., 1976; Stoel-Gammon & Cooper, 1984; Vihman et al., 1986) have concentrated on consonant inventories, Ingram (1976) has attempted to grapple with the acquisition of vowels. Using the data from four case studies (Ingram, 1974; Leopold, 1947; Menn, 1971; Velten, 1943), he compared the vowels in the first 50 words. General trends could be noted, and most children seemed to follow the acquisitional pattern of [a] preceding [i] and [u].

Consonant inventories follow the same pattern. Although certain similarities have been verified, several investigations have pointed out the wide range of variability among individual subjects (e.g., Ferguson & Farwell, 1975; Stoel-Gammon & Cooper,

CLINICAL EXERCISES

Consider the vowel and consonant data that were just presented and make a list of the consonants, vowels, and syllable structures you might see in the beginning words of children.

Based on your list, formulate 15 words that contain these vowels, consonants, and syllable shapes (and would be age appropriate) that you could use when working with a child who is just beginning to say first words.

It should be noted that the Vihman, Ferguson, and Elbert (1986) data in Table 5.3 reduce the individual variation among children considerably. For example, if child A produces two words with word-initial [n] whereas child B produces 43 words with [n], both of those children are counted for [n] use in this table. However, the use of this particular sound in the two children's inventories is hardly comparable.

1984; Vihman, 1992; Vihman et al., 1986). If one wants to generalize, the marked use of voiced labial and dental stops and nasals ([b], [d], [m], [n]) has to be underlined. Ferguson and Garnica (1975) make the point that [h] and [w] are also among the first consonants acquired. For a summary of findings substantiating these generalizations from five different investigations, see Table 5.3. The data in Table 5.3 compare the consonant inventory of 7 children labeled "Stanford" (Vihman et al., 1986) to 19 other children from research studies noted in the table. As can be seen, all the children have words containing [b] and [m]. More than half of the children in the studies produced [p], [t], [d], [k], [g], [ʃ], [n], [w], and [h] consonants as well.

TABLE 5.3 Initial Consonant Productions within the First-Fifty-Word Vocabularies of Seven Stanford Subjects and Nineteen Other English-Speaking Children

	Stanford	Others		Stanford	Others[1]
p	×	+	ʃ	+	+
b	×	×	ʒ	0	0
t	×	+	tʃ	–	–
d	×	+	dʒ	–	–
k	×	+	m	×	×
g	+	+	n	×	+
f	+	–	ŋ	–	–
v	–	0	l	–	–
θ	+	–	r	+	–
ð	+	–	w	+	+
s	–	–	j	+	–
z	–	–	h	+	+

Note: × = all children in study; + = more than half but not all children in study; – = more than than one but less than half the children in study; 0 = none of the children.

[1]Data derived from Ferguson and Farwell (1975); Shibamoto and Olmsted (1978); Leonard, Newhoff, and Mesalam (1980); and Stoel-Gammon and Cooper (1984).

Source: Reprinted by permission from M. M. Vihman, C. A. Ferguson, and M. Elbert, *Phonological Development from Babbling to Speech: Common Tendencies and Individual Differences.* Copyright © 1986 by Cambridge University Press.

Longitudinal Findings. Longitudinal research follows a child or a group of children over a specific time frame. Such research has the advantage of observing the acquisition process of individual children. However, longitudinal research is often limited in that only one child or a small group of subjects is evaluated. Stoel-Gammon (1985) presented a longitudinal investigation that not only used spontaneous speech but also included a sizable number of children.

Thirty-four children between 15 and 24 months of age participated in the Stoel-Gammon (1985) study. The investigation was constructed to look at meaningful speech only; therefore, the subjects were grouped according to the age when they actually began to say at least 10 identifiable words within a recording session. This resulted in three groups of children: Group A children, who had 10 words at 15 months; Group B, who had 10 words at 18 months; and Group C, who had 10 words at 21 months. The data from the Stoel-Gammon (1985) study provide information about early consonant development and can be summarized as follows:

1. A larger inventory of sounds was found in the word-initial than in the word-final position.

2. Word-initial inventories contained voiced stops prior to voiceless ones; the reverse was true for word-final productions.

3. The following phones appeared in at least 50% of all the subjects by 24 months of age:

   [h, w, b, t, d, m, n, k, g, f, and s] word-initially:
   [p, t, k, n, r, and s] word-finally

CLINICAL APPLICATION

Comparing Jakobson's Results to the First Words of Two Children

The following are the first words of Joan Velten (Velten, 1943) and Jennika lngram (Ingram, 1974).

	Joan			Jennika	
Age	Words	Actual Production	Age	Words	Actual Production
;10	up	[ap]	1;3	blanket	[ba], [babi]
	bottle	[ba]		byebye	[ba], [baba]
;11	bus	[bas]		daddy	[da], [dada], [dadi]
	put on	[baza]		dot	[dat], [dati]
	that	[za]		hi	[haⁱ]
1;0	down	[da]		mommy	[ma], [mami], [mama]
	out	[at]			
	away	['ba ba]		no	[no]
	pocket	[bat]		see	[si]
				see that	[si æt]
1;1	fuff	[af], [faf]		that	[da]
	put on	[baˈda]			
1;2	push	[bus]	1;4	hot	[hat]
	dog	[uf]		hi	[haⁱ], [haⁱdi]
	pie	[ba]		up	[ap], [api]
1;3	duck	[dat]		no	[nodi], [dodi], [noni]
	lamb	[bap]			
1;4	M	[am]			
	N	[an]			
	in	[n̩]			

If the month increments are seen as later phases of development, the following order occurs in the first words for Joan and Jennika:

	Joan	Jennika
Vowels	[a] → [u]	[a], [i], [o], [æ], [aⁱ]
Consonants	[p], [b] → [s], [z] → [t], [d] → [f] → [m], [n]	[b], [d], [t], [h], [m], [n], [s] → [p]
Syllable shapes	VC, CV → CVC, CVCV	CV, CVCV, CVC → VC, VCV
	CVCVs are not reduplications	Most CVCVs are reduplications
Phonetic variability	Fairly stable forms	More variability

Both Joan's and Jennika's vowel development follows Jakobson's findings: [a] is followed by, or co-occurs with, [i] and/or [u]. Joan's order of consonant development, however, shows clear differences from the order described by Jakobson. For example, she does seem to use the fricatives [s] and [z] before the homorganic stops [t] and [d]. Both children demonstrate rather late development of specific bilabial sounds that, according to Jakobson, are the earliest consonants: For Joan [m] and for Jennika [p] are later than certain fricatives.

CLINICAL APPLICATION

Developmental Research and Therapeutic Implications

It is often stated that speech-language pathologists follow a developmental model in therapy; that is, the model targets sounds or processes that are developmentally earlier before those that are later. Stoel-Gammon's (1985) data support techniques that are typically used in therapy:

1. *Sounds first appear in the word-initial position.* In therapy, a newly acquired sound is normally placed in the word-initial position. Developmental data give evidence that this is indeed easier for a child.
2. *Anterior stops and nasals are acquired earlier.* In therapy, this is often used as a guiding principle. These sounds are very early and should, therefore, be in the speech of children. Even most children with phonemic-based disorders have these sounds in their consonant inventories.

There are also some interesting results from the Stoel-Gammon (1985) study that are not often employed in therapy:

1. *The liquid [r] nearly always appeared in word-final position.* Based on this finding, words such as *more* and *bear* might be easier than *red* or *rope* for children with [r] difficulties (assuming that a specific child has difficulty with the central vowels with r-coloring *and* the approximant [r]).
2. *Word-initial inventories contained voiced stops first; word-final inventories contained voiceless stops first.* According to this finding, children with [k] and [g] problems might benefit from first working on [g] in the word-initial position before [k] in the word-final position. (This is based on the earlier result that sounds appear first in the word-initial position followed by later use in the word-final position.)

Because of the limited number of subjects, this application of Stoel-Gammon's (1985) results to therapeutic practice is probably premature. The intent here is to demonstrate how research findings can directly impact therapy.

4. The "r" as a rhotic vowel [ɚ] or a rhotic diphthong [ɑɚ] nearly always appeared first in a word-final position.
5. If the mean percentage of norm consonant productions was calculated (Shriberg & Kwiatkowski, 1982b), 70% accuracy was achieved. Because there is obviously a large difference between the inventory produced by 2-year-olds and that produced by adults, the author states that this accuracy level suggests that children are primarily attempting words that contain sounds within their articulatory abilities.
6. The order of appearance of initial and final phones was relatively constant across the three groups of children tested. Individual differences existed in the appearance of phones related to fricatives/affricates and liquids.

Although individual variability was observed in the Stoel-Gammon (1985) investigation, the ability to follow the children in a longitudinal manner from the same point (10 identifiable words in a recording session) regardless of their age seemed to reduce the extreme variability noted in other cross-sectional research. Although this study did not contain a large number of subjects, it certainly suggests some clinical implications.

Individual Acquisition Patterns. Throughout this discussion, individual variability has been stressed. The next question follows automatically: Do children show individual acquisition patterns or strategies? In other words, do children build their phonological inventory around certain sounds? If so, do these sounds represent the children's preference for a particular sound or set of sounds? Ferguson and Farwell (1975) referred to *salience* and *avoidance* factors. *Salience* implies that children will acquire words that contain sounds within their phonological inventories. The **salience factor** is defined as children's active selection in early word productions of sounds that are important or remarkable (salient) to the children. The **avoidance factor** is defined as the avoidance of words that do not contain sounds within a specific child's inventory. (This principle seems to apply only to the production of words; investigations relative to comprehension have not produced similar results [see Hoek, Ingram, & Gibson, 1986]). Production selection and avoidance have often been observed; for example, Schwartz and Leonard (1982) have added experimental support to this claim.

Individual strategies employed may include preferences for certain sounds, certain syllable structures, and/or sound classes or sound features. Individual preference can also refer to those objects and contexts that a child enjoys more than others. A child's preference and environment will most certainly have an effect on which words are acquired and which phonetic inventory is established during the production of the first 50 words.

Prosodic Feature Development

As children move from the end of the babbling period to first words, the previously noted intonational contours continue. The falling intonation contour still predominates, although both a rise–fall and a simple rising contour have also been observed (Kent & Bauer, 1985).

An important aspect of communication during the first-50-word stage is *prosodic variation*. Examples of children's speech during this time have included pitch variations to indicate differences in meaning. For example, a falling pitch on the first syllable, [da↓ da], as daddy entered the room versus [da↑ da], a rising pitch on the first syllable, was realized when a noise was heard outside when daddy was expected (Crystal, 1986). Prosodic features are also used to indicate differences in syntactical function. Bruner (1975) labels these prosodic units *place-holders*. A demand or question, for example, is often signaled first by prosody; words are added later. For example, a child aged 1;2 first used the phrase "all gone" after dinner by humming the intonation. Approximately a month passed before the child's segmental productions were somewhat accurate (Crystal, 1986). One widely held view is that these prosodic units fulfill a social function. They are seen as a means of signaling joint participation in an activity shared by the child and the caregiver. Several authors suggest that prosodic features are evidence of developing speech acts (Dore, 1975; Halliday, 1975; Menn, 1976). A word with a specific intonation pattern might indicate requesting, calling, or demanding, for example. The following prosodic features associated with intentional communication have been observed (Marcos, 1987):

CLINICAL EXERCISES

You are trying to note salience and avoidance factors in the speech of a 2;6-year-old child. Would it be better to use spontaneous speech or an articulation test? Or would both be necessary to determine these factors? Why?

Why are salience and avoidance factors important to consider when assessing a young child? Can you think of some ways to get information on salience and avoidance from the child's caregivers to supplement your assessment?

10 to 12 Months

First words, naming, labeling

Begin with a falling contour only. A flat or level contour is usually accompanied by variations such as falsettos or variations in duration or loudness. Example: At 10 and 11 months, Hildegard (Leopold, 1947) lengthened the vowels of words such as [de:] for there.

13 to 15 Months

Requesting, attention getting, curiosity, surprise, recognition, insistence, greeting

Rising contour. High falling contour that begins with a high pitch and drops to a lower one. This is noted in the previous example of [da↑ da].

Prior to 18 Months

Playful anticipation, emphatic stress

High rising and high rising–falling contour.

> Example: A child might use a high rising intonation pattern on *ball* to indicate that the game is about to begin.

Around 18 Months

Warnings, playfulness

Falling–rising contour. Rising–falling contour.

> Example: A child might use a falling–rising contour on *no* to indicate that he or she has been warned not to do that, that is, to repeat this warning. The same *no* with a rising–falling contour could be used during a game to indicate that daddy is not going to get the ball.

As can be noted, intonational changes seem to develop prior to stress. Although various pitch contours appear earlier than the first meaningful words, contrastive stress is first evidenced only at the beginning of the two-word stage or at the age of approximately 1;6. During the first-50-word stage, the observed pitch variations can be said to represent directional sequences (rising versus falling, for example) or range patterns (high versus low within the child's pitch range). For a more detailed analysis of early intonational development, see Crystal (1986) and Snow (1998a, 1998b, 2000).

The Preschool Child

This section stresses information on the developing phonology of children from approximately 18 to 24 months, the end of the first-50-word stage, to the beginning of the sixth year. During this time, the largest growth within the phonological system takes place. However, not only is a child's phonological system expanding but also large gains are seen in other language areas. From 18 to 24–30 months of age, a child's expressive vocabulary has at least tripled from 50 to 150–300 words (Lipsitt, 1966; Mehrabian, 1970), and the receptive vocabulary has grown from 200 to 1,200 words (Weiss & Lillywhite, 1981). The transition from one-word utterances to two-word sentences, a large linguistic step, is typically occurring at this time. With the production of two-word sentences, a child has entered the period of expressing specific semantic relationships: the beginning of syntactical development.

Around a child's fifth birthday, the expressive vocabulary has expanded to approximately 2,200 words, and about 9,600 words are in a child's receptive vocabulary (Weiss & Lillywhite, 1981). Almost all of the basic grammatical forms of the language—such as questions, negative statements, dependent clauses, and compound sentences—are now present as well (Owens, 2008). More important, the child knows now how to use language to communicate in an effective manner. A five-year-old talks differently to babies than to their friends, for example. The child also knows how to tell jokes and riddles and is quite able to handle the linguistic subtleties of being polite and rude.

A child's phonological development at 18 to 24 months still demonstrates a rather limited inventory of speech sounds and phonotactic possibilities. At this time, perception seems to somewhat precede production. By the end of the preschool period, around the child's fifth birthday, an almost complete phonological system has emerged.

All these changes occur in less than 4 years. Although this section focuses on phonological development, such a discussion must always be seen within the context of the equally large expansions in morphosyntax, semantics, and pragmatics that occur during this time.

Segmental Form Development: Vowels

One area of sound acquisition that has been widely neglected in most discussions of phonological development is the acquisition of vowels. This neglect has been at least partially justified with the statement that children have acquired all vowels within the General American English sound inventory by the age of 3 (Templin, 1957). Little information is available on the development of vowels. This section on vowel development in preschool children will use the data presented by Irwin and Wong (1983) and Velten (1943). Although several methodological problems with Irwin and Wong's investigation have been pointed out (see Smit, 1986), it nevertheless examines the vowel productions in spontaneous conversations of children from 18 to 72 months of age. The Velten (1943) data come from a diary study of Joan Velten.

According to the Irwin and Wong (1983) data, the children show the acquisition of [ɑ], [ʊ], [i], [ɪ], and [ʌ] at 18 months if the criterion is set at 70% accuracy. For the individual subjects at this age level, the correct production of vowels ranged from 23% to 71%. By 24 months, the only vowels that did not reach 70% group accuracy were [ɝ] and [ɚ]. By the age of 3, all the vowels were accounted for with virtually no production errors. Interestingly enough, at age 4, the accuracy for [ɚ], [u], and [ə] dropped again to less than 90%. More recently data from the Memphis Vowel Project (Pollock, 2013; Pollock and Berni, 2003) seem to support Irwin and Wong (1983). Pollock and Berni (2003) noted that between 18 to 35 months of age, the percentage of nonrhotic vowel errors was relatively high. However, after 36 months, nonrhotic vowel errors were minimal (0 to 4%). However, in relationship to rhotic vowels Pollock (2013) notes that at 30 to 35 months of age accuracy was only 61%. It is not until 48-53 months of age that accuracy of rhotic vowels is above 90% (36-41 months of age, accuracy is 80%; 42-53 months of age, accuracy is 78%).

Another view of vowel acquisition is offered by diary studies. Velten's (1943) data show that prior to the age of 21 months, her daughter used the [a] vowel. After a surge in vocabulary at 21 months, the vowel [u] was added. When this child is compared to Irwin and Wong's (1983) data, large discrepancies between the two become obvious. Again, the previously discussed concepts of salience and avoidance may apply to the described differences. Some children possibly select, for the most part, words that consist of sounds within their repertoire, avoiding those words and sounds that are not. Salience and avoidance in conjunction with individual phonetic preference could account for the noted differences.

Far more information is needed in the area of vowel acquisition. From the data presently available, it appears that nonrhotic vowels are indeed generally mastered by the age of 3. Whether individual variation plays a large role in this acquisition process still needs to be documented. This is an interesting area of research, especially in light of the deviant vowel systems that can be noted in children with speech sound disorders.

Segmental Form Development: Consonants

Cross-Sectional Results. It appears that no chapter on phonological development can be complete without looking at the large sample studies that began in the 1930s (Wellman, Case, Mengert, & Bradbury, 1931) and have continued periodically since that time. However, it seems appropriate to preface such a discussion with the problems inherent in these studies.

Large sample studies on phonological development were initiated to look at a large number of children in order to examine which sounds were mastered at which age levels. To this end, the studies evaluated most of the speech sounds within a given native language. With a few exceptions (Irwin & Wong, 1983; Olmsted, 1971; Stoel-Gammon, 1985, 1987a), these studies have used methods similar to articulation tests to collect their data; that is, the children were asked to name pictures and certain sounds that were then judged productionally as "correct" or "incorrect."

In this type of procedure, general as well as specific problems arise. First, the fact that a child produces the sound "correctly" as a one-word response does not mean that the sound can also be produced "correctly" in natural speech conditions. Practitioners have always been aware of the often large articulatory discrepancies between one-word responses and the same sounds used in conversation. Second, the choice of pictures/words will certainly affect the production of the individual sounds within the word. Not only a child's familiarity with the word plays a role but also factors such as the length of the word, its structure, the stressed or unstressed position of the sound within the word, and the phonetic context in which the sound occurs are involved. These factors help or hinder production. Therefore, strictly speaking, the only conclusion that can be drawn from cross-sectional studies is that a child could or could not produce that particular sound in that specific word.

The third point is a theoretical issue. As stated repeatedly in this text book, there has been an adoption of certain newer concepts and terminology within the field of speech-language pathology. This chapter's title, for example, focuses on phonological development, not speech sound development. With the inclusion of the terms *phonology* and *phonological development*, certain conceptual changes have been accepted. These cross-sectional studies are perhaps indicative of the inventory of speech sounds that children typically possess at certain ages, but they do not document a particular child's phonological system.

Specific methodological differences among various cross-sectional studies are also important factors when interpreting the results including the criteria used to determine whether a child has "mastered" a particular sound. Although this has been elaborated on in several articles and books (e.g., Smit, 1986; Vihman, 2004), it is worth mentioning again. Table 5.4 provides a comparison of several of the larger cross-sectional studies.

Looking at age comparisons in Table 5.4, we can observe a difference in reported mastery of 3 or more years for some sounds. For example, note the difference in the ages of mastery for the [s] in the more recent Prather, Hedrick, and Kern (1975) and in the older Poole (1934) studies. The Poole investigation has a mastery age of 7½ years, whereas the Prather and associates investigation shows an age level of 3 years. A 3-year difference can be found for [z] acquisition when the Prather data are compared to the Templin (1957) results. Again, Prather and colleagues assign a much earlier level of mastery. One question that is often asked in this context is: Does this mean that children are now producing sounds "correctly" at an earlier age? The answer is no; many of these differences result from the way *mastery* was defined. Poole, for instance, stated that 100% of the children must use the sound correctly in each of the positions tested. Prather and

The lack of response from the younger children could reflect the aforementioned avoidance factor: Words that contain sounds not in the child's inventory will be avoided.

TABLE 5.4 Age Levels for Speech Sound Development According to Six Studies

	Wellman et al. (1931)	Poole (1934)	Templin (1957)	Prather et al. (1975)	Arlt & Goodban (1976)	Smit (1993b)
m	3	3½	3	2	3	2
n	3	4½	3	2	3	2
ŋ	not tested	4½	3	2	3	4
p	4	3½	3	2	3	2
b	3	3½	4	2;8	3	2
t	5	4½	6	2;8	3	2
d	5	4½	4	2;4	3	3
k	4	4½	4	2;4	3	2
g	4	4½	4	2;4	3	2
w	3	3½	3	2;8	3	2
j	4	4½	3½	2;4	not tested	3½
l	4	6½	6	3;4	4	5½
r	5	7½	4	3;4	5	7
h	3	3½	3	2	3	2
f	3	5½	3	2;4	3	3
v	5	6½	6	4	3½	4
s	5	7½	4½	3	4	6
z	5	7½	7	4	4	6
ʃ	not mastered by age 6	6½	4½	3;8	4½	3½
ʒ	6	6½	7	4	4	not tested
θ	not mastered by age 6	7½	6	4	5	5;6
ð	not mastered by age 6	6½	7	4	5	4½
tʃ	5		4½	3;8	4	3½
ʤ	not mastered by age 6		7	4	4	3½

Source: Based on studies by Wellman, Case, Mengert & Bradbury (1931); Poole (1934); Templin (1957); Prather, Hedrick, & Kern (1975); Arlt & Goodban (1976); and Smit 1993b.

associates and Templin, on the other hand, set this level at 75%. In addition, rather than using the 75% cutoff level for all three positions (initial, medial, and final) as Templin had done, Prather and associates used only two positions (initial and final) for the calculations. The Smit data (1993b) noted in Table 5.4 did not report a mastery age. However, this has been calculated from the results of the study and set at 75%. The Smit (1993b) study used primarily initial- and final-word positions. Only [l] and [r] were tested in the medial position. This clearly changes the ages to which mastery can be assigned. A shift to earlier acquisition noted in the Prather and associates study could be accounted for by these methodological changes. Also, as Smit (1986) points out, the Prather results are based on incomplete data sets, especially at the younger age groupings.

CLINICAL EXERCISES

Based on the various methodologies, which of the six studies presented might you choose for determining "mastery" age? Why?

Although data from vowel acquisition suggest that children can master vowels, including [ɝ] and [ɚ], by age 4 to 5, children with r-problems often have difficulties with these central vowels with r-coloring. Based on the rhotic vowel acquisition data and Table 5.4, when would you begin working on r-sounds in therapy? Why?

Although Prather and associates began with 21 subjects in each age group, several of these children did not respond to many of the words. Thus, at times, only 8 to 12 children were used to calculate the norms. The children who did not respond to some words may have been avoiding them because they felt that they could not pronounce them "correctly."

Ingram (1989a) points out problems related to the Templin study, summing them up as follows:

> Templin's study provides a useful descriptive overview of English phonological acquisition. Here, however, we will conclude with a caution about using large sample data such as these for anything more than the most general of purposes, setting out a series of problems with Templin's study in particular and large sample studies in general. The limitations of such studies need to be emphasized because their results may be inappropriately used both for theoretical and practical purposes, the latter including cases where a child might be misidentified as being speech-delayed because of his performance on a Templin-style articulation test. (p. 366)

What, then, is the alternative? Several investigators (e.g., Irwin & Wong, 1983; Stoel-Gammon, 1985) have attempted to improve the situation by using spontaneous speech and/or longitudinal investigations. Although spontaneous speech samples are in some respects better than the picture-naming tasks, several problems remain. Speech samples can also give us a biased picture. We actually probe into only a small portion of a child's conversational abilities and then generalize, assuming that this is representative of the child's overall performance. Also, factors outside our control might determine which words and sounds the child does produce and which ones he or she does not. As a result, the sample obtained will probably not contain all the sounds in the particular child's phonetic inventory.

Longitudinal data, on the other hand, can give us a real insight into the individual acquisition process, an important aspect missing in cross-sectional studies. The following discussion examines data from longitudinal studies on consonant development in children.

Longitudinal Results. Several longitudinal studies of consonant development exist, but they report on either a single child or a small group of children (e.g., Leopold, 1947; Menn, 1971; Vihman et al., 1985). Therefore, the data cannot be readily generalized. However, Vihman and Greenlee (1987) used a longitudinal methodology to examine the phonological development of ten 3-year-old children with the following results:

1. Stops and other fricatives were substituted for [ð] and [θ] by all children.
2. More than half of the children also substituted sounds for [r] and [l] (gliding) and employed palatal fronting, in which a palatal sound is replaced by an alveolar ([ʃ] becomes [s]).
3. Two of the 10 children demonstrated their own particular "style" of phonological acquisition.
4. On the average, 73% of the children's utterances were judged intelligible by three raters unfamiliar with the children. However, the range of intelligibility was broad, extending from 54% to 80%. As expected, children with fewer errors were more intelligible than those with multiple errors. Another factor also played a role: The children who used more complex sentences tended to be more difficult to understand.

> The avoidance factor may also influence spontaneous speech. Words might be avoided that contain sounds that the child cannot say.

This last finding is significant. It documents the complex interaction between phonological development and the acquisition of the language system as a whole. The simultaneous acquisition of complex morphosyntactic and semantic relationships could well have an impact on the growth of the phonological system. In addition, it has been hypothesized that **phonological idioms** (Moskowitz, 1971) or **regression** (Leopold, 1947) occurs as a child attempts to master other complexities of language. Both terms refer to accurate sound productions that are later replaced by inaccurate ones. When trying to deal with more complex morphosyntactic or semantic structures, the child's previously correct articulations appear to be lost, replaced by inaccurate sound productions.

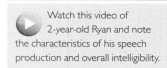
Watch this video of 2-year-old Ryan and note the characteristics of his speech production and overall intelligibility.

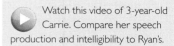
Watch this video of 3-year-old Carrie. Compare her speech production and intelligibility to Ryan's.

Phonological Processes

Within the last decade, the study of phonological development has shifted from examining the mastery of individual sounds to the acquisition and ordering of the phonological system. According to natural phonology, there seems to be a time frame during which normally developing children do suppress certain processes. This approximate age of suppression is helpful when determining normal versus disordered phonological systems and can be used as a guideline when targeting remediation goals. The following section addresses some developmental aspects of syllable structure, substitution, and assimilation processes.

Syllable Structure Processes. Syllable structure processes address the general tendency of young children to reduce words to basic CV structures. These processes become evident between the ages of 1;6 and 4;0 when there is a rapid growth in vocabulary and the onset of two-word utterances (Ingram, 1989b).

Reduplication is an early syllable structure process. Ingram (1989b) notes that it is a common process during children's first-50-word stage. There was no evidence of this process, however, in the youngest group of children (1;6 to 1;9) in the Preisser, Hodson, and Paden (1988) study.

Final consonant deletion is a relatively early process. Preisser and associates (1988) state that it was extremely rare in the utterances of the children in the 2;2 to 2;5 age group. Ingram (1989b) and Grunwell (1987) note the disappearance of this process around age 3.

Unstressed syllable deletion, sometimes called *weak syllable deletion*, lasts longer than final consonant deletion, until approximately 4 years of age (Ingram, 1989b). This is also confirmed by Grunwell's (1987) data. However, Preisser and associates (1988) noted that most of the children in their sample appeared to have suppressed this process by around their second birthday. (Only 3% of the 20 children over age 2;2 demonstrated unstressed syllable deletion.)

Definitions and examples of phonological processes are given in the "Natural Phonology" section of Chapter 4.

CLINICAL APPLICATION

Using Cross-Sectional Mastery Level Charts: Yes or No?

This textbook points out some of the problems inherent in large cross-sectional studies that provide ages of sound mastery. Should these charts then be discarded? Probably not. Sound mastery charts give useful information about the general ages and order in which speech sounds develop. They can provide a broad framework for comparison, especially for beginning clinicians.

Clinicians should remember, however, that varying methodologies and criteria for sound mastery across investigations have produced a wide range of acquisition ages. Differences in ages of mastery for some sounds are often 3 to 4½ years apart. Based on the results of the Prather et al. (1975) study, a clinician could justify doing [s] therapy with a 3-year-old, but according to the Poole (1934) investigation, the clinician should wait until the child is 7½ years old. These sound mastery charts should never be the single deciding factor for intervention. Clinical decision making involves much more than comparing a child to the mastery ages provided by cross-sectional research. Most public schools, for example, require standardized articulation tests, which use standard scores and percentile ranks to document a child's abilities, not sound mastery charts.

Cluster reduction is a syllable structure process that lasts for a relatively long time. Haelsig and Madison (1986) noted cluster reductions that still occurred in 5-year-old children, whereas Roberts, Burchinal, and Footo (1990) evidenced rare instances of this process in their 8-year-old children. The Smit (1993a) study presented some evidence of cluster reduction in the 8;0- to 9;0-year-old children for specific initial consonant clusters (approximately 1–4% of the 247 children for primarily three-consonant clusters). Greenlee (1974) describes four developmental stages of consonant reduction: (1) deletion of the entire cluster: [it] for *treat*, (2) reduction to one cluster member: [tit] for *treat*, (3) cluster realization but one member substitution: [twit] for *treat*, and (4) norm articulation: [trit]. The Smit (1993a) and McLeod, van Doorn, and Reed (2001) data support Stages 2 through 4, whereas Stage 1, complete deletion of a cluster, was very rare or not seen at all even in the 2-year-old subjects.

Epenthesis refers to the insertion of a sound segment into a word, thereby changing its syllable structure. The intrusive sound can be a vowel as well as a consonant, but most often, it is restricted to a schwa insertion between two consonants. This schwa insertion—for example, [pəliz] for *please*—is used to simplify the production difficulty of consonant clusters. Smit (1993a) and Smit, Hand, Freilinger, Bernthal, and Bird (1990) report that between the ages of 2;6 and 8;0, schwa insertion in clusters is a common process.

Substitution Processes. *Stopping* refers most frequently to the replacement of stops for fricatives and affricates. Because of the fact that fricatives and affricates are acquired at different ages, stopping is not a unified process but should be broken down into the individual sounds for which this process is employed. Table 5.5 summarizes the ages at which stopping is suppressed for the different fricative sounds.

Fronting denotes the tendency of young children to replace palatals and velars with alveolar consonants. Frequently occurring fronting processes consist of [ʃ] → [s], palatal fronting, and [k] → [t] and [d] → [g] velar fronting. Palatal fronting may also occur in affricate productions, [tʃ] → [ts] and [dʒ] → [dz]. Lowe, Knutson, and Monson (1985) found velar fronting to be more prevalent than palatal fronting. They also found that fronting rarely occurred in normally developing children after the age of 3;6. Based on the Smit (1993b) data, both velar fronting and palatal fronting were still noted until approximately age 5;0, although the frequency of occurrence was very limited (less than 5% of the 186 children).

TABLE 5.5 Age of Suppression of Stopping

	2;0	2;6	3;0	3;6	4;0	5;0	
[f]----- ---------|--------------------|--------------------|				|	|	|	
[v]---- ---------|--------------------|--|							
[s]-------------|--------------------|--------------------| Distortions more frequent than stopping							
[z]-------------|--------------------|--------------------- -------------------------| Distortions more frequent							
[ʃ]-------------|--------------------| Distortions more frequent than stopping							
[tʃ]------------|--------------------|----------------------| Relatively frequent							
[dʒ]------------|--------------------|--------------------|-- -------------------|--------------------| Very frequent							
							Occasional process
[θ]-------------|--------------------|--------------------|-- -------------------|--------------------|--------------------|-------------------------|							
							Very frequent process in 2–4-year-olds
[ð]-------------|--------------------|--------------------|-- -------------------|--------------------|--------------------|-------------------------|							

Source: Summarized from Smit (1993b).

Gliding of [r] and [l] seems to extend beyond 5;0 years of age (Grunwell, 1987; Smit, 1993b) and can be infrequently found even in the speech of children as old as age 7 (Roberts et al., 1990; Smit, 1993b). The suppression of these and other common processes are summarized in Tables 5.5 and 5.6.

Assimilation Processes.   Many different assimilation processes occur in the speech of children. Children at different stages of their speech development tend to use assimilation processes in systematic ways. One of the most frequently occurring assimilatory processes is *velar harmony* (Smith, 1973). Prominent examples are:

Assimilation is discussed in some detail in Chapters 2 and 4.

[gɔk]	for	"dog"
[keʰk]	for	"take"
[kɑk]	for	"talk"

However, regressive assimilation processes are not limited to velar consonants. Smith (1973) reported similar regressive assimilations in which bilabials influenced preceding nonlabial consonants and consonant clusters. Among his examples are:

[bebu]	for	"table"
[bɔp]	for	"stop"
[mibu]	for	"nipple"

TABLE 5.6   Age of Suppression for Several Processes

	2;0	3;0	4;0	5;0	6;0	7;0	8;0	9;0
Labialization[1]	--							
Alveolarization[1]	---							
Affrication[1]	----------------------------							
Deaffrication[1]	-------------------------------------							
Vowelization[1]	--							
Derhotacization[2]	----------------------------------							
Denasalization[3]	---------							
Epenthesis[4]	--						
Consonant cluster substitution[2]	--						
Voicing Changes								
Context sensitive[5]	-------------------							
Initial voicing[6]	--						
Final devoicing[7]	---							

[1]Suppression for 75% of the children tested (Lowe, 1996).
[2]Suppression for 90% of the children tested (Smit, 1993b).
[3]The most common error for [m] and [n] but only occasional use (less than 10%) by age 2;0 (Smit, 1993a).
[4]From Smit (1993a).
[5]Grunwell (1987).
[6]Suppression for 85% of the children tested (Khan and Lewis, 2002).

CLINICAL EXERCISES

In Table 5.5, you see that stopping of [s], [z], and [ʃ] seems to be suppressed around age 3 to 3½. After that, distortions become more frequent. Does this suggest anything in the way of a developmental process? In other words, would your assessment results differ if a child is still stopping these sounds at age 4 and beyond?

The data in Table 5.6 suggest that r-problems such as derhotacization and vowelization are suppressed at around age 4 to 4½. Presently these difficulties are not being treated until children are in first or second grade. What would be your opinion of the relatively late age for treating r-problems?

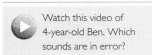 Watch this video of 4-year-old Ben. Which sounds are in error?

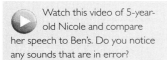 Watch this video of 5-year-old Nicole and compare her speech to Ben's. Do you notice any sounds that are in error?

Although not all children display these types of assimilation processes, they may be part of the normal speech development in 1;6- to 2-year-olds. If they persist beyond age 3;0, they begin to constitute a danger sign for a disordered phonological system (Grunwell, 1987).

Prosodic Feature Development

At the time when children begin to use two-word utterances, a further development in the usage of suprasegmentals occurs: *contrastive stress.* This term indicates that one syllable within a two-word utterance becomes prominent. The acquisition process seems to proceed in the following order.

First, within a child's two-word utterance, a single prosodic pattern is maintained; the two words have a pause between them that becomes shorter and shorter. The next step in the acquisition process appears to be the prosodic integration of the two words into one tone-unit. A **tone-unit**, or what is often called a *sense-group,* is an organizational unit imposed on prosodic data (Crystal, 2010). Such a tone-unit conveys meaning beyond that implied by only the verbal production. When the two words become one tone-unit (i.e., without the pause between them and with one intonational contour), one of these words becomes more prominent, usually louder and associated with an identifiable pitch movement (Crystal, 2010). At the end of this process, there exists a unifying rhythmic relationship between the two items; thus, pauses become less likely. The following developmental pattern could be observed:

Daddy (pause) eat

Daddy (pause shortens) eat

'Daddy 'eat (no pause, both stressed)

'Daddy eat (first word stressed)

The use of contrastive stress in the two-word stage may be used to establish *contrastive meaning* (Brown, 1973). It is assumed that the meaning of the combined one-tone utterance is different from the meaning of the two words in sequence. Later, we see that this contrastive stress is used to signal differences in meaning with similar words. Thus, "'Daddy eat" could indicate that "Daddy is eating," whereas "Daddy 'eat" could indicate, perhaps, that "Daddy should sit down and eat."

The existing studies of prosodic feature development agree that the acquisition of intonation and stress begins at an early age. Adultlike intonational patterns are noted prior to the appearance of the first word, whereas the onset of stress patterns seems to occur clearly before the age of 2. However, true mastery of the whole prosodic feature system does not seem to take place until children are at least 12 years old (Atkinson-King, 1973; Malikouti-Drachman & Drachman, 1975).

English as a Second Language: Considerations for Phonological Development in Children

There is an increasing number of English language learners within the United States. Within less than 20 years, it is estimated that 40% of the entire school-age population will be

English language learners. Certain areas of the United States have already exceeded these estimates. For example, in California, 60–70% of school-age children are not native speakers of English (Roseberry-McKibbon and Brice, 2010). In addition, the number of children in the United States who speak a language other than English at home has more than doubled since 1980. Statistics estimate that 21% of children ages 5 to 17 do not speak English in their home environment (National Center for Children in Poverty, 2010). With these statistics in mind, it is important that we understand the differences in speech development that occur in children who are attempting to learn English as their second language.

First, within the developmental process, there may be **interference** or **transfer** from their first language (L1) to English (L2) (Roseberry-McKibbon, 2007). Thus, children may make an error in English because of the direct influence of their first language. This may impact phonological development in several ways. The most direct influence is the phonological inventory. Therefore, if a phoneme does not exist in the first language, children may substitute another phoneme that is somewhat comparable. Both vowels and consonants are typically affected because of the differences in the phonemic systems between L1 and L2. For example, in the Vietnamese phonological system, the [ɪ] and [ʊ] vowels do not exist; however, [i] and [u] are present. Therefore, children may substitute [i] for [ɪ], saying [hit] for "hit" or [u] for [ʊ] as in [luk] for "look." Consonantal inventories are also transferred. Staying with the Vietnamese language, certain dialects do not have "th"-sounds, but [s] and [z] are present. The child learning English may transfer [s] and [z] to English, replacing [θ] and [ð]. Examples of resulting substitutions are "those" that becomes [zoz] or "think" that is pronounced as [sɪŋk].

Not only do the differences between the phonological inventories of L1 and L2 transfer or interfere but also the phonotactic differences will be noticeable within the developmental process. To review, *phonotactics* refers to the arrangement of sounds within a given language; examples include which consonants can be arranged to form consonant clusters and the number and type of consonants that can begin and end a syllable. In Spanish, the [v] at the end of a word is devoiced and transfers to English as [lʌf] for "love." In addition, in Spanish consonant clusters are reduced in the word-final position; thus in English, the word "start" may become [staɚ] (Penfield & Ornstein-Galacia, 1985; Perez, 1994). There are no consonant clusters in Vietnamese or Cantonese (Cheng, 1994; Ruhlen, 1976), and no word-final consonants in Hmong (Matisoff, 1991; Mortensen, 2004). These phonotactic differences may all transfer from L1 to L2.

In addition, rhythmic differences (stress, intonation, and duration) may exist in a child's first learned language. If these transfer to English, the overall speech pattern may somehow sound different and be more difficult to understand. For a more complete account of the phonology of several languages, refer to Chapter 8. The phonological inventories, phonotactic possibilities, and rhythmical differences are provided for several languages.

The transfer or interference from L1 to L2 is not limited to the phonological development. Morphology—for example, the plural -s production when an [s] (and/or [z]) is not present in L1 or the consonant clusters formed by past tense "ed" as in "walked" or "listened"—may present difficulties for the learner of English. Of course, syntax, semantics, and pragmatics may also be influenced by the transfer or interference of L1 to L2.

Although not directly related to the phonological development, many English language learners have been noted to experience a **silent period**. These children are very quiet, speaking very little as they focus on understanding the new language. Within the classroom, this may be interpreted as the children are being extremely "shy" or not able to meet the demands there. The younger a child is, the longer the silent period may last. Older children may stay in this silent period for a few weeks or months, whereas preschoolers may be relatively silent for a year or more. Again, this is a normal phenomenon and a portion of the developmental process (Roseberry-McKibbon & Brice, 2010).

A first-grader, Jessica, is very quiet both in the class-room and in speech-language therapy. Her teacher thinks she is extremely shy. She will often shake her head, which is interpreted as "she doesn't know the answer." She is learning English as a second lan-guage; her first language is Spanish. You hypothe-size that she might be going through a silent period.

What could you do to help the teacher under-stand this developmental process?

What could you do as a clinician in speech-language therapy to aid in this transition, remem-bering that Jessica is trying to understand English as best as she can?

In addition, **code switching** or **code mixing** may occur. In this developmental process, speakers alternate between L1 and L2. This may occur within a phrase or between sentences (Pence & Justice, 2008). Zentella (1997) gives the following examples of code switching between Spanish and English: "It's already full, mira" ("It's already full, look") or "Because yo lo dije" ("Because I said it").

As a portion of this developmental process, English language learners may demonstrate a phe-nomenon referred to as *language loss*. As these children become more proficient in English, they lose skills and fluency in their native language if that language is not reinforced and maintained. This is called *subtractive bilingualism* and can be very detrimental to the chil-dren's learning of the native language and family life (Roseberry-McKibbon & Brice, 2010). This may cause difficulties within the family if the parents only speak L1 and no English. As noted earlier, more than 20% of young children do not speak English in their home environment. Clinicians should be sensitive to these issues and reassure the families that this is a normal developmental process. From personal experi-ence, families often voice the opinion that it is harmful to the children to be learning two languages. Families accept the fact that the children's first learned language is not as profi-cient as before and, therefore, do not reinforce that language. Bilingualism has many advan-tages for children both cognitively and linguistically. In our world, which is becoming more and more international, bilingualism is a valuable resource. Families should be encouraged to nurture their children's native language so that language loss of L1 does not occur.

The School-Age Child

By the time children enter school, their phonological development has progressed consid-erably. At age 5;0, most of them can converse freely with everyone and make themselves understood clearly to peers and adults alike. However, their pronunciation is still recogniz-ably different from the adult norm. Phonologically, they still have a lot to learn. Although their phonological inventory is nearly complete, this system must now be adapted to many more and different contexts, words, and situations. Other phonological features are obvi-ously not mastered at all at this time. Certain sounds are still frequently misarticulated, and some aspects of prosodic feature development are only beginning to be incorporated.

Most of the research in child phonology has centered on the development of pho-nological skills in the first 5 years of life. However, recent interest in later phonological acquisition has evolved in part because of the established relationship between learning to speak and learning to read.

Segmental Form Development

The development of children's phonological system includes both perceptual and pro-ductional maturation. Although the focus of this chapter is on production, it should be emphasized that school-age children's perceptual skills are still very much in the process of growing. The gradual establishment of phonemic categorization skills, for example, continues well beyond 5 years of age. It is not until 14 years of age that children can reliably give categorical responses to certain types of synthetic stimuli (Fourcin, 1978).

Tallal, Stark, Kallman, and Mellits (1980) reported that the perceptual constancy of children's phonemic categorizations still changes between 5 and 9 years of age. Also, the recognition of isolated words under quiet and noisy environmental conditions demonstrates improvement until at least age 10 (Elliott et al., 1979). The processing ability of specific continuous speech samples is still measurably slower for fifth-graders than for adults (Cole & Perfetti, 1980), and the ability to understand specifically structured sentences under difficult listening conditions continues to develop until the age of 15 (Elliott, 1979). Perceptually, children are still fine-tuning, certainly during the beginning school years, and in some respects far beyond.

Productionally, children are also fine-tuning during the school years. Most of the information on children's production abilities is based on the results of articulation tests, i.e., based on responses to picture naming. If we look at these investigations (e.g., Lowe, 1986, 1996; Templin, 1957), we find that acceptable pronunciation of certain sounds is not achieved until between age 4;6 and 6;0. The most common later sounds are [θ, ð, ʒ] (Sander, 1972). Other findings (Ingram, Christensen, Veach, & Webster, 1980) include one or more of these consonants: [r, z, v]. Based on single-item pronunciation, most investigators agree that children complete their phonemic inventory by the age of 6;0 or, at the latest, 7;0. However, data from the Iowa-Nebraska Articulation Norms (Smit, 1993b) found dentalized [s] productions in 10% of the 9-year-old children tested.

Consonant clusters also prove difficult for school-age children. The acquisition of clusters usually takes place anywhere from age 3;6 to age 5;6. During this time, children may demonstrate consonant cluster reduction, lengthening certain elements of the cluster, for example [s:no], or epenthesis. In epenthesis, children insert a schwa vowel between two consonantal elements of a cluster, as in [səno], for example. The Iowa-Nebraska data (Smit, 1993a) offer interesting insight into 27 different initial clusters. In this study, 1,049 children between the ages of 2;0 and 9;0 were screened using an articulation test format. The data can be summarized as follows:

1. On 14 of the 27 initial clusters tested, a small percentage of children in the *8;0- to 9;0-year-old group* (N = 247, frequency of occurrence = approximately 2%) reduced two consonant clusters to a single element. These clusters included [pl], [kl], [gl], [sl], [tw], [kw], [tr], [dr], [fr], [sw], [sm], [sn], [st], and [sk].

2. The consonant clusters [br] and [θr] demonstrated a higher frequency of consonant cluster reduction (5–15%) for children from *ages 5 to 9.*

3. For the *5;6- to 7;0-year-olds*, the consonant clusters that fell at 75% or below group accuracy included [sl], [br], [θr], [skw], [spr], [str], and [skr].

4. Epenthesis, or schwa insertion in consonant clusters, occurs frequently up to *age 8;0.* The 9-year-olds rarely exhibited schwa insertion.

These data demonstrate that consonant cluster realizations are not adultlike for all children even at age 9.

In addition, children's timing of the sounds within consonant clusters is not yet comparable to adult performance (Gilbert & Purves, 1977; Hawkins, 1979). When the temporal relationships between the elements of a cluster were compared for children and adults, differences, particularly in voice onset time, were still present at 8;0 years of age.

Although this information indicates that phonological development extends past the age of 7, most of the available research has focused on the development of the phonological inventory. Unfortunately, other features of the phonological system are still relatively uncharted territory. For example, the development of allophonic variations in older children should also be addressed. How do children learn the acceptable range of phonetic variation in different contexts within their speech community? Local (1983) exemplified this development process by tracing the acquisition of one vowel produced by a boy between the ages of 4;5 and 5;6. The variability of sound production and the learning of its acceptable allophonic limitations are decisively important tasks for the developing school-age child.

The intricate interrelation of normal phonological development with other areas of language growth, which has been previously emphasized, demands attention at this point in children's development as well. The acquisition of vocabulary, for example, is a monumental task that is accomplished in a relatively short time. When children begin kindergarten, they are said to have an expressive vocabulary of approximately 2,200 words (Weiss & Lillywhite, 1981). New sound sequences occurring in new words require not only increased oral-motor control and improved timing skills but also the internalization of new phonological rules. For instance, the conditions under which voiceless stops in English need to be aspirated might become a new achievement.

The acquisition of morphology is also related to phonological growth. The learning of specific morphological structures implies the learning of phonological rules. The children have to understand under which conditions the plural suffix -*s* is voiced [z] ("boys") or a voiceless [s] ("hats"), for example. This interconnection between morphology and phonology has been termed **morphophonology**, which refers to the study of the different allomorphs of the morpheme and the rules governing their use. For example, children's production of [əz] to indicate the plural form for *glass* versus [s] as the plural of *boat* falls within the study of morphophonology as do the rules governing the productional changes from *divide* to *division* and from *explode* to *explosion*. Research findings (e.g., Atkinson-King, 1973; Ivimey, 1975; Myerson, 1978) document that children who are as old as 17 are still acquiring certain morphophonological patterns. The complex interrelationship among the phonological system and other components of language continues into children's later school years.

Phonological Awareness, Emerging Literacy, and Phonemic-Based Disorders

One other important aspect that needs to be addressed in this section pertains to the interconnections between learning to speak and learning to read. Although a general consensus has not been reached as to which variables are indispensable for acquiring reading, there does seem to be a close relationship between early speech and emerging literacy. Thus, a strong correlation between the phonological development, especially segmentation skills, and later reading achievement has been found (e.g., Clarke-Klein & Hodson, 1995; Lundberg, Olofsson, & Wall, 1980). Moreover, early language development, specifically the perceptual processing of sounds, has been found to be one of the strongest predictors of later reading acquisition (Lundberg, 1988). Some of these skills develop during the early school years.

Metaphonological skills are also related to reading. A subcategory of metalinguistics, **metaphonology**, involves children's conscious awareness of the sounds within a particular language. It includes how those sounds are combined to form words. Therefore, metaphonological skills pertain to children's ability to discern how many sounds are in a word or which sound constitutes its beginning or end. Phonological awareness abilities are one important metaphonological skill. A growing body of knowledge documents the relationship between phonological awareness and emerging literacy. The following section briefly summarizes these results.

Research over at least two decades has affirmed the importance of phonological awareness and its relationship to reading acquisition (e.g., Blachman, 2000; Foy & Mann, 2012; Lonigan, Burgess, & Anthony, 2000; Stanovich, 2000). Reviews of the literature have noted that strong phonological awareness skills are characteristics of good readers, whereas children with poor phonological awareness skills in kindergarten and early school years are far more likely to become poor readers (e.g., Catts, Fey, & Zhang, 2001; Leafstedt, Richards, & Gerber, 2004; Torgesen, 2000). This section defines phonological awareness, discusses the various levels of phonological awareness, and examines the impact that speech sound disorders have on developing phonological awareness skills and early literacy.

Phonological awareness is an individual's awareness of the sound structure or phonological structure of a spoken word in contrast to written words (Gillon, 2004). It is a child's conscious ability to detect and manipulate sound segments, such as moving sounds around in a word, combining certain sounds together, or deleting sounds. Phonological awareness should be examined in the broader scope of phonology because we find that long before a child becomes aware of the phonological structure of words, he or she has specialized phonological knowledge. This knowledge allows the child to make a judgment about whether a word is part of his or her native language, to self-correct any speech errors or mispronunciations, and to discriminate between acceptable and unacceptable variations of a spoken word.

Phonological awareness uses a single modality—the auditory one. It is the ability to hear sounds in spoken words in contrast to recognizing sounds in written words, which accesses a child's coding abilities. **Coding** is translating stimuli from one form to another—for example, from auditory to written form or from written to auditory. Phonological awareness should also be separated from phonemic awareness. *Phonological awareness* is a more general term that refers to all sizes of sound units, such as words (e.g., How many words are in the sentence *He hit the ball*?); syllables (e.g., How many syllables does *banana* have?); onset-rimes (e.g., Which one of these words rhymes with *bed: man, lock,* or *head*?); and phonemes (e.g., What is the first sound in *dog*?). **Phonemic awareness**, however, refers only to the phoneme level and necessitates an understanding that words comprise individual sounds. Examples would include a child's ability to segment and match sounds (e.g., What is a word that starts with the same sound as *Cathy*?) and the ability to manipulate sounds (e.g., What would *mean* be without the final *n* sound?). The concepts of phonological and phonemic awareness should also be separated from phonological processing.

Phonological processing is the use of sounds of a language to process verbal information in oral or written form that requires working and long-term memory. Research provides strong support that phonological processing includes two broad dimensions: coding and awareness (Hurford et al., 1993; Liberman & Shankweiler, 1985). Coding, which contains two dimensions, phonetic and phonological, includes multiple processes that require memory and coding from one form of representation to another. An example might be that a child learns that the letters *sh* sound a certain way. This knowledge is stored in memory, which the child must access when trying to sound out a new word, *shelf*. The distinction between the two coding dimensions is the type of memory that is accessed. In other words, phonetic coding takes place in working memory for such processes as sounding out unfamiliar words.

In contrast, phonological coding is related to the semantic lexical abilities in long-term memory. This seems to involve a three-step process. First, written symbols are matched to the pronunciation of the written word. Second, the pronunciation of the written word is matched with the pronunciation of words in memory. Third, pronunciations of words in memory are linked with meaning for retrieval of meaning and pronunciation (Wesseling & Reitsma, 2000). At least four types of phonological processing skills demonstrate differences between norm readers and poor readers: memory span (retention of new strings of verbal items), recall of verbal information (in contrast to recall of nonverbal items), articulation rate, and rapid naming (Cornwall, 1992; Torgesen, 2000; Torgesen, Wagner, Simmons, & Laughon, 1990).

Thus, phonological awareness is a subdivision of phonological processing; however, phonological awareness is less complex: coding puts more demands on memory and processing of information. Phonological awareness is a multilevel skill of breaking down words into smaller units and can be described in terms of syllable awareness, onset-rime awareness, and phoneme awareness (Gillon, 2004). A variety of measures can be used to evaluate a child's knowledge of these three levels.

Syllable Awareness. Awareness at the syllable level requires that a child understands that words can be divided into syllables. For example, the word *baby* has two syllables: "ba" and "by." Tasks used to evaluate syllable awareness include (1) syllable segmentation (How many syllables, or beats, are in *banana*?), (2) syllable completion (Here is a picture of a rainbow. I'll say the first part of the word and you can complete it. Here is a rain____), (3) syllable identity (Which part of "rainbow" and "raincoat" sound the same?), and (4) syllable deletion (Say "rabbit." Now say it again without the "ra").

Onset-Rime Awareness. This awareness involves recognition of the onset of the syllable (all sounds prior to the vowel nucleus) and the rime, or the rest of the syllable, that includes the syllable peak and coda.(See Chapter 2 for a review of syllable structure.) Onset-rime awareness is typically measured by using some type of rhyming tasks. To be able to rhyme, children must be able to separate the onset from the rime of the word. Thus, a child knows that *cat, bat,* and *hat* rhyme as the onset changes in each; however, the rime stays the same: "at." Tasks that measure onset-rime awareness include (1) spoken rhyme recognition (Do these words rhyme: *hop* and *top*?), (2) recognition of words that do not rhyme (Which word does not rhyme: *cat, sat, car*?), (3) spoken rhyme production (Tell me a word that rhymes with *dog.*), and (4) onset-rime blending ("c" "at" is blended to "cat.").

Phonemic Awareness. This skill can be measured in a number of ways. For each of the tasks, a child's ability to manipulate sounds is tested. Examples include (1) phoneme detection (Which one of the following words has a different first sound: *rose, red, bike, rabbit*?), (2) phoneme matching (Which word begins with same sound as "rose"?), (3) phoneme isolation (Which sound do you hear at the beginning of "toad"?), (4) phoneme completion (Here is a picture of a ball. Can you finish the word for me? "ba____."), (5) phoneme blending (I am going to say a word in a funny way. Can you tell me what the word is? b—i—g.), (6) phoneme deletion (Can you say "toad" without the "d" sound?), (7) phoneme segmentation (How many sounds are in "jeep"?), (8) phoneme reversal (Say "bat." Now say "bat" backwards: "tab."), (9) phoneme manipulation (Say "meat." Now say it again but this time change the "m" and the "t" around: "team."), and (10) spoonerisms (for example, *hot dog* becomes *dot hog.*).

CLINICAL EXERCISES

For each of the 10 skills listed under the section "Phonemic Awareness," identify two different examples for each skill.

Explain why skills numbered 8, 9, and 10 are more complex. Think about what a child must do to complete the task. Does memory play more of a role for these skills?

There seems to be a developmental progression in the acquisition of phonological awareness skills. First, an awareness of larger units, such as words and syllables, precedes awareness of smaller units, such as individual sounds. In a comprehensive study by Lonigan, Burgess, Anthony, and Barker (1998), which tested several levels of phonological/phonemic awareness in 356 children between the ages of 2 and 5, the following results emerged. First, age influenced the performance on all tasks. Although accelerated growth was evident between the ages of 3 and 4 years, it was not until around age 5 that children were able to consistently perform phoneme detection tasks. Second, the linguistic complexity of the task influenced performance. Children across age groups showed stronger performance on blending and deleting at the word level (*dog + house = doghouse*), followed by success at the syllable level (*win + dow = window*), and the weakest performance at the phoneme level (*d + o + g = dog*). Third, performance on the phonological awareness tasks was moderately correlated to scores on receptive and expressive language tasks at the 4- and 5-year-old levels, but not at the younger ages.

Although stable performance of phonological awareness tasks may not be evident until 4 years of age, some 2- and 3-year-old children can demonstrate phonological awareness knowledge. Maclean, Bryant, and Bradley (1987) appear to be among the earliest investigators who found that a moderate percentage of 3-year-old children can perform competently on a rhyme detection task. When Lonigan and colleagues (1998) reduced the load on memory by having the children look at three pictures and point to the picture that did not rhyme, nearly 25% of the 2½-year-old children scored above chance on the task.

It must be noted that some researchers have questioned the progressive nature of phonological development. In other words, the seemingly noted fact that syllable awareness emerges before rhyme awareness and rhyme awareness before phoneme awareness was not evidenced in all children. For example, individual reports of older poor readers document children who performed better on phoneme manipulation tasks as opposed to performance on rhyme tasks (Duncan & Johnston, 1999). These findings are contrary to the trends noted in most other children.

The next question that arises is whether phonological awareness abilities are predictive of later reading and spelling competencies. In a large number of studies that attempted to control for variables such as memory, intellectual ability, and home and preschool environments (e.g., Lundberg, Olofsson, & Wall, 1980; Share, Jorm, Maclean, & Matthews, 1984; Torgesen, Wagner, & Rashotte, 1994; Torneus, 1984), the following findings are suggested:

1. There is a positive relationship between phonological awareness and reading. Children with phonological awareness skills learn to read more easily than children who do not have these skills (Snow, Burns, & Griffin, 1998).
2. Performance on phonological awareness tasks in kindergarten and first grade is a strong predictor of later reading achievement (Hecht, Burgess, Torgesen, Wagner, & Rashotte, 2000; Torgesen, Wagner, Rashotte, Burgess, & Hecht, 1997).
3. Direct training of phonological awareness and sound-letter correspondence with children who are not yet reading improves their reading and spelling skills (Adams, Foorman, Lundberg, & Beeler, 1997; Swank, 1997).
4. Phonological awareness teaching works best when combined with instruction in sound-letter correspondence (Bradley & Bryant, 1983).

Finally, the relationship among phonological awareness, developing literacy, and speech disorders is relevant to this discussion. Approximately 4% of 6-year-old children will approach reading with a speech sound disorder (Shriberg, Tomblin, & McSweeney, 1999). Are their phonological awareness skills impacted by their speech problems? If so, will these children be at a greater risk for developing reading and spelling difficulties? It appears that children with articulation-based disorders—and, therefore, motor-based problems that affect the mechanics of actually producing the sound—are not at high risk for literacy problems (e.g., Bishop & Adams, 1990; Catts, 1993; Dodd, 1995). However, those children who have a phonemic-based disorder are potentially at risk for written language difficulties. The extent of this problem is probably determined by their patterns of linguistic strengths and weaknesses (Gillon, 2004). The specific findings from children with expressive phonemic-based difficulties and their phonological awareness skills may be summarized as follows:

1. As a group, children with phonemic-based difficulties show deficits on a variety of phonological awareness tasks (e.g., Bird & Bishop, 1992; Bird, Bishop, & Freeman, 1995; Gillon, 2000; Marion, Sussman, & Marquardt, 1993; Preston, Hull, & Edwards, 2013; Webster & Plante, 1992).

2. Without intervention, these difficulties with phonological awareness persist over time. Difficulties have been especially noted in acquiring phonemic level skills (e.g., Gillon, 2002; Snowling, Bishop, & Stothard, 2000).

3. Children with additional spoken language problems (morphosyntactic or semantic) generally experience poorer long-term outcomes in reading and writing when compared to children with isolated phonemic-based production difficulties (Bishop & Adams, 1990; Catts & Kamhi, 1999; Hodson, 1994; Lewis, Freebairn, & Taylor, 2000; Preston, Hull, & Edwards, 2013; Snowling, Goulandris, & Stackhouse, 1994; Stackhouse, 1993, 1997; Wells, Stackhouse, & Vance, 1996).

4. In addition to phonological awareness difficulties, children with expressive phonemic-based problems display weaknesses in other areas that appear to be important for literacy development, including letter-name knowledge and verbal working memory (e.g., Webster, Plante, & Couvillion, 1997).

5. The type of phonemic-based disorder is relevant to predicting reading outcomes. Thus, children who show consistent use of unusual or idiosyncratic errors (as opposed to normal developmental processes) may evidence more severe difficulties in acquiring literacy skills (e.g., Dodd et al., 1995; Leitao, Hogben, & Fletcher, 1997; Preston, Hull, & Edwards, 2013).

6. The severity of a child's phonemic-based disorder influences literacy outcomes. Children with severe phonemic-based disorders, significant phonological processing difficulties, and other language impairments are very likely to have persistent reading and spelling difficulties (e.g., Bird et al., 1995; Bishop & Robson, 1989; Larrivee & Catts, 1999; Stackhouse, 1982, 1997). However, for the most part, these children respond positively to phonological awareness instruction, which can prevent the long-term effects (Gillon, 2000).

To summarize, phonological awareness is a subcategory of phonological processing. It contains many different levels of skills and seems to demonstrate a systematic developmental sequence. It is highly correlated to later reading and spelling abilities. Children with phonemic-based difficulties demonstrate more problems with phonological awareness and, consequently, difficulties with reading acquisition. These reading and spelling deficits may persist, especially in children with idiosyncratic errors and those with severe phonemic-based problems.

Prosodic Feature Development

As prosodic features evolve, they begin to assume grammatical function. For example, specific intonation patterns are employed to differentiate between statements and certain questions in English ("He is coming."↘ versus "He is coming?"↗). Contrasting stress realizations signal different word classes ('construct versus con 'struct). On the sentence level, the combined effects of higher pitch and increased loudness usually convey communicatively important modifications of basic meaning ("This is a 'pen" versus " 'This is a pen"). This section examines the grammatical function of prosodic features in school-age children and their relationship to phonological development.

As previously noted, children begin to use intonational patterns toward the end of the first year of life. As these grammatical abilities develop, new uses of intonation emerge. For example, the contrast between rising and falling pitch differentiates the two grammatical functions of a tag question in English ("asking" as in "We're ready, aren't we?" ↗ and "telling" as in "We're ready, aren't we!" ↘). Differences in intonation patterns such as these appear to be learned during children's third year (Crystal, 2010). However, the learning of intonation goes on for a long time. Studies report that children as old as 12 years were still acquiring some of the fundamental functions of English intonation, especially those for signaling grammatical contrast (Cruttenden, 1985; Ianucci & Dodd, 1980; Wells, Peppé, & Goulandris, 2004). As Crystal reported, even teenagers have been shown to have difficulty understanding sentences in which intonation and pausing are used to differentiate meanings. His example: "She *dressed*, and fed the baby" (indicating she dressed herself and then fed the baby) versus "She *dressed* and *fed* the baby" (indicating she dressed as well as fed the baby). Thus, although certain intonational features seem to be among the earliest phonological acquisitions, others may be some of the last.

Several studies have examined the use of contrastive stress both on the word level ('record versus re'cord) and on the sentence level (determining whom Mary hit in the following sentences: "John hit Bill and then *Mary* hit him" versus "John hit Bill and then Mary hit *him*") (e.g., Atkinson-King, 1973; Chomsky, 1971; Hornby & Hass, 1970; Myers & Myers, 1983). Although the ages differ depending on the type and design of the research, results suggest that children are still learning certain aspects of contrastive stress until the age of 13.

The acquisition of prosodic features is a gradual process that in some respects extends into the teens. It is closely connected to the new phonological, morphosyntactic, semantic, and pragmatic demands placed on developing children. As the complexity of the linguistic environment and the children's interaction with that environment increase, so do the subtle intricacies of each of these language levels.

SUMMARY

First, this chapter provided an overview of structural and functional development in infancy and early childhood. At birth, the infant's respiratory, phonatory, resonatory, and articulatory systems are not fully developed. Many changes must occur before the systems are ready to support sound and voice production for speech. In addition, children's perceptual abilities are developing. The second portion of this chapter summarized early perceptual skills, including categorical perception and phonemic awareness. The third section of this chapter traced the segmental form and prosodic feature development of children from vocalizations prior to babbling to the time when their speech sound inventory has reached an adultlike form. The prevalence of certain sounds and syllable shapes was traced from babbling to the first words. As the number of words in children's vocabularies increases, inventory and complexity of syllables grow as well. During this early stage of expansion, the prosodic feature, intonation, begins to be used to signal different intentions.

The linguistic development of preschool children is characterized by a large growth in all aspects of language; the acquisition of new phonological features is a portion of this quickly maturing system. Although cross-sectional studies have attempted to provide so-called mastery ages for sounds, these results cannot be easily generalized. Longitudinal data that document individual variability in sound acquisition as well as the influence of other language areas on phonological skills were then summarized. This section included a brief summary of the speech sound and phonological difficulties that children learning English as a second language may encounter. The suppression of many phonological processes is occurring within this time interval as well. Based on research findings, approximate ages were given for the suppression of several common phonological processes.

Both segmental form and prosodic features continue to mature during children's school years. Although the sound inventory is approaching adult-like form, many aspects of the phonological system are still maturing. Children need to learn morphophonemic variations as well as metaphonological skills. Metaphonological skills were briefly discussed in relationship to the emerging literacy of children. During the school years, phonological development often impacts children's abilities to learn reading and writing. The close interdependencies among phonology, language development, and literacy learning point to the importance of normal phonological development in children.

CASE STUDY

Diagnostic Implications of Phonological Process Suppression

Approximate ages of suppression have been provided for several common phonological processes. This information can be helpful during our diagnostic assessment. The following phonological processes were identified in Clint, age 3;6.

Word	Production	Phonological Process
house	[haʊ]	Final consonant deletion
cup	[kʌ]	Final consonant deletion
gun	[gʌ]	Final consonant deletion
shovel	[ʃʌbəl]	Stopping of [v]
vacuum	[bækju]	Stopping of [v], final consonant deletion
vase	[beɪ]	Stopping of [v], final consonant deletion
scratching	[krætʃɪŋ]	Consonant cluster reduction
skunk	[kʌŋk]	Consonant cluster reduction
star	[taɚ]	Consonant cluster reduction
jumping	[dʌmpɪŋ]	Stopping of [dʒ]
jelly	[dɛli]	Stopping of [dʒ]
jeep	[dip]	Stopping of [dʒ]
that	[dæt]	Stopping of [ð]
bath	[bæt]	Stopping of [θ]
feather	[fɛdɚ]	Stopping of [ð]

Similar processes were also noted in conversational speech.

Which of the noted processes should be suppressed by age 3;6? Final consonant deletion is usually suppressed by around age 3;0, whereas stopping of [v], [θ], [ð], and [dʒ] extends to age 3;6 or beyond. Consonant cluster reduction is also a process that is suppressed at a relatively late age. Based on these results, the only process that might cause concern at Clint's age would be final consonant deletion. Again, discretion must be exercised when using these approximate ages of suppression as the sole criterion for determining the necessity for intervention.

THINK CRITICALLY

1. Lori is a 20-month-old toddler who is brought to your clinic by her parents who are concerned that she has not begun to say real words. Although she babbles strings of babbles, such as [baba], [maba], [toto], and [dada], she does not evidence true words

nor does she impose intonation or rhythmic patterns on the babbles. The parents report that just recently (within the last 2 to 3 weeks), Lori occasionally imitates a babble that she has just produced if the parents have her attention and immediately say her babble back to her. What prelinguistic stage is Lori in? Approximately how delayed is she in respect to speech development?

2. The following results of an articulation test are from Ryan, age 6;6. We noted his phonological processes in Chapter 4.

horse	[hoᵘɚθ]	pig	[pɪk]	chair	[ʃɛɚ]
wagon	[wægən]	cup	[kʌp]	watch	[waʃ]
monkey	[mʌŋki]	swinging	[ṣwɪŋɪŋ]	thumb	[fʌm]
comb	[koᵘm]	table	[teˈbəl]	mouth	[maᵘf]
fork	[foɚk]	cat	[kæt]	shoe	[su]
knife	[naˈf]	ladder	[læsɾɚ]	fish	[fɪs]
cow	[kaᵘ]	ball	[bal]	zipper	[ðɪpɚ]
cake	[keˈk]	plane	[pweˈn]	nose	[noᵘθ]
baby	[beˈbi]	cold	[koᵘd]	sun	[θʌn]
bathtub	[bæftəb]	jumping	[dʌmpən]	house	[haᵘθ]
nine	[naˈn]	TV	[tivi]	steps	[stɛp]
train	[tweˈn]	stove	[θtoᵘv]	nest	[nɛt]
gun	[gʌn]	ring	[wɪŋ]	books	[bʊkθ]
dog	[dag]	tree	[twi]		
yellow	[wɛloᵘ]	green	[gwin]		
doll	[dal]	this	[dɪθ]		
bird	[bɝd]	whistle	[wɪθəl]		
carrots	[kɛɚət]				

Based on Ryan's age, compare which sounds might be considered in *error* if the ages of speech sound development from the Poole (1934) versus the Templin (1957) investigations are used (page 125). (Actually any two studies could be used for comparison.) Discuss the problems when using these sound mastery age levels.

3. Use the results generated in Chapter 4 (pages 93–94) that identified the phonological processes noted for Ryan. Based on his age (6 years, 6 months), identify which phonological processes are age appropriate, which ones might be considered borderline, and which ones should be suppressed at his age.

TEST YOURSELF

1. *Prelinguistic behavior* refers to
   a. the development of an infant's vocal tract
   b. the ability to perceive speech sounds prior to birth
   c. all vocalizations prior to a child's first words
   d. prosodic feature development

2. Infants begin to learn about voice and speech
   a. prior to birth (in the womb)
   b. at birth when others begin talking to them
   c. when they start babbling
   d. when they say their first word

3. Canonical babbling includes
   a. reduplicated babbling
   b. nonreduplicated babbling
   c. reflexive babbling
   d. a and b
   e. none of the above
4. Which prosodic feature seems to be the first to develop?
   a. contrastive stress
   b. intonation
   c. syllable stress
   d. durational variations
5. Which stage typically is the beginning of the linguistic phase of language development?
   a. canonical babbling
   b. nonreduplicated babbling
   c. first-50-word stage
   d. two-word stage
6. What syllable shapes predominate the first-50-word stage of language development?
   a. CV, VC, and CVC
   b. CVCC
   c. CCVC
   d. CVCVCC

7. Which one of the following is among the later developing sounds?
   a. [f]
   b. [j]
   c. [s]
   d. [k]
8. Which of the following is *not* a syllable structure process?
   a. cluster reduction
   b. final consonant deletion
   c. gliding
   d. reduplication
9. If a child says [tip] for *keep*, this is an example of which type of process?
   a. stopping
   b. gliding
   c. fronting
   d. epenthesis
10. Which one of the following refers to a child's conscious awareness of sounds within his or her native language?
    a. morphophonology
    b. metaphonology
    c. phonetic coding
    d. phonotactics

FURTHER READINGS

Gillon, G. (2004). *Phonological awareness: From research to practice.* New York: Guilford Press.

Hua, Z., & Dodd, B. (Eds.). (2006). *Phonological development and disorders: A multilingual perspective.* North Somerset, UK: Multilingual Matters.

Lowe, R. (2002). *Workbook for the identification of phonological processes and distinctive features.* Austin, TX: PRO-ED.

McGuinness, D. (2005). *Language development and learning to read: The scientific study of how language development affects reading skill.* Cambridge, MA: MIT Press.

Assessment and Appraisal
Collection of Data

LEARNING OBJECTIVES

When you have finished this chapter, you should be able to:

- Compare and contrast "screening" and a "comprehensive assessment."
- Identify the advantages and disadvantages of articulation tests and stimulability testing.
- Identify specific assessment measures that can be used to supplement articulation testing.

- Evaluate structures and functions of the speech mechanism within the appraisal process.
- Define and know how to assess emerging phonology.
- Identify the specific procedures that can be used to aid in the evaluation of an unintelligible child.

THE PREVIOUS CHAPTERS have provided a foundation that can now be applied to the diagnosis and treatment of impaired articulation and phonology. Before our diagnosis begins, two questions should be asked: (1) What information do we actually need? and (2) How should we gather that information? Consider a child coming to speech/language services whose parents are concerned because the child's speech is virtually unintelligible. On the other hand, consider an adolescent who seeks therapy because of a somewhat conspicuous [s]-production. These two individuals present completely different situations, ages, and degrees of impairment, and we would need different information to effectively evaluate the situation. How, then, do we assess these diverse situations? The first step is to look at the various parts of an assessment.

Assessment is one of the most important tasks clinicians perform; it is the basis for treatment decisions. **Assessment**, the clinical evaluation of a client's disorder, can be divided into two phases: appraisal and diagnosis (Darley, 1991). **Appraisal** refers to the collection of data, whereas **diagnosis** represents the end result of studying and interpreting these data.

Therefore, the appraisal portion of our assessment would answer the two questions previously stated concerning what information we actually need and how we gather that information. Appraisal is a very important aspect of our assessment. The collection of too little or unspecific information will not provide enough data for an adequate diagnosis. At the other extreme, collecting too much or unnecessary data is wasting the client's and clinician's valuable time. Therefore, professional assessment demands qualified (and verifiable) decisions throughout the appraisal process.

This chapter deals with the collection of data for an assessment. Its first goal is to identify the different types of data needed for a comprehensive diagnosis. These parts are identified and procedures outlined for each method. The second goal is to emphasize clinicians' roles in choosing among available measures—that is, the clinical decision-making process leading to the selection of instruments serving each individual client maximally. Effective assessments are essential for clinical procedures; they lead us through the entire diagnostic and therapeutic process.

> **BOX 6.1**   Interviewing and Obtaining Case History Information: Bibliographical Sources
>
> Haynes, W. O., & Pindzola, R. H. (2004). *Diagnosis and evaluation in speech pathology* (6th ed.). Boston: Allyn & Bacon.
>
> Rollin, W. (2000). *Counseling individuals with communication disorders* (2nd ed.). Boston: Butterworth-Heineman.
>
> Ruscello, D. M. (2000). *Tests and measurements in speech language pathology*. Woburn, MA: Butterworth-Heinemann.
>
> Shipley, K. G., & McAfee, J. G. (2004). *Assessment in speech-language pathology: A resource manual* (3rd ed.). San Diego, CA: Singular Thomson Learning.
>
> Shipley, K. G., & Roseberry-McKibbin, C. (2006). *Interviewing and counseling in communicative disorders: Principles and procedures*. Austin, TX: Pro-Ed.
>
> Tomblin, J. B., Morris, H. L., & Spriestersbach, D. C. (2000). *Diagnosis in speech-language pathology* (2nd ed.). San Diego, CA: Singular Thomson Learning.
>
> Westby, C., Burda, A., & Mehta, Z. (2003). Asking the Right Questions in the Right Ways: Strategies for Ethnographic Interviewing. Retrieved from www.asha.org/about/publications/leader-online/archives/2003/q2/f030429b.htm.

The data collection involves at least four different areas: (1) case history, (2) interviews with parents and other professionals, (3) school and medical records, and (4) evaluation by the clinician. Procedures and information important for the first three areas are covered in many texts. Selected sources are given in Box 6.1. This chapter covers only the fourth and most specific task, the evaluation by the clinician.

Evaluation by the Clinician

Clinicians collect data in two different ways: through a procedure known as *screening* or a more comprehensive evaluation. A **screening** consists of activities or tests that identify individuals who merit further evaluation. A screening procedure does not collect nearly enough data to establish a diagnosis; it only demonstrates the need for further testing. Screening measures can be formal or informal. Formal measures include elicitation procedures, which often have normative data and cutoff scores. Informal measures are typically devised by the examiner and may be directed toward a particular population or age level. Screenings are typically used to give the clinician an initial impression of a client. However, many states are moving away from using screening measures in the public schools. In these states, a complete assessment battery is administered using standardized tests to document the presence or absence of a specific disorder. This author uses a spontaneous language sample (see page 153) in addition to information supplied by the teacher and/or parent to "screen" whether a child demonstrates specific speech sound or language issues. If there is a concern, the child is then referred for a comprehensive evaluation. Screenings are beneficial for those individuals who "fail" the procedure and are later more comprehensively evaluated. Screenings are not always reliable in that some individuals may "pass" the procedure but still demonstrate impairments. Screenings were not devised to serve as a database for a diagnosis; they are too limited in their scope. In contrast, a **comprehensive evaluation** is a series of activities and tests that allows a more detailed and complete collection of data. A *comprehensive phonetic-phonemic evaluation* is the core of the appraisal for articulatory/phonological impairments. It includes data from the following sources:

- An articulation test and stimulability measures
- Conversational speech assessment in varying contexts
- Hearing testing

- Speech mechanism examination
- The possible selection of additional measures such as language testing, perceptual performance, contextual testing, and/or cognitive assessment (Bernthal, Bankson, & Flipsen, 2009; Lowe, 1994)

The following section examines each of the activities of this process, beginning with an initial impression and its usefulness in the collection of data.

Initial Impression

Clinicians can start collecting data even before the formal appraisal actually begins—for example, by closely observing the conversation between a caregiver and a child, a teacher and a child in a classroom situation, or a child communicating with his or her peers. This initial contact will provide an important first impression. The task is to notice certain features of the conversation and put them onto a simple form such as the one in Figure 6.1. Although additional variables have to be considered later, this record of the initial impression is meant to aid in planning and organizing the remainder of the assessment.

If the initial impression is that a child is partly or totally intelligible, the next step, the collection of data from an articulation test, could be initiated. If, on the other hand, the initial impression yields an unintelligible child, additional procedures for data collection may need to be considered, especially for the spontaneous speech sample. Very young children, adults with dysarthria or apraxia of speech, and individuals with English as a second language all require additional considerations. Guidelines for these populations are found later in this chapter and in Chapter 8 and 11.

Name _____ Age _____

Conversational partner _____ Date _____

Intelligibility

Good _____ Partly intelligible _____ Unintelligible _____

Single-word responses and continuous speech show comparable intelligibility _____

Single-word responses are more intelligible than continuous speech _____

General overview of misarticulations

Affects consonants _____

Affects consonants and vowels _____

Noted misarticulations _____

_____

_____

Other factors affecting intelligibility (for example, hyper- or denasality, vocal loudness or quality, rate of speech)

_____

Caregiver's/teacher's/peer's response to misarticulations

No response _____ Asks for repetition _____ Tries to correct _____

Child's response to parent's/caregiver's intervention _____

_____

_____

FIGURE 6.1 Sample Form for the Initial Impression

In some states and public schools, observation of children in their classroom or school environment is the only "screening" measure allowed by law. If a child is pulled from the classroom and in any way informally or formally tested, a parent signature is required. Check with your school district to find out the procedure in your particular school and state.

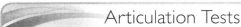

Articulation Tests

Articulation tests are typically designed to elicit spontaneous naming based on the presentation of pictures. Most consonants of General American English are tested in the initial, medial, and final positions of words.

Some Advantages and Disadvantages of Articulation Tests

Use of articulation tests has several advantages. First, these tests are relatively easy to give and score; the necessary time expenditure is usually minimal. This is an attractive feature for those who feel limited in the time they can spend with appraisal procedures. Second, the results provide the clinician with a quantifiable list of "incorrect" sound productions in different word positions. This is clearly relevant to further assessment and therapy planning. Third, the use of norm-referenced, standardized, single-word tests is typically considered to be a necessary part of an evaluation for a speech sound disorder (Skahan, Watson, & Lof, 2007). Scores from these tests allow the clinician to compare an individual client's performance with the performance of others of a similar age. In addition, these scores could be used to document the client's need for, and progress in, therapy.

There are, however, also several problems inherent in articulation tests. They can be summarized as follows:

1. An articulation test examines sound articulation in selected isolated words. However, eliciting sounds based on single-word responses can never give adequate information on the client's production realities in connected speech. Sound articulation within selected words may not be representative of a client's ability to produce a particular sound under natural speech conditions.

2. Articulation tests do not give enough information about a client's phonological system. Articulation tests are measures of speech sound production. As such, they were never meant to provide enough assessment data for a phonological analysis. Although some spontaneous naming measures analyze sounds in error according to phonological processes, the information they provide is not enough for a comprehensive phonological analysis.

3. Articulation tests do not test all sounds in all the contexts in which they occur in General American English. Although this would admittedly be a rather large task, some articulation tests do not even test the total inventory of speech sounds of General American English. If scored according to the directions provided, most articulation tests do not test vowels, for example, and very few consonant clusters are sampled.

4. The sounds actually tested do not occur in comparable phonetic contexts; that is, they are not context controlled. For example, the sounds before and after the tested consonants are different from word to word. The words used also vary in lengths and complexities. This presents the client with a task that changes in the production difficulty from word to word. An analysis by Eisenberg and Hitchcock (2010) found that only 4 of the 11 articulation tests they reviewed demonstrated a controlled environment for a large number of the word-initial consonants. In this same

study, none of the tests demonstrated a controlled word environment for a large number of the word-final consonants tested.

5. Articulation tests, like all standardized tests, are selected probes into rather limited aspects of an individual's total articulatory behavior and/or abilities. An articulation test examines only a very small portion of a person's articulatory behavior—it explores her or his speech performance with particular test items, on a certain day, in a unique testing situation. It would not be realistic to generalize that such limited results represent a reliable measure of the client's articulatory abilities, let alone the client's phonological system.

Pick one articulation test that you have available. Consider that you are testing a child with [s] and [z] problems. How many words does the test contain that would identify these sounds? Count also those words that are not specifically testing [s] or [z] for the articulation score but do contain these sounds. Do you think you have an adequate number of words?

There are 13 word-initial and 13 word-final [s] clusters in General American English. How many consonant clusters does the articulation test you have chosen include?

Factors to Consider When Selecting a Measure of Articulation

In selecting a measure of speech sound competency, several factors are important. In addition to the test's construct and its technical characteristics, the following should be considered: (1) its appropriateness for the client's age or developmental level, (2) its ability to supply a standardized score, (3) its analysis of the sound errors, and (4) its inclusion of an adequate sample of the sound(s) relevant to the individual client at hand.

Appropriateness for the Age or Developmental Level of the Client. Although the age ranges vary, most tests can be administered to children from approximately 3 years to school age. Selection becomes a troublesome issue for very young and older adolescent or adult clients. Younger clients, who may include 2-year-olds or delayed 3- and 4-year-olds, may not respond well to a formal articulation test. Some younger children might react better to those tests that contain large colored pictures or realistic manipulatable objects. For other children, the naming of actual objects or spontaneous speech may be the only way to assess sound production skills. For the evaluation of adolescent or adult clients, two problems exist. First, many of the tests are not standardized for children beyond the ages of 12 or 13. In addition, most articulation tests are oriented toward a much younger population. This may prove demeaning for older adolescents and adults and, therefore, is inappropriate. Certain articulation tests contain printed sentences that can be read by clients. Although the sentence content and the reading level are designed for early school-age children, articulation tests that provide sentences to be read might prove less of a problem for older clients.

Later in this chapter, the section on "Special Considerations" examines alternative ways to assess younger clients with emerging phonological systems.

Ability to Provide a Standardized Score. Some articulation tests are not standardized; that is, standardized scores are not available as outcome measures. Although this is seldom the case in newer tests, older tests—although worthwhile probes—do not give standardized measures. Therefore, the results obtained from a client cannot be compared to the performance of other individuals of a similar age. Many sites, especially public school settings, require that the test provide standardized measures for assessment purposes; therefore, tests should be selected correspondingly.

Analysis of the Sound Errors. Many different tests are available. Some are labeled articulation tests, whereas others purport to be tests of *phonology*. Most articulation tests and tests of phonology do not differ in their examination format (both use the same format: spontaneous picture naming) but in their analysis of the results. Typically, tests of phonology categorize misarticulations according to phonological processes. Although the clinician could go through any articulation test noting the number and type of phonological processes used, those tests that already contain such a procedure will probably allow the clinician a more expedient assessment.

See Table 6.1 for an overview of a few articulation tests that can be used to assess preschool and school-age children.

CLINICAL APPLICATION

Using Articulation Tests to Examine Phonological Processes

The evaluation of phonological processes is a portion of several articulation tests (e.g., Assessment Link between Phonology and Articulation [ALPHA], Lowe, 1996; Bankson-Bernthal Test of Phonology, Bankson & Bernthal, 1990; and Khan-Lewis Phonological Analysis (Khan & Lewis, 2002), which uses the responses from the Goldman-Fristoe Test of Articulation. See Table 6.1 for additional tests that provide analysis procedures for phonological processes. Phonological processes can be determined from the results of any articulation test. The clinician examines the results of the articulation test and notes the phonological processes employed. The following is an example from the PAT-3: Photo Articulation Test (Lippke, Dickey, Selmar, & Soder, 1997):

Word	Child's Response	Phonological Process
saw	[tɑ]	stopping [s] → [t]
pencil	[pɛnθəl]	consonant cluster substitution [ns] → [nθ], fronting [s] → [θ]
house	[haʊ]	final consonant deletion [s] → ∅
spoon	[pun]	consonant cluster reduction [sp] → [p]
skates	[keˈtθ]	consonant cluster reduction [sk] → [k]
		consonant cluster substitution [ts] → [tθ], fronting
stars	[tɑɚ]	consonant cluster reduction [st] → [t]
		final consonant deletion [z] → ∅[1]
zipper	[dɪpɚ]	stopping [z] → [d]

[1]In this example, the production is characterized as a final consonant deletion because [ɑɚ] is considered a centering diphthong.

Which phonological processes are operating and how often they occurred could then be analyzed.

TABLE 6.1   Selected Examples of Articulation and Phonological Tests

Name	Age Range	Word Positions Tested	Scores Provided	Comments
Articulation Tests				
Arizona 3: Arizona Articulation Proficiency Scale (3rd ed.). Fudala, J. (2000). Los Angeles: Western Psychological services.	1;6 to 18;11 years	Initial- and final-word positions.	Standardized, gives standard score, Z-score, percentile, speech intelligibility values, and level of articulatory impairment.	Gives weighted scores for each consonant. Tests vowels. A 4th edition that offers phonological process analysis is being developed.
Goldman-Fristoe 2 Test of Articulation (2nd ed.). Goldman, R., & Fristoe, M. (2000). Circle Pines, MN: American Guidance Service	2 to 16+ years	Initial-, medial-, and final-word positions.	Standardized, gives standard score, and percentile rank; a confidence interval can be calculated.	Can be used with the Khan-Lewis test (Khan, L., & Lewis N. [2002]. Circle Pines, MN: American Guidance Service) to assess phonological processes

Name	Age Range	Word Positions Tested	Scores Provided	Comments
Photo Articulation Test: PAT-3 (3rd ed.). Lippke, S., Dickey, S., Selmar, J., & Soder, A. (1997). Danville, IL: Interstate Printers and Publishers	3 to 12 years	Initial-, medial-, and final-word positions.	Standardized, gives standard scores, age equivalents, and percentiles.	Uses actual photographs to test sounds; tests vowels and diphthongs.
Structured Photographic Articulation Test-II (2nd ed.). Dawson, J. I., & Tattersall, P. J. (2001). DeKalb, IL: Janelle Publications.	3 to 9 years	Initial-, medial-, and final-word positions.	Standardized scores including standard scores, percentile score ranks, percentile band scores, test-age equivalent scores.	Uses photographs of Dudsberry, a cute golden retriever puppy, interacting with various objects. It does not test vowels although the manual provides a probe for imitation of each vowel in one word. The aim is to test articulation although seven common phonological processes are provided.
Phonological Tests				
Assessment Link between Phonology and Articulation—Revised. Lowe, R. (1996). Mifflinville, PA: Speech and Language Resources	3 to 8;11 years	Initial- and final-word positions.	Standardized, gives standard scores, percentile ranks.	The manual provides several analyses and gives analysis forms that can be used to document phonological processes, vowel errors, and consonant clusters.
Bankson Bernthal Test of Phonology. Bankson, N., & Bernthal, J. (1990). Austin, TX: Pro-Ed.	3 to 6 years	Initial- and final-word positions.	Standardized, gives standard score, percentile rank, and standard error of measurement.	Provides various ways to analyze results, phonological processes included.
Clinical Assessment of Articulation and Phonology: CAAP (2nd ed.). Secord, W. A., & Donohue, J. S. (2002). Greenville, SC: Super Duper Publications.	2;6 to 11;11 years	Pre- and postvocalic consonants.	Standard scores, percentile rank scores, age equivalent scores.	Consonant clusters tested are only words containing [s], [r], and [l] clusters. Vowels are not tested. Sentences are provided which can be used with children who can read.
Diagnostic Evaluation of Articulation and Phonology (DEAP). Dodd, B., Hua, Z., Crosbie, S., Holm, A., & Ozanne, A. (2006). San Antonio, TX: Pearson.	3 to 8;11 years	Initial- and final-word positions.	Standardized, provides standard scores and percentile ranks for several measures.	Subtests include Sounds in Words, Phonological Process Use, Single Words vs. Connected Speech Agreement Criterion. Contains a diagnostic screen and articulation, phonology, and oral motor screening.
HAPP-3 Hodson Assessment of Phonological Patterns (3rd ed.). Hodson, B. (2004). Austin, TX: Pro-Ed.	Preschool	Initial-, medial-, and final-word positions.	Standardized, gives percentile rank and severity rating.	Assesses phonological processes, can be used as a direct link to the cycles approach.
Khan-Lewis Phonological Analysis (2nd ed.). Khan, L., & Lewis, N. (2002). Circle Pines, MN: American Guidance Service.	2 to 21;11 years	Initial-, medial- and final-word positions.	Ten developmental phonological processes yield standard scores, percentile rank scores, test-age equivalent scores, and percentage of occurrence for individual processes by age.	This test uses the words from the Goldman-Fristoe Test of Articulation and translates errors into more common phonological processes. As with the Goldman Fristoe, vowels are not tested.

Note: All standardized measures have used the latest U.S. Census reports to determine gender, race/ethnicity, and geographical percentages that are used in direct proportion for their standardization population.

Inclusion of an Adequate Sample of the Sound or Sounds Relevant for the Individual Client. Articulation tests typically contain words that sample the sound inventory of General American English. Thus, most of the consonants of General American English are examined within the articulation test. However, most articulation tests do not sample the most frequently misarticulated sounds in a large number of different contexts. For example, the [s] may be tested in only two or three different words. An adequate number of words containing the sound in various word positions is often not available. Supplemental testing with additional words can always be achieved later, but a test that provides adequate goal-directed material for individual clients uses our diagnostic time more efficiently.

Assessment Procedures to Supplement Articulation Tests

Which assessment strategies, then, can be employed to minimize the previously mentioned shortcomings of articulation tests?

1. *If a word contains any aberrant vowel or consonant productions, transcribe the entire word.* This gives valuable additional information about the client's sound production skills. For example, assume that the tested word is *yellow*, that the initial [j] is being evaluated, and that the client says [jɛwoᵁ]. According to the scoring instructions, the initial [j] would be noted as being "correct," and the clinician would continue on to the next item. However, if the entire word has been transcribed, the clinician can later evaluate the [l] production and compare it to the other words on the test that contain [l]. (In addition, some articulation measures test only sounds in the initial and final word positions; however, some clients demonstrate difficulties with medial productions.) Transcribing the entire word complements the test information considerably and supplies insights into vowels and consonant cluster productions as well.

2. *Supplement the articulation test with additional utterances that address the client's noted problems.* The target sound(s) should be sampled in various vowel contexts and word positions, for example. There are several ways to do this. One is to develop a list of words containing the needed sound(s). This has the advantage of tailoring the supplemental materials to exactly fit the client's needs. One could also use commercially prepared materials. Two examples are McDonald's Deep Test of Articulation (McDonald, 1964) and Secord's Clinical Probes of Articulation Consistency (C-PAC) (Secord, 1981a). McDonald's Deep Test uses pictures to elicit a compound word, such as *hot + dog = hotdog*. The words formed are not typical compound words of General American English; however, a variety of phonetic contexts can be sampled this way. The C-PAC assesses the targeted consonant before and after various vowels (in one-syllable words, consonants initiating and terminating the word) in consonant clusters, in sentences, and during storytelling. For children who cannot read, the elicitation mode is imitative. These commercially available protocols have the advantage of assessing a sound in a variety of contexts without any preparation on the part of the clinician.

Articulation tests are often referred to as citation-form testing. *Citation form* refers to the spoken form of a word produced in isolation as distinguished from the form it would have when produced in conversational speech. Both citation-form testing and spontaneous speech sampling should be used to collect data for a comprehensive evaluation.

3. *Always sample and record continuous speech.* Although it has been well documented that production differences exist in clients between single-word tasks (citing) and spontaneous speech (talking) (e.g., Andrews & Fey, 1986; Bernhardt & Holdgrafer, 2001; Morrison & Shriberg, 1992), many practitioners continue to use articulation tests as the sole basis for their analysis procedures. Morrison and Shriberg state that "citation-form testing yields neither typical nor optimal measures of speech performance" (p. 271). An articulation test is not good enough for the appraisal and diagnosis of clients with speech sound disorders. See the section "Spontaneous Speech Sampling" for further information.

4. *Determine the stimulability of the error sounds.* This task can be easily and relatively quickly accomplished at the end of an articulation test. See the following section on "Stimulability Testing."

Organizing Articulation Test Results: Describing the Error

Most articulation tests include a form that can be used to record a client's responses. By completing this form, the clinician obtains information about the accuracy of the sound articulation and the position of this sound within the test word. Each articulation test gives directions on how to record accurate and inaccurate sound realizations. At least three different scoring systems describe sound errors (Shriberg & Kent, 2013). The following scoring systems are available.

Two-Way Scoring. A choice is made between a production that is "right" (accurate articulation of the sound in question) and "wrong" (inaccurate articulation). Two-way scoring can be used effectively to give feedback to the client and to document therapy progress. However, because of its limitations and its inability to render any usable information about the type of aberrant articulation taking place, the two-way scoring system is not appropriate for scoring articulation tests.

Five-Way Scoring. This system uses a classification based on the type of error. "Correct," or norm, productions constitute one category. The other four categories are (1) deletion or omission—that is, a sound is deleted completely, (2) substitution—a sound is replaced by another sound, (3) distortion—the target sound is approximated but not closely enough to be considered a norm realization, and (4) addition—a sound or sounds are added to the intended sound. The five-way scoring system is commonly suggested in the manuals of articulation tests.

However, this system has several inherent problems. First, articulation tests often do not define, or give examples of, which articulatory patterns are considered within normal limits. The many dialectal and contextual variations could result in a somewhat different but entirely acceptable pronunciation. For example, the alveolar flap [ɾ] is a common pronunciation for [d] in *ladder*. Should this variation be considered "correct" if the medial d-sound is being tested? Clinicians should be aware of these common variations and how they may impact their scoring. Second, the category of deletion or omission may include the presence, rather than the absence, of a sound. Normally, deletion implies that a sound segment has been eliminated, as in [mu] for *moon*, for example. However, Van Riper and Irwin (1958) include glottal stops, unvoiced articulatory placements, and short exhalations under omissions as well. If the production of [wæʔən] for *wagon* is considered, according to these authors, the [g] would be classified as a deletion. Actually, it would be more accurate to label this as a substitution of a glottal stop for [g]. This ambiguous definition of deletion can detract from the accuracy of the results when sound realizations are later analyzed. Third, the terms *substitution* and *distortion* have a long history of defi-nitional unclarity. Some authors (Van Riper, 1978; Van Riper & Irwin; Winitz, 1975) state that a more precise way to consider distortions is to regard them as substitutions of non-English sounds. For example, a child produces [ʃ] in which the active and passive articula-tors are too far back; that is, rather than prepalatal, it has a palatal placement. There is a palatal fricative, transcribed as [ç], that is a regular speech sound in many languages. Therefore, this palatal [ʃ] production could be designated either as a distortion of [ʃ] or as a substitution of [ç] for [ʃ]. Such vagueness in regard to what constitutes a distortion versus a substitution can also impact the scoring of many articulation tests.

Phonetic Transcription. Transcription systems describe speech behavior. The goal of any phonetic transcription is to represent spoken language by written symbols. Of the three scoring systems mentioned, phonetic transcription requires the highest degree of clinical skill. The goal is not to *judge* specific misarticulations but to *describe* them as accurately as possible. Phonetic transcription has several advantages over the other two systems: (1) it is far more precise, (2) it gives more information about the misarticula-tion, which is helpful for both assessment and intervention, and (3) among professionals, it is the most universally accepted way to communicate information about articulatory features. Phonetic transcription uses broad and narrow transcriptions including diacrit-ics, which are indispensable for a comprehensive evaluation. This system is used for the following analyses of citation articulation tests as well as spontaneous speech sampling.

Stimulability Testing

Another assessment procedure often used by clinicians during the assessment process is stimulability testing. **Stimulability testing** refers to testing the client's ability to produce a misarticulated sound in an appropriate manner when "stimulated" by the clinician to do so. Many variations in this procedure exist, but commonly, the clinician asks the client to "watch and listen to what I am going to say, and then you say it" (Bernthal, Bankson, & Flipsen, 2009). Although there is no standardized procedure for stimulability testing, an isolated sound is usually first attempted. If a norm articulation is achieved, the sound is placed within a syllable and subsequently in a word context. The number of models pro-vided by the clinician typically varies from one to five attempts.

For many clinicians, stimulability testing is a standard procedure concluding the administration of an articulation test. It gives a measure of the consistency of a client's performance on two different tasks: the spontaneous naming of a picture and the imitation of a speech model provided by the clinician. Such information is very helpful in appraising the articulatory capabilities of a client. (See Bleile, 2002; Hodson, Scherz, & Strattman, 2002; Khan, 2002; Lof, 2002; Miccio, 2002; and Tyler & Tolbert, 2002.)

Children's articulatory stimulability has been used to determine therapy goals and to predict which children might benefit more from therapy. It has been suggested that sounds that were more stimulable would be easier to work on in therapy; therefore, highly stimu-lable sounds would be targeted first (Rvachew & Nowak, 2001). When used as a means of predicting which children might benefit from therapy, high stimulability was correlated with more rapid therapeutic success (Miccio, Elbert, & Forrest, 1999). It was also proposed that high stimulability might mean that children were on the verge of acquiring the sounds and would not even need therapeutic intervention (Khan, 2002). Although stimulability testing seems to be one type of data collected by most clinicians, its effect on treatment targets is still questionable. In her article on treatment efficacy, Gierut (1998) points out that two studies (Klein, Lederer, & Cortese, 1991; Powell, Elbert, & Dinnsen, 1991) have documented that targeting nonstimulable sounds prompted change in those sounds and other untreated stimulable sounds. In comparison, treatment of a stimulable sound did not necessarily lead to changes in untreated stimulable or nonstimulable sounds. Gierut concludes that treatment of nonstimulable sounds may be more efficient than treatment of stimulable sounds because of the widespread change that seems to occur. However, a second study (Rvachew, Rafaat, & Martin, 1999) noted lack of treatment progress on nonstimulable sounds when compared to stimulable ones. To summarize, stimulability testing gives useful information. However, it should not be the only source when deciding whether a client receives services or which therapy sequence to choose.

Spontaneous Speech Sample

Over the years, a number of authors have documented the differences that exist in children's speech when single-word citing responses are compared to spontaneous speech (e.g., Andrews & Fey, 1986; Bernhardt & Holdgrafer, 2001; Masterson, Bernhardt, & Hofheinz, 2005; Morrison & Shriberg, 1992; Wolk & Meisler, 1998). However, assessment and treatment protocols continue to be based primarily on the results of citation articulation tests. Some clinicians may argue that they do not have time to complete the transcription and analysis of a spontaneous speech sample. However, these samples can serve many different functions. For example, conversational speech samples can supply additional information about the language, voice, and prosodic capabilities of the client. Based on the data from the spontaneous speech sample, specific semantic, morphosyntactical, and pragmatic analyses could supplement language testing when required. However, the conversational speech sample is not optional but a basic necessity for every professional assessment.

Although any conversational speech sample is more representative of a client's production capabilities than a one-word citation-form test, the type of sampling situation also plays a role. Several authors have found an increase or decrease in errors depending on the production task required. First, more complex linguistic contents generally cause an increase in misarticulations (Panagos & Prelock, 1982; Schmauch, Panagos, & Klich, 1978). Second, different communicative needs can also influence production accuracy. For example, improvement of speech patterns was noted in five children when they were trying to relate information that was important to them.

CLINICAL EXERCISES

More complex linguistic contexts generally cause an increase in misarticulations. For a 5-year-old, what would be a simple versus a more complex linguistic situation? How would you structure a simple linguistic situation?

In the five-way scoring system for articulation testing, why would those sounds listed as "distortions" need further delineation? Give an example of a distortion in which further information might be helpful in therapy.

Organization of the Continuous Speech Sample

A continuous speech sample should be planned and executed in a systematic manner to minimize the time investment and maximize the results. Here are some suggestions.

Begin with the Articulation Test. One goal of a continuous speech sample in a comprehensive assessment is to compare a client's productions on a single-word citation task to those in continuous speech. Errors that have been noted in single words can be helpful in planning the continuous speech sample. For example, if a child demonstrates error productions for [s], [ʃ], [tʃ], [dʒ], and [l] on the articulation test or if the articulation test does not sample particular sounds, these could be targeted.

Provide Objects or Pictures That May Elicit Targeted Sounds. Objects and pictures containing the targeted sounds can then become a portion of the spontaneous speech procedure. Speech-language specialists could increase comparability between citing and talking tasks by attempting to trigger some of the same words that were on the articulation test.

Plan the Length of the Sample. There has been a lot of discussion about which sample length furnishes adequate information for a comprehensive assessment. Grunwell (1987) states that "100 different words is the minimum size of an adequate sample; 200–250 words is preferable" (p. 55). On the other hand, Crary (1983) found that 50-word samples for process analysis provided as much information as 100-word speech samples. More recently Heilmann, Nockerts, & Miller (2010) found that the results of a 1-minute sample were as consistent as 3- and 7-minute samples.

It should be kept in mind that in normal conversation, children articulate between 100 and 200 syllables per minute (Culatta, Page, & Wilson, 1987). Therefore, based on the findings of Heilmann et al. (2010), a 1-minute sample of conversational speech should render approximately 100–200 words, depending on the length of each word. In most cases, if the sample is organized, this will probably constitute an adequate sample. With most children, much of the transcription can be attained spontaneously. For example, a clinician could write what the client says and use only phonetic transcription for sounds in error. Assuming that another 10 minutes is required later to transcribe portions of the sample, the total recording and transcribing time amounts to around 15 minutes. In light of the acquisition of needed information for goal-directed therapy, this is not a large time investment. Perhaps a lack of the necessary transcription skills deters clinicians more than the actual time involvement. The bottom line for clinicians is that a spontaneous speech sample is not an option but is a necessity.

Plan Diversity into the Sample. Various communicative situations should be a portion of the recorded speech sample. A variety of situations will ensure that the sample adequately represents the client's phonetic and phonemic skills. This may include several talking situations, such as picture description, storytelling, describing the function of objects, and problem solving. Communicative diversity could also include the client talking with caregivers or siblings. Varying communicative situations also allow for articulatory differences that occur between pragmatically and linguistically diverse samples.

Monitor the Recording and Gloss Any Utterances That Might Later Be Difficult or Impossible to Understand from the Recording. Diligent monitoring will ensure that the quality of a recording remains constant. This can mean anything from readjusting the device being used if the client moves to asking the client to repeat an utterance if it is not completely intelligible. It is helpful and often necessary to gloss the word or phrase, especially if later transcription difficulties are anticipated. **Glossing** means repeating with normal pronunciation what the client has just said for easier identification later. This can be done quite naturally so that it will not interfere with the structured situation.

Transcribe As Much of the Spontaneous Speech Sample as Possible during the Recording. Live transcriptions have the advantage of capturing phonetic detail that may be lost with a recording. They also decrease the subsequent transcription time. In addition, listening to 1 or 2 minutes of conversation before actually recording the sample may dramatically increase transcription effectiveness because of the clinician's adjustment to the client's pronunciation patterns. Unintelligible utterances should be clearly marked (language sampling techniques use a series of *X*s to note unintelligibility). It is not necessary to spend time trying to decipher these responses. Instead, it is better to gloss the utterance whenever the intelligibility of the response might be later questioned.

Record the Continuous Speech Sample. Many currently used devices can record a language sample. Most individuals have a cell phone, which, depending on its sound quality, could be used to video record the client. Also the use of portable devices, such as iPads, whose sound and video quality is far superior to that of most cell phones, has become more popular. Whatever device you use, be sure to test its sound quality *before* you make the recording. Know how to utilize the sound volume control and where the built-in microphone on the device is located. The author missed a complete sample by allowing a child to hold the iPad but had a finger directly over the microphone. (Also be aware of covers that may fit too closely to the microphone and thus, impede its functioning.) Children typically like to see and hear the recordings that you have made of them. One idea is for the child or you to hold the device and make a short 10-second segment. Play this back and see whether it is loud enough and can be easily understood. If your cell phone's sound quality is not adequate, use another device. Most clinicians are provided a computer in their workplace. An adequate sound sample can be recorded using your computer and typically a small plug-in external microphone. Microphones are relatively inexpensive and can deliver a good-quality audio signal. Again, be careful placing the microphone and always test beforehand. For portable microphones, the best distance from the child is approximately 6 to 8 inches. The microphone should be slanted slightly toward the client's nose to eliminate distortions because of the expiratory release of certain consonants.

> ## CLINICAL EXERCISES
>
> You are planning a language sample with a 6;3-year-old boy who has difficulties with [l], [r], [ʃ], [tʃ], and [ʤ].
>
> What objects could you use to elicit a language sample containing these sounds?
>
> How would you build diversity into the spontaneous speech sample? Can you think of different situations, tasks, or pictures that you could use?

Evaluation of the Speech Mechanism

An evaluation of both the structure and the function of a client's speech mechanism is a prerequisite for any comprehensive assessment. Its intent is to assess whether the system appears adequate for regular speech sound production. At first glance, the examination of the speech-motor system looks like a relatively simple procedure that has often been described. However, the interpretation of the results is not necessarily as straightforward as it would seem.

It might be beneficial to view the results of the evaluation of the speech mechanism as being along a continuum in which one end indicates normal structure and function and the other end indicates grossly deviant structural and/or functional inadequacies. At the normal end of the continuum, assume that the client has passed all required procedures. This is commonly the case, and no further speech-motor testing appears to be necessary—the client has passed the oral-speech assessment.

At the other end of the continuum, results could show such a pronounced structural or functional aberration from norm that an organic cause of the speech difficulty needs to be considered. If organicity is noted, further testing and/or referral to a medical expert is warranted.

Between the endpoints of this continuum exists a broad range of structural and functional deviations that may or may not directly impact the adequate production of speech sounds. Often clinicians find minor structural and/or functional inadequacies that do not appear severe enough to be considered "organic" yet certainly do not qualify as "passing." Interpreting such results is often difficult. Our evaluation of the speech mechanism is actually just a screening measure requiring more testing and possible referral when any functional and/or structural inadequacies are found. One possible screening form for the evaluation of the speech-motor system is summarized in Appendix 6.1.

What to Look for When Evaluating the Speech Mechanism

Examining the Head and Facial Structures. One of the first impressions is obtained by simply observing the client's face and head. Sitting opposite the client, first evaluate the size and the shape of the head. Relative to the body size, the head should appear normal—not too large and not too small. In addition, its shape should be considered. The relationship between the cranium (the upper portion of the skull containing the brain) and the facial skeleton (the lower portion of the skull containing, among other structures, the articulators) should be evaluated. The cranial portion should not appear too large nor the facial area too small or vice versa. Micrognathia, for example, is marked by an unusually small jaw. Next, the symmetry of the facial features should be inspected. Do the right and left sides of the face appear fairly similar both in proportion and in overall appearance? *Proportion* refers to the structures on both sides being on corresponding planes and their dimensions being similar. For example, right and left eyes are level and both appear to be about the same size. *Appearance* refers to the overall shape of the structures in question and to the normal state of resting muscle—that is, to the muscular tone. Oddly shaped eyes, nose, or mouth would be a deviancy within this category. In addition, any drooping of the structures or lack of muscle tone on one side of the face should be noted. At rest, the right and left sides of the lips should be even, the red of the lips, or vermilion, forming a smooth curve. Appearance and proportions of the nares (the nostrils), the nasal septum (the structural division of the nose, dividing the nasal cavity into right and left halves), the philtrum (the vertical groove between the upper lip and the nasal septum), and the columella (the vertical ridges on either side of the philtrum) should be evaluated. In short, any striking features of the head and face should be noted. This would include a fairly common syndrome called *adenoid facies,* the result of chronic or repeated infections that lead to enlarged adenoids, mouth breathing, a shortening of the upper lip, and an elongated face (Zemlin, 1998).

Examining Breathing. Respiration can be indirectly observed by examining breathing patterns. The clinician should observe and evaluate the client's breathing patterns at rest (silent breathing) and during speech. During silent breathing, the client's mouth should be closed with no noticeable clavicular breathing (excursions in the clavicular area that cause the shoulders to move up and down during breathing). In addition, during silent breathing, the amount of time between the inspiratory and expiratory phases should be fairly equal. Therefore, an approximately one-to-one relationship exists between the time for inspiration and for expiration. During speech production, the normal time relationship between inspiratory and expiratory phases is somewhere between one and two+; that is, depending on the length of the utterance, the expiratory phase should be at least twice as long as the inspiratory. Any irregularities in breathing patterns should be noted. This includes irregular breathing patterns, muscular jerks or spasms during breathing, forced inhalations or exhalations, or any other (especially recurrent) conspicuous respiratory movements.

Examining the Oral and Pharyngeal Cavity Structures. The structures involved in this area of the speech mechanism examination include the teeth, the tongue, the palate, and the pharyngeal areas.

The Teeth. First, the occlusion of the teeth is important. Normal occlusion (Class I) is characterized by the lower molars being one-half of a tooth ahead of the upper molars. There are different types of malocclusions, including Class II (overbite), Class III (underbite), open bite, and cross bite. (Definitions of these malocclusions are given in Appendix 6.1.) Next, the clinician should check to see whether all teeth are present and that their spacing and axial orientation appear adequate. The *axial orientation* of the teeth refers to the positioning of the individual teeth. Abnormalities in this respect would pertain to irregularly "tipped" or rotated teeth. Malocclusions of the teeth and missing teeth may affect the production of specific speech sounds.

The Tongue. First, examine the size of the tongue in its relationship to the size of the oral cavity. Does it appear too large, overfilling the oral cavity (macroglossia), or does it seem too small for the cavity size (microglossia)? Either of these conditions would signal a deviancy. In addition, the tongue's appearance is examined to see whether the color appears normal and the muscular dorsum of the tongue demonstrates a healthy muscle tone. Any "shriveled" tongue appearance might signal a paralytic condition. Next, the surface of the tongue needs to be observed. It should be relatively smooth. Any fissures (grooves or cracks in the dorsum of the tongue), lesions (wounds or abrasion), and fasciculations (any visible "bundling" of muscles) would indicate a deviancy. Finally, the tongue needs to be examined in its resting position. It should look symmetrical without any muscular twitching or movements.

The Hard and Soft Palates. Until this point, the clinician has observed just structures. Examination of the hard and soft palate goes beyond observation. It necessitates feeling structures with a finger and evaluating structures within the pharyngeal cavity. Therefore, it is necessary that the clinician wear examining gloves and be equipped with a small penlight to carry out the task. The hard palate's color; the size and shape of the palatal vault; and the presence or absence of clefts, fissures, and fistulas (openings or holes in the palate) should be determined. The midline of the hard and soft palates is usually a pink and whitish color; a blue tint may suggest a submucous cleft. To exclude this possibility, the clinician should feel along the midline of the hard palate to ensure that the underlying bony structure is intact. The uvula should be examined and its length and any structural abnormalities noted. A bifid uvula (a uvula that is split into two portions), for example, may indicate

---

CLINICAL APPLICATION

Diadochokinetic Rates

The following data on diadochokinetic rates are summarized from Fletcher (1972, 1978), Kent, Kent, and Rosenbek (1987), and St. Louis and Ruscello (2000):

Age	Repetition Rates/Second	Stimulus
6	4.2	[pʌ]
	4.1	[tʌ]
	3.6	[kʌ]
	1.0	[pʌ]-[tʌ]-[kʌ]
7	4.7	[pʌ]
	4.1	[tʌ]
	3.8	[kʌ]
	1	[pʌ]-[tʌ]-[kʌ]
8+	5–6	[pʌ]
	5–6	[tʌ]
	5–6	[kʌ]
	2	[pʌ]-[tʌ]-[kʌ]

Although these rates have been found for children as young as 5 years old, counting diadochokinetic rates is not suggested for younger children. In addition, Kent and associates (1987) state that there is much variability in the performance of children and that across the life span, normative data are limited. Therefore, the use of such tasks and their interpretation should be carried out with caution. In addition, Weismer (1997) questions the role of using these types of procedures in the evaluation of speech disorders. He concludes that these rates may not furnish important diagnostic data: These tasks do not simulate speech production, and the rapid repetition of syllables are not consistent with speaking rates or with articulatory movement patterns found in conversational speech.

This is a video of 3-year-old Elizabeth doing a short portion of the functional assessment of the speech mechanism. Watch how this 3-year-old reacts to the various tasks. Remembering that these are not normed for children under 5 years of age, note also her attempts at the diadochokinetic rates . youtube .com/watch?v=TWNWVrcTyEk

a submucous cleft. Finally, the fauces (the passage between the oral and the pharyngeal cavities) and the pharyngeal area itself need to be assessed. Excessive redness or a swollen appearance of the tonsils and/or adenoids might indicate an inflammation and warrants medical referral.

Functionally Assessing the Speech Mechanism. The functional integrity of the speech mechanism is as important as adequate structures. In this portion of the assessment, the movement patterns of the lips, mandible, tongue, and velum are examined. For the purpose at hand, proper function means not only that the client can move the structures on command but also that the range, smoothness, and speed of the movements are adequate. As the client is performing the various tasks, the clinician should pay attention to the following:

1. Can the client adequately perform the task?
2. Is the range of movements adequate?
3. Are the movements integrated and smooth?
4. Given the age of the client, is the speed of movement within normal limits?

Diadochokinetic rates have often been used to test the speed of movement of the articulators. These rates refer to the maximum repetition rate of the syllables [pʌ], [tʌ], and [kʌ] alone and in various combinations. The rate is measured by either a (1) *count by time* procedure in which the examiner counts the number of syllables spoken in a given interval of time or (2) a *time by count* measurement in which the tester notes the time it takes to perform a specific number of repetitions.

In general, it can be said that diadochokinetic rates increase with age (Fletcher, 1972, 1978; St. Louis and Ruscello, 2000). St. Louis and Ruscello's data show that from about 8 years of age until adulthood the rates remain very similar. The Clinical Application on page 157 outlines these data.

If the client cannot move individual structures on command but has movements during involuntary tasks—for example, the client cannot stick out the tongue when asked to do so but can stick out the tongue to lick a postage stamp—this could indicate an apraxic condition. Further testing becomes necessary.

The sections "Childhood Apraxia of Speech: A Disorder of Speech Motor Control" and "Motor Speech Disorders: Acquired Apraxia of Speech" in Chapter 11 offer further suggestions in determining an apraxic condition. The major goal of this portion of the speech motor assessment is to determine whether the functional integrity of the articulators appears adequate. Isolated functional deviancies only suggest motor problems but do not necessarily translate into an inability to articulate certain speech sounds. Such functional difficulties should be evaluated considering the client's articulatory performance, articulatory limitations, and intelligibility. Several functional tasks for lips, mandible, tongue, and velum are indicated in Appendix 6.1.

CLINICAL EXERCISES

You are testing diadochokinetic rates with a 7-year-old child. Can you think of two or three words or short phrases that would incorporate [pʌ], [tʌ], and [kʌ] that you could use?

Make a list of three comprehensive language tests (not screening measures) that could be used for preschool children and three that could be used for school-age children.

Selection of Additional Assessment Measures

Approximately 80% of the clinical population with "delayed speech" has associated language problems (Keating, Turrell, & Ozanne, 2001; Shriberg, 1991; Shriberg, Kwiatkowski, Best, Hengst, & Terselic-Weber, 1986; Shriberg, Kwiatkowski, & Rasmussen, 1990;

Toppelberg, Shapiro, & Theodore, 2000). Therefore, language testing is recommended for every child who has an articulation and/or a phonological disorder. In addition, a hearing screening is essential. Other measures may include testing specific auditory discrimination skills and appraising the client's cognitive abilities. Selection of additional tests largely depends on an evaluation of the background information, medical and/or school records, and the clinical impression of the individual client.

Hearing Screening

A hearing screening is a portion of every assessment procedure. According to the revised set of "Guidelines for Identification Audiometry" (American Speech-Language-Hearing Association [ASHA], 1985) and the "Guidelines for Audiologic Screening" (ASHA, 1997), the following procedures should be part of the audiologic screening:

1. Taking a history, which includes noting recent episodes of ear pain (otalgia) and/or ear discharge (otorrhea)
2. Visually inspecting to determine the presence of structural defects as well as ear canal and eardrum abnormalities
3. Using identification audiometry
4. Taking acoustic immittance measurements

Referral criteria for each are included in Table 6.2.

Especially with children, a clinician should know of any developmental history that could affect their hearing status. This would include a history of episodes of otitis media, "earaches," or the placement of tubes. Shriberg and Kwiatkowski (1982a) verified that one-third of children enrolled in speech or language intervention had histories of recurrent middle ear disease. Although controversy exists surrounding the exact role that chronic otitis media plays in the acquisition of phonology, it may at least interact with other risk factors in some children. This interaction could easily lead to a greater risk of delayed or impaired communication skills.

Language Testing

Because of the high percentage of language problems in children with speech disorders, language testing belongs to the evaluation process. This should be done using formal, standardized assessment measures. There are many standardized language measures. Speech and language treatment sites, including public school settings, hospitals, and private organizations, all have access to standardized measures. These standardized measures could

TABLE 6.2 Referral Criteria for Audiologic Screening

History Information	
Recent history of earaches, ear pain (otalgia)	Refer
Recent history of ear discharge (otorrhea)	Refer
Visual Inspection of the Ear	
Structural defect of the ear, head, or neck	Refer
Ear canal abnormalities, including blood or effusion, occlusion, inflammation, excessive cerumen, tumor, and/or foreign material	Refer
Eardrum abnormalities, including abnormal color, bulging eardrum, fluid line or bubbles, perforation, retraction	Refer
Identification Audiometry	
Procedure: Air conduction screening at 20 dB HL at 1,000, 2,000, and 4,000 Hz[1]	
Failure to respond at one frequency in either ear	Refer
Tympanometry	
Procedure: Static admittance, equivalent ear canal volume, and tympanometric width used in the screening protocol	
Flat tympanogram and equivalent ear canal volume (V_{ec}) outside normal range	Refer
Low static admittance (Peak Y) on two successive occurrences in a 4–6 week interval	Refer
Abnormally wide tympanometric width (TW) on two successive occurrences in a 4–6 week interval	Refer

[1]According to ASHA (1985, 1997), these criteria may require alteration for various clinical settings and populations.

Source: Copyright 1990 by the American Speech-Language-Hearing Association.

include the Preschool Language Scale – 5th edition (PLS-5) (Zimmerman, I. L., Steiner, V. G., and Evatt Pond, R., 2011. Boston: Pearson.), the Clinical Evaluation of Language Fundamentals – 5th edition (CELF-5) (Semel, E., Wiig, E. H., and Secord, W. A., 2013. Boston: Pearson) or the Comprehensive Assessment of Spoken Language (CASL) (Carrow-Woolfolk, E., 1999. Circle Pines, MN: American Guidance Service), for example.

Specific Auditory Perceptual Testing

For many years, the appraisal of auditory perceptual skills, specifically speech sound discrimination testing, was a standard procedure for all clients with speech sound difficulties. The reasoning was that faulty speech sound perception often caused, or was linked to, the production problems. This was promoted by earlier works such as Van Riper's (1939b) *Speech Correction* in which discrimination training was seen as a necessary portion of every therapy sequence.

Investigations into the relationship between auditory discrimination abilities and the production of speech sounds have extended from the 1930s (e.g., Anderson, 1941; Hall, 1938; Lapko & Bankson, 1975; Locke, 1980a, 1980b; Monnin & Huntington, 1974; Travis & Rasmus, 1931; Williams & McReynolds, 1975; Winitz, 1969; Winitz, Sanders, & Kort, 1981). The results of these and many other studies were inconclusive: Some investigators found a positive relationship between auditory discrimination and articulation skills, whereas others did not. Several reasons for the variation of these results have been suggested (Schwartz & Goldman, 1974; Winitz, 1984). These different outcomes, however, did not support the cause–effect relationship earlier hypothesized. As a result of these findings, auditory discrimination testing seemed to lose much of its value as a standard assessment procedure.

Currently, speech sound discrimination testing is typically performed only with those clients who demonstrate a collapse of two or more phonemic contrasts into a single sound (Bernthal, Bankson, & Flipsen, 2009). If a child substitutes [w] for [r] and [l], this would exemplify the collapse of three phonemic contrasts into a single sound: The phoneme /w/ would represent /w/, /r/, and /l/. Auditory discrimination testing is a means to ascertain whether clients who do not use phonemic contrasts might also not perceive the difference between these contrasts.

Within the last few years, auditory discrimination testing has departed from testing general discrimination skills. Both Locke (1980b) and Winitz (1984) advocate the use of specific auditory discrimination testing that (1) is tailored to the individual client, (2) considers the client's speech sound difficulties or the collapse of the particular phonemic contrasts, and (3) includes the productionally problematic phonetic environment in words and in more meaningful sentence contexts.

Discrimination Testing and the Phonological Performance Analysis (Winitz, 1984). Winitz offers additional suggestions that could be incorporated into the assessment of auditory discrimination skills of clients:

1. *The test items should be relevant and client oriented.* General auditory discrimination tests are not a good measure of a client's difficulties. If a client produces [r] incorrectly, for example, tasks should concentrate on her or his discrimination of [r], not of [l] or [t]. However, if a client substitutes [w] for [r], the task should reflect differentiating between these two sounds.

2. *The specific aberrant productions of the client should be targeted.* A client's production should be contrasted to the norm production of the sound in question. The abilities of a client who lateralizes [s] to discriminate between a lateral [s] and a regular [s]

should be examined. Therefore, the clinician must be able to replicate any of the client's distortions.

3. *The phonetic context in which the incorrect productions occur must be considered.* The clinician must know whether the client's production occurs in the word-initial, -medial, or -final position; in singletons or in consonant clusters; or with specific vowels, for example. If a client evidences deletion of [z] at the end of a word, the discrimination testing should emphasize the presence versus the absence of [z] in this position—for example, *toe* versus *toes*. Similarly, a client who produces an unrounded [ʃ] preceding front vowels should be tested with words with front vowels—for example, *ship, sheep,* and *sheet.*

Winitz (1984) also proposes a phonological performance analysis to supplement the aforementioned auditory discrimination tasks. The purpose of such an analysis is to determine whether clients perceive the distinction among contrastive sounds that they misarticulate. Although the previous suggestions are guidelines for appraising all clients with speech sound difficulties, the phonological performance analysis is appropriate for those who demonstrate the collapse of two (or more) phonemic contrasts. Minimal pairs containing the respective phoneme contrasts are embedded in sets of sentences with a somewhat connected topic.

Although the phonological performance analysis attempts to test minimal pairs in connected sentences rather than in isolated word productions, the development of such a battery for each client would not only be time consuming but also probably tax a clinician's artistic and creative skills. To aid in this task, several examples of sentences contrasting commonly substituted sounds in minimal pairs are provided in Appendix 9.1 of Chapter 9.

Cognitive Appraisal

Speech-language pathologists are not qualified to perform formal IQ testing. However, the results of a cognitive appraisal may be important when developing further assessment and treatment goals. IQ testing might then be initiated by referring a client to appropriate professionals. Often such test results may be obtained through medical, school, or client records.

Caution should be exercised, though, when interpreting the results of IQ measures of children demonstrating phonetic-phonemic disorders. First, a large percentage of children with speech disorders also demonstrate language difficulties. Some cognitive assessment tools use tasks very similar to those used to assess language. Therefore, IQ scores may be affected by children's language incompetence. This is particularly a problem with full-scale IQ scores (Nelson, 1998). For this reason, some authors have suggested using nonverbal cognitive measures (Paul, 2007), although tests designed to evaluate nonverbal cognitive skills may appraise only a limited aspect of cognition (Kamhi, Minor, & Mauer, 1990). Second, intelligibility may play a role in the assessment of children with moderate to severe phonemic difficulties, particularly if verbal IQ measures are used. Nonverbal measures would be helpful with unintelligible children; however, as previously noted, these tests appear restricted. Third, cognitive measures, similar to other standardized tests, do not adequately reflect the abilities of children from culturally and linguistically diverse backgrounds. Although the sample used to norm a particular test typically contains a percentage of children from culturally and linguistically diverse backgrounds (usually the same percentage as these minorities are represented within the U.S. population), this percentage is so small that the inherent test bias for these populations is not eliminated. The presence of language and/or phonetic-phonemic impairments may further compound the interpretation of IQ scores of children from culturally or linguistically diverse backgrounds.

Although the results of a cognitive appraisal may give helpful guidelines for planning subsequent assessment and remediation strategies, the interpretation of the results is not without its problems. Clinicians should be aware of the type of cognitive assessment instrument used to appraise the individual (e.g., verbal versus nonverbal) and the limitations of each measure. *Extreme care should be exercised when interpreting the scores of children from linguistically and culturally diverse background.*

Special Considerations

Children with Emerging Phonology

The period of **emerging phonology** is the time span during childhood in which conventional words begin to appear as a means of communication. Although this level of development usually occurs when children are toddlers, it may also occur in older children with more severe deficits in language learning. Within the assessment process, special consideration must be given to children with an emerging phonological system. Both the diagnostic procedures themselves and the analysis of the results will be different for this population.

Characteristics of Children with Emerging Phonological Systems. Children with emerging phonology are referred for speech-language services for several reasons. First, some may have been born with known risk factors. Identifiable developmental disorders include Down syndrome and other genetic disorders, known hearing impairments, and cerebral palsy. Second, some children will have early acquired disorders secondary to diseases or trauma such as encephalitis, closed head injury, or abuse. Third, children will be brought by parents who are concerned about their child's development: Parents might have observed differences in the expressive communication abilities and/or intelligibility of their child compared to those of other children of a similar age. Fourth, various sources will refer children because they are "late talkers" and their expressive language is slow to emerge.

The group of children with developmentally delayed emerging phonology is typically characterized by small expressive vocabularies showing a reduced repertoire of consonants and syllable shapes (Nathani, Ertmer, & Stark, 2006; Paul & Jennings, 1992; Pharr, Ratner, & Rescorla, 2000; Rescorla, Mirak, & Singh, 2000). Often their words are unintelligible. The limited phonological system may also impact further semantic and morphosyntactic development. Therefore, it is important to appraise the phonological system within the broader framework of children's developing language system. In addition to hearing screening, assessment procedures should always include language testing for this group of children.

Procedural Difficulties with Emerging Phonological Systems. Previously noted assessment procedures encompass several tasks that provide useful and necessary information. However, for children at this level of development, several of these tasks may be difficult to complete.

1. *Articulation tests and stimulability measures.* Depending on the children's developmental level, the administration of standardized articulation tests and stimulability measures might not be possible because these children are not yet skilled at following directions or at imitating. An alternative method might include the naming of objects. However, because of the limited expressive vocabulary of most of these children, this adaptation may have severe limitations.

What to Do? With caregivers' help, a clinician can usually procure a fairly complete sample of words a child is using. Based on the production of these words, the child's consonant and vowel inventory as well as syllable shapes can be established. Such words can be obtained in a number of ways. The following possibilities are given as suggestions:

a. Have the family record the child saying specific spontaneous and elicited words at home.

b. Have the caregiver bring a few objects that the child can name from home.

c. Have the caregiver keep a log of the intended words that the child can produce as well as the approximate way in which each word was pronounced.

Although a recording is a good idea, the quality must be ensured so that the productions can be accurately evaluated. Based on personal clinical experience, asking a caregiver to bring familiar objects from home and keeping a log of utterances usually provide more diagnostic information than recordings. Bringing in familiar objects from the home environment is especially productive in the initial session. For a young child in an unfamiliar setting, this might provide a small comfort zone that will open communication doors. Caregiver logs of the child's spoken words become a necessity when attempting to assess the shy child who does not communicate at the first or even second meeting. Clinicians need to keep in mind that caregivers are not skilled in phonetic transcription and have limited abilities to write down how the child pronounced a certain word. Explanations and examples should be given to the caregiver on how to proceed with this task.

2. *Spontaneous speech sample.* Children with emerging phonological systems who are being evaluated for a possible communication disorder probably do not talk a lot. When they talk, their utterances may contain only one or two words, and these may be partially unintelligible. Collecting a spontaneous speech sample may, therefore, be a challenge. However, spontaneous samples not only provide data for establishing sound and syllable inventories but also establish communicative situations that elicit spontaneous utterances. If children are using primarily single words, a one-word utterance analysis such as Bloom's (1973) or Nelson's (1973) will quantify the types of words being used. As mentioned earlier, children's emerging phonological systems should be examined and evaluated within the broader parameters of their emerging language as a whole.

What to Do? Techniques described in the previous section on articulation testing can also be used to obtain a conversational speech sample. With shy children who do not respond in an unfamiliar setting, observations of their communicative interaction with the caregivers before or after the session may give valuable information.

3. *Examination of the oral-facial structures and the speech-motor system.* Important diagnostic information will be gained if a relationship between the speech-motor abilities and the slow speech development of these children can be verified. However, the assessment of the structure and function of the speech-motor system is often very difficult to obtain from younger children. This is in part because of their intolerance of the procedures needed to complete an oral examination as well as their limitations in imitating sounds and movements on command.

What to Do? Several fun situations can be initiated to assist in the examination of the speech-motor system. Paul (2007) suggests pretending to make clown or fish faces together, letting a child first look inside your mouth with a small flashlight, and then pretending to look for a dinosaur or elephant in the child's mouth. However, even with the best ideas,

CLINICAL EXERCISES

You are evaluating a 2;6-year-old child, Laura, with emerging phonology. When she speaks spontaneously, you are having a hard time understanding her. What type of materials could you use, and how would you structure this portion of your assessment to get some type of spontaneous speech but at the same time be able to target some individual words?

Laura only uses single words and you have asked the caregivers to write down the words that she uses at home. Why is this important for your phonological evaluation and your preliminary analysis of Laura's language skills?

clinicians often fail to get the cooperation of a young child. One possibility would be to wait until the child becomes better acquainted with the clinician and then attempt the procedure again. A second possibility is to gather information about the child's feeding and babbling behaviors. Questions about the child's feeding behavior might help discover related developmental disorders. See Box 6.2 for some sample questions about feeding that could be used to indirectly gather information about the child's speech-motor system. Babbling history could be used in attempting to establish the quantity and diversity of the child's babbling. Both quantity and diversity of babbling behaviors have been correlated to measures of language.

The relationship between babbling and language development is discussed in Chapter 5.

4. *Hearing screening.* A hearing screening is indispensable for children with emerging phonological systems for a number of reasons (the high prevalence of otitis media and its impact on hearing is only one). Speech-language specialists equipped with a portable audiometer typically use a screening procedure that has the client signaling, by raising a hand, for example, when a tone is heard. This type of screening procedure may not be possible with children at this age. However, conditioned response audiometric screening may yield results.

What to Do? Children who have failed screening attempts need to be referred for a comprehensive audiological evaluation.

5. *Additional tests.* It is well documented that children with phonological disorders often have language problems as well (e.g., Keating et al., 2001; Shriberg, 1991; Webster, Majnemer, Platt, & Shevell,

---

BOX 6.2	Questions to Use to Assess the Feeding Behavior in the Child with an Emerging Phonological System

During sucking of liquids, did any of the following occur?

- Tongue thrusting (abnormally forceful protrusion of the tongue from the mouth)
- Lip retraction (drawing back the lips so that they form a tight line over the mouth)
- Jaw thrusting (abnormally forceful and tense downward extension of the mandible)
- Lip pursing (a tight purse string movement of the lips)
- Jaw clenching (abnormally tight closure of the mouth)
- Tonic bite reflex (abnormally strong jaw closure when the teeth or gums are stimulated)

During swallowing, did/do any of the following occur?

- Drooling

- Having excessive mucus present
- Coughing, choking, gagging
- Hyperextending the head or neck

During biting and chewing, do any of the following occur?

- Abnormal movements of the jaws, lips, and tongue with solid foods of different consistencies
- Munching versus chewing motions (munching is the earliest form of chewing and involves a flattening and spreading of the tongue combined with up-and-down jaw movement, whereas chewing is characterized by spreading and rolling movements of the tongue and rotary jaw movements)
- Abnormal patterns

Source: Summarized from Jaffe (1989).

2005). Therefore, the language abilities of these children need to be assessed. For young children between 2 and 3 years of age, the language assessment instrument must be selected with care. Because of these children's limited attention spans, difficulties in following directions, and their relatively poor imitation skills, even some standardized language tests normed for these ages might not be successfully administered.

What to Do? Numerous developmental tests rely partially or totally on the information supplied by the caregiver about a child's level of functioning. The analysis of language in naturalistic contexts can also be used to assess a child's pragmatic, morphological, syntactical, and semantic competencies.

Analysis of Children's Emerging Phonological System.

Several authors suggest that an independent analysis be used with children who are at the emerging level of phonological development (Bernthal, Bankson, & Flipsen, 2009; Paul & Jennings, 1992). An independent analysis considers only a child's productions but does not compare them to the adult norm model. Because only a relatively limited number of consonants and vowels are typically present in a child's inventory, a comparison to the adult norm model would not be helpful for later assessment and intervention. At this stage of children's development, more information can be gained by seeing which sounds and syllable shapes are present. The children's inventory must first be expanded before comparisons to the adult model can be made.

Three types of data are collected for the independent analysis: the inventory of speech sounds, the syllable shapes a child uses, and any constraints noted on sound sequences. The inventory of speech sounds includes all vowels and consonants found in a child's accumulated word productions. Data on syllable shapes would pertain to single sound productions to signify a word (V = vowel, C = consonant) and to the use of both open and closed syllable forms (CV, CVCV, CVC). Sound production constraints would include any sound or sound combinations that are used only in certain word or context positions. Examples of this category would include [p] used only word-initially or [d] in CVCV structures.

Mean Babbling Level and Syllable Structure Level.

For children with emerging language skills, Morris (2010) suggests a procedure used to obtain mean babbling level and syllable structure level. These measures were based on studies by Stoel-Gammon (1987); Fasolo, Majorano, & D'odorico (2008); Paul & Jennings (1992); Pharr, Ratner, & Rescorla (2000); and Thal, Oroz, & McCaw (1995). The measures provide a metric that summarizes phonetic and syllable shape information for babble into one score that can be used to show progress over time. The mean babbling level restricts analysis to babbling while the syllable structure level focuses on productive words.

CLINICAL APPLICATION

Inventory of Speech Sounds, Syllable Shapes, and Constraints

Ted is a 1;8-year-old child with Down syndrome who is being followed in the early intervention program. His mother and the speech-language pathologist have recorded these 12 words.

"yes"	[jɛ]	"pig"	[pɪ]
"mom"	[mʌm]	"hug"	[hʌk]
"daddy"	[dædi]	"bike"	[baɪ]
"hello"	[hoʊ]	"duck"	[dʌk]
"grandpa"	[dapa]	"truck"	[tʌk]
"bye"	[bɪ]	"cow"	[daʊ]

Vowel inventory: [i, ɪ, ɛ, æ, a, oʊ, aɪ, aʊ, ʌ]

Consonant inventory: [m, p, b, t, d, k, j, h]

Syllable shapes: CV, CVC, CVCV

Constraints: [k] is used only in a postvocalic position after the central vowel [ʌ].

Refer to Table 6.3 for a description of the procedures and subsequent results that can be used to examine the severity of phonological delay.

TABLE 6.3 Mean Babbling Level and Syllable Structure Level

Mean Babbling Level: Total Number of Consonants		
Procedure:	Unstructured parent–child play sample using age-appropriate toys. In the first analysis, the total number of different consonants is counted.	
Results:	Children	Age in Months	Number of Consonants

Children	Age in Months	Number of Consonants
Norm	18–24	14
Small expressive vocabulary	18–24	6
Norm	24–36	18
Small expressive vocabulary	24–36	10

The child's number of different consonants can be compared to that of the average for children in the norm group and to the average for children with small expressive vocabularies to determine which group average it is closer to.

Mean Babbling Level and Syllable Structure Levels	
Procedure:	Unstructured parent–child play sample using age-appropriate toys. Approximately 50 utterances are recorded during a 30-minute session.
	The mean babbling level examines only babbled responses: The vocalization was judged by the parent and the examiner/observer to be non-meaningful if it contained minimally a voiced vocalic or a voiced syllabic consonant, was produced with an egressive airstream, and was judged to be "speechlike," not a cry, scream, cough, or vegetative sound.
	Based on the content, each utterance is assigned a certain level.
	A percentage is calculated based on the number of utterances produced at each level.
	The following levels (1–3) are used for calculating both mean syllable structure level and mean babbling level. Mean babbling level examines non-meaningful utterances while mean syllable structure level examines both meaningful and non-meaningful utterances.
Levels:	*Level 1:*, Vocalization is composed of only a voiced vowel (V syllable shape [ɑ], [u]), a voiced syllabic consonant (C syllable shape [l̩], [m̩]), or CV syllable in which the consonant is a glottal stop, glide, or [h] ([wi], [hɑ]). The following are examples of Level 1 vocalizations: [i], [oᵘ], [l̩], [m̩], [n̩], [hɑ], [wa], [ʔa], [ʔa], [ju].
	Level 2: Vocalization is composed of a VC ([ʌp], [ɪk]), CVC with a single consonant ([bab], [mam]), or a CV shape that contains consonants other than those noted at Level 1 ([tu], [mu]). Voicing differences are disregarded; therefore [bip] or [toᵘd] would be considered Level 2. The following are examples of Level 2 vocalizations: [ʌk], [um], [ab], [papa], [baba], [noᵘ], [tɛdi], [kaka], [lala].
	Level 3: Vocalization is composed of syllables with two or more different consonant types that differ in place and manner ([dɑli], [kɪti]). Only voicing differences would be considered Level 2. The following are examples of Level 3 vocalizations: [bati], [boᵘno], [dʌk], [hɛlo], [jʌki], [hat], [koᵘt].
	Count all r-colored vowels and diphthongs as vowels, not consonants.
	Include phonetic variants of the same word if the variation includes a consonant or syllable structure change.
	Include only one instance of each unintelligible word.
Results:	Norm children at 24 months of age SSL = 2.2
	Children with small expressive vocabularies at 24 months of age SSL = 1.7
	The child's SSL average can be compared to that of the average for children in the norm group and to the average for children with small expressive vocabularies to determine which group average it is closer to.

Unintelligible Children

The speech of unintelligible children is so disordered that the speaker's message cannot be understood. Unintelligible children are not limited to any specific age group. For example, Hodson and Paden (1981) report children who at 8 years of age were considered unintelligible.

Characteristics of Unintelligible Children. Hodson and Paden (1993) evaluated the speech of 60 unintelligible children ranging in age from 3 to 8 years. All of these highly unintelligible children evidenced varying degrees of difficulty with the production of liquids, stridents, and consonant clusters. Prevalent phonological processes in the speech of these children were cluster reduction, stridency deletion, stopping, gliding and vocalizations of liquids, and labial and nasal assimilations. Hodson (1992) notes that the least intelligible children were those who omitted entire classes of sounds. A few of the children produced no obstruents, either before or after the vowel nucleus (*bed* was realized as [ɛ] or [wɛ]), and a small number of the children did not produce sonorant consonants (*run* was pronounced [ʌ]).

Procedural Difficulties with Unintelligible Children. Children 3 years and older usually have no difficulty completing an articulation test, stimulability testing, or the speech-motor assessment. Even with reduced intelligibility, a single-word articulation test will probably render transcribable results that can be used for a phonetic-phonemic analysis. The major difficulty for the clinician when evaluating unintelligible children is being able to understand and transcribe a spontaneous speech sample. With careful structuring, an understandable spontaneous speech sample may be possible even with unintelligible children.

What to Do?

1. *Choose the topic and attempt to structure the situation as much as possible.* If the context is unknown—that is, if unintelligible children are talking about a self-generated topic—the clinician will have even more difficulty understanding the sample. Scripts of action events, scripts of routine events, and scripted events (Lund and Duchan, 1993) will give structure and predictability to the conversation. *Scripts of action events* depict everyday occurrences with predictable

> Watch and listen to the following short video of a 15-month-old child. Transcribe the words she uses and apply the syllable structure level analysis to them. Based on this very short sample, what is this child's SSL? youtube.com/watch?v=xwglVbilvtc

---

CLINICAL APPLICATION

Syllable Structure Levels

Further utterances were gathered from Ted, who was presented in the previous Clinical Application. The syllable structure level is noted for each vocalization.

"yes"	[jɛ]	Level 1	"pig"	[pɪ]	Level 2
"mom"	[mʌm]	Level 2	"hug"	[hʌk]	Level 3
"daddy"	[dædi]	Level 2	"bike"	[baɪ]	Level 2
"hello"	[hoʊ]	Level 1	"duck"	[dʌk]	Level 3
"grandpa"	[dapa]	Level 3	"truck"	[tʌk]	Level 3
"bye"	[baɪ]	Level 2	"cow"	[daʊ]	Level 2

Additional nonconventional vocalizations used to calculate mean babbling level:

[ha]	Level 1	[oʊ]	Level 1
[dɪdɪ]	Level 2	[bubu]	Level 2
[pu]	Level 2	[i]	Level 1
[bæbæ]	Level 2	[pabi]	Level 2
[bʌpi]	Level 2	[ja]	Level 1
[m̩]	Level 1	[ʌ]	Level 1

Total number of consonants: 8
Mean babbling level: 1.5
    Percentage of level 1: 50% Level 2: 50% Level 3: 0%
Syllable structure level: 1.83
    Percentage of level 1: 33.3% Level 2: 50% Level 3: 16.7%

Ted is 20 months of age. His total number of consonants is much closer to the average found for children with small expressive vocabularies. Although Ted's syllable structure is slightly higher than those found in such children, it is still closer to the average for that group when compared to the norm children at 24 months of age.

elements. Therefore, if children are asked to explain what they do at McDonald's to get a hamburger, the predictability of the events should aid comprehension. *Routine events* begin, progress, and end in essentially the same way each time they occur. If the topic is baseball and the children should explain what the person coming up to bat must do, the known progression of events will again help the clinician understand the conversation. *Scripted events* are activities that have been performed previously, and, therefore, all participants have expectations of how they will progress. For example, a child and a clinician could fix the wheel on a broken toy truck. The clinician would then ask the child to explain what they had just done. If the clinician models sentences, for example, "First, we saw that the truck had a missing wheel. Next, we looked for the wheel," the child might use similar sentence patterns. Again, the predictability of the utterances should increase the clinician's ability to understand what the child is attempting to say.

2. *Gloss the utterances the children say as much as possible.* The clinician should gloss any utterances that may later be difficult to understand from a recording. *Glossing* means repeating the child's utterance according to norm pronunciation. If the child says [aⁱ oᵘ oᵘm] for "I go home," the clinician repeats the utterance in a regular manner so that it is recorded with the sample.

Tables 6.4 and 6.5 can be useful in organizing data for later analysis.

TABLE 6.4   Considerations When Collecting Data

Hearing screening		
Does not pass screening	⟶	Referral
Examination of speech mechanism		
Not passing, deviancies	⟶	Additional testing, referral
Initial impression		
Poor intelligibility	⟶	Need careful planning of further evaluation, especially spontaneous speech sample; see section "Unintelligible Children"
Articulation test		
Few errors	⟶	Stimulability, contextual testing
Many errors	⟶	Attempt stimulability
Speech sample		
Poor intelligibility	⟶	Choose topic, structure situation, gloss utterances
Language testing		
Not within normal limits	⟶	Note language difficulties. May need further evaluation of language skills.
Auditory discrimination testing		
Noted collapse of phoneme oppositions	⟶	Do auditory discrimination testing
Cognitive appraisal		
Necessary	⟶	Referral, obtain records

TABLE 6.5   Check Sheet for Data Collection

Hearing screening	Pass _____ Not Passing _____
Examination of speech mechanism	Pass _____ Not passing _____
	Noted deviancies _____
	_____
Initial impression	Intelligibility
	Good _____ Fair _____ Poor _____
	Error productions noted
	_____
Articulation test	Error productions noted
	_____
	Stimulability testing
	Sound _____
	Sound level: Yes _____ No _____
	Syllable level: Yes _____ No _____
	Word level: Yes _____ No _____
	Sound _____
	Sound level: Yes _____ No _____
	Syllable level: Yes _____ No _____
	Word level: Yes _____ No _____
	Sound _____
	Sound level: Yes _____ No _____
	Syllable level: Yes _____ No _____
	Word level: Yes _____ No _____
Contextual testing	Sound _____
	Word contexts that elicit norm production
	_____
	Sound _____
	Word contexts that elicit norm production
	_____
	Sound _____
	Word contexts that elicit norm production
	_____
Speech sample	Intelligibility
	Good _____ Fair _____ Poor _____
	Error productions noted
	_____
Language testing	Specific areas of deficiency
	_____
	_____
Auditory discrimination testing	Sound _____
	Does _____ Does not _____ discriminate
	Sound _____
	Does _____ Does not _____ discriminate
Information on cognitive appraisal	Necessary _____ Not necessary _____

SUMMARY

First, this chapter summarized the various areas of data collection in the appraisal portion of the assessment process. These include (1) an articulation test, (2) a spontaneous speech sample, (3) an evaluation of the oral mechanism, and (4) additional measures exemplified by a hearing screening, language testing, auditory perceptual testing, and cognitive appraisal. Methods and goals for each of these areas as well as the limitations that might be inherent in the procedures were discussed. For example, an articulation test provides a relatively time-efficient way to evaluate articulation skills; however, it does not provide the clinician with any information about the client's abilities to use these skills in naturalistic contexts. In the second part of this chapter, special assessment considerations were examined for children with an emerging phonological system and unintelligible speakers. Each of these groups of clients presents the clinician with challenges that will necessitate changes in the assessment process and the evaluation of the results. This chapter is seen as a guide to assist the clinician in selecting procedures that will maximize clinical decision making within the diagnostic process.

CASE STUDY

You have just given Ashley, age 4;5, an articulation test. Consistent use of the following errors were noted.

[s̠], [z̠] for [s] and [z] on all words

[t], [d] for [θ] and [ð] on all words

[w] for [l]

[w] for [r] for the consonantal [r] and lack of r-coloring on central vowels with r-coloring

[p], [b] for [f] and [v]

Based on the data supplied by Smit (1993b) on page 125, which of the misarticulations would be considered age-appropriate errors?

Which of the difficulties would be problems that you might want to target in therapy?

How could you structure a spontaneous speech sample to include objects that might stimulate production of these sounds and promote various communicative situations?

THINK CRITICALLY

The following selected words are from the HAPP-3 (Hodson, 2004).

1. basket
2. glasses
3. spoon
4. zip
5. boats
6. cowboy hat
7. green
8. feather
9. fork
10. mask
11. star
12. toothbrush
13. three
14. mouth
15. screwdriver
16. truck
17. thumb
18. music box

19. watch
20. rock
21. shoe

22. string
23. crayons
24. hanger

The child that you are assessing has s- and r-problems.

How many words are tested with these sounds, and in which word position do they occur?

Make a list that you could use to supplement the results of the articulation testing for r- and s-sounds.

TEST YOURSELF

1. All of the following pertain to the collection of data in the assessment *except for* the
   a. interview with parents and other professionals
   b. selection of therapy targets
   c. school and medical records
   d. evaluation by the clinician

2. In an assessment, you begin collecting data about your client
   a. as you greet and observe the client interacting with family
   b. when you begin administering an articulation test
   c. during the spontaneous speech sample
   d. after the speech mechanism evaluation

3. When selecting a measure of articulation for assessment, you should consider
   a. the age and development level of the child
   b. whether the test is able to provide standardized scores
   c. how the test analyzes speech sound errors
   d. whether the test includes an adequate sample of sounds relevant to the client
   e. all of the above

4. Of the three different scoring systems for sound errors, which is considered to be the most precise and most universally accepted among professionals?
   a. two-way scoring
   b. five-way scoring
   c. phonetic transcription

5. Approximately 80% of the clinical population with "delayed speech" also have associated problems with
   a. hearing
   b. language
   c. vision
   d. oral structure

6. What are diadochokinetic rates?
   a. rates used to measure the number of fricative sounds articulated per second
   b. measures used to examine the rate of movement of the articulators
   c. the number of children in a given sample who have both articulation- and phonemic-based impairments
   d. measures used to assess the dentition of a client

7. You observed a clinician who administered an articulation test, completed a speech mechanism evaluation, and administered a language test to a child. You most likely were observing a
   a. comprehensive evaluation
   b. screening
   c. cognitive evaluation

8. Which of the following is a disadvantage to articulation tests?
   a. the time needed to administer a test is usually minimal
   b. results from these tests usually yield a list of "incorrect" sound productions in different word positions
   c. examination of errors in isolated words
   d. tests provide standardized scores

9. Taking a history, visual inspection, screening audiometry, and acoustic immittance are all portions of a
   a. speech screening
   b. cognitive screening
   c. language screening
   d. hearing screening
10. Because it is often difficult to administer an articulation test to a young child with emerging phonology, you

a. ask the family for additional information (recorded speech from home, a log of words from home, etc.)
b. do not evaluate the child for services
c. examine only the oral structure
d. evaluate language instead

FURTHER READINGS

Hegde, M. N. (2007). *Pocketguide to assessment in speech-language pathology* (3rd ed.). Clifton Park, NY: Delmar.

Ruscello, D. (2001). *Tests and measurements in speech-language pathology*. Woburn, MA; Butterworth-Heinemann.

McAfee, J. G., & Shipley, K. G. (2009). *Assessment in speech-language pathology: A resource manual* (4th ed.). Clifton Park, NY: Delmar Cengage Learning.

Smit, A. B. (2004). *Articulation and phonology: Resource guide for school-age children and adults*. Clifton Park, NY: Thomson Delmar Learning.

APPENDIX 6.1   Speech-Motor Assessment Screening Form

Each of the following parameters is assessed using the following system:

Pass	Within normal limits
Deviant	Deviant from norm, divided into "slight" or "marked" deviancy
Not passing	Clearly outside of normal limits

Structure				
Head/Face				
Sitting opposite the client, evaluate head and facial structures according to the categories provided.	Pass	Deviant		Not Passing
		Slight	Marked	
Size, shape of head				
Symmetry of facial features				
Left half vs. right half				
Absence of drooping or spasticity				
Mandible/maxilla relationship				
Appearance of lips (contact at rest; vermilion)				
Appearance of nose (septum; nares)				
Appearance of philtrum/columella				
Absence of any striking features (e.g., adenoid facies, facial dimensions)				
Comments				

Breathing		Deviant		Not
Observe and evaluate the client's breathing behavior (as "structural" prerequisite for speaking and voice production) during normal (silent) breathing and during speaking. During silent breathing, the client's mouth should be closed and no clavicular movement should be noticeable.	Pass	Slight	Marked	Not Passing
Silent breathing				
Mouth closed (mouth open would indicate a deviancy)				
Relationship for the time of inspiration versus expiration is about 1:1				
Lack of clavicular breathing				

Breathing		Deviant		Not
	Pass	Slight	Marked	Not Passing
Breathing during speaking				
Breathing through nose (exclusive mouth breathing is a deviancy)				
Relationship for the time of inspiration versus expiration is 1:2 +				
Lack of clavicular breathing				

Comments

Oral/Pharyngeal Cavity

The head should be bent back slightly for inspection of the palatal areas. A few reminders:

Missing frontal teeth might have a direct effect on sibilant production.

Dentition:

Class I (normal) occlusion: lower molars (or canine for children without molars) appear one-half a tooth ahead of upper molars.

Class II malocclusion (overbite): Maxilla protruded in relation to mandible, measured by the positions of the first (maxillary and mandibular) molars.

Class III malocclusion (underbite): Mandibular molar more than half a tooth ahead of maxillary molar.

Open bite: Gap between biting surfaces. Especially frontally open bites might influence articulation negatively.

Cross bite: Misalignment of the teeth characterized by a crossing of the rows of teeth.

Macroglossia = tongue appears too large

Microglossia = tongue appears too small

Shrinkage (i.e., a "shriveled" tongue area) might indicate a paralytic condition.

The midline of the hard and soft palates appears normally pink and white; a blue tint suggests a submucous cleft.

Redness of fauces and pharynx might indicate inflammation.

	Pass	Deviant		Not Passing
		Slight	Marked	
Dentition				
Front teeth present				
Spacing of teeth adequate				
Axial orientation of teeth is adequate				
Dentition				
Class I normal occlusion				
If a malocclusion is noted, indicate the type:				

Oral/Pharyngeal Cavity	Pass	Deviant		Not Passing
		Slight	Marked	
Tongue				
Normal size in relationship to oral cavity				
Normal color				
No shrinkage				
Absence of fissures, lesions, fasciculations				
Normal resting position				
Palate (hard and soft)				
Normal color				
Normal width of vault				
Absence of fistulas, fissures				
Absence of clefts				
If cleft, circle one: Repaired Unrepaired				
Normal uvula				
If abnormal, circle one: Bifid Other deviations				
Normal length of uvula				
Appearances of fauces, pharynx				

Comments:

Function				
For older children and adults, these tasks can be elicited by asking the client to complete the task. For younger children (preschool age and below), imitation may be required.				
Head/Face	Pass	Deviant		Not Passing
		Slight	Marked	
Eyes/facial appearance				
Raising of eyebrows is symmetrical				
Can smile, frown on command				
Smiling, frowning symmetrical				
Lips				
Can protrude lips with mouth closed				
Can protrude lips with mouth slightly open				
Can protrude lips to left/right side				

Head/Face	Pass	Deviant Slight	Deviant Marked	Not Passing
Can protrude and spread lips ([u]–[i])				
Demonstrates rapid lip movements				
("pa-pa-pa")				
Mandible				
Can lower mandible on command				
Can move mandible to left/right side				

Comments

Oral/Pharyngeal Cavity	Pass	Deviant Slight	Deviant Marked	Not Passing
Tongue				
Can stick out tongue				
Can move tongue upward (try to touch nose with tip of tongue)				
Can move tongue downward (try to touch chin with tip of tongue)				
Can move tip of tongue from the left to the right corner of the mouth				
Can move tongue quickly and smoothly from right to left corner of mouth				
Can move tongue smoothly around vermilion of lips (lick around lips) clockwise and counterclockwise				
Can move tongue from left to right on outside/inside of upper teeth				
Can move tongue from left to right on outside/inside of the lower teeth				
Can say "pa-pa-pa" quickly, smoothly				
Can say "ta-ta-ta" quickly, smoothly				

Oral/Pharyngeal Cavity	Pass	Deviant Slight	Deviant Marked	Not Passing
Tongue				
Can say "ka-ka-ka" quickly, smoothly				
Can alternate between quick repetitions of "pa-ta" and "ta-pa"				
Can alternate between quick repetitions of "pa-ta-ka," "ka-ta-pa," and "ta-pa-ka"				
Velopharyngeal function				
During short, repeated "ah" phonation, adequate velar movement is noted				
Can puff up cheeks				
Can maintain intraoral air (puffed cheeks) when slight pressure is applied to cheeks				
Absence of nasal emission				

Breathing	Pass	Deviant		Not Passing
		Slight	Marked	
Silent breathing				
During quick inspiration breath intake is through nose				
During quick inspiration breath intake is thoracic/abdominal				
Breathing during speaking				
Can sustain "ah" for 5 seconds				

Comments:

Diagnosis

Articulation- versus Phonemic-Based Speech Sound Disorders

LEARNING OBJECTIVES

When you have finished this chapter, you should be able to:

- Describe how to evaluate the inventory and distribution of speech sounds.
- Distinguish speech sound disorders based on articulatory versus phonemic characteristics.
- Explain what signals the primary features of a speech sound disorder that is primarily articulation- versus phonemic-based.
- Identify the areas that are analyzed for a comprehensive phonemic analysis.

- Specify the guidelines for beginning therapy based on the diagnosis of a speech sound disorder.
- Explain how you would analyze error patterns according to place-manner-voicing features and phonological process analysis.
- Distinguish between least and most phonological knowledge.
- Differentiate severity from intelligibility, and list factors that affect intelligibility of an utterance.
- Determine the percentage of consonants correct.

CHAPTER 6 outlined different assessment procedures that would inform clinicians about a client's speech sound abilities in several areas. These procedures include both citation form and spontaneous speech sound performance as exemplified by the gathering of data from an articulation test and a spontaneous speech sample. Supplemental tests that would screen the adequacy of the oral mechanism, hearing, language, auditory perception, and cognitive abilities were also suggested. The next step in the assessment process is to *organize, analyze, and interpret the collected data.* The end product of this assessment portion not only provides clinicians with a solid foundation for diagnostic decisions but also leads directly to treatment goals.

One of the first diagnostic decisions facing clinicians is *how* to organize and analyze the available data. There are many possibilities, which all lead to somewhat different interpretations. Choosing the organization and analysis that best suit an individual client is important. Above all, a client's type and degree of speech sound difficulties play a major role in this selection process.

The first goal of this chapter is to present some general organizational methods that can be used to give clinicians an overview of the speech sound problems noted on the articulation test and spontaneous speech sample. This organization is suitable for any dependent analysis, regardless of age of the client or the type and degree of impairment. The chapter's second goal is to provide an analysis procedure that will aid clinicians in determining whether a client has primarily an impairment of speech sound form or deficiencies in phonemic function. This analysis will first consider the preservation or collapse of phonemic contrasts in a client's speech. Although a clear division into an articulatory- versus a phonemic-based disorder is not always possible (a client may demonstrate characteristics of both), clinicians need to be aware of the important differences between the two. A tentative decision as to primarily articulatory versus phonemic difficulties will guide clinicians in further analyses and intervention decisions. The third goal of this chapter is to present additional analysis procedures. For a client with primarily an articulatory-based disorder, the author offers suggestions for further testing and guidelines on integrating diagnostic results into beginning therapy goals. For a client with primarily a disorder of phonemic function, a specific assessment battery is introduced. Organizational categories for this battery include (1) the inventory and distribution of sounds, (2) syllable shapes and constraints, (3) phonological contrasts, and (4) phonological rules or patterns. Analyzing the patterns or phonological rules of a particular client's speech can be achieved in a number of ways. Several contemporary methods for this analysis are described.

It should be emphasized that the overall aim of this chapter is to provide information to aid in clinical decision making. There are no prescribed answers. Based on all assessment data collected, each clinician needs to determine for each and every individual client which analysis procedures need to be completed for a valid diagnosis. This chapter is seen as an aid to making those decisions.

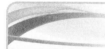

Preliminary Analysis: Inventory and Distribution of Speech Sounds

One way to organize the results of the articulation test and spontaneous speech sample is to look at the inventory and distribution of speech sounds. The **inventory of speech sounds** are all speech sounds a client articulates. However, for many clients, this is not a simple dichotomy between norm and aberrant productions. Some clients show a regular production of a speech sound in one context but not in another. This is exemplified by a child who substitutes [t/s] within a word and at the end of a word but realizes the target sound correctly when the word begins with [s]. Such inconsistencies should be duly noted because they provide important clinical information. In addition, some clients normally realize a sound in contexts in which it does not belong but consistently mispronounce it in contexts in which it should be used. For example, an analysis revealed that a child had no accurate productions of [s] in all words that contained s-sounds. However, in the word *brush*, [ʃ] was replaced by an accurate [s]. This phenomenon has often been reported and frequently occurs in children with phonemic-based disorders (Fey, 1992). Examples such as these demonstrate that norm articulation of the sound in question is within a client's capabilities; however, the client does not seem to understand the language-specific function and/or organization of specific phonemes. Such information aids considerably in determining which clients show evidence of a phonemic-based disorder.

The **distribution of speech sounds** refers to where within a word the norm and aberrant articulations occur. Articulation tests often categorize according to three word positions: initial, medial, and final. As previously noted, *word-medial position* is an imprecise term. This lack of precision has bothered many practitioners who were interested in looking more closely at the client's error patterns.

Some of the problems inherent in using the term medial to refer to all sounds between the first and last sounds of a word were discussed in the "Syllable Structure" section of Chapter 2.

In an attempt to introduce more structure and to reflect the hierarchical relationship of the syllable to the word, Grunwell (1987), for example, adopted a categorization that divides each multisyllabic word into its syllables. The sounds within the syllable are then further classified according to whether they initiate or terminate syllables. Although this system is clearly superior to the three-position method used by most articulation tests, dividing words into syllables poses its own problem: where to place the syllable boundaries. There is no clear-cut way to predict where a particular speaker will divide the syllables of a word. For example, does one say "roo-ster" or "roos-ter"? Ask several people how *telephone* is divided: *te-le-phone* or *tel-e-phone*? The problem of where and how to syllabify words is not a new one. For decades, many scholars have wrestled with the problem (e.g., Jespersen, 1913; Ladefoged, 2006; Rosetti, 1959; Scripture, 1927; Sievers, 1901; Stetson, 1936, 1951). To date, it still cannot be said with any certainty exactly where syllables begin and end.

More recently, syllabication guidelines for General American English have been offered (e.g., French, 1988; Grunwell, 1987; Lowe, 1994). These guidelines are based on where the majority of a given set of normal speakers syllabified specific words. However, these guides are often based on subjective feelings of where syllables can and cannot be divided. Although most syllabication guidelines contain the warning that syllable divisions may vary from speaker to speaker, they do not solve the problematic aspects of the syllable and its division.

It seems plausible that children with phonological difficulties syllabify words quite differently from what is normally the case. By imposing predetermined syllabication guidelines on words, which may or may not be accurate in a specific case, any subsequent analysis could be faulty and could lead to wrong conclusions.

Therefore, the following analysis procedure is based not on where the syllable supposedly begins and ends but rather on where the consonants occur relative to the vowel nuclei. This procedure eliminates the necessity of establishing syllable divisions and can be used on words from an articulation test or from a spontaneous speech sample. The consonants can be divided into three categories:

1. *Prevocalic consonants.* Consonants that occur before a vowel. These may be singletons (i.e., single consonants) or consonant clusters at the beginning or within the word or utterance.
2. *Postvocalic consonants.* Consonants that occur after a vowel. These may be singletons or consonant clusters at the end or within a word or utterance.
3. *Intervocalic consonants.* Consonants that occur between two vowels. These may be singletons or consonant clusters at the juncture of two syllables.

CLINICAL EXERCISES

Divide the following words into prevocalic, nucleus (vowel), intervocalic, or postvocalic.

hat	shoe	tiger	yellow
umbrella	jumping	banana	pajamas

Which word(s) do not have a postvocalic consonant? Which word(s) do not have a prevocalic consonant?

Using a Matrix to Examine the Inventory and Distribution of Speech Sounds

Appendix 7.1 is an example of a matrix that can be used to record the utterances from both articulation tests and spontaneous speech samples. The entire word is written in the left-hand column. Next, the word is divided into individual sound realizations. Using phonetic transcription, *first*, the target production (the intended sound) and *then* the client's realization (what was actually produced) are recorded for each sound within the word. This is a different notation than when a clinician uses a / to indicate "is substituted for". For example, on an articulation test one might see θ/s, indicating [θ] was substituted for [s]. When applicable, prevocalic, syllable nucleus, and postvocalic sounds are recorded for one-syllable words, whereas multisyllable words would contain intervocalic sounds. The word *chicken* [tʃɪkən] for which the client says [tɪtə] is used to demonstrate the process:

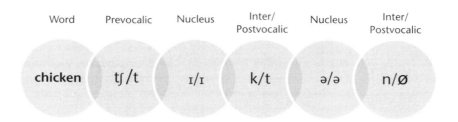

In this example, the symbol ∅ is used to indicate deletions. In addition, clinicians can circle any type of aberrant productions.

This information is then transferred to the matrix for summarizing phones according to pre-, inter-, and postvocalic word positions, found in Figure 7.1. For the purpose at hand, a checkmark (✓) is used to indicate a norm realization, ∅ to record deletions, and the appropriate phonetic symbols with diacritics to document substitutions and distortions. Therefore, this matrix is used to record both the norm and the aberrant productions of the client. As can be noted in Figure 7.1, singleton consonant productions are recorded separately from clusters. Using the *chicken* example, [t] would be recorded in the prevocalic matrix under tʃ ([tʃ] → [t]), [t] would be recorded under intervocalic [k] ([k] → [t]), and a ∅ would be placed in the postvocalic box under [n]. If a clinician would like to consolidate the results even further, Figure 7.2 could be used as a matrix to record pre-, inter-, and postvocalic realizations on a single form. Results from Figures 7.1 and 7.2 give clinicians (1) the inventory of consonants, (2) the distribution of phones, and (3) the number of times each consonant occurred.

Appendix 7.2 presents the results of the Goldman-Fristoe Test of Articulation (Goldman & Fristoe, 2000) for H. H., a 7;4-year-old child who was introduced in Chapter 4. It provides a list of words from the articulation test that have been transcribed. Although spontaneous speech results should also be included in the assessment, for simplification, this introduction analyzes only the results of the articulation test. (A spontaneous speech sample that could be analyzed according to these procedures is at the end of Chapter 4 in Appendix 4.1.) See Appendices 7.2–7.5 at the end of this chapter. In these appendices, the Single Word Responses from the articulation test (Appendix 7.2), the Preliminary Matrix for Recording Utterances (Appendix 7.3), the Matrix for Recording Phones According to Pre-, Inter-, and Postvocalic Word Positions (Appendix 7.4), and the Matrix for Recording the Overall Inventory of Phones (Appendix 7.5) have been filled out for H. H.

FIGURE 7.1 Matrix for Recording Phones According to Pre-, Inter-, and Postvocalic Word Positions

Phonemic Contrasts: Differentiating Articulation- from Phonemic-Based Disorders

Clients with phonemic-based disorders are characterized by impaired phonemic systems; they show difficulties using phonemes contrastively to differentiate meaning. Therefore, two or more phonemes represented by the same sound production indicate that the contrastive phonemic function has not been realized; *the meaning differentiating contrast has been neutralized.* The emphasis in this phase of the analysis is on the *contrastive use of sounds*, not on their accurate production. Loss of phonemic contrast is the central problem of clients with phonological impairments.

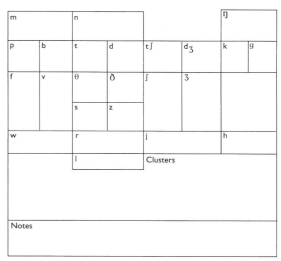

FIGURE 7.2 Matrix for Recording the Overall Inventory of Phones

Depending on the client, the neutralization of specific phonemic contrasts can be consistent or inconsistent. A *consistent loss* is indicated by the exact same realization (the same distortion, substitution, and/or deletion) occurring every time in a client's realizations. Consistent loss of a phonemic contrast can be exemplified by a child who, regardless of the position of the sound in the word, realizes all [s] sounds as [t] ([s] → [t]). The child has neutralized the contrast between /s/ and /t/. Also, a child who always deletes the intended phoneme ([s] → ∅) would demonstrate a consistent loss of phonemic contrast as well. *Inconsistent* realizations refer to substitutions or deletions that occur only in certain contexts. The sounds produced by a child who realizes [t] for [s] before a vowel but produces [s] accurately in specific words after the vowel nucleus indicate an inconsistent loss of the phonemic contrast. If we examine H. H.'s productions, we see several inconsistent losses of phonemic contrast. One example is [f]. At the beginning of a word, H. H. realizes [f] as [b] ([f] → [b]) in such words as *fishing*, *feather*, and *finger*. However, between two vowels (intervocalic position) in *telephone*, H. H. produces [f] correctly. At the end of the word, such as in *knife*, H. H. deletes [f]. This is an example of an inconsistent loss of a phonemic contrast. The final decision on which speech sounds are indeed employed as contrastive phonemes often requires the clinician to check sound oppositions through minimal pairs, for example.

What to Do? The analysis of phonemic contrasts can begin with the matrices presented in Figures 7.1 and 7.2. These provide an overview, which can be used to fill out Figure 7.3, the Neutralization of Phonemic Contrasts Summary Form.

1. Look for those sounds that are *consistently* used for another phoneme. For example, [k] was consistently realized as [t] in H. H.'s productions (Appendices 7.4 and 7.5). There were no instances (including consonant clusters) in which [t] was not substituted for /k/.

2. Look for those sounds that are *inconsistently* used—that is, occurring only in certain contexts. Inconsistencies are exemplified by (a) norm productions in some instances and the collapse of the phoneme contrast in others, or (b) the production of two or more different sound realizations for one phoneme, or (c) the use of substitutions in certain contexts together with sound deletions in other contexts. Another inconsistent collapse of phonemic contrasts occurs for H. H. with [θ]. In the prevocalic position, [θ] → [b] (see "thumb"); postvocalically, [θ] is deleted (see "bath"). Also, check to see

List all target sounds together and the substitution(s) used. By examining the Overall Inventory Matrix, determine whether the substitution is consistent (occurs every time) or inconsistent (occurs only in certain contexts). Circle the appropriate word.

Target	→	Substitution		Target	→	Substitution	
_____	→	_____	Consistent / Inconsistent	_____	→	_____	Consistent / Inconsistent
_____	→	_____	Consistent / Inconsistent	_____	→	_____	Consistent / Inconsistent
_____	→	_____	Consistent / Inconsistent	_____	→	_____	Consistent / Inconsistent
_____	→	_____	Consistent / Inconsistent	_____	→	_____	Consistent / Inconsistent
_____	→	_____	Consistent / Inconsistent	_____	→	_____	Consistent / Inconsistent
_____	→	_____	Consistent / Inconsistent	_____	→	_____	Consistent / Inconsistent
_____	→	_____	Consistent / Inconsistent	_____	→	_____	Consistent / Inconsistent
_____	→	_____	Consistent / Inconsistent	_____	→	_____	Consistent / Inconsistent

Collapse of Contrasts
List all target sounds that have the **same** substitution.

Targets	Substitution
_____	_____
_____	_____
_____	_____
_____	_____
_____	_____

Sound Preferences
List any speech sounds that are used for a wide range of target phonemes.

FIGURE 7.3 Neutralization of Phonemic Contrasts Summary Form

whether any pattern can be noted in the pre-, inter- and/or postvocalic positions. From Appendix 7.4, we see that H. H. does seem to demonstrate a pattern with [tʃ]: In pre- and intervocalic positions, a [t] is realized; in the postvocalic position, [tʃ] is deleted.

CLINICAL EXERCISES

Why is it important to know whether or not a child has "sound preferences" for therapy?

Could there be a relationship between the sound preferences and the collapse of phonemic contrasts? Examine the data from H. H. and see whether you notice any patterns.

3. Summarize the collapse of contrasts. The purpose of this overview is to discover any substitutions that represent more than one target phoneme. Therefore, all target phonemes with the same substitution are grouped together. For H. H., [k], [s], [z], and [tʃ] are replaced by [t], for example. In addition, [d] replaced [g], [dʒ], [ð], and [ʃ]. These are summarized for H. H. in Appendix 7.6.

4. Look for any *sound preferences*. A sound or sound combination representing different phonemes exemplifies this. Sound preferences should be checked to see whether any patterns exist, for example, one phone used for a whole class of consonants. For H. H., [t] and [d] seem to represent sound preferences; both were employed as substitutions for four different phonemes. The summary of H. H.'s phonemic contrasts is provided in Appendix 7.6. Only consonant singletons were entered in this form, but it could also be used to record consonant cluster productions.

Further testing may be warranted for sounds that show inconsistent contrasts. This could be easily achieved by having the client name pictures or read minimal pair words.

CLINICAL APPLICATION

Neutralization of Phonemic Contrasts for H. H

See Appendix 7.6. For H. H., the following neutralization of phonemic contrasts for singleton consonants was established:

1. Consistent neutralization of contrasts:	[k] → [t]
	[ʤ], [ð] → [d]
2. Inconsistent contrast neutralization:	[r] → [w]; [tʃ], [z], [s] → [t] (note: [tʃ], [z], and [s] are deleted in the postvocalic position)
	[ʃ] → [s] (note: occurs only in postvocalic position)
	[ʃ] → [d] (note: occurs in pre- and intervocalic positions)
	[g] → [d] (note: [g] is deleted in the postvocalic position)
	[f], [θ] → [b] (note: [f] is realized correctly one time in intervocalic position)
	[l] → [w] (note: [l] is deleted in the postvocalic position)
3. Sound preferences:	[d] is used to represent four other phonemes
	[t] is used to represent four other phonemes

Decision Making: Speech Sound Difficulties That Are Primarily Articulation-Based

It is important to analyze all existing data, possibly supplementing them with additional information, before arriving at the tentative decision that a client does show evidence of a speech sound disorder that is articulation-based. In doing this, speech-language specialists must always keep in mind that articulation and phonemic-based speech sound disorders can co-occur. "It would be a mistake to adopt an either/or dichotomy" (Elbert, 1992, p. 242). The following section outlines the factors that help clinicians in the process of decision making when considering a speech sound disorder that is primarily articulation-based.

Signals of Articulation-Based Disorders

1. *Preservation of phonemic contrasts.* Substitution of one phoneme for another suggests the collapse of phonemic contrasts and, therefore, a phonemic-based disorder. However, if one sound is being used as a substitution for several phonemes, the client's realizations should be carefully examined to determine whether even minimal production differences are being used to signal phonemic contrasts. For example, a child might be using a palatalized [s], [sʲ], as a substitution for [ʃ]. The palatalized [s] is articulated with the tongue in a more posterior position than is normally the case for the [s] but too far forward for a typical sh-production. In addition, this same child could be using a dentalized [s] for [θ]. The dentalized [s̪] demonstrates a more anterior tongue position than is normally the case. Both substitutions would be labeled as [s] distortions; however, in this case, the child is demonstrating production variations to signal the phonemic contrasts: [sʲ] for [ʃ] and [s̪] for [θ]. Even minimal form differences, if used consistently, could indicate the preservation of phonemic contrasts. Omissions of sounds should also be carefully

CLINICAL APPLICATION

Speech Sound Disorder: Primarily Articulation- or Phoneme-Based Difficulties?

Tommy's parents requested an evaluation of his speech sound skills. They were concerned that he had some misarticulations that were not age appropriate. The initial impression of Tommy, age 7;1, was that of an alert child who was fairly intelligible but seemed to have problems with [s], [z], [r], [θ], and [ð]. Tommy passed a hearing screening, an examination of the speech mechanism, and language testing fell within the norm range. A spontaneous speech sample and an articulation test revealed the following:

1. Substitution of w/r ([r] → [w]) in all word positions. The r-coloring of central vowels was also not realized. Results were consistent in single-word tasks and spontaneous speech.
2. Substitution of θ/s and ð/z ([s, z] → [θ, ð]) in all word positions with the exception of [st] blends at the beginnings or end of words. In these blends, [s] was accurate. Such an accurate production of [s] in blends was noted only in one-word samples, not in conversational speech.
3. Substitution of t/θ and d/ð ([θ, ð] → [t, d]) in all word positions, consistent in one-word samples and spontaneous speech.

Initial Analysis

Tommy did not seem to fit the typical picture of a child with a phoneme-based disorder. Because of his age, the clinician was not too concerned about the th-problems. However, she was concerned that Tommy's errors constituted a collapse of phonemic contrasts. Further testing was warranted.

Preservation of Phonemic Contrasts

Minimal pairs were used to test Tommy's productions of [w] versus [r]. The clinician noticed subtle differences in attempted [r]-productions when contrasted to his realization of [w]. For example, there was not as much lip rounding when he tried to say a word beginning with [r] when compared to his [w] realization. Tommy was not stimulable for [r] at the sound level. When he was asked to produce minimal pairs with [s] and [θ], his [s] sounded like a [θ] in certain contexts and like a dentalized [s] ([s̪]) in others. He was stimulable for [s], [z], [θ], and [ð] at the sound and word levels.

Peripheral Motor-Based Difficulties

Errors were consistent across word positions. The accurate production of [s] in [st] blends was thought to be the effect of coarticulation. Discrimination of minimal pairs with [s] versus [θ] and [z] versus [ð] demonstrated an accuracy of more than 90%. Discrimination of [w] versus [r] was 70% accurate.

Clinical Decision Making

The clinician decided that Tommy showed more evidence of a motor-based articulation disorder than of a phoneme-based disorder. Further testing did not indicate perceptual or cognitive-linguistic-based difficulties. In certain contexts, Tommy distinguished productionally and perceptually between the target sounds and his substitutions.

evaluated to determine whether articulatory changes can be discovered between minimal pairs with and without the deleted sound. Several investigators have demonstrated that omitted sounds may be represented by some other articulatory gesture to preserve the phonemic contrasts (Bauman-Waengler, 2002a, 2002b; Smit & Bernthal, 1983; Weismer, 1984). Noted changes included variations in vowel duration and a final gliding articulation of the vowel preceding the deleted sound.

What to Do? Use pictures or words representing minimal pairs of the target sound and the substitution or omission. Have the client spontaneously produce each word. If a distinguishable articulatory contrast is realized between the two sounds, use narrow transcription to document the variation. Different articulatory gestures might indicate that the client is differentiating between the two phonemes but not in a conventional manner.

2. *Peripheral, motor-based problems.* By definition, articulation-based disorders are characterized by misarticulations—that is, aberrant speech sound forms. Speech sound errors within this framework are also relatively consistent; that is, inadequate motor learning of the particular sound is generalized throughout the system. Therefore, consistent inventory constraints are noted regardless of the position of the sound within the word (Elbert, 1992). In addition, articulation-based disorders are not cognitive-linguistic (organizational) or perceptually based problems (Kamhi, 1992). Organizational difficulties would be reflected in disturbed phonotactics, whereas clients with perceptually based problems may not be able to discriminate between the target sound and its inaccurate production.

What to Do? Examine a client's irregular productions relative to their occurrence in the pre-, inter-, or postvocalic positions. If the production remains relatively consistent, this would suggest an articulation-based disorder. However, if positional constraints are discovered, the organization or phonotactics may not be intact, pointing to a phonemic-based disorder (Elbert, 1992).

Often no pattern can be discovered; that is, the client produces the sound correctly in some words and incorrectly in others. In this case, two additional factors should be considered: (1) the phonetic context and (2) the possibility of an emerging sound. Because of the possible influence of coarticulation, specific phonetic contexts may enhance or hinder the production of the target sound. Words that contain accurate sound realizations should be examined to determine whether a common phonetic context exists. Emerging sound patterns in children's speech can also result in inconsistent realizations. Support for this possibility includes the appearance of the sound in "easy" contexts (e.g., single syllables or supporting coarticulatory conditions) and its stimulability at the sound or word level. If the production is influenced by the phonetic context or the sound seems just to be emerging, this would suggest an articulation-based disorder.

Guidelines for Beginning Therapy: Articulation-Based Speech Sound Disorder

The gathering of data is completed and diagnostic decisions have been made. Any diagnosis should also lead directly to the selection of intervention goals and strategies. Although goals and strategies will constantly change, depending on the client and the noted difficulties, specific diagnostic information should aid in deciding where to begin with therapy.

Stimulability. Although stimulability is not an absolute predictor of which error sounds will improve in therapy and at which level therapy should begin (sound, syllable, word level), stimulability can be used as a probe to find out which sounds might be somewhat easier for a client to realize. If a client is stimulable for a particular sound, the clinician could attempt this sound in therapy for a trial period.

Correct Production of the Sound in a Specific Context. The collected data often give evidence of a typically misarticulated sound produced *accurately* within a specific word context. Such a word might appear on an articulation test or in the spontaneous speech sample. It was also suggested that articulation test results be supplemented with additional word lists. These probes could yield such a context as well. Norm productions of a word or words containing a usually misarticulated sound verify that, under certain contextual conditions, a client is able to realize its regular articulation. These words, therefore, offer themselves as a therapeutic beginning point.

Minimal pair words for the most frequently misarticulated sounds are in Chapter 9.

CLINICAL EXERCISES

Frequently occurring misarticulations include [s], [z], r-sounds, and [θ], [ð]. You have just assessed a child who is at the end of first grade with all of these misarticulations. Rank order these sounds from highest to lowest according to their frequency of occurrence using the information in Appendix 7.7, page 208.

List two variables other than the frequency of occurrence that you would want to consider when planning where to begin therapy.

CLINICAL APPLICATION

Decision Making: Where to Begin Therapy

The previous Clinical Application with Tommy can be used as an example to illustrate these guidelines for making decisions concerning where to begin therapy.

Sound	Stimulable	Correct Word Context	Intelligibility	Development
[r]	No	No	High frequency	Earlier than [s], [z], [θ], [ð]
[s], [z]	Yes, sound/word	Yes, st-blends	High frequency	Relatively late
[θ], [ð]	Yes, sound/word	No	[ð] high, [θ] low	Later sound

Given these variables, it would appear that in this case, [s] and [z] were good choices for initiating a trial probe in therapy. They were stimulable, appeared correctly in certain word contexts, and had a high frequency of occurrence in General American English. Therefore, they will have a definite impact on Tommy's speech intelligibility. In addition, [s] and [z] are typically developmentally earlier than [θ] and [ð]. However, because of the high frequency of occurrence of [r] in General American English and relative early mastery in the acquisition process, [r] should probably be targeted before [θ] and [ð].

Sounds Affecting Intelligibility. Certain sounds affect intelligibility more than others. One main reason is their relatively high frequency of occurrence in conversational contexts. Refer to Appendix 7.8 for a chart displaying the frequency of occurrence of General American English consonants. Other sounds may affect intelligibility because of their conspicuous aberrant articulation. Therapeutically, high priority should be given to sounds that most affect a client's intelligibility.

Developmentally Earlier Sounds. Under comparable clinical circumstances, sounds that are acquired developmentally earlier should be considered first targets. The term *comparable clinical circumstances* means that both sounds were stimulable to the same degree and that the sounds in question seemed to have a comparable impact on the client's intelligibility.

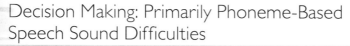

Decision Making: Primarily Phoneme-Based Speech Sound Difficulties

If a phonemic-based difficulty is suspected, a thorough *phonological assessment* becomes necessary. Data for a phonological assessment can be organized in a number of ways. The following organizational scheme is one that has been described either partially or totally by several authors (e.g., Elbert & Gierut, 1986; Fey, 1992; Grunwell, 1987; Howell & Dean, 1994; Ingram, 1989b; Lowe, 1994). This organization will help clinicians to answer important assessment questions and to plan therapy goals. The categories found in this organizational scheme are:

1. Inventory of speech sounds
2. Distribution of speech sounds
3. Syllable shapes and constraints
4. Phonological contrasts
5. Phonological error patterns

Inventory and Distribution of Speech Sounds

The inventory and distribution of speech sounds were discussed earlier in this chapter. Figures 7.1 and 7.2 on pages 180–181 are provided to aid in organizing and analyzing these parameters.

Syllable Shapes and Constraints

The term **syllable shape** refers to the structure of the syllables within a word. Therefore, the unit of analysis is the word; that is, each word is described according to occurring vowels, designated as *V*, and consonants, *C*, within that word. Syllable shapes vary with open syllables such as *eye* or *go* being the easiest to produce. Syllable shapes in General American English can be very complex, containing up to three consonants in the prevocalic and four in the postvocalic positions. Syllable shapes are important because clients with phonemic-based disorders may delete syllables, use predominantly open syllables, or demonstrate specific consonant preferences in the production of syllables (Crystal, 1981; Hodson & Paden, 1991; Pollock & Schwartz, 1988).

A **syllable constraint** refers to any restriction or limitation established in the production of syllable shapes. Children acquiring speech in a normal manner use many different syllable shapes at an early age. When Stoel-Gammon (1987) analyzed the speech of 32 two-year-olds, she found that 31 of them produced two different types of closed syllables, and more

More information can be found in the "Syllable Structure" section of Chapter 2.

than half of them demonstrated CVCVC structures and word-initial clusters. Approximately
half of the 2-year-olds in this investigation were
also realizing word-final clusters. Therefore, even
children with an emerging phonological system
should demonstrate both open and closed syllable
structures.

The information about syllable shapes
and any possible constraints can be obtained
from the articulation test and the spontaneous
speech sample. Both the type and frequency of
occurrence of the syllable shapes of each word
should be noted. Worthwhile information is
also gained by determining whether discrepancies exist between the responses on the articulation test and the conversational speech sample.
Specific syllable constraints in the speech sample
could in part explain a decrease in the client's
intelligibility.

See Table 7.1 for some of the most frequent
one-syllable word shapes. Several two-syllable
shapes are included; more could be added. According to Shriberg and Kent (2013),
approximately 77% of the words of General American English spoken by adults are one-
syllable words, and both one- and two-syllable words compose almost 94% of the total
words used. The main goal of our analysis is to determine whether the client has basic
syllable structures and, if so, which ones. Simple open and closed syllable shapes of one-
and two-syllable words should be a portion of the client's repertoire.

TABLE 7.1 Common One- and Two-Syllable Shapes

Shape	Examples
One-Syllable	
V	a, I
CV	go, he
CCV	grow, tree
VC	up, on
VCC	ask, oops
CVC	hop, doll
CCVC	trees, brush
CVCC	hopped, lamp
CCVCC	stopped, drink
Two-Syllable	
CVCVC	wagon, shovel
CVCCV	window, candy
CVCCVC	bathtub, jumping

What to Do?

1. Analyze the client's sample to determine whether one-, two-, and, when
   appropriate, three- or more syllable
   words exist. Note whether there is a
   large proportion of any single syllable
   type. For example, it is remarkable
   if the client uses primarily only one-
   syllable words.
2. Analyze any reductions in the syllable
   number or syllable shapes. Reductions
   in the number of syllables include mul-
   tisyllablic words in which syllable deletions occur. For example, *telephone*, a
   three-syllable word, might be reduced
   to [tɛfoʊn]. Changes in the syllable
   shape are exemplified by words in
   which deletion of consonants has
   altered the original syllable shape. For
   example, *house*, a CVC shape, might
   become [haʊ], a CV shape.

CLINICAL APPLICATION

Syllable Shapes with H. H.

The following results were found after analyzing the data
from the Goldman-Fristoe test for H. H. in Appendix 7.2 on
page 204:

1. One- and two-syllable words were present.
2. Three-syllable words (*telephone, pajamas*) were reduced
   to two syllables; however, H. H. could produce three syllables (see *Santa Claus* and *Christmas tree*).
3. Syllable shapes of one-syllable CVC words were frequently reduced to a CV structure, although in the
   majority of cases the CVC structure was maintained.
4. The majority of two-syllable words were reduced in
   shape by final consonant deletion.

Based on this sample, H. H. can produce one- and two-
syllable words; however, the syllable shapes were often
reduced; that is, they were produced as open syllables in
two-syllable words.

Phonological Contrasts

The organization and analysis of data for determining phonological contrasts were discussed earlier in this chapter. See the section "Phonemic Contrasts: Differentiating Articulatory-Based from Phonemic-Based Disorders" on page 181 and Figure 7.3 on page 182.

Phonological Error Patterns

Phonological assessment attempts to evaluate the phonological system of each client as accurately as possible. An accurate assessment leads to both an effective diagnosis and successful subsequent therapy. Although a client's productions must be compared to the adult model, it should also be kept in mind that the client's realizations represent a system in themselves. A **system** refers to an orderly combination of parts forming a complex unity. A central goal of any phonological assessment is to understand a client's phonological system. Identifying and categorizing the error patterns are important aspects of this understanding. Knowledge of existing patterns within the system will lead directly to important therapeutic decisions. On the other hand, a lack of this knowledge can easily result in interpreting a client's "system" as just random. This leads to therapy procedures that may not be as goal directed.

A number of methods are available for analyzing error patterns. Whereas some techniques are based more on production features—analyzing the speech sound form—others attempt to analyze the client's phonemic system. Recalling that articulation- and phonemic-based disorders can, and often do, occur together, the following form- and function-based frameworks are offered: (1) place-manner-voice, (2) phonological process, and (3) assessing phonological knowledge.

Place-Manner-Voice Analysis. The place-manner-voice analysis is a production-based system; it depicts speech sound form. As its name implies, this analysis describes error patterns according to a rather broad phonetic feature classification system. Place, manner, and voicing characteristics of each error sound are compared to those representing the norm production features. This comparison can then be examined to determine whether any patterns emerge within the sound system. In this context, *patterns* are defined as a client's frequent use of a specific place-manner-voicing feature. The place-manner-voice analysis is designed only to classify substitutions of one sound for another; it does not account for distortions and deletions. The following place-manner-voice categorization system is taken from Howell and Dean (1994):

CLINICAL EXERCISES

A child reduces two-syllable words to one syllable and consistently deletes the final consonant in one-syllable words. Do you think this is evidence of an articulation- or a phonemic-based disorder? Explain your choice.

Place-manner-voicing analysis does not account for distortions or deletions. Why is it important to know about a child's distortions and deletions when you are planning therapy?

Place of Articulation	
Labial	[p], [b], [f], [v], [m], and [w]
Dental	[θ] and [ð]
Alveolar	[t], [d], [s], [z], [n], and [l]
Postalveolar	[ʃ], [ʒ], [tʃ], and [ʤ]
Palatal	[j], [r]
Velar	[k], [g], and [ŋ]
Glottal	[h]

Manner of Articulation	
Stop-plosives	[p], [b], [t], [d], [k], and [g]
Fricatives	[f], [v], [θ], [ð], [s], [z], [ʃ], [ʒ], and [h]
Affricates	[tʃ] and [dʒ]
Nasals	[m], [n], and [ŋ]
Liquids	[l] and [r]
Glides	[w] and [j]
Voicing	
Voiced	[b], [d], [g], [v], [ð], [z], [ʒ], [dʒ], [m], [n], [ŋ], [l], [r], [w], and [j]
Voiceless	[p], [t], [k], [f], [θ], [s], [ʃ], [tʃ], and [h]

Figure 7.4 is a graph of the consonants of General American English according to the place-manner-voicing analysis system, and Figure 7.5 is a Place-Manner-Voicing Summary Sheet. A summary sheet filled out for H. H. can be found in Appendix 7.7, pages 207–208.

What to Do? Transfer the information from the Overall Inventory of Phones Matrix (Figure 7.2) to the Place-Manner-Voicing Summary Sheet (Figure 7.5) in the following way:

1. Write target sound and substitution in the left-hand column.
2. Compare the substitution to the target sound, noting any place, manner, and/or voicing features that were affected. Circle the appropriate change in feature(s). Some substitutions will be only one-feature changes; others could be changes in place, manner, *and* voicing characteristics.
3. List the specific place, manner, and/or voicing change that occurred in the column marked Specific Changes. For example, if a child substituted a [t] for [k] ([k] → [t]), "place" would be circled and "velar → alveolar" recorded in the blank after the place feature.
4. List the number of times this particular feature change occurred in the Number of Errors column.
5. List each single-sound substitution according to the prescribed directions. After all substitutions and feature changes have been listed, look for patterns of errors by using the summary at the bottom of the sheet.

	Labial		Dental		Alveolar		Postalveolar	Palatal	Velar		Glottal	
Stops	p	b			t	d			k	g		
Nasals		m				n				ŋ		
Fricative	f	v	θ	ð	s	z	ʃ	ʒ			h	
Affricative							tʃ	dʒ				
Liquids						l		r				
Glides		w						j				

FIGURE 7.4 Place-Manner-Voice Features of General American English Consonants

Target	→	Substitution	Circle Differences	Specific Changes	No. of Errors
_____	→	_____	Place Manner Voicing	_____ _____ _____	____ ____ ____
_____	→	_____	Place Manner Voicing	_____ _____ _____	____ ____ ____
_____	→	_____	Place Manner Voicing	_____ _____ _____	____ ____ ____
_____	→	_____	Place Manner Voicing	_____ _____ _____	____ ____ ____
_____	→	_____	Place Manner Voicing	_____ _____ _____	____ ____ ____

Summary

PLACE		MANNER		VOICING	
Change	No. of Occ.	Change	No. of Occ.	Change	No. of Occ.
_____	____	_____	____	_____	____
_____	____	_____	____	_____	____
_____	____	_____	____	_____	____
_____	____	_____	____	_____	____
_____	____	_____	____	_____	____
_____	____	_____	____	_____	____

Distortions _____

Deletions _____

FIGURE 7.5   Place-Manner-Voicing Summary Sheet

CLINICAL APPLICATION

Place-Manner-Voicing Analysis for H. H.

Using the summary sheet in Appendix 7.7, pages 207–208, H. H.'s place, manner, and voicing substitutions could be summarized as follows:

Place: High occurrence of alveolars being substituted for postalveolar and velar phones (postalveolar and velar → alveolar)

Manner: High occurrence of stops being substituted for fricatives (fricatives → stops)

Voicing: Errors of both voiced → voiceless and voiceless → voiced consonants

In summary, place-manner-voice analyses are production based. They provide clinicians with information about specific production changes that occur in a client's speech when compared to norm realizations. Although the system evaluates actual phonetic features of speech sounds, it is rather broad based. Some important features, such as the active articulator, and secondary features, such as lip rounding of [ʃ], are not accounted for. Only substitutions of one sound for another can be classified according to place-manner-voicing parameters. Sound deletions, distortions, assimilations, and syllable structure changes are not assessed.

Phonological Process Analysis. This type of analysis procedure was introduced in Chapter 4. A phonological process analysis is a means of identifying substitutions, syllable structure, and assimilatory changes that occur in clients' speech. Each error is identified and classified as one or more of the phonological processes. Patterns of errors are described according to the frequency of noted phonological processes and/ or those that affect a class of sounds. The processes used to identify substitutions are again primarily production based; however, they do account for sound and syllable deletions as well as several assimilation processes.

Certain processes seem to occur more frequently in the speech of children developing their phonological systems in a normal manner. Others, labeled *idiosyncratic processes*, occur infrequently in the norm population (Stoel-Gammon & Dunn, 1985). On most protocols, substitution processes are limited to consonants, but vowel processes have been identified as well (Ball & Gibbon, 2002; Pollock & Keiser, 1990; Reynolds, 1990; Stoel-Gammon & Herrington, 1990). For examples of idiosyncratic processes found in the speech of children with phonological disorders, see Figure 7.6. Phonological processes used to identify vowel errors are summarized in Figure 7.7.

FIGURE 7.6 Idiosyncratic Processes Found in the Speech of Children with Phonological Disorders

The following are a few examples of the relatively uncommon processes that have been found in the speech of children with phonological disorders:

Process	Example		
Initial consonant deletion	"duck"	[dʌk] →	[ʌk]
Backing of stops	"tub"	[tʌb] →	[kʌb]
Backing of fricatives	"sun"	[sʌn] →	[ʃʌn]
Glottal replacement	"gun"	[gʌn] →	[ʔʌn]
Denasalization	"knee"	[ni] →	[di]
Fricatives replacing stops	"toe"	[toʊ] →	[soʊ]
Stops replacing glides	"yarn"	[jɑɚn] →	[dɑɚn]
Metathesis (reversal of two sounds)	"nest"	[nɛst] →	[nɛts]
Affrication (a nonaffricate becomes an affricate)	"top"	[tɑp] →	[tʃɑp]
Migration (movement of a sound from one position in the word to another position)	"soap"	[soʊp] →	[oʊps]
Unusual cluster reduction	"plane"	[pleɪn] →	[leɪn]
Unusual substitution processes	"plane"	[pleɪn] →	[reɪn]
Vowel processes, for example, centralization of vowels	"bed"	[bɛd] →	[bʌd]

Source: Summarized from: Bauman-Waengler and Waengler (1988, 1990); Dodd and Iacano (1989); Leonard and McGregor (1991); Roberts, Burchinal, and Footo (1990); Stoel-Gammon and Dunn (1985); Waengler and Bauman-Waengler (1989).

FIGURE 7.7   Phonological Processes Used to Identify Vowel Errors

Several common and idiosyncratic substitution processes that describe changes in consonant productions have been identified. However, children with phonological disorders may also evidence impaired vowel systems. The following processes have been used to describe vowel substitutions in children (Ball & Gibbon, 2002; Bauman-Waengler, 1991; Pollock & Keiser, 1990):

1. *Vowel backing.* A front vowel is replaced by a back vowel of a similar tongue height. Example: [ɪ] → [ʊ].
2. *Vowel fronting.* A back vowel is replaced by a front vowel of a similar tongue height. Example: [u] → [i].
3. *Centralization.* A front or back vowel is replaced by a central vowel. Example: [ɛ] → [ʌ].
4. *Decentralization.* A central vowel is replaced by a front or back vowel. Example: [ʌ] → [ɛ].
5. *Vowel raising.* A front vowel is replaced by a front vowel with a higher tongue position, or a back vowel is replaced by a back vowel with a higher tongue position. Example: [æ] → [ɛ].
6. *Vowel lowering.* A front vowel is replaced by a front vowel with a lower tongue position, or a back vowel is replaced by a back vowel with a lower tongue position. Example: [u] → [ʊ].
7. *Diphthongization.* A monophthong is realized as a diphthong. Example: [ɛ] → [ɛ^I]
8. *Monophthongization (or diphthong reduction).* A diphthong is realized as a monophthong. Example: [a^I] → [a].
9. *Complete vowel harmony.* A vowel change within a word that results in both vowels being produced the same. Example: [tɛdi] → [tɛdɛ]
10. *Tenseness harmony.* A lax vowel becomes tense when there is another tense vowel in the same word. Example: [mɛni] → [meni]
11. *Height vowel harmony.* A vowel is replaced with a vowel that is closer in tongue height to another vowel in the same word. Example: [bæskɪt] → [bɛskɪt]

Treatment implications of Stampe's (1979) theory of natural phonology include suppression or decrease of the aberrant phonological processes to increase the complexity of children's phonological patterns. The suppression of these phonological processes occurs naturally in the speech of normally developing children, but for children with phonological disorders, treatment must focus on helping to reduce the use of age-inappropriate processes as well as processes that are not acceptable for the adult language being learned. Typically, several sounds that demonstrate active use of a specific phonological process are selected. These sounds are trained in close succession to aid children in decreasing the use of this particular phonological process. Therapy emphasizes the meaningful use of speech, and words are seen as the smallest units to be contrasted and practiced.

A phonological process analysis was completed for Ryan, age 6;6, who was introduced in Chapter 4. This analysis, is summarized for Ryan in Table 7.2. Ryan demonstrates a high frequency of occurrence of the processes fronting, gliding, cluster substitution, and cluster reduction. The following transcriptions are the results of the articulation test from Ryan.

Phonological processes provide a means of classifying error patterns noted in disordered speech and suggest a direct and simple way to handle intervention. Although these processes have been labeled phonological, they are based to a large extent on phonetic

TABLE 7.2 Phonological Process Analysis Summary Sheet for Ryan

Processes	Number of Occurrences
Syllable Structure Changes	
Cluster reduction	*4*
Cluster deletion	
Reduplication	
Weak syllable deletion	*1*
Final consonant deletion	
Initial consonant deletion	
Other _____	
Substitution Processes	
Consonant cluster substitution	*7*
Fronting	*11*
Labialization	*3*
Alveolarization	*1*
Stopping	*2*
Affrication	
Deaffrication	*2*
Denasalization	
Gliding of liquids	*6*
Gliding of fricatives	
Vowelization	
Derhotacization	
Voicing	
Devoicing	*2*
Other	
Assimilation Processes	
Labial assimilation	
Velar assimilation	
Nasal assimilation	
Liquid assimilation	
Other _____	
_____	
_____	

horse	[hoᵘɚθ]	cold	[koᵘd]
wagon	[wægən]	jumping	[dʌmpən]
monkey	[mʌŋki]	TV	[tivi]
comb	[koᵘm]	stove	[θtoᵘv]
fork	[foɚk]	ring	[wɪŋ]
knife	[nɑˈf]	tree	[twi]
cow	[kɑᵘ]	green	[gwin]
cake	[keˈk]	this	[dɪθ]
baby	[beˈbi]	chair	[ʃɛɚ]
bathtub	[bæftəb]	watch	[wɑʃ]
nine	[nɑˈn]	thumb	[fʌm]
train	[tweˈn]	mouth	[mɑᵘf]
gun	[gʌn]	shoe	[su]
dog	[dɑg]	fish	[fɪs]
yellow	[wɛloᵘ]	zipper	[ðɪp]
doll	[dɑl]	nose	[noᵘθ]
pig	[pɪk]	sun	[θʌn]
cup	[kʌp]	house	[hɑᵘθ]
swinging	[swɪŋɪŋ]	steps	[stɛp]
table	[teˈbəl]	nest	[nɛt]
cat	[kæt]	books	[bʊkθ]
ladder	[læɾɚ]	bird	[bɝd]
ball	[bɑl]	whistle	[wɪθəl]
plane	[pweˈn]	carrots	[kɛɚət]

production features. For example, substitution processes are named after the differences between the production of the target and the error sound. Phonological processes do not give concrete information about the neutralization of specific phonemic contrasts, nor do they account for phonological rules that might be operating. Even more important, the presence of phonological processes in the speech of an individual *does not* necessarily indicate the presence of a phonemic-based disorder. In their contemporary usage, phonological processes are descriptive terms; the existence of a particular process neither explains the problem nor denotes its etiology (e.g., Butcher, 1990; Fey, 1992). Kamhi (1992) has identified the practice of using phonological processes to *imply* a phonemic-based disorder as being the most serious problem associated with this type of analysis.

To summarize, phonological processes, a central aspect of natural phonology, have been extensively used to describe disordered speech patterns and to select treatment goals. The speech of children with disordered phonological systems may show differences in type and use of phonological processes when compared to the speech of children with normally

CLINICAL APPLICATION

Using Phonological Processes

Lillian, age 5;6, was screened by the speech-language pathologist in her kindergarten class. The classroom teacher said that Lillian was at times hard to understand. The speech-language pathologist summarized her screening results according to phonological processes:

Process	Examples	Total Number of Times Used
Velar fronting	[k] → [t] [kʌp] → [tʌp] [g] → [d] [gʌn] → [dʌn]	14 times, all words tested
Final consonant deletion	[beɪk] → [beɪ] [lɑg] → [lɑ]	5 times, only on words ending with [k] and [g]
Cluster reduction and cluster substitution	[klaʊn] → [taʊn] [græs] → [dæs]	5 times, only on words with [k] and [g] clusters

Lillian was still using the early process velar fronting. In addition, inconsistent use of processes was noted. When [k] or [g] was produced in the word-initial position or in consonant clusters, fronting was demonstrated. In the word-final position, the sounds were deleted.

CLINICAL EXERCISES

You assess Grace, a kindergartener, and find that she dentalizes [t], [d], [s], [z], and [l]. You can see that her tongue is projecting between her teeth on all these productions. You also notice that in general she has a tendency to have her tongue with a more frontal position than is normally the case.

What phonological process could you give to these productions?

Because of the fact that you can assign a phonological process to all these articulations, do you think that this child has a phonemic-based disorder? Discuss why or why not.

developing systems. However, caution should be exercised when descriptions of phonological processes are used to imply the presence of a phonemic-based disorder.

Assessment of Productive Phonological Knowledge. Elbert and Gierut (1986) present an approach to analyzing a child's *productive phonological knowledge*. The authors postulate that "the way in which the child *uses* the sound system allows us to determine what the child *knows* about the sound system" (p. 50). This approach emphasizes first that a child's performance must be described independently of the adult norm system. It is only *after* the child's phonological knowledge is assessed that his or her phonological system can be compared to the adult model. The analysis procedures seem to be particularly useful with children who have severe phonemic-based disorders or complex patterns of errors. This analysis may not be necessary for children who exhibit only one or two sound errors or for those who produce sound distortions.

A child's productive phonological knowledge is determined by (1) the breadth of the distribution of sounds and (2) the use of phonological rules. The breadth of the distribution of sounds consists of the phonetic inventory, the phonemic inventory, and the distribution of sounds in the phonemic inventory.

Based on information gained from the breadth of distribution of sounds, the use of phonological rules, and the nature of a child's lexical representations, six different levels of productive phonological knowledge were hypothesized (Elbert & Gierut, 1986; Elbert, 2001, Elbert & Morrisette, 2010). Type 1 knowledge represents the most productive knowledge (adult-like) and Type 6 the least.

Type 1. This involves adult-like lexical representation for target morphemes in all word positions. Type 1 knowledge is signaled by norm production of sounds. Children generally have Type 1 knowledge of nasals and glides. Using /s/ as an example, a child with Type 1 knowledge would produce [s] correctly in all word positions and for all morphemes. This /s/ would never be produced incorrectly.

Type 2. Adult-like lexical representation for target morphemes in all word positions; however, phonological rules would apply to account for specific variations. Keeping our example with /s/, words with /s/ initially would be correct as well as /s/ in the medial-word position. However, in some words there would be variable pronunciation. Therefore, for this example, "toss" and "goose" would demonstrate norm [s] productions, but if a high-front vowel preceded the [s], it could be produced correctly or as a [t]. Here an example would be "peace" that could be pronounced as [pis] or [pit] and "kiss" that would be pronounced as [kɪs] or [kɪt].

Type 3. This is adult-like lexical representation for target in all word positions but only for some morphemes. However, there are some words—it is presumed that these were early acquired words—in which the sound is still incorrect. This type of knowledge can be described by "fossilized forms"—that is, forms that were produced incorrectly at an early age and are now resistant to change. Using the /s/ example, the brother's name "Sam" is pronounced as [tæm].

Type 4. This is adult-like lexical representation in some word positions for target morphemes. Type 4 knowledge is signaled by positional constraints. Irregular sound realizations are noted but only in certain word positions. Using the /s/ example, a Type 4 knowledge might demonstrate correct production of [s] word initially. However, this [s] is incorrect in the medial- and final-word positions.

Type 5. Adult-like lexical representation in some word positions for some target morphemes. Type 5 knowledge is signaled by those representations that were noted in both Type 3 and Type 4 levels. Thus, positional constraints and fossilized forms are both operating on a sound. Using /s/ as an example, the child can produce [s] correctly in some instances when they are word initial. In other words, the [s] is still incorrect; thus, "see" [si], "seal" [sil], and "sit" [sɪt] are correct, yet "soup" is [tup] and "song" is [tɑŋ].

Type 6. Nonadult-like lexical representation in all word positions of all target morphemes. These sounds reflect inventory constraints; they are always produced in an aberrant manner relative to the target sound. Using the /s/ example, this sound would be produced incorrectly in all words.

Measures of Intelligibility and Severity

Measures of intelligibility and severity can be especially helpful in documenting the necessity for or progress in therapy. Measures of severity and intelligibility that meet the specific needs of the age and the speech status of the particular client can be selected.

Measures of Intelligibility

Intelligibility refers to a judgment made by a clinician based on how much of an utterance can be understood. Measurements of the degree of speech intelligibility are based on a subjective, perceptual judgment that is generally related to the percentage of words that the listener understands. Factors influencing speech sound intelligibility include the number, type, and consistency of speech sound errors (Bernthal, Bankson, & Flipsen, 2009). Clearly, the number of errors is related to the overall intelligibility. However, just adding up the errors does not yield an adequate index of intelligibility. For example, Shriberg and Kwiatkowski (1982a, 1982b) reported a low correlation between the percentage of consonants correct and the intelligibility of a speech sample.

The intelligibility of an utterance is influenced by several factors. Connolly (1986) lists the following:

1. The loss of phonemic contrasts
2. The loss of contrasts in specific linguistic contexts

3. The number of meaning distinctions that are lost because of the lack of phonemic contrasts
4. The difference between the target and its realization
5. The consistency of the target-realization relationship
6. The frequency of abnormality in the client's speech
7. The extent to which the listener is familiar with the client's speech
8. The communicative context in which the message occurs

Although intelligibility remains essentially a subjective evaluation, many authors have attempted to quantify it and to apply their results to a wide array of children and adults with communication disorders (e.g., Gordon-Brannan & Hodson, 2000; Hodson & Paden, 1981; Kent, Miolo, & Bloedel, 1994; Shriberg & Kwiatkowski, 1982a; Webb & Duckett, 1990; Wilcox, Schooling, & Morris, 1991). A summary of intelligibility measures is outlined in Box 7.1.

BOX 7.1   Measures of Intelligibility

In spite of the fact that there is not a general procedure for measuring intelligibility, the percentage of words understood in a speech sample is a common way to calculate intelligibility (Gordon-Brannan, 1994). Therefore, an unfamiliar listener puts a (+) mark for every word understood in a speech sample and a (–) for every word not understood. A percentage of intelligibility can then be calculated.

Intelligibility can be categorized according to several indices. The following is based on the frequency of occurrence of misarticulated sounds (Fudala, 2000):

Level 6. Sound errors are occasionally noticed in continuous speech.

Level 5. Speech is intelligible, although noticeably in error.

Level 4. Speech is intelligible with careful listening.

Level 3. Speech intelligibility is difficult.

Level 2. Speech is usually unintelligible.

Level 1. Speech is unintelligible.

A number of procedures have been used, or could be used, to assess intelligibility. The following are selected for the purpose at hand.

The Beginner's Intelligibility Test (BIT), a sentence-level test that was originally designed for children who are hearing impaired but can be used with very young or very unintelligible children, Osberger, Robbins, Todd, and Riley, 1994.

CID Word Speech Intelligibility Evaluation (Word SPINE), for children and adolescents with severe and profound hearing impairments, Monsen, 1981.

CID Picture Speech Intelligibility Evaluation (Picture SPINE), for children and adolescents with severe and profound hearing impairments, Monsen, Moog, and Geers, 1988.

Ling's Phonologic and Phonetic Level Speech Evaluation (PPLSE), for individuals who are hearing impaired, Ling, 1976.

Children's Speech Intelligibility Measure (CSIM), a word-level test for ages 3–10, Wilcox and Morris, 1999.

Children's Speech Intelligibility Test (CSIT), for children of any age, especially for very young children or children with cognitive or motor limitations, Kent, Miolo, and Bloedel, 1994.

Procedures that emphasize phonological process analysis:

Hodson Assessment of Phonological Patterns (HAPP-3), for children with object-naming competence, Hodson, 2004.

Functional Loss (FLOSS), for children with limited phonological systems, Leinonen-Davis, 1988.

The RULES Phonological Evaluation, for children with phonological disorders, Webb and Duckett, 1990.

Vihman-Greenlee Phonological Advance Measure, for children, especially those with phonological disorders, Vihman and Greenlee, 1987.

Procedures that emphasize word-level intelligibility:

Assessment of Intelligibility of Dysarthric Speech, for adults and older children, Yorkston and Beukelman, 1981.

Preschool–Speech Intelligibility Measure (P–SIM), for preschool children but could be used with older children, Wilcox, Schooling, and Morris, 1991.

Phonological Mean Length of Utterance (PMLU) and the *Proportion of Whole-Word Proximity* (PWP), for children primarily, Ingram and Ingram, 2001.

Coplan and Gleason (1988) suggest the following guidelines for the percentage of conversation that is intelligible in typical children.

2 years of age	50% intelligible
3 years of age	75% intelligible
4 years of age	100% intelligible although speech sound errors are possible, speech is intelligible

Measures of Severity

Articulatory competency can also be measured by different severity classifications. Severity measures are attempts to quantify the degree of involvement. Shriberg and Kwiatkowski (1982a, 1982b) originally developed a metric for measuring the severity of involvement in children with phonological disorders. They suggest calculating the *percentage of consonants correct* (PCC). Based on research, this type of calculation was found to correlate most closely to listeners' perceptions of severity. This concept was later expanded to other measures (Shriberg, Austin, Lewis, McSweeny, & Wilson, 1997). Quantitative estimates of severity using the PCC give clinicians an objective measure to establish the relative priority of those who might need therapy, for example. The PCC calculations can be translated into the following severity divisions:

90% mild

65–85% mild–moderate

50–65% moderate–severe

50% severe

Box 7.2 provides the procedure for determining the PCC according to the Shriberg et al. data.

Watch this video and listen to these two short speech samples of three-year-olds Elizabeth and Sandy. Mark the words with + if you could understand them and – if you could not. Figure a percentage of intelligibility and compare it to the Coplan and Gleason (1988) guidelines. Is the percentage higher or lower than the guidelines provided? youtube.com/watch?v=PYxM229pAzw and youtube.com/watch?v=EBM854BTGL0

Listen to the first 2 minutes of the following video of Evan who is 4 years old. Do you think that he is 100% intelligible? If not, which speech sounds are still in error? youtube.com/watch?v=3jHD-7Bc2rM Now listen to the video of this 4-year-old who has been described as having apraxia of speech. If you disregard what the father is saying to help in comprehension of his speech, what would be his level of intelligibility?

BOX 7.2   Determining the Percentage of Consonants Correct (PCC)

What is measured? | A 5- to 10-minute conversational sample is recorded and analyzed.

What to score? | Only consonants are scored using this metric. The examiner is required to make correct versus incorrect judgments on individual consonant productions. The following sound changes are considered incorrect:

1. Deletion of a target consonant
2. Substitution of a target consonant, including the substitution of a glottal stop or a cognate
3. Partial voicing of a prevocalic consonant
4. Any distortions
5. Addition of a sound to a correct or incorrect target sound
6. Initial [h] deletion and final n/ŋ substitutions in stressed syllables only. For example [ɪt] for *hit* and [rɪn] for *ring* would be incorrect. However, in unstressed syllables—for example, saying [fɪʃən] for *fishing*—would be considered correct. Acceptable allophonic variations are considered correct. For example, the intervocalic allophonic variation of [t] in *water* [wɑɾɚ] is considered correct.
7. Postvocalic [ɚ], such as in "farm" [fɑɚm] are considered consonants and are counted as such, [ɝ] and unstressed [ɚ] are classified as vowels and not counted.

What not to score? | Do not score utterances that are unintelligible or consonants in the second or successive repetitions of a syllable. For example, if the child says [bə bə lun], score only the first [b]. Also, do not score target consonants in the third or successive repetitions of adjacent words unless the articulation changes. For example, if the child says [trit], [trit], [trit], only the consonants in the first two words are counted. However, if the child changes the articulation saying [trit], [twit], [trit], then the consonants in all three utterances are counted.

Calculation: | The percentage of consonants correct is calculated in the following manner:

$$\frac{\text{Number of correct consonants}}{\text{Number of correct plus incorrect consonants}} \times 100$$

Shriberg, Austin, Lewis, McSweeny, and Wilson (1997) have expanded the original concept of percentage of consonants correct (PCC) to other measures that examine the percentage of vowels correct (PVC) and a matrix that weights distortion errors, the articulation competence index (ACI), to mention just 2 of the 10 total indexes. A conversational speech sample is the basis for all calculations. For information on the various metric values, see Shriberg and colleagues.

SUMMARY

The goal of this chapter was to show how the data gathered in the appraisal section of our speech sound assessment could be used for different types of analyses. The first portion of this chapter demonstrated how to organize the data collected from the appraisal portion outlined in Chapter 6. A preliminary analysis of speech sounds produced correctly versus those in error included an introduction to forms and procedures to determine the distribution of speech sounds. These procedures were exemplified using a case study of the child H. H. The next step in the diagnostic process examined the data to determine whether a neutralization of phonemic contrasts existed. Based on the definitions of primarily articulation- versus phonemic-based impairments, differentiating characteristics of these two disorders were discussed.

The remaining portion of this chapter outlined the procedures for a comprehensive phonological

assessment. These included the inventory and distribution of speech sounds, analysis of the syllable shapes and constraints, phonological contrasts, and analysis of phonological error patterns. There are several ways to analyze the patterns of errors in a phonological assessment. The following means were exemplified: place-manner-voicing, phonological process, and assessment of productive phonological knowledge. Each of these analyses offers differing results. For each one, sample forms and procedures as well as a continued implementation of each analysis using the case study of H. H. were provided. Finally, measures of severity and intelligibility were described. These measures can be used to document the need for, and progress in, therapy as well as to serve as a basis for clinical research.

CASE STUDY

Spontaneous Speech Sample for H. H.

The following spontaneous speech sample is from H. H. Using the directions from Box 7.2, determine the PCC.

Looking at Pictures	
[dæ ə pɪtə əv ə ta]	[oᵘ dæt ə tɪti]
That a picture of a dog.	Oh, that a kitty.
[hi ə bɪ dɑ]	[wi hæf ə tɪti]
He a big dog.	We have a kitty.
[hi baᵘ ən hæ ə tawə]	[wi dat aᵘ tɪti ə wɑːŋ taˈm]
He brown and has a collar.	We got our kitty a long time.
Conversation with Mom	
[tæn wi do tu mədanoᵘ]	[hi tʌm tu mədanə wɪt ʌt]
Can we go to McDonald?	He come to McDonald with us?
[aˈ wʌ ə ti bɜdə]	[xxxxx mɑˈ haᵘ]
I want a cheeseburger.	Xxxx My house.
[aˈ wʌ fɛnfaˈθ]	[mɑmi lɛ do]
I want french fries.	Mommy let go.
[wɛ ɪt bɪwi]	[lɛ do naᵘ]
Where is Billy?	Let go now.

Talking about Summer Vacation	
[wi doᵘf tu dæma]	[si hæt wɑtə taᵘt]
We drove to Grandma.	She has lot'a cows.
[si wɪf ɪn oᵘ +haⁱo]	[taᵘt ju noᵘ mu taᵘ]
She live in Ohio.	Cows, you know, moo cow.
[si hæt ə fɑm]	[deⁱ it ə ho wɑt]
She has a farm.	They eat a whole lot.

	Correct Consonants	Incorrect Consonants
That a picture of a dog.	2	6
He a big dog.	3	2
He brown and has a collar.	4	6
Oh, that a kitty.	2	2
We have a kitty.	3	2
We got our kitty a long time.	6	4
Can we go to McDonald?	6	5
I want a cheeseburger.	2	5
I want french fries.	4	6
Where is Billy?	2	3
He come to McDonald with us?	7	6
My house.	2	1
Mommy let go.	3	2
Let go now.	2	2
We drove to Grandma.	4	4
She live in Ohio.	2	3
She has a farm.	3	3
She has lot'a cows.	2	5
Cows, you know, moo cow.	3	3
They eat a whole lot.	3	3

Number of correct consonants = 65

Divided by:

Number of correct plus incorrect consonants = 138

= 71 × 100 = 7.1%

PCC = 7.1% <50% = severe

THINK CRITICALLY

The following results are from Brandon, age 5;6:

house	[haᵘs̩]	matches	[mætəs̩]	thumb	[tʌm]
telephone	[tɛfoᵘn]	lamp	[wæmp]	finger	[fɪnə]
cup	[tʌp]	shovel	[tʌvoᵘ]	ring	[wɪŋ]
gun	[ɣʌn]	car	[tɑə]	jumping	[djʌmpən]

knife	[naɪˈf]	rabbit	[wæbət]	pajamas	[djæməʂ]
window	[wɪnoᵘ]	fishing	[fɪtsʲən]	plane	[pweˈn]
wagon	[ʌæɣən]	church	[tsʲɜtsʲ]	blue	[bwu]
wheel	[ʌiə]	feather	[fɛdə]	brush	[bwʌsʲ]
chicken	[tsʲɪtən]	pencils	[pɪntoʂ]	drum	[dwʌm]
zipper	[ʐ ɪpə]	this	[dɪʂ]	flag	[fwæɣ]
scissors	[sʲɪtə]	carrot	[tewət]	Santa	[ʂænə]
duck	[dʌ]	orange	[ɔwɪntsʲ]	tree	[twi]
yellow	[jɛwoᵘ]	bathtub	[bæftʌb]	squirrel	[twɜwoᵘ]
vacuum	[væɣum]	bath	[bæf]	sleeping	[ʂwipən]
bed	[bɛd]	stove	[ʂtoᵘf]		

1. Which sounds are in the phonetic inventory and which ones are in the phonemic inventory for Brandon?
2. Use Figure 7.3, Neutralization of Phonemic Contrasts Summary Form, to list the neutralization of phonemic contrasts for Brandon. Do you notice the collapse of contrasts or any sound preferences?
3. Do you think that Brandon has an articulation- or a phonemic-based speech sound disorder, or do you see characteristics of both? State your reasoning.
4. Do you notice any idiosyncratic processes in the results of Brandon's articulation test?

TEST YOURSELF

1. Clients with phonemic-based disorders show difficulty using
   a. appropriate stress in words
   b. phonemes to contrastively differentiate meaning
   c. s-sounds in a word
   d. articulatory motor movements to produce speech sounds
2. Which one of the following factors is *not* important when considering the guidelines for beginning therapy?
   a. stimulability
   b. sounds affecting intelligibility
   c. whether the sound is a fricative
   d. developmentally earlier sounds
3. A comprehensive phonological assessment includes all of the following *except*
   a. inventory of speech sounds
   b. distribution of speech sounds
   c. syllable shapes
   d. stimulability
4. Which of the following is an example of an open syllable shape?
   a. VCC   c. CCV
   b. CVC   d. CCC
5. A child substitutes a [t] for a [θ] ([θ] → [t]). According to place-manner-voicing analysis, this would be the following:
   a. dental → labial, fricative → stop
   b. dental → alveolar, fricative → stop

c. dental → postalveolar, fricative →
stop, voiceless → voiced

d. dental → alveolar, fricative → stop,
voiceless → voiced

6. Phonological process analysis is a
means of identifying all of the following *except*

a. substitutions

b. contrastive use of phonemes

c. syllable structure changes

d. assimilatory changes

7. Which one of the following would be
considered an idiosyncratic process?

a. [k] → [t]

b. [t] → [s]

c. [ʃ] → [s]

d. [tʃ] → [ʃ]

8. A subjective judgment made by a clinician based on how much of an utterance can be understood is referred to as

a. severity

b. intelligibility

c. percentage of consonants correct

d. articulatory competency

9. Articulation- and phonemic-based
disorders

a. can co-occur

b. always co-occur

c. never co-occur

d. are unrelated

10. Least phonological knowledge would
be represented by which of the
following?

a. adult-like lexical representation for
target morphemes, but some irregular productions occur

b. nonadult-like lexical representation in all word positions of all target words

c. adult-like lexical representations
with positional constraints and fossilized forms

d. adult-like lexical representation,
but positional constraints are noted

FURTHER READINGS

Bernthal, J., Bankson, N., & Flipsen, P. (2009). *Articulation and phonological disorders* (6th ed.). Boston: Allyn & Bacon.

Bleile, K. (2004). *Manual of articulation and phonological disorders: Infancy through adulthood* (2nd ed.). Clifton Park, NY: Thomson-Delmar Learning.

Gierut, J. (1986). On the assessment of productive phonological knowledge. *Journal of the National Student Speech-Language-Hearing Association*, 14, 83–100. Available at www.indiana.edu/~sndlrng/papers/Gierut%2086.pdf

Halle, M. (2002). *From memory to speech and back: Papers on phonetics and phonology, 1954–2002*. Berlin: Walter de Gruyter.

Williams, A. L. (2003). *Speech disorders: Resource guide for preschool children*. Clifton Park, NY: Thomson-Delmar Learning.

APPENDIX 7.1   Preliminary Matrix for Recording Utterances

Word	Prevocalic	Nucleus	Inter-/Post-Vocalic	Nucleus	Inter-/Post-Vocalic	Nucleus	Inter-/Post-Vocalic	Nucleus	Postvocalic
___	/	/	/	/	/	/	/	/	/
___	/	/	/	/	/	/	/	/	/
___	/	/	/	/	/	/	/	/	/
___	/	/	/	/	/	/	/	/	/
___	/	/	/	/	/	/	/	/	/
___	/	/	/	/	/	/	/	/	/
___	/	/	/	/	/	/	/	/	/
___	/	/	/	/	/	/	/	/	/

APPENDIX 7.2 Single-Word Responses to Goldman-Fristoe Test of Articulation for Child H. H.

Target Word	Child's Production
1. house	[hɑᶷ]
2. telephone	[tɛfoᶷ]
3. cup	[tʌp]
4. gun	[dʌn]
5. knife	[nɑᶦ]
6. window	[wɪnoᶷ]
7. wagon	[wædən]
wheel	[wi]
8. chicken	[tɪtə]
9. zipper	[tɪpə]
10. scissors	[tɪtə]
11. duck	[dʌt]
yellow	[jɛwoᶷ]
12. vacuum	[ætu]
13. matches	[mætət]
14. lamp	[wæmp]
15. shovel	[dʌvə]
16. car	[tɑə]
17. rabbit	[wæbɪ]
18. fishing	[bɪdɪn]
19. church	[tɜ]
20. feather	[bɛdə]
21. pencils	[pɛntə]
this	child would not say
22. carrot	[tɛwə]
orange	[oᶷwɪn]
23. bathtub	[bætə]
bath	[bæ]
24. thumb	[bʌm]
finger	[bɪnə]
ring	[wɪŋ]
25. jump	[dʌmp]
26. pajamas	[dæmi]
27. plane	[beᶦn]
blue	[bu]
28. brush	[bʌs]
29. drum	[dʌm]
30. flag	[bæ]
31. Santa Claus	[tænə dɑ]
32. Christmas	[tɪtmə]
tree	[ti]
33. squirrel	[twɜə]
34. sleeping	[twipɪn]
bed	[bɛd]
35. stove	[doᶷ]

APPENDIX 7.3   Preliminary Matrix for Recording Utterances with Examples from H. H.

Word	Prevocalic	Nucleus	Inter-/Postvocalic	Nucleus	Inter-/Postvocalic	Nucleus	Inter-/Postvocalic	Nucleus	Postvocalic
house	h/h	aʊ/aʊ	s/ø	/	/	/	/	/	/
telephone	t/t	ɛ/ɛ	l/ø	ə/ø	f/f	aʊ/aʊ	n/ø	/	unstressed syllable deletion /
cup	k/t	ʌ/ʌ	p/p	/	/	/	/	/	/
gun	g/d	ʌ/ʌ	n/n	/	/	/	/	/	/
knife	n/n	aɪ/aɪ	f/ø	/	/	/	/	/	/
window	w/w	ɪ/ɪ	nd/nø	oʊ/oʊ	/	/	/	/	/
wagon	w/w	æ/æ	g/d	ə/ə	n/n	/	/	/	/
wheel	w/w	i/i	l/ə	/	/	/	/	/	/

APPENDIX 7.4   Matrix for Recording Phones According to Pre-, Inter-, and Postvocalic Word Positions for Child H. H.

Prevocalic

m ✓		n ✓					
p ✓	b ✓✓ ✓	t ✓	d ✓	tʃ [+] [t]	dʒ [d] [d]	k [+] [+] [t]	g [d]
f [b] [b] [b]	v Ø	θ [b]	ð	ʃ [d]	Clusters [pl]→[b] [bl]→[b] [br]→[b] [dr]→[d]	[fl]→[b] [kr]→[+] [skw]→[tw] [sl]→[+w] [st]→[d]	
		s [+] [+]	z [+]				
w ✓✓✓		r [w] [w] l [w]		j ✓		h ✓	
Notes:							

Intervocalic

m ✓		n ✓				ŋ	
p ✓✓	b ✓	t	d	tʃ [+]	dʒ	k [+]	g [d]
f ✓	v ✓	θ	ð [d]	ʃ [d]	ʒ	Clusters [nd]→[n] [ŋg]→[n] [kj]→[+] [kl]→[d] [ns]→[nt] [sm]→[tm] [θt]→[+] [st]→[+]	
		s	z [+]				
w		r [w] [w] l [w]		j		h	
Notes:							

Postvocalic

m Ø ✓ ✓		n Ø ✓✓ Ø ✓				ŋ ✓	
p ✓	b Ø	t Ø Ø	d ✓	tʃ Ø	dʒ	k [+]	g Ø
f Ø	v Ø	θ Ø	ð	ʃ [s]	ʒ	Clusters [mp] ✓✓ [lz] → Ø [ndʒ] → [n]	
		s Ø	z Ø [+] Ø				
Notes:		r l Ø Ø Ø		[ɚz] → [ə] scissors			

APPENDIX 7.5   Overall Inventory of Phones for Child H. H.

m 4✓ 1 Ø		n 5✓ 2 Ø				ŋ 1✓	
p 4✓	b 4✓ 1 Ø	t 1✓ 2 Ø	d 2✓	tʃ 3[t] 1 Ø	dʒ 2[d]	k 5[t]	g 2[d] 1 Ø
f 1✓ 1 Ø 3[b]	v 1✓ 2 Ø	θ 1 Ø 1[b]	ð 1[d]	ʃ 2[d] 1[s]	ʒ not tested		
		s 2[t] 1 Ø	z 3[t] 2 Ø				
w 3✓		r 4[w]		j 1✓		h 1✓	
•Prevocalic 1[pl]→[b] 1[bl]→[b] 1[br]→[b] 1[dr]→[d] 1[fl]→[b] 1[kr]→[t]	l 2[w] 3 Ø 1[skw]→[tw] 1[sl]→[tw] 1st→[d]	Clusters •Intervocalic 1nd→[n] 1[kj]→[t] 1[ns]→[nt] 1[θt]→[t] 1[ŋg]→[n] 1[kl]→[d]		1[sm]→[tm] 1[st+]→[t] •Postvocalic 2[mp]✓ 1[lz]→Ø 1[ndʒ]→[n]			
Notes *Vowel nucleus* 5 [ɚ]→[ə] 2 [ɝ]→[ɜ]							

APPENDIX 7.6   Neutralization of Phonemic Contrasts Summary Form: Application for Child H. H.

List all target sounds together and the substitution(s) used. By examining the Overall Inventory Matrix, determine whether the substitution is consistent (occurs every time) or inconsistent (occurs only in certain contexts). Circle the appropriate word.

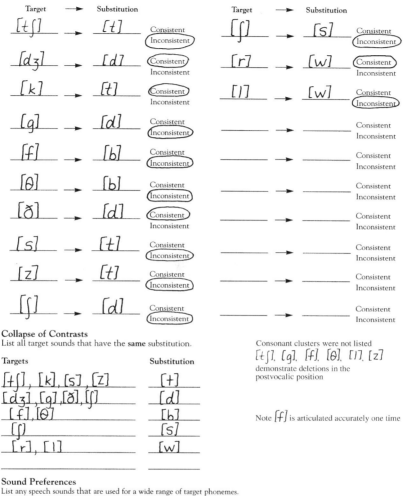

Collapse of Contrasts
List all target sounds that have the **same** substitution.

Targets	Substitution
[tʃ], [k], [s], [z]	[t]
[dʒ], [g], [ð], [ʃ]	[d]
[f], [θ]	[b]
[ʃ]	[s]
[r], [l]	[w]

Consonant clusters were not listed
[tʃ], [g], [f], [θ], [l], [z]
demonstrate deletions in the postvocalic position

Note [f] is articulated accurately one time

Sound Preferences
List any speech sounds that are used for a wide range of target phonemes.

[d] and [t]

APPENDIX 7.7 Place-Manner-Voicing Summary Sheet for Child H. H.

Target	→	Substitution	Circle Differences	Specific Changes	No. of Errors
[tʃ]	→	[t]	(Place) (Manner) Voicing	postalveolar → alveolar / affricate → stop	3 / 3
[dʒ]	→	[d]	(Place) (Manner) Voicing	postalveolar → alveolar / affricate → stop	2 / 2
[k]	→	[t]	(Place) Manner Voicing	velar → alveolar	5
[g]	→	[d]	(Place) Manner Voicing	velar → alveolar	2
[f]	→	[b]	Place (Manner) (Voicing)	fricative → stop / voiceless → voiced	3 / 3

Summary

PLACE		MANNER		VOICING	
Change	No. of Occ.	Change	No. of Occ.	Change	No. of Occ.
postalveolar → alveolar	8	affricate → stop	5	voiceless → voiced	6
velar → alveolar	7	fricative → stop	12	voiced → voiceless	3
dental → labial	1	liquid → glide	5		
dental → alveolar	1				
palatal → labial	3				
alveolar → labial	2				

Distortions ___[ʊ]___

Deletions ___[m], [n], [b], [t], [tʃ], [g], [f], [v], [θ], [s], [z], [l]___

Target	→	Substitution	Circle Differences	Specific Changes	No. of Errors
[θ]	→	[b]	(Place) (Manner) (Voicing)	dental → labial fricative → stop voiceless → voiced	1 1 1
[ð]	→	[d]	(Place) (Manner) Voicing	dental → alveolar fricative → stop	1 1
[ʃ]	→	[d]	(Place) (Manner) (Voicing)	postalveolar → alveolar fricative → stop voiceless → voiced	2 2 2
[ʃ]	→	[s]	(Place) Manner Voicing	postalveolar → alveolar	1
[s]	→	[t]	Place (Manner) Voicing	fricative → stop	2
[z]	→	[t]	Place (Manner) (Voicing)	fricative → stop voiced → voiceless	3 3
[r]	→	[w]	(Place) (Manner) Voicing	palatal → labial liquid → glide	3 3
[l]	→	[w]	(Place) (Manner) Voicing	alveolar → labial liquid → glide	2 2
―――	→	―――	Place Manner Voicing		

APPENDIX 7.8   Proportional Occurrence of Consonant Phonemes in First-Grade, Third-Grade, and Fifth-Grade Children's Speech[1]

	Percent of All Consonants					
	1st Grade		3rd Grade		5th Grade	
Rank	Consonant	Percent	Consonant	Percent	Consonant	Percent
1	n	13.63	n	13.46	n	12.59
2	r	8.20	r	8.73	r	9.01
3	t	7.91	t	7.77	t	7.69
4	m	7.49	s	7.48	s	7.31
5	s	6.94	d	6.53	d	6.81
6	d	6.31	m	6.30	m	5.43
7	w	5.57	w	5.22	l	5.33
8	l	4.96	l	5.05	w	5.05
9	k	4.96	ʔ[2]	4.92	k	4.82
10	z	4.58	k	4.76	z	4.62
11	ʔ[2]	4.49	ð	4.58	ð	4.52
12	ð	4.42	z	4.28	ʔ	3.65
13	h	3.37	b	3.13	h	3.04
14	b	3.18	h	3.07	b	2.94
15	g	2.90	g	2.52	g	2.56
16	f	2.21	p	2.34	j	2.53
17	p	2.12	f	2.18	p	2.49
18	v	1.64	j	1.88	f	2.30
19	j	1.41	v	1.58	v	2.12
20	ŋ	1.05	ŋ	1.19	ŋ	1.38
21	θ	1.03	θ	.96	ʃ	1.33
22	ʃ	0.84	ʃ	.94	θ	1.04
23	ʤ	0.53	tʃ	.57	tʃ	0.74
24	tʃ	0.51	ʤ	.57	ʤ	0.69
25	ʒ	0	ʒ	0	ʒ	0

[1]These data are adapted from Carterette and Jones (1974).
[2]/ʔ/ is included as a "phoneme" of English in the original data.
Source: Lawrence D. Shriberg, Raymond D Kent, *Clinical Phonetics* (2nd ed.). Allyn & Bacon, Pearson Education, Inc., 1995, 358.

Dialects and English as a Second Language

CHAPTER
8

LEARNING OBJECTIVES

When you have finished this chapter, you should be able to:

- Differentiate between Standard English and Vernacular English.
- Differentiate between a regional and a cultural dialect.
- Describe the features of African-American Vernacular English, Appalachian English and Ozark English.

- Evaluate the role that speech-language therapists can play when assessing a child with limited English proficiency.
- Describe the speech sound and specific prosodic characteristics of Spanish, Vietnamese, Cantonese, Korean, Filipino, Hmong, and Arabic American English.
- Identify the procedures that should be considered when evaluating an English language learner.

LANGUAGE variations are quite normal in a society composed of a multitude of social groups that have become quite diversified. Most individuals in the United States have ancestors from other countries and geographic regions have established their own language variations. In addition, immigrants to this country very often do not speak English as their primary language. These and many other factors contribute to a growing diversity in cultural norms, lifestyles, and, of course, speech and language distinctions. The goal of this chapter is to examine a few of these variations that are important as speech-language professionals work with this diverse population.

The purpose of this chapter is, first, to define *dialect* and to compare technical and professional viewpoints concerning this term. The second section examines regional dialects, those variations that are primarily related to geographical areas, and social/ethnic diversities. Phonological characteristics of African-American Vernacular English, Appalachian English, and Ozark English are provided to illustrate three dialects within the United States. The last section of this chapter focuses on the phoneme system of several foreign dialects by noting differences in phonological systems and their patterns as well as exemplifying common problems. Clinical implications for these speech variations are outlined.

Dialects

Dialect is a neutral label that refers to any variety of a language that is shared by a group of speakers. Although this section focuses on the variations in speech sounds represented by a dialect, readers should keep in mind that dialects also encompass specific use of vocabulary, word forms (such as plural endings), sentence structure, and melodic patterns.

The technical use of *dialect*, as a neutral term, implies no particular social or attitudinal evaluations; that is, there are no "good" or "bad" dialects. Dialects are simply those language variations that typify a group of speakers in a language. The factors that might correlate with a particular dialect usage can be as simple as geographical locality or as complex as a person's notion of cultural identity. It is important to remember that socially acceptable or so-called standard versions of a language constitute dialects as much as those varieties that are considered socially isolated or stigmatized language differences. General American English (GAE) also has a dialect referred to as *Standard English.*

There appear to be two sets of representations of Standard English: formal and informal (Wolfram & Schilling-Estes, 2006). **Formal Standard English**, which is applied primarily to written language and most formal spoken language situations, tends to be based on the written language and is exemplified in usage guides and grammar texts. When there is a question as to whether a form is considered Standard English, these texts would be consulted. **Informal Standard English** considers the assessment of the members of the American English–speaking community as they judge the "standardness" of other speakers. This notion exists on a continuum ranging from standard to nonstandard speakers of American English and relies far more heavily on grammatical structure than pronunciation patterns (Wolfram & Schilling-Estes). In other words, listeners accept a range of regional variations in pronunciation but are not as accepting of specific grammatical structures. For example, a rather pronounced Boston or New York regional dialect would be accepted, but structures such as double negatives would not be considered Standard English. On the other hand, **vernacular dialects** refer to those varieties of spoken American English that are considered outside the continuum of informal Standard English (Wolfram & Schilling-Estes). Vernacular dialects are signaled by the presence of certain structures. Therefore, a set of nonstandard English structures marks them as being vernacular. For example, the presence of double negation, lack of subject-verb agreement, and use of variations from standard verb forms would constitute features that could label the speaker as using a vernacular dialect. Although a core of features might exemplify a particular vernacular dialect, not all speakers display the entire set of structures. Therefore, differing patterns of usage exist among speakers of one particular vernacular dialect.

Dialects can vary along several parameters. First, one can describe a dialect according to its hypothesized causative agent. If one examines causation, two main categories are formed: those dialects that (1) correspond to various geographical locations, which are considered **regional dialects** and (2) are generally related to socioeconomic status and/or ethnic background, labeled **social** or **ethnic dialects.** In addition, dialects are classified according to their linguistic features including the phonological, morphological, syntactical, semantic, and pragmatic differences that are distinctive when that dialect is compared to Informal Standard English. It appears that regional dialects typically demonstrate at least distinctive phonological and semantic features. On the other hand, social and ethnic dialects can vary along *all* of the previously stated linguistic features.

Regional Dialects

Individuals who have studied dialect (dialectologists) traditionally have listed three main dialect groups in the United States: northern, midland, and southern. More recent scholars prefer a simple north–south distinction, although there are still significant differences in the boundaries of each proposed area. Many researchers believe that there are no discrete dialect boundaries and no clear-cut dialect divisions in American English. However, data from the Telsur Project show clear and distinct dialect boundaries with a high degree of similarity in each dialect. The Telsur Project of the Linguistics Laboratory of the University of Pennsylvania is one of the largest and most extensive ongoing collections of data related to the dialect regions of the United States. The home page for this project is located within the linguistics department at the University of Pennsylvania. The data consist of phonetic transcriptions and acoustic analyses of informants' vowel systems. These data have been recently compiled in the *Atlas of North American English* (Labov, Ash, & Boberg, 2005) and represent the active processes of change and diversification that the authors have been tracing since 1968 (Labov, 1991, 1994, 1996; Labov, Yaeger, & Steiner, 1972). Their results document four major dialect regions: the North, the South, the West, and the Midland (see Figure 8.1). The first three demonstrate a relatively uniform development of General American English sound shifts, each moving in somewhat different directions. The fourth region, the Midland, has considerably more diversity, and most of its individual cities have developed dialect patterns of their own. The following is a brief summary of these four major dialect regions.

North. The area referred to as North is divided into the North Central region, the Inland North, Eastern New England, New York City, and Western New England. For the short

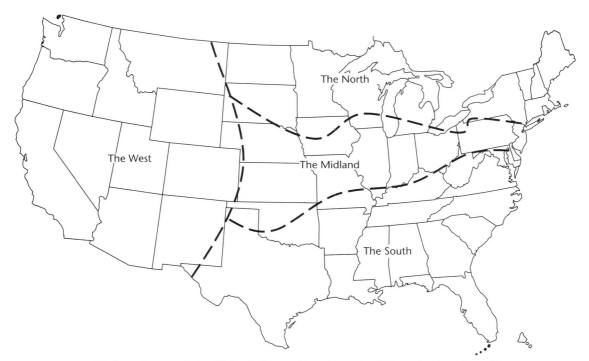

FIGURE 8.1 Dialect Areas of the United States Based on the Telsur Project Results
Source: Summarized from Labov, Ash, and Boberg (1997).

vowels [ɪ], [ɛ], [æ], [ʊ], [ʌ], and [ɑ-a-ɔ], all these areas evidence a specific vowel shift (the Northern Cities Vowel Shift, which is discussed in Labov, 1991, for example). For the long vowels, which include the diphthongs, the North Central and the Inland North regions maintain a long high position, which is typical of the vowel quadrilateral that has been presented in this text. The r-coloring of postvocalic r-productions, such as in *farm* [fɑɚm], is also maintained in these areas.

On the other hand, the Eastern New England area demonstrates r-lessness in which (1) rhotic diphthongs such as those noted in *farm* [fɑɚm] and *porch* [poᵘɚtʃ], (2) stressed central vowels with r-coloring such as in *bird* [bɝd] and *shirt* [ʃɝt], and (3) unstressed central vowels with r-coloring such as in *mother* [mʌðɚ] and *over* [oᵘvɚ] lose the r-coloring, resulting in possible pronunciations such as [fɑəm] or [fɑm] for *farm*, [poᵘətʃ] or [poᵘtʃ] for *porch*, [bɜd] for *bird*, [ʃɜt] for *shirt*, [mʌðə] for *mother,* and [oᵘvə] for *over*.

In addition, the two vowels [ɑ] and [ɔ] are merged into an intermediate vowel, typically [ɑ] or more frequently [a]. Thus, distinct pronunciations for words such as *caught* [kɔt] and *cot* [kɑt] are not realized. Instead, one similar vowel is used for both words. The exception to this is the city of Providence, Rhode Island, which has the characteristic r-lessness but does not merge the [ɑ] and [ɔ] vowels.

New York City has a distinctive dialect that is not reproduced farther west and, therefore, does not fit neatly into any larger regional group. The long vowels maintain a high position similar to that noted for the North Central and Inland North areas. There is consistent r-lessness of postvocalic "r" except for (1) the central vowel with r-coloring [ɝ] and (2) when a final "r" is followed by a vowel in the next word, such as *The car is here.* In addition, the /æ/ vowel splits into lax and tense forms, and the production differences between [ɑ] and [ɔ] are maximal, the [ɔ] vowel being raised to a mid-high position. No clear patterns of sound change seem to occur in Western New England.

South.   The South demonstrates a vowel shift referred to as the Southern Shift (see Labov, 1991). However, a small area of the Southeast—the two cities of Charleston, South Carolina, and Savannah, Georgia—is distinct from the rest of the South. In these cities, the vowel changes are minimal when compared to the rest of the South. A characteristic of the southern region is the [ɑ]–[ɔ] distinction. With the exception of the margins of the South—western Texas, Kentucky, Virginia, and the city of Charleston—this distinction is marked not by a change in the vowel quality but by a back upglide for [ɔ]. Thus, the nuclei of the vowels are acoustically very similar; however, [ɔ] is productionally signaled by a back upgliding movement of the tongue somewhat similar to [ɔᵒ].

Listen to the following two speakers, one from the Northeast (Maine) and one from the South (North Carolina). Try to transcribe their speech and note the variations according to the dialectal variations identified.

Midland.   Speakers in the Midland area do not seem to participate in the vowel shifts that are noted in the South and North. Labov and colleagues (2005) divide the Midland into two sections: South and North. The consistently noted feature of the South Midland is the fronting of [oᵘ], resulting in a [ʌ]-like quality. Exceptions are Louisville, Kentucky, and Savannah, Georgia. Using this criterion, Philadelphia is a member of the South Midland, and Pittsburgh and St. Louis are considered North Midland.

West.   The diversity of dialects declines steadily as one moves westward, resulting in a diffusion of northern, midland, and southern characteristics. Although there are exceptions, characteristics of the West are aligned with those of the Midland. The most prominent feature of western phonology is the merger of [ɑ] and [ɔ]; however, as noted previously, this is not restricted to the West. The second feature that emerges is the fronting of the vowel [u] as in *two* or *do*, which is produced with a tongue position that is more anterior than typical, for example. Although these two characteristics are also noted in the South Midland, their occurrence appears to be much higher in the West.

Regional dialects are related to geographical regions in the United States. These regional boundaries have shifted over the years, and different researchers have described the regions somewhat differently.

Appalachian versus Ozark English

Broadly speaking, *Appalachia* refers to that part of the United States that encompasses the Appalachian Mountain range. However, if the area where Appalachian English is spoken is more narrowly defined, it refers to parts of Kentucky, Tennessee, Virginia, North Carolina, and all of West Virginia. West Virginia is the only state that is included as a whole in this region, although Appalachian English is most often associated with rural populations, not the few metropolitan centers. Speech patterns are most often associated with rural sections of Kentucky, Tennessee, West Virginia, and, to a lesser extent, bordering regions of Virginia and the Carolinas. There are differences from one community to another, but many features are shared in these areas.

On the other hand, Ozark English is spoken in a parallelogram-shaped area that includes the Ozark plateaus, Boston Mountains, Arkansas River Valley, and Ouachita Mountains. It includes a portion of northern Arkansas, southern Missouri, southeast Kansas, and southeast Oklahoma and seems to be bounded roughly by the Arkansas, Grand, Missouri, and Black Rivers. Again, differences have been noted in communities; however, this area is generally considered the area where Ozark English is spoken.

Appalachian and Ozark English are closely related and share many similarities. However, this does not indicate that there is one "mountain dialect" with Ozark English simply being an extension of Appalachian English. It appears historically that these two dialects could descend from a single dialect that was developing in the southern Appalachians in the late 1800s and early 1900s. However, as migration to the Ozark area occurred, the dialect has developed independently since the 1900s into what is now termed *Ozark English.*

Many phonological and grammatical variations are present in these dialects relative to Standard American English. Table 8.1 is a summary of phonological features that vary in respect to the two dialects. It is based on the findings of Christian, Wolfram, and Nube (1988).

Watch this video and listen to the first 2–3 minutes of Appalachian English. Which features do you see that are comparable to Ozark English? youtube.com/watch?v=03iwAY4KIIU

TABLE 8.1 Differences Noted between Appalachian English and Ozark English

Feature	Appalachian English	Ozark English
Epenthesis following clusters: Those with [s] + stop are followed by [ɪz].	"across the <u>desks</u>" [dɛskɪz] Relatively infrequent, more common with plurals	"it <u>lasts</u> for three days" [læstɪz] Relatively infrequent
Intrusive [t]: Items ending with [s]; sometimes [f] has a [t] added.	"<u>once</u> a day" [wʌnsət] More extensive in Appalachian English	"<u>twice</u> a month" [twɑsət]
Fricative stopping: Preceding nasals, voiced fricatives could be stopped, are particularly prevalent with [z], and can occur with [ð] and [z] as well.	"<u>isn't</u> he?" [ɪdn̩t] Found in both dialects	They <u>wasn't</u> raising nothing" [wʌdn̩t] Found in both dialects
Initial [w] reduction: In unstressed position in the sentence, [w] could be deleted.	"a good <u>one</u>" [ən] Fairly prevalent	"<u>they was</u> there" [ðe ʾəz] Fairly prevalent

(Continued)

TABLE 8.1 (Continued)

Feature	Appalachian English	Ozark English
Initial unstressed syllables: Initial unstressed syllables are deleted.	"I don't remember" [mɛmbɚ] Prevalent	"between the two" [twin] Prevalent
[h] addition can occur on "it" and "ain't."	"I said I ain't a gonna do it" [haˈnt] Occurs to some extent	"it was bigger" [hɪt] Occurs to some extent
r-lessness (postvocalic "car," intraword vocalic "carry," and following [θ], especially preceding a round vowel, for example "throw."	Following [θ], [r] absence "throw" [θo] Quite prevalent	Following [θ], [r] absence "throwed" [θod] quite prevalent; other forms present but to a limited degree
Loss of [l] preceding labial consonants occurs.	"wolf" [wʊf]	"help" [hɛp]
Words with final [oᵘ], a [r] and possibly [r] + schwa [ə] replace the [oᵘ].	"yellow" [jɛlɚ] More common in Appalachian English	"tomato" [təmetɚə] Occurs
Final unstressed schwa is raised to high front vowel.	"soda" [soʊdi] Occurs	"extra" [ɛkstri] Occurs
"ire" collapse: The sequence "ire" (which is usually two syllables) is reduced to one syllable without the diphthong.	"fire" [fɑr] Stable in Appalachian English	"iron" [ɑrn] Similar to Appalachian English
Lowering of [ɛɚ]: Mid-vowel is lowered so that "bear" sounds similar to "bar."	"bear" [bar] Mostly in older speakers, more common in Appalachian English	"there" [ðar] Occurs in older speakers

Source: Christian, Wolfram, and Nube (1988).

CLINICAL EXERCISES

In what regional area were you raised? Do you notice characteristics of your speech that seem to coincide with that particular dialect?

Which regional dialects have some degree of "r-lessness"? Why would this be important to know in your clinical practice?

Data in Table 8.2 provide a somewhat different view of regional dialects evidenced in the United States. It includes the geographic areas where these dialects can be heard. Certain phonological changes are associated with each dialect. However, they are not mutually exclusive but demonstrate considerable overlap of several features.

See Table 8.3 for some of the productional overlap in the regional dialects as well as those in African-American English.

TABLE 8.2 Additional Regional Dialects with Notable Changes in Pronunciation

Dialect	Geographical Area(s)
New York	Metropolitan New York
New England	Upper Maine, the Narragansett Bay region, and metropolitan Boston
Southern	Coastal plains from Virginia to eastern Texas, including most of North Carolina, South Carolina, Georgia, Alabama, Mississippi, and Louisiana
Ozark English	Parts of northern Arkansas, southern Missouri, southeast Kansas, and southeast Oklahoma
Appalachian English	Areas of Kentucky, Tennessee, Virginia, North Carolina, and all of West Virginia (urban centers of West Virginia excluded)

Sources: Carver (1987); Christian, Wolfram, & Nube (1988).

TABLE 8.3 Specific Phonological Features of Regional and Cultural Dialects

Phonological Feature	Example	Dialects
Changes in r-Sounds		
Loss of r-coloring on central vowels	*bird* = [bɜd] *father* = [faðə]	New York, New England, Southern, African-American Vernacular English
Neutralization of [r] in postvocalic clusters	*farm* = [fɑm]	New York, New England, Southern, possibly Ozark English
Neutralization of [r] in an intervocalic word position	*Carol* = [kɛəl]	African-American Vernacular English, possibly Ozark English
Neutralization of [r] after a consonant	*throw* = [θoᵘ]	Appalachian, Ozark, African-American Vernacular English
Changes in Individual Consonants		
Initial [w] reduction	*will* = [ɪl]	Appalachian, Ozark English
Substitution of t/θ and d/ð initiating a word	*that* = [dæt] *think* = [tɪŋk]	African-American Vernacular English
Substitution of f/θ and v/ð intervocalic and in final word position	*bathtub* = [bæftʌb] *mouth* = [maᵘf]	African-American Vernacular English
Aspirated vowels initiating a word, sounds like an [h] sound	*it* = [hɪt]	Appalachian, Ozark English
Intrusive [t]	*cliff* = [klɪft]	Appalachian English, can occur in Ozark English
Devoicing of final [b], [d], and [g]	*lid* = [lɪt]	African-American Vernacular English
Changes in Consonant Clusters		
Epenthesis	*ghosts* = [gostəs]	Appalachian, Ozark English
Metathesis	*ask* = [æks]	African-American Vernacular English
Word-final reduction of consonant cluster (especially prominent if one of the consonants is an alveolar)	*test* = [tɛs]	African-American Vernacular English
Deletion of [l] in word-final consonant clusters	*help* = [hɛp]	African-American Vernacular English, also noted in Appalachian and Ozark English before labial consonants
Deletion of word-final consonants with nasalization of preceding vowels	*man* = [mæ̃]	African-American Vernacular English

Sources: Summarized from Christian, Wolfram, & Nube (1988); Fasold & Wolfram (1975); Seymour & Miller-Jones (1981); Wolfram (1994).

Other important variables of dialect have also been recognized in the study of General American English. Among these variables are ethnicity, race, and cultural dimensions of dialect. This next section examines these aspects as they relate to phonological variations in the United States.

Ethnicity, Race, Culture

Often, the terms *race, culture,* and *ethnicity* are used interchangeably in professional literature and informal conversations. However, there are distinctions between each of these terms. **Race** is a biological label that is defined in terms of observable physical features (such as skin color, hair type and color, head shape and size) and biological characteristics (such as genetic composition). **Culture** is a way of life developed by a group of individuals to meet psychosocial needs. It consists of values, norms, beliefs, attitudes, behavioral styles, and traditions. **Ethnicity** refers to commonalities such as religion, nationality, and region. Although race is a biological distinction, it can take on ethnic meaning if members of a biological group have evolved specific ways of living as a subculture.

Several types of relationships could exist between ethnicity and language variation. For ethnic groups that maintain a language other than English, language transfer is possible. *Transfer* indicates incorporating language features into a nonnative language based on the occurrence of similar features in the native language (see also Chapter 5 for information on *transfer*). In some Hispanic communities in the Southwest, the use of "no" as a generalized tag question (You go to the movies a lot, no?) could be attributable to the transfer from Spanish as could phonological features such as the merger of /ʃ/ and /tʃ/ (*shoe* sounds like *chew*), the devoicing of /z/ to /s/ (*lazy* becomes [leˈsi]), and the merger of /i/ and /ɪ/ (*pit* and *peat* sound similar or *rip* and *reap* are pronounced with the same vowel quality).

If one looks through the publications of ethnic dialects, it appears that African-American Vernacular English is one of the most publicized dialects. The next section examines some of the general and phonological characteristics of this dialect.

African-American Vernacular English

Sometimes called *Black English* or *African-American English,* African-American Vernacular English is a systematic, rule-governed dialect spoken by many but not all African-American people in the United States. Although it shares many commonalities with Standard American English and Southern English, certain differences distinguish this dialect. These differences affect the phonological, morphological, syntactical, semantic, and pragmatic systems. This section addresses only the phonological variations.

Not all African-Americans use African-American Vernacular English, and among those who do, the degree of use differs significantly. Several variables influence the use of this dialect: age, gender, and socioeconomic status being the most noted. Relative to age, evidence suggests that the use of this dialect decreases as the individual ages. Elementary school children use a type of dialect that varies the most from mainstream language, whereas dialect features that appear prominently in adolescence level off in adulthood (Washington, 1998).

Gender differences in the use of African-American Vernacular English have also been reported. Males often exhibit increased use of vernacular, nonstandard forms relative to females. This increase in use in the male population possibly represents differential socialization along gender lines. More positive values of masculinity are associated with more frequent use of vernacular forms, whereas women, particularly middle-class women, use standard forms more frequently (Labov et al., 1972).

Socioeconomic status also seems to contribute to differences in the use of this dialect. Low- and working-class African-Americans reportedly use this dialect more frequently than do middle- or upper-middle-class African-Americans. This distinction could also reflect differences in educational background. Terrell and Terrell (1993) suggest that there is a continuum of dialect use from those who do not use the dialect at all to those who use this dialect in almost all communicative contexts. This continuum is significantly influenced by social status variables. African-Americans from middle- and upper-middle-class backgrounds appear to be more adept at code switching, changing back and forth between African-American Vernacular English and Standard American English, than their lower- and working-class counterparts.

A comparison of the documented phonological features of African-American Vernacular English to other dialects in the United States notes four types of phonological distinctions. First those features that can occur in all dialects of General American English but are either more frequent in African-American Vernacular English or in a wider range of communicative contexts. The first four items in Table 8.4 belong to this category. Second, some phonological variations are common to African-American Vernacular English and other nonstandard vernacular dialects but these features are not present in formal or informal standard dialects. Items 5–8 in Table 8.4 represent these features. Third, some of the phonological features represent those noted in the phonology of the South. Often these distinctions (items 9–12) are features of older speakers of southern phonology and are rapidly disappearing in present-day speech. Others (items 13–17) do not or only rarely appear in earlier records of African-American Vernacular English or southern dialect but emerged during the last quarter of the nineteenth century and are expanding rapidly in the speech of both dialects. The last set of features (items 18–24) seems to be distinctive of African-American Vernacular English.

TABLE 8.4 Frequently Cited Features of African-American Vernacular English

Feature	Example
Features in Most Dialects of American English That Appear to Be Most Prevalent in African-American Vernacular English	
1. Final consonant cluster reduction	*first girl* → firs' girl
Loss of second consonant	*cold* → col; *hand* → han
2. Unstressed syllable deletion	*about* → bout
Initial and medial syllables	*government* → gov'ment
3. Deletion of reduplicated syllable	*Mississippi* → miss'ippi
4. Vowelization of postvocalic [l]	*bell* → [bɛə]; *pool* → [puə]
Features in Vernacular Dialects of American English but Not in Standard Dialects	
5. Loss of "r" after consonants	*throw* → [θoᵘ]
After [θ] and in unstressed syllables	*professor* → [pəfɛsɚ]
6. Labialization of interdental fricatives	*bath* → [bæf]; *teeth* → [tif]
7. Syllable-initial fricatives replaced by stops	*those* → [doᵘz]; *think* → [tɪŋk]
Especially with voiced fricatives	*these* → [diz]
8. Voiceless interdental fricatives replaced by stops	*with* → [wɪt]
Especially when close to nasals	*tenth* → [tɪnt]
Features in Old-Fashioned Southern Dialects	
9. Metathesis of final [s] + stop	*ask* → [æks]; *grasp* → [græps]
10. Loss of r-coloring of stressed central vowel [ɝ]	*bird* → [bɜd]; *word* → [wɜd]
11. Loss of r-coloring of centering diphthongs with [ɚ]	*four* → [foə]; *farm* → [fɑəm]
12. Loss of r-coloring of unstressed central vowel [ɚ]	*father* → [faðə]; *never* → [nɛvə]
Features Recently Evolving in Southern and African-American Vernacular English Dialects	
13. Reduction of diphthong [ɑⁱ] to [ɑ] before voiced obstruents and in the final syllable position	*tied* → [tɑd]; *lie* → [lɑ]
14. Offglide centering in [ɔⁱ] to [ɔə]	*oil* → [ɔəl]; *boil* → [bɔəl]
15. Merger of [ɛ] and [ɪ] before nasals	*pen* → [pɪn]; *Wednesday* → [wɪnzdi]
16. Merger of tense and lax vowels before [l]	*bale and bell* → [bɛl];
([i] → [ɪ]; [e] → [ɛ])	*feel* and *fill* → [fɪl]
17. Fricatives that become stops before nasals	*isn't* → [ɪdn̩]; *wasn't* → [wʌdn̩]
Features Apparently Restricted to African-American Vernacular English	
18. Stress of initial syllables, shifting the stress from the second syllable	*police* → [ˈpoᵘ.lis]; *Detroit* → [ˈdi.trɔᵊt]
19. Deletion of final nasal consonant but nasalization of preceding vowel	*man* → [mæ̃]; *thumb* → [θʌ̃]

(Continued)

TABLE 8.4 (Continued)

Feature	Example
20. Final consonant deletion (especially affects nasals)	*five* → [fɑ:]; *fine* → [fɑ:]
21. Final stop devoicing (without shortening preceding consonant)	*bad* → [bæ:t]; *dog* → [dɔ:k]
22. Coarticulated glottal stop with devoiced final stop	*bad* → [bæ:tʔ]; *dog* → [dɔ:kʔ]
23. Loss of [j] after specific consonants (loss of palatalization in specific contexts)	*computer* → [kɑmputə]; *Houston* [hustn̩]
24. Substitution of [k] for [t] in [str] clusters	*street* → [skrit]; *stream* → [skrim]

Sources: Summarized from Wolfram (1994); Stockman (1996).

CLINICAL APPLICATION

African-American American English: More Than Phonological Changes

Although several phonological features of African-American Vernacular English have been introduced in this section, semantic, morphological, syntactic, and pragmatic variations are also a part of this dialect (see, for example, Van Keulen, Weddington, & DeBose, 1998, or Terrell & Terrell, 1993). Children could use these dialect features during language assessment; it is, therefore, important that clinicians be aware of these variations. The following is a summary of African-American Vernacular English features noted in the grammatical structure of preschoolers (e.g., Washington & Craig, 1994).

Morphological and Syntactic Form[1]	Examples
Zero Copula or Auxiliary *Is, are,* and modal auxiliaries *will, can,* and *do* not consistently used	"the bridge out" "how you do this"
Subject-Verb Agreement Use of a subject and verb that differ in either number or person	"what do this mean"
Fitna/Sposeta/Bouta Abbreviated forms for "fixing to," "supposed to," and "about to"	*fitna:* "she fitna a backward flip"
Ain't Use as a negative auxiliary	"why she ain't comin?"
Undifferentiated Pronoun Case Interchange of nominative, objective, and demonstrative cases of pronouns	"him did and him"
Multiple Negation Two or more negative markers in one utterance	"I don't got no brothers"
Zero Possessive Possession coded by word order that deletes the possessive -*s* marker or uses the nominative or objective case of pronouns rather than the possessive	"he hit the man car" "kids just goin' to walk to they school"

[1] Other morphological and syntactic variations were noted, but the previously noted forms were used by at least one-third of the children in the Washington and Craig (1994) study.

Implications for Appraisal. For the speaker who primarily is speaking a dialect or learning English as a second language, several issues need to be considered during an assessment process. The first and foremost factor is determining which phonological characteristics constitute dialectal differences. When contrasted to General American English, the noted variations in pronunciation could be dialectal differences, not signs of a disordered phonological system.

> Watch this video and listen to the first 2½ minutes of it. Note the variations in phonology, morphosyntax, and semantics of the various individuals. Which of the previously presented phonological features do you hear? youtube .com/watch?v=RTt07IVDeww

What to Do?

1. Be sensitive to local dialect patterns and to any regional or cultural dialects that could impact the client's speech. Make an unbiased assessment of an individual's phonology to account for the norms of the particular dialect. In other words, are these phonological variations also represented in individuals with whom this client interacts? In addition, in a society in which the mobility level is high, expect certain regional dialects to appear outside their associated geographical areas.

2. Choose assessment instruments that account for dialectal variations, or consider dialect features when scoring any standardized measure. Some articulation tests—the Goldman-Fristoe (Goldman & Fristoe, 2000), for example—has guidelines for scoring certain dialect features. However, many instruments do not. A clinician's knowledge of dialect features (see Table 8.3) is helpful in scoring these measures.

3. Evaluate not only the presence of specific dialect features but also their frequency. Research results indicate that a judgment of disordered versus different phonological systems is often influenced by the relative frequency rather than just the categorical presence or absence of certain patterns (Bauman-Waengler, 1993a, 1993b, 1994b, 1995, 1996; Kercher & Bauman-Waengler, 1992; Seymour, Green, & Hundley, 1991; Stockman, 1996; Wolfram, 1994).

4. Assess a client's communicative effectiveness in the regional or cultural dialect. If the dialect is unfamiliar, ask other professionals or members of the community about the client's communication skills. The client's teachers are often a good source of information.

CLINICAL EXERCISES

The following is a partial list of words from the Arizona Articulation Proficiency Scale, 4th edition (Fudala, 2000):

horse	baby	bathtub	pig	cup	nine	train
monkey	comb	cake		wagon	dog	table	red

Based on the features that are distinctive to African-American Vernacular English (see Table 8.4, pages 219–220), describe what dialect variations you might hear in those word productions if you were assessing a child who is speaking African-American Vernacular English.

The Speaker of English as a Second Language

The number of immigrants to the United States has increased, averaging more than one million a year between 1990 and 2003 (*Yearbook of Immigration Statistics, 2003*). These individuals come from a wide array of countries and backgrounds and bring a wealth of different languages to the United States. One way to examine the types and numbers of non-English language backgrounds of a **limited English proficient student** is by reviewing the statistics provided by the Department of Education Office of English Language Acquisition, Office of English Language Acquisition, Language Enhancement, and Academic Achievement for limited English proficient students (2013), the U.S. Census Bureau, American Community Survey (2010), and the Migration Policy Institute, National Center on Immigrant Integration Policy (2010).

According to the Migration Policy Institute (2010) more than 460 languages are spoken by limited English proficient students nationwide. The data submitted indicate that Spanish is the native language of the great majority of these students (65.8%), followed by Chinese

The term *limited English proficient* is used for any individual between the ages of 3 and 21 who is enrolled or preparing to enroll in an elementary or secondary school, who was not born in the United States, or whose native language is other than English. This term also applies to individuals who are Native Americans or Alaska Natives and those who come from an environment in which a language other than English has had a significant impact on them. The difficulties in speaking, writing, or understanding the English language compromise the individual's ability to successfully achieve in classrooms where the language of instruction is English or to participate fully in society (PL 107-110, The No Child Left Behind Act [Title III] of 2001). Title III funds are provided to ensure that limited English proficient students (LEPS), including immigrant children and youth, develop English proficiency and meet the same academic content and achievement standards that other children are expected to meet.

(6.0%), Vietnamese (3.2%), Korean (2.5%), and Tagalog (2.0%). Languages with more than 10,000 speakers include Hmong, Arabic, Armenian, Chuukese, French, Haitian Creole, Hindi, Japanese, Khmer, Lao, Mandarin, Marshallese, Navajo, Polish, Portuguese, Punjabi, Russian, Serbo-Croatian, and Urdu. It is interesting to note that the total number of limited English proficient students has increased from more than 4 million in 2002 to more than 25 million in 2010.

Spanish is the dominant language among limited English proficient students in 46 states. Tagalog represents the majority of limited English proficient students in Alaska and Hawaii, French is the predominant language in Maine, and German is found in North Dakota. Refer to Table 8.5 for the three top languages spoken by limited English proficient students by state (2010 statistics).

The following section contrasts the vowel, consonant, and suprasegmental systems of Spanish, Vietnamese, Hmong, Chinese (Cantonese), Korean, Tagalog (Filipino), and Arabic to the phonological system of General American English. This contrast is provided as a possible way to predict which features might be difficult for individuals whose native language is one of those listed and who are learning English as a second language. Although other factors play a role in second language acquisition, it appears that a primary cause of difficulty

TABLE 8.5 Top Three Languages Spoken by Limited English Proficient Students (LEPS) by U.S. State

State	Number of LEPS	1st Language	%	2nd Language	%	3rd Language	%
Alabama	106,089	Spanish	75.70	Chinese	4.80	Korean	2.60
Alaska	38,675	Tagalog	21.00	Spanish	16.50	Korean	6.50
Arizona	616,400	Spanish	80.90	Navajo	3.80	Chinese	2.10
Arkansas	87,142	Spanish	79.90	Vietnamese	3.20	Laotian	2.60
California	6,851,824	Spanish	67.90	Chinese	8.20	Vietnamese	4.40
Colorado	326,788	Spanish	75.10	Vietnamese	30.00	Chinese	2.60
Connecticut	273,392	Spanish	53.90	Portuguese	6.40	Polish	6.00
Delaware	38,760	Spanish	66.00	Chinese	6.60	Gujarati	2.70
District of Columbia	23,553	Spanish	59.70	African Languages	10.20	French	5.50
Florida	2,083,631	Spanish	76.80	French Creole	8.20	Vietnamese	1.70
Georgia	525,251	Spanish	68.00	Korean	5.10	Vietnamese	4.80
Hawaii	152,709	Tagalog	17.60	Japanese	13.10	Chinese	12.90
Idaho	56,551	Spanish	77.20	Russian	2.00	African Languages	1.60
Illinois	1,155,639	Spanish	62.90	Polish	8.60	Chinese	3.80

State	Number of LEPS	1st Language	%	2nd Language	%	3rd Language	%
Indiana	190,052	Spanish	64.80	Chinese	5.90	German	4.50
Iowa	82,533	Spanish	60.10	Vietnamese	7.40	Serbo-Croatian	5.10
Kansas	119,909	Spanish	72.00	Vietnamese	5.60	Chinese	4.80
Kentucky	85,884	Spanish	59.10	Vietnamese	4.20	Chinese	4.00
Louisiana	116,485	Spanish	52.90	French	17.50	Vietnamese	12.80
Maine	21,716	French	41.70	Spanish	12.40	African Languages	9.90
Maryland	343,696	Spanish	49.30	Chinese	8.00	Korean	6.10
Massachusetts	541,648	Spanish	38.30	Portuguese	16.50	Korean	9.60
Michigan	298,059	Spanish	33.30	Arabic	13.90	Chinese	5.90
Minnesota	211,735	Spanish	41.40	Hmong	12.20	African Languages	11.90
Mississippi	44,761	Spanish	69.50	Vietnamese	6.80	Chinese	4.90
Missouri	127,477	Spanish	45.90	Chinese	7.00	Vietnamese	6.40
Montana	8,778	Spanish	26.00	German	23.60	Russian	5.80
Nebraska	75,974	Spanish	73.70	Vietnamese	4.70	African Languages	4.10
Nevada	327,292	Spanish	74.70	Tagalog	6.70	Chinese	4.50
New Hampshire	30,452	Spanish	30.60	French	16.10	Chinese	7.30
New Jersey	1,009,085	Spanish	57.50	Chinese	4.80	Portuguese	4.20
New Mexico	179,836	Spanish	84.50	Navajo	7.70	Vietnamese	1.40
New York	2,432,688	Spanish	50.60	Chinese	13.40	Russian	5.40
North Carolina	432,983	Spanish	76.90	Vietnamese	2.90	Chinese	2.80
North Dakota	8,565	German	20.80	Spanish	14.70	African Languages	12.50
Ohio	249,360	Spanish	35.90	Chinese	7.80	German	6.00
Oklahoma	131,577	Spanish	76.50	Vietnamese	6.20	Chinese	2.60
Oregon	223,302	Spanish	65.40	Vietnamese	7.30	Chinese	5.40
Pennsylvania	451,034	Spanish	43.60	Chinese	8.00	Vietnamese	4.90
Rhode Island	89,537	Spanish	57.50	Portuguese	16.30	Chinese	3.70
South Carolina	133,548	Spanish	76.40	Chinese	2.90	Vietnamese	2.80
South Dakota	14,906	Spanish	38.10	African languages	13.20	German	12.80
Tennessee	167,943	Spanish	66.50	Chinese	4.00	Arabic	3.70
Texas	3,310,492	Spanish	87.40	Vietnamese	3.20	Chinese	2.00
Utah	134,760	Spanish	73.10	Chinese	4.10	Vietnamese	2.30
Vermont	9,793	Spanish	20.80	French	18.70	Chinese	10.60
Virginia	421,444	Spanish	52.40	Korean	7.50	Vietnamese	6.40
Washington	496,622	Spanish	47.30	Chinese	8.00	Vietnamese	6.70
West Virginia	11,385	Spanish	46.90	Chinese	8.30	Arabic	5.90
Wisconsin	170,796	Spanish	61.80	Hmong	9.40	Chinese	4.00
Wyoming[1]	29,037	Spanish	90.40	Vietnamese	6.00	Russian	3.60
U.S. Total	25,051,952	Spanish	65.80	Vietnamese	3.20		

[1]Wyoming was not summarized in the 2010 data; therefore, the numbers for Wyoming are from 2002.

Source: Summarized from Migration Policy Institute (2010). State immigration data profiles. Migration Policy Institute tabulations of the U.S. Bureau of the Census' American Community Survey (ACS) and Decennial Center.

is transfer or interference between the native language and General American English (Yeni-Komshian, Flege, & Liu, 2000).

Spanish American English

Many dialects and language variations of Spanish fall under this one large categorization. Immigrants in the United States who speak Spanish seem to come from (1) Mexico, (2) Central and South America, (3) Puerto Rico, (4) Cuba, (5) the Dominican Republic, and (6) other coutries not specifically identified in the 2010 U.S. census (United States Census Bureau. [2010] *Census 2010*). Washington, D.C.: United States Department of Commerce. See Figure 8.2 for an estimate of the distribution of Spanish speakers in the United States according to this census.

This discussion first examines some basic qualities of the vowel and consonant system of Hispanic Spanish and then attempts to note those differences that might occur in the various dialects of Spanish, such as Puerto Rican and Nicaraguan.

Spanish has five vowels: [i], [e], [u], [o], and [a]. It has no central vowels with or without r-coloring. In addition, all Spanish vowels are long and tense. Thus, for the Spanish student of English, the contrasts between *beat* and *bit, pool* and *pull, boat* and *bought,* and *cat, cot,* and *cut* are difficult. In addition, the [e] and [o] vowels are monophthongs in Spanish. So, although easily recognizable, they sound somewhat different. There is some comparability between the diphthongs of Spanish and English: [aɪ], [aᵘ], and [ɔɪ]. However, the gliding action between onglide and offglide in Spanish for each of these vowels is quicker and reaches a higher, more distinct articulatory position than those of General American English (González, 1988).

Spanish consonants show many similarities. The voiced and voiceless stop-plosives are present ; however, [t] and [d] are articulated as dentals as opposed to the alveolar production of [t] and [d] in General American English. For the Spanish productions, the tip of the tongue is against the edges of the inner surfaces of the upper front teeth. The production is symbolized as [t̪] and [d̪]. Other shared consonants include [j, w, f, m, l, s, tʃ, and n]; [θ] could occur in some dialects but not in others. The consonants [v, z, h, ð, ʃ, dʒ, ʒ, ŋ] are present in General American English but not in Spanish. Although [ŋ] and [ð] are allophones of other phonemes, they do not form minimal pairs in Spanish. In addition, the letter *r* is pronounced differently in Spanish. Spanish has two *r* phonemes: [ɾ] and [r̄]. The [ɾ], which was introduced in Chapter 3, is a flap, tap, or one-tap trill that is an allophonic variation of [t] or [d] in General American English when [ɾ] is produced between two vowels. For example, in casual conversation in General American English, the word *ladder* or *better* can be pronounced [lærɚ] or [bɛrɚ]. The second symbol [r̄] is an alveolar trill (which, according to the International Phonetic Association [2005], is transcribed [r], but to eliminate confusion, it is symbolized here as [r̄]) in which the apex of the tongue flutters rapidly against the alveolar ridge with either two or three vibrations. Therefore, the transference of the Spanish "r" to English produces a somewhat qualitatively different "r" sound. See Table 8.6 for a comparison of the vowel and consonant sounds in General American English to those in Hispanic Spanish.

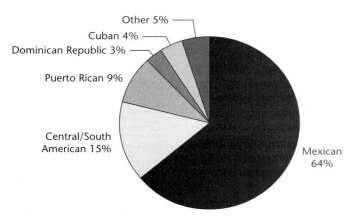

FIGURE 8.2 Distribution of Spanish-Speaking Individuals in the United States

Other 5%
Cuban 4%
Dominican Republic 3%
Puerto Rican 9%
Central/South American 15%
Mexican 64%

Cuban American English. Cuban Americans are considered the oldest population of Hispanic immigrants in the United States. Most of them

TABLE 8.6 Phonological Inventory: A Comparison of Hispanic Spanish to General American English (GAE)

Spanish Vowels	Vowel Differences: Spanish and GAE
[i, e, u, o, a]	■ [ɪ, ɛ, æ, ʊ, ʌ, ə, ɝ, ɚ] and diphthongs are not present in Spanish. ■ Spanish speaker could substitute similar vowels in GAE (e.g., *could* → [kud]) ■ Spanish speaker could substitute [eɪ̄] for [ɝ], *bird* → [beɪ̄d]
Spanish Consonants	**Consonant Differences: Spanish and GAE**
[p, t, k, b, d, g]	■ Because voiceless stops are unaspirated in Spanish, speaker could produce GAE voiceless stops as unaspirated. ■ In GAE [t] and [d] are alveolar production, they are dentalized in Spanish.
[f, x, ɣ, s, β] ([x] is a voiceless velar fricative, [ɣ,] is a voiced velar fricative, and [β] is a voiced bilabial fricative)	■ The GAE [v, z, ð, θ, ʃ, ʒ] are not present in Spanish.
[tʃ]	■ The GAE [dʒ] is not present in Spanish, variable production of [tʃ].
[w, j, l, r, r̄]	■ The production of "r" in GAE may be replaced by the [r̄] which is a trilled vibrant production in Spanish.
[m, n, ɲ]	■ The GAE [n] is an alveolar production while the [n] in Spanish is a dentalized production. ■ The GAE production of [ŋ] is not present in Spanish, the [ɲ], which is present in Spanish, is a palatalized nasal.

Shared consonant blends: [pl, pr, bl, br, tr, dr, kl, kr, gl, gr, fl, and fr] Consonant blends not in Spanish [st, sp, sk, sm, sl, sn, sw, tw, kw, skr, spl, spr, str, skw]

Note: Because Spanish does not allow the letter *s-* in any blend to begin a sentence, this may become a phonotactic constraint. Spanish speakers learning English may try to maintain that phonological aspect of Spanish (e.g., *snake* becomes *esnake*).

Sources: Summarized from Goldstein (1995); Perez (1994); Ruhlen (1976).

CLINICAL APPLICATION

Phonological Changes—Hispanic Spanish

Differences between General American English and Hispanic Spanish lead to the following problems, which Goldstein (2007) and Perez (1994) have noted.

1. Variable production of [tʃ] and [ʃ] in Spanish, thus [tʃoᵘ] for show and [ʃɛk] for check may result in General American English.
2. There is no [z] in Spanish, devoicing of [z] to [s] may occur in General American English.
3. Lack of [v] in Spanish may lead to devoicing of [v] especially in word-final position, thus [hæf] for *have* in General American English.
4. Since there is no [v] in Spanish, in General American English [v] may be realized as [β] (a voiced bilabial fricative) or [b] especially between two vowels, thus, [aβan] for *oven* (the General American English central vowels [ʌ] and [ə] might be replaced by the Spanish [a] vowel).
5. Realization of General American English [θ] and [ð] by the Spanish [t] and [d], thus [tɪŋk] for *think* and [deɪ] for *they*
6. Realization of the General American English [j] for [dʒ] in word-initial position, thus [jas] for *just*
7. Devoicing of General American English [dʒ] between two vowels and in word-final positions, thus, [tineˈtʃɚ] for *teenager* and [læɲwɪtʃ] for *language*
8. Realization of the Spanish [a] vowe for the General American English [ʌ] in stressed syllables, thus [drag] for *drug*
9. Tensing of [ɛ] to [e] in General American English, especially preceding nasals, thus [frend] for *friend*

10. Inconsistent realizations of General American English [i] – [ɪ], [e] – [ɛ], [ɛ], and [æ], and [u] – [ʊ] oppositions, thus, *sick* could be pronounced [sik]
11. Velarization of the General American English [h] to the Spanish [x] (a voiceless velar fricative), thus [xi] for *he*
12. Reduction of consonant clusters in General American English in word-final position, thus *war* for *ward* or *bar* for *bark*
13. Deletion of intervocalic flaps and occasionally other consonants in General American English, thus [lɪl] for *little* and [læɚ] for *ladder*, resulting in syllable reduction in General American English
14. Trilling of the "r" in General American English, which could result in [ɾ] or [r̄] for *r*, thus, [əɾaʊnd] or [ər̄aʊnd] for *around*
15. Intrusive [h] in General American English, thus [hændhɪt] for *and it*
16. Unstressed syllable deletion in General American English such as [sɛpt] for *accept*
17. Shift of major stress on noun compounds from the first word to the second word in General American English, thus, *mini ˈskirt* instead of *ˈmini-skirt*
18. Shift of major stress on verb particles from the second word to the first word in General American English, for example, *ˈshow up* instead of *show ˈup*
19. Shift of stress on specific General American English words such as *ˈac cept* for *ac ˈcept*

Watch the following video of a Spanish American speaker. Listen as she says the following words and sentences: "have, jeep, think, check, teenager: How are you today? I am fine, thank you. It is wonderful weather. There is sunshine and not rain. It is simply marvelous." Transcribe and note the differences in pronunciation.

live today in New York, New Jersey, California, and Florida. Cuban American Spanish is categorized as a variety of Caribbean Spanish, which includes the three Antillean islands as well as the coastal areas of Mexico, Panama, Colombia, and Venezuela (Otheguy, Garcia, & Roca, 2000).

Puerto Rican American English.   Before the invasion of Puerto Rico by the United States in 1898, the island had belonged to Spain for approximately 400 years (Zentella, 2000). Since then, Puerto Rico has experienced intense Americanization. New York presently has the largest population of Puerto Ricans, although a considerable number also live in Massachusetts, Florida, and Pennsylvania (Zentella). The use of Spanish and English varies according to the situation; however, generation also plays an important role. For example, parents who grew up in Puerto Rico speaking Spanish and moved to the United States tend to use Spanish at home with their children, whereas their children speak both English and Spanish.

CLINICAL APPLICATION

Phonological Changes—Cuban American

According to Hidalgo (1987), the following phonological features are problematic for speakers of Cuban American Spanish.

1. Before consonants, [s] is typically aspirated, and in word-final position, [s] is deleted in Cuban Spanish. This could lead to deletion of the final [s] if a transfer is made between Cuban Spanish and General American English.
2. The consonants [l] and [r̄] are frequently interchanged before consonants and in word-final position in Cuban Spanish. This could lead to inconsistent realizations of [l] and [r] in General American English.
3. Deletion of intervocalic and word-final [d]-production in Cuban Spanish could lead to a similar deletion pattern for [d] in General American English.
4. The [r̄] in Cuban Spanish can be pronounced like [h] or as a uvular approximate. This could impact the quality of the r-productions in General American English.
5. In Cuban Spanish the labio-dental [v] is used as a variant of [b], particularly in words spelled with *v*. This could positively impact the production of General American English as the previously noted [b] for [v] substitution, often seen in Spanish speakers, would not be present,

CLINICAL APPLICATION

Phonological Changes—Puerto Rican Spanish

Zentella (2000) noted the following pronunciation problems in General American English for native Puerto Rican Spanish speakers:

1. The use of [s] for [z] and [tʃ], especially before [i] and [e] in Puerto Rican Spanish, could lead to pronunciation differences such as [sip] for *cheap* or [sen] for *chain*.
2. Similarities are noted in items 2, 4, and 5 from the Goldstein (2007) and Perez (1994) list for native speakers of Hispanic Spanish and those noted for Puerto Rican Spanish speakers: problems with devoicing of [z] in all environments, especially in word-final position; realization of [v] as [β] (a voiced bilabial fricative) or [b] especially between two vowels, thus [aβan] or [aban] for *oven*, and realization of [θ] and [ð] as [t] and [d], thus [tɪŋk] for *think* and [deⁱ] for *they*.
3. The consonants [l] and [r̄] are frequently interchanged before consonants and in word-final position in Puerto Rican Spanish. Inconsistent realizations of [l] and [r] could result in General American English.
4. The Spanish [r̄] could be pronounced as an uvular approximant in the middle of words and in the word-initial position. This could impact the quality of the r-productions in General American English.

Nicaraguan American English. Most of the immigration of Nicaraguans to the United States took place during the Somoza regime in the middle of the 1970s with the uprising of the Sandinista group (Lipski, 2000). Nicaraguan populations are primarily concentrated in New York City, Los Angeles, New Orleans, and Miami. In the Nicaraguan population, a group of individuals speaks one of two indigenous languages from this area—Miskito or Caribbean Creole English. Because of their English language skills, this last group of Nicaraguans was able to integrate almost immediately into the job market of the United States (Lipski). The Spanish of the Nicaraguans shares many similarities with the other noted phonemic variations of Spanish speakers in the United States.

Vietnamese General American English

With the end of the Vietnam War in 1975 and the subsequent rule of Vietnam by a communist government, an influx of immigrants came from Indochina to the United States in search of political asylum. Vietnamese is part of the Viet-Muong grouping of the Mon-Khmer branch of the Austroasiatic language family. This family also includes Khmer, which is spoken in Cambodia, and Munda languages spoken in northeastern India and in parts of southern China. Vietnamese is a tone language; the variations in tones signify different meanings. Three dialects of Vietnamese are mutually intelligible: North Vietnamese (Hanoi dialect), Central Vietnamese (Hué dialect), and Southern Vietnamese (Saigon dialect). The tones in each of these dialects vary slightly, although the Hué dialect is more markedly different from the others. Refer to Table 8.7 for a summary of the vowels and consonants of Vietnamese (Hanoi dialect) according to Cheng (1994), Hwa-Froelich (2007), and Tang and Barlow (2006).

CLINICAL APPLICATION

Phonological Changes—Nicaraguan Spanish

According to Lipski (2000), the following phonological features of Nicaraguan Spanish could influence pronunciation of General American English:

1. Weak production of the intervocalic [j] occurs in Nicaraguan Spanish. In General American English words such as *yoyo* and *oh yes,* the [j] sound could be impacted and could be perceived as a sound deletion.
2. Due to the velarization of word-final [n] to [nˠ] or [ŋ] in Nicaraguan Spanish an inconsistent distinction between [n] and [ŋ] at the end of words in General American English could occur; thus, *sun* could be produced as *sung*.
3. The Nicaraguan Spanish [r̄] may be pronounced as a velar approximate in the middle of words and in the word-initial position. This could impact the quality of the r-productions in General American English.

TABLE 8.7 Phonological Inventory: A Comparison of Vietnamese to General American English (GAE)

Vietnamese Vowels	Vowel Differences: Vietnamese and GAE
[i, u, e, ɛ, o, ɔ, a, ɯ, ɤ] ([ɯ] is a high-back vowel without lip rounding; [ɤ] is a mid-back vowel without lip rounding.)	■ [ɪ, ʊ, ɝ, ɚ] and most diphthongs do not exist in Vietnamese; [ie], [ɯɤ], and [uo] are diphthongs in the southern dialect. ■ Vowels which do not exist in Vietnamese speakers (such as [ɪ] and [ʊ]) may lead to a substitution of similar vowels in GAE (e.g., *hit*→[hit]).
Vietnamese Consonants	**Consonant Differences: Vietnamese and GAE**
[p, b, t̪, tʰ, ʈ, d, c, k, ʔ] ([ʈ] is a voiceless retroflex stop, whereas [c] is a voiceless palatal stop.)	■ The [t] consonant is dentalized, and one /t/ has aspiration in Vietnamese. These may replace the alveolar production of [t] in GAE. ■ There is no [g] in Vietnamese, therefore, the voiceless [k], which is present in Vietnamese may be used to replace [g] in GAE.
[f, s, z (or z̧), x,ɣ, h] ([x] is a voiceless velar fricative, [ɣ] is the voiced velar fricative, and [z̧] is a retroflex fricative.)	■ [z] seems to be limited to the northern dialect speakers of Vietnamese, therefore, this could create the use of the voiceless [s] in GAE. ■ [v, ʃ, ʒ] appear only in certain dialects of Vietnamese. Therefore, these consonants may be absent in some Vietnamese natives speaking GAE. ■ [ð, θ] do not exist in Vietnamese. Substitutions for these sounds by [s] or possibly [f] may be used by the Vietnamese speaker speaking GAE. ■ [tʃ, dʒ] appear only in certain dialects of Vietnamese. Therefore, production may be variable in GAE, another fricative being used by the Vietnamese speaker of GAE.
[j, w, l, r, ɽ] ([ɽ] is a tap/flap retroflex sound.)	■ Depending on the dialect, r-sounds are variable in Vietnamese. The tap/flap retrofex [ɽ] is noted in northern and southern dialect speakers of Vietnamese, whereas central dialect speakers produced [r]. This could lead to qualitative differences in GAE pronunciation of "r" by the native Vietnamese speaker.
[m, n, ŋʔ, ɲ] ([ɲ] is a palatal nasal.)	■ Postdorsal-velar nasals exist in Vietnamese, however it is [ŋʔ] a nasal combined with a glottal stop. The palatal nasal of Vietnamese could be substituted for the postdoral-velar nasal of GAE.
Vietnamese is a tone language.	■ Vietnamese has no consonant blends. This will present difficulties for the Vietnamese speaker learning GAE with its many consonant clusters. ■ Final consonants in Vietnamese are limited to [p, t, k, m, n, ŋ].

CLINICAL APPLICATION

Phonological Changes—Vietnamese

Based on the absence of certain consonants and the discussion by Cheng (1994) and Hwa-Froelich (2007), the following possible pronunciation difficulties could arise in a Vietnamese speaker of GAE.

1. The long vowel [i] in Vietnamese could be used for the [ɪ] vowel in GAE. Thus, "pick" sounds like [pik]. Either [e] or [ɛ] could be used as a substitute for [æ]; thus, "tap" sounds like [tep] or [tɛp].
2. There are no central vowels with r-coloring in Vietnamese. This sound, especially its prevalence in GAE, might be problematic for Vietnamese speakers of GAE.
3. The affricates [tʃ] and [dʒ] do not exist in certain dialects of Vietnamese and could be productionally difficult for a Vietnamese speaker of GAE.
4. Vietnamese has a limited number of final consonants. The consonants [p, t, k, m, n, ŋ] are the only final consonants used by all three Vietnamese dialects. Therefore, a Vietnamese speaker might have problems realizing other consonants in the word-final position.

5. Vietnamese has no consonant combinations. A Vietnamese speaker could either reduce the combination to a singleton production or insert a schwa sound between the blend. Thus, the word *stew* might become [sətu].

6. [θ] and [ð] are not present in Vietnamese. There is a tendency to substitute the [t] or [s] for [θ] and [d] or [z] for [ð]. The consonants [d, s, z] do not exist in word-final position in Vietnamese; therefore, [t] could be a common substitution.

Korean American English

In 1903, the first Korean immigrants arrived in Honolulu, Hawaii, then a U.S. protectorate. Today, more than one million Korean Americans live throughout the United States, representing one of the largest Asian American populations in the country. The largest concentrations—about one-quarter of all the Korean Americans—are found in the five-county area of Los Angeles, Orange, San Bernardino, Riverside, and Ventura. The next largest area of concentration is the New York region, including New York City, northern New Jersey, and the Connecticut–Long Island area. This area constitutes about 16% of the entire Korean American population in the United States. The Baltimore–Washington metro area also has a large number of Korean Americans.

The Korean language belongs to the Altaic language group but contains many words of Chinese origin (Ball & Rahilly, 1999). It has 19 consonants and 8 vowels that occur distinctively long or short. Table 8.8 summarizes the vowels and consonants of Korean (Pae, 2007; Ladefoged and Maddieson, 1996; and Lee, 1999).

> Watch the following videos. The first one is of a Vietnamese American speaker, and the second is of a Korean American speaker. The Vietnamese speaker says the following words: *cheese, watch, scratch, father, yellow,* while the Korean speaker says these words: *with, thumb, letter, really, first.* They both say the following sentences: "How are you today?" "I am fine, thank you." "It is wonderful weather." "There is sunshine and not rain." "It is simply marvelous." Transcribe their speech and note the differences in pronunciation.

TABLE 8.8 Phonological Inventory: A Comparison of Korean to General American English (GAE)

Korean Vowels	Vowel Differences: Korean and GAE
[i, e, ø, ɛ, a/ɑ, ɯ, u, o, ʌ] ([ɯ] is a high-back vowel without lip rounding, and [ø] is a close-mid-vowel similar to [e] but with lip rounding.)	■ Korean has a set of short vowels and long vowels that, according to Lee (1999), demonstrate slightly different tongue positions. ■ Korean has several diphthongs that begin with [j], ([ja/jɑ, jʌ, jo, ju, jɛ,]) and [w] ([wa/ɑ, wʌ, wɛ, wi]), and [ɯ] ([ɯi]). ■ The vowels [ɪ, æ, ʊ] as well as the central vowels with r-coloring are not present in Korean.
Korean Consonants	**Consonant Differences: Korean and GAE**
[p, pʰ1, t, tʰ, k, kʰ, d1]	■ Voicing is context dependent in Korean; when initiating a syllable, stop-plosives are voiceless; intervocalically, they are voiced. This could cause difficulties with voiced and voiceless stop-plosives in GAE.
[s, z, h]	■ [f, v, ʃ, ʒ, θ, ð] are not present in Korean leading to substitution of another fricative in GAE.
[tʃ tʃʰ, dʒ, dʰʒ]2	■ Affricates in Korean appear similar to those of GAE; however, aspiration has phonemic value in Korean and could lead to difficulties understanding specific words in GAE.
[m, n, ŋ]	

(Continued)

TABLE 8.8 (Continued)

Korean Consonants	Consonant Differences: Korean and GAE
[l, ɾ, w]	■ The consonants [r, j] are not present in Korean. The [l] in Korean is in allophonic variation with [ɾ], which has certain similarities to [r], but leads to the typical mix-up of these consonants. ■ The syllable structure of Korean is C, VC, or CVC. ■ Syllable-final sounds in Korean consist only of [p, t, k, m, n, ŋ, l]. Other final consonants may be difficult for the Korean speaking GAE. ■ There are no syllable-initial or final consonant clusters in Korean, although intersyllabic clusters are possible. Therefore, consonant clusters may prove problematic for the Korean speaker when using GAE.

[1]Initiating a word, these sounds are voiceless unaspirated or slightly aspirated whereas intervocalically, they are voiced.

[2]Lee (1999) describes the affricate dʰʒ as containing palatal stops ([c] and [ɟ]), whereas Ladefoged and Maddieson (1996) use the symbols [tʃ tʃʰ, dʒ, dʰʒ] that are noted above. Kim and Pae (2007) transcribe the affricates as [tɕ] and [tɕʰ], i.e., stops followed by alveolo-palatal fricatives.

CLINICAL APPLICATION

Phonological Changes—Korean

The following are considered problematic for Korean speakers of GAE.

1. Korean differs considerably from GAE in the phonetic realization of word-final stops. Korean word-final stops are always unreleased—that is, produced without audible aspiration—whereas GAE stops can be either released or unreleased. This and the differences in voicing and aspiration initiating a word versus intervocalically can lead to confusion of [p] – [b], [t] – [d], and [k] – [g] pairs of words such as *cap* and *cab*.

2. Several GAE consonant sounds do not exist in the Korean speech sound system. These include the fricatives /f/, /v/, /θ/, and /ð/. These sounds are typically produced as /p/, /b/, /t/, and /d/, respectively, and the /p/ – /f/ and /b/ – /v/ sound distinctions are very often confused.

3. Korean speakers make no distinction between /r/ and /l/ because [l] is an allophonic variation of [ɾ] that may sound somewhat like an r-sound. Combined with the fact that there are no central vowels with r-coloring, leads to problems with r-sounds and the stereotyped [r] – [l] mix-up.

4. The structure of syllables in Korean and English differs. In Korean, consonants are not released unless they are followed by a vowel in the same syllable, and word-final consonants are never released. This may cause the insertion of a vowel at the end of GAE words that ends with a consonant. For example, *Mark* becomes [maku] and *college* becomes [kaɭədʒi]. This is a strong characteristic of the speech of Korean speakers just beginning to learn GAE.

5. Because syllable-initial and -final consonant clusters do not exist in Korean, Korean learners of GAE could have difficulty realizing these clusters.

6. Korean is a syllable-timed language, and Korean learners of GAE are not accustomed to the patterns of stressed and unstressed syllables in GAE words.

7. Korean learners of English have little or no experience in using GAE in communicative situations in which emphasizing and deemphasizing words takes on a meaning in context. Also, Korean has a very different syntactic structure when compared to GAE. Because of these factors, Korean learners of GAE tend to pronounce each word in a sentence with equal emphasis. They have difficulty producing and perceiving forms with weak stress in GAE and have problems knowing where to speed up, slow down, add stress, or deemphasize words in their sentences for communicative effect.

Cantonese American English

The majority of Chinese Americans are from the Canton Province in southern China. They originally settled in California; according to the U. S. Census Bureau, Statistical Abstract of the United States (2012) more than 300,000 Chinese Americans live in the San Jose–San Francisco–Oakland–Greater Los Angeles area. More than 500,000 Chinese Americans now reside in New York City.

As one of the Chinese languages, Cantonese belongs to the Sino Tibetan language family, which also includes Tibetan, Lolo Burmese, and Karen (the latter two are also spoken in Burma). The major languages in Chinese are Mandarin, Wu, Min, Yue (Cantonese), and Hakka (Li and Thompson, 1987). Because Cantonese has so many dialects, the language is sometimes referred to as a group of *Cantonese dialects*, not just Cantonese. Oral communication is virtually impossible among speakers of some different Cantonese dialects. For instance, there is as much difference between the dialects of Taishan and Nanning as there is between Italian and French. According to its linguistic characteristics and geographical distribution, Cantonese can be divided into four main dialects: Yuehai (including Zhongshan, Chungshan, Tungkuan) as represented by the dialect of Guangzhou City, Siyi (Seiyap) as represented by the Taishan city (Toishan, Hoishan) dialect, Gaoyang as represented by the Yangjiang city dialect, and Guinan as represented by the Nanning city dialect, which is widely used in Guangxi province. If not otherwise specified, the term *Cantonese* often refers to the Guangzhou dialect, which is also spoken in Hong Kong and Macao. See Table 8.9 for the vowels and consonants of this dialect.

TABLE 8.9 Phonological Inventory: A Comparison of Cantonese (Hong Kong) to General American English (GAE)

Cantonese Vowels	Vowel Differences: Cantonese and GAE
[i, y, ɛ, œ, ɔ, u, ɐ, a] + [ɪ, ɵ, ʊ] are allophonic variations of [i, œ, u], respectively. ([y] is a high-front vowel with lip rounding, [ɵ] is a central vowel with lip rounding, and [œ] is a vowel similar to [ɛ] but with lip rounding.)[1] Diphthongs: [ai, ei, ɐi, ui, ɔi, au, ɐu, ou, ɵy, ɛu]	■ Although there are many vowel similarities between Cantonese and GAE, [æ, ɑ, ɝ, ɚ, ʌ, ə] are not present in Cantonese. These may be difficult vowel sounds for the Cantonese speaker of GAE. ■ Although Cantonese has long and short vowels, they do not differ qualitatively. Therefore, long and short vowels such as [e] and [ɛ] in GAE, which do differ qualitatively, can be difficult for the Cantonese speaker of GAE. ■ Diphthongs of Cantonese, whereas not exactly the same, sound fairly close to those represented in GAE.
Cantonese Consonants	**Consonant Differences: Cantonese and GAE**
[p, pʰ,[2] t, tʰ, k, kʰ, kʷ[3]]	■ Stop-plosives, with the exception of [b, d, g] exist in Cantonese. These voiced stop-plosives may be difficult for Cantonese speakers of GAE. ■ In Cantonese, phonemic oppositions are signaled by the presence and absence of aspiration whereas aspiration in GAE does not have phonemic value. Cantonese speakers can have distributional difficulties with aspirated and unaspirated productions in GAE.
[f, s, h]	■ Voiced fricatives [v, z] as well as [ʃ, ʒ, θ, ð] are not present in Cantonese, therefore, may be difficult for the Cantonese speaker of GAE.
[ts, tʰs, dz, dʰz]	■ Affricates are somewhat different in Cantonese. There is phonemic opposition between aspirated and unaspirated [t, d] in affricate productions. In GAE, aspiration does not have phonemic value and the fricative portion of the affricate is more posteriorly articulated. ■ [r] is not present in Cantonese but is a fairly frequent consonant in GAE.

(Continued)

TABLE 8.9 (Continued)

Cantonese Consonants	Consonant Differences: Cantonese and GAE
Cantonese, a tone language	■ In Cantonese final consonants are limited to [p, t, k, m, n, ŋ]. Therefore, other final consonants may be difficult for Cantonese speakers of GAE ■ Consonant clusters do not exist in Cantonese unless [kʷ] and [kʷʰ] are considered. In GAE consonant clusters are very frequent. ■ Six possible syllable shapes in Cantonese are C, V, CV, VC, CVV, and CVC. There are many other possible syllable shapes in GAE. ■ Syllables are equally stressed, and each syllable carries a tone in Cantonese. Stressing is variable in GAE and may prove problematic for the Cantonese speaker learning GAE.

[1]There are long and short variants of many vowels and diphthongs in Cantonese. Officially Cantonese counts fifty-two vowels (Cheng, 1994).

[2]The raised [ʰ] indicates that these sounds have an aspirated and a nonaspirated variation, which is phonemic, and therefore distinguishes meaning between words.

[3]The [kʷ] is a coarticulated consonant; because the [k] and [w] are articulated together, some refer to it as a *consonant cluster*.

Source: Summarized from Lee (1999); To, Cheung, & McLeod (2013).

CLINICAL APPLICATION

Phonological Changes—Cantonese

Chan and Li (2000) outline the following learner difficulties regarding GAE for Cantonese speakers.

1. Cantonese has no voiced syllable-final plosives; therefore, GAE learners tend to substitute [p, t, k] for [b, d, g] in the word-final position. In addition, Cantonese speakers tend not to release the voiceless plosives, which is transferred to GAE. Thus, *rope* and *robe* or *mate* and *maid* are practically indistinguishable. Cantonese learners of GAE also tend to devoice plosives in syllable-initiating position.
2. Because of the absence of voiced [v] and [z], Cantonese speakers of GAE tend to substitute their voiceless counterparts, [f] and [s].
3. Because [ʃ] and [ʒ] do not exist in Cantonese, [s] is often used in GAE as a substitute for these sounds.
4. Cantonese does not have "th" sounds, and Cantonese GAE speakers often substitute [t] or [f] for [θ] ([tɪn] for *thin*) and [d] or [f] for [ð] ([feɪ] for *they*).
5. The affricates [tʃ] and [ʤ] do not exist; Cantonese GAE speakers tend to substitute [ts] and [dz] for [tʃ] and [ʤ].
6. Cantonese GAE speakers often have trouble distinguishing [l], [n], and [r]. When the [r] is in a word-initial position, these speakers tend to substitute an l-like sound for [r]. Other speakers might substitute [w] for [r]. In word-initial position, [n] could be substituted for [l], whereas in final position, the [l] could be deleted or a [u] sound used, rendering *wheel* as [wiu].
7. Long and short vowels are problematic for Cantonese speakers of GAE. Thus, word pairs with [i] – [ɪ] and [u] – [ʊ] could be difficult.
8. When [i] or [ɪ] occur at the beginning of a word, Cantonese speakers of GAE tend to add a [j] sound; thus, *east* and *yeast* could sound the same. This is a transfer from Cantonese as the vowel [i] in word-initial position is preceded by [j].
9. Because Cantonese contains no consonant clusters, Cantonese speakers of GAE tend to delete these clusters in words or insert a schwa vowel between the consonant sounds of the cluster.

Filipino/Tagalog American English

Filipino has been the national language of the Philippines since 1937. It is based on Tagalog, which is a Malayo-Polynesian language. Filipino is primarily Tagalog with borrowed words from several languages, such as Old Javanese, Malay, Sanskrit, Arabic, Spanish, Chinese, and English. Foreign words that have been introduced have impacted the Filipino lexicon and phonology, but the morphosyntax has stayed basically the same.

The Philippines has 171 indigenous languages; Filipino is the second language of 70–90% of the population. Since 1973, the Philippines has implemented a bilingual Filipino–English educational policy, and the mass media report in both Filipino and GAE. The U.S. Census Bureau, 2011 American Community Survey estimated the U.S. population of Filipinos at 4 million. Filipino Americans are the second largest population of Asian Americans and represent the largest population of overseas Filipinos (69% of Filipinos who are foreign born). Significant numbers of Filipino-Americans reside in California, Hawaii, Texas, Illinois, and the New York metropolitan area. See Table 8.10 for the vowels and consonants of Filipino.

TABLE 8.10 Phonological Inventory: A Comparison of Filipino (Tagalog) to General American English (GAE)

Filipino/Tagalog Vowels	Vowel Differences: Filipino/Tagalog and GAE
[a, e, i, o, u] all vowels short	■ [ɪ, ɛ, æ, ʊ, ʌ, ə, ɝ,ɚ] are not present in Tagalog. Long vowels do not exist in Tagalog, and speakers could have difficulty with the long versus short vowel oppositions
Diphthongs: [iw, iy/ ey, ɑy, ɑw, uy/oy]	■ The diphthongs of Tagalog are close to the articulations of the diphthongs in GAE.
Filipino/Tagalog Consonants	**Consonant Differences: Filipino/Tagalog and GAE**
[p,b, t, d, t̪, d̪, k, g, ʔ]	■ In Filipino all stop-plosives are represented which occur in GAE.
	■ The glottal stop is used in Tagalog to differentiate pronunciations that are the same in spelling "bata" [bata] = bathrobe, "bata"[baʔa] = child. As the glottal stop is not a consonant of GAE, this may be perceived as an intrusive sound.
[s, ʃ, h]	■ The fricatives [f, v, z, ʒ, θ, ð] do not exist in Tagalog/Filipino, however, are frequent consonants in GAE.
[tʃ, dʒ]	■ Affricates in Tagalog/Filipino are the same as GAE.
[w, j, r]	■ In Tagalog/Filipino the [r] is similar to the Spanish trilled [r], either a flap or a trill. This may be noticeable in "r" productions of GAE.
	■ In Tagalog/Filipino, [d] and [r] are allophones, therefore, confusion may exist between [d] and [r] in GAE.
	■ There is no [l] in Tagalog/Filipino, however, is fairly frequent in GAE.
[m, n, ŋ]	■ In Tagalog/Filipino [ŋg] can occur anywhere in a word, including the beginning. However, in GAE, [ŋ] is only in the word- or syllable-final position.
	■ There are no native root words in Tagalog/Filipino with initial consonant clusters. Words with initial consonant clusters are borrowed words in Tagalog/Filipino.
	■ The most common syllable structures in Tagalog/Filipino are CV and CVC. In syllables where the vowel is in the initial position, a glottal stop acts as the onset. GAE has many more syllable shapes and glottal stops are not used phonemically in GAE.

Sources: Himmelmann, ed. Booij, Lehmann, Mugdan, & Skopeteas (2000). Malabonga and S. Marinova-Todd (2007).

CLINICAL APPLICATION

Phonological Changes—Filipino/Tagalog

Differences between GAE and Filipino English can lead to the following problems noted by Malabonga and Marinova-Todd (2007) and Ryan (2009).

1. The central vowel [ʌ] does not exist in Filipino/Tagalog. Substitution of [a] for it will occur in GAE, thus [kap] for "cup." In unstressed syllables, the substitution of [a] for [ə] are probably not noticeable.
2. Inconsistent realizations of [i] – [ɪ], [e] – [ɛ]/ [æ], and [u] – [ʊ]. Thus, "ten" in GAE could be pronounced [ten].
3. The "r" that is a tap or trill in Filipino/Tagalog is substituted for GAE central vowels with r-coloring [ɝ], [ɚ] and the consonantal-r. This is productionally different but is still perceived as an "r" that is somewhat "off." In Tagalog, the [d] and [r] are allophones; they could be used interchangeably. However, because both [d] and [r] exist in GAE and Tagalog, this should not create problems.
4. The th-sounds [ð, θ] do not exist in Tagalog. Substitutions of [d]/[z] (possibly [s] in GAE because [z] does not exist in Filipino) for [ð] and [t]/[s] for [θ] are common. Thus, "thought" becomes [tat] or [sat], and "they" becomes [de] or [ze] or possibly [se].
5. Tagalog has no [f] or [v]. Sound substitutions in GAE are typically [p] and [b]. Thus, the word "Filipino" is typically pronounced [pilopino].
6. Although initial consonant clusters do exist in Filipino/Tagalog, initial consonant clusters are present but they are from borrowed words. Therefore, initial- and final-word consonant clusters in GAE pronunciations could be reduced or a schwa inserted; "stop" becomes [sap] or [tap], possibly [sətap].

Watch the following video and listen to this Filipino girl read a "very difficult word list." Note the speech sound differences, especially the stress difficulties as she tries to say these GAE words. Also note the differences between her reading of individual words (and how the written word could change her pronunciation) and her spontaneous speech between the readings. youtube .com/watch?v=RTt07IVDeww

Hmong General American English

Many Hmong people have immigrated to the United States to escape the death and horror of a genocidal war against them. The long campaign of the Laotian and Vietnamese governments to destroy the Hmong is vengeance for Hmong support of the United States in the Vietnam War. According to the United States Census Bureau, *Statistical Abstract of the United States: 2012* (131st Edition), more than 260,000 Hmong people live in the United States and are largely concentrated in California, Wisconsin, and Minnesota. Several million Hmong people remain in China, Thailand, and Laos, speaking a variety of Hmong dialects. The Hmong language group is a monosyllabic, tonal language (7 to 12 tones, depending on the dialect). Hmong appears to have two basic dialects: Mong Leng and Hmong Der. These two dialects are mutually intelligible. In Table 8.11, the consonant and vowel inventories are based on the Mong Leng dialect as identified by Mortensen (2004), and the phonology of Hmong Der can be found in Ratliff (1992). Table 8.11 depicts the vowels and consonants of Hmong Mong Leng dialect; information is summarized from Matisoff (1991), McCurdy (2010) and Mortenson (2004).

Arabic American English

Arabic is the largest group of the Semitic language family with 206 million speakers. Classified as a Central Semitic language, it is closely related to Hebrew and Aramaic. More than 300 million people across much of the Middle East, North Africa, and the Horn of Africa speak a collection of Semitic languages. Modern Standard Arabic has its historical basis in Classical Arabic, which has documented inscriptions since the sixth century and has been a literary and liturgical language of Islam since the seventh century. See Table 8.12 for an overview of the Standard Arabic vowels and consonants.

TABLE 8.11 Phonological Inventory: A Comparison of Mong Leng Hmong to General American English (GAE)

Hmong Vowels	Vowel Differences: Hmong and GAE
[i, ɨ, e, æ, a, u, ɔ] ([ɨ] is a rounded centralized vowel with a high tongue position. The tongue position is moved horizontally so that the maximum elevation of the tongue is mediopalatal rather than prepalatal as it is with [i].)	■ In Hmong, [æ] and [a] are variants of one /a/-type vowel; they can be used interchangeably. Hmong speakers might have trouble realizing the distinctions between these two vowels in GAE.
Three nasalized vowels exist: [ĩ], [ũ], and [ã].	■ The short vowels [ɪ, ɛ, ʊ, o] and the central vowels of GAE are not part of the Hmong inventory. Hmong speakers of GAE may have difficulty realizing these vowels or may substitute similar vowels.

Hmong Consonants	Consonant Differences: Hmong and GAE
[p, pʰ, pˡ, pˡ, t, tʰ, t, tʰ, c, cʰ, k, kʰ, q, qʰ, ʔ, d, dʰ] Note: the superscript [ʰ] indicates aspiration which has phonemic value in Hmong, while the superscript elevated [ˡ] or [ˡ] indicates lateral release of the consonant in question.	■ The voiced stops [b, g] do not exist in Hmong, however are consonants in GAE.
[ᵐb ᵐbʰ, ᵐbˡᵐbˡ, ⁿd ⁿdʰ, ⁿdⁿdʰ, ⁿɟⁿɟʰ, ᵑgᵑgʰ, ᴺɢᴺɢʰ] ([d] is a retroflexed voiced plosive, [ɢ] a voiced uvular plosive, [ɟ] a voiced palatal plosive.)	■ The voiced stops [b, d, g] are prenasalized stops which is indicated by the [ᵐ, ⁿ, ᵑ, ⁿ, ᴺ] before the sound in question. This indicates that the nasal is produced prior to the stop. This could create qualitative difficulties in GAE in which the stop-plosives are without nasalization.
[f, v, s, ʂ, z̧, ç, ʝ, h]¹	■ [ʂ, z̧, ç, ʝ] are retroflexed and palatalized fricatives of Hmong that could be used as substitutions for [ʃ,ʒ]. The GAE consonants [θ, ð] do not exist in Hmong.
[ⁿdz,ⁿdz, ⁿḑ, ⁿdz̧ʰ]	■ All affricates are prenasalized in Hmong. This is not the case in GAE.
[l, j] [m, mˡ mɬ, n, ɲ, ŋ] Hmong is a tone language.	■ [r] and [w] are not part of the Hmong inventory but are consonants of GAE.
	■ Hmong has only open syllables and there are no syllable-final consonants. Although spelling looks like the word has a final consonant, those consonants indicate tone, "pab" = "ball" pronounced [pɔ] + high tone. GAE has many different types of syllable shapes and has many words with syllable-final consonants.

¹For "s", some speakers of Hmong produce an aspirated [s]. The ʝ sound is a voiceless palatal fricative that is similar (but with a narrower opening between the active and passive articulators) to a voiceless [j].

CLINICAL APPLICATION

Phonological Changes—Hmong

Based on the absence of certain consonants, the following pronunciation difficulties are possible for the Hmong speaker of GAE.

1. Voiced stop-plosives are prenasalized in Hmong. In this context, prenasalized consonants are phonetic sequences of a nasal (one with the same active and passive articulators as the voiced stop-plosive) that behave phonologically like single consonants. There is the possibility of transferring these prenasalized stop-plosive productions to GAE.
2. The voiced fricative [z] does not exist in Hmong. Hmong speakers of GAE might substitute the voiceless fricative [s] in words containing [z].
3. The consonant [w] is not in the inventory of Hmong. Hmong learners of GAE may need to learn this sound.
4. An *r* sound is not present in Hmong. In addition, there are no central vowels with r-coloring. This sound, especially its prevalence in GAE, might be problematic for Hmong speakers of GAE.

5. The affricates in Hmong are prenasalized. GAE learners might tend to substitute the pre-nasalized affricates for [tʃ] and [ʤ]. In addition, the lack of [ʃ] and [ʒ] in Hmong could cause problems.
6. The Hmong language has many stop-plosives with a lateral release such as [pˡ] and [pʰˡ]. Hmong learners of GAE might substitute these for [pl], as in "play" for example.
7. Hmong has no word-final consonants. Thus, word-final consonants, especially those with consonant clusters in GAE, could be difficult for Hmong speakers to realize.
8. Most words are monosyllabic in Hmong. This could pose difficulties when Hmong speakers try to pronounce multisyllabic GAE words and manipulate word stress.

In terms of speakers, Arabic is the largest group of the Semitic language family with 206 million speakers. Classified as a Central Semitic language, it is closely related to Hebrew and Aramaic. The Semitic languages are a collection of languages spoken by more than 300 million people across much of the Middle East, North Africa, and the Horn of Africa. Modern Standard Arabic has its historical basis in Classical Arabic, which has documented inscriptions since the sixth century. Classical Arabic has been a literary and liturgical language of Islam since the seventh century. There are several discussion points when proposing a phonological system of Standard Arabic. The following vowel and consonant categorization is based on Huthaily (2003), Newman (2002), and Thelwall and Akram Sa'Adeddin (1999). See Table 8.12 for an overview of the Standard Arabic vowels and consonants.

TABLE 8.12   Phonological Inventory: A Comparison of Arabic to General American English (GAE)

Standard Arabic Vowels	Vowel Differences: Arabic and GAE
[i, a, u]	■ Arabic has three vowels, which appear in long and short variations. Tongue position for short vowels is somewhat low, resembling [ɪ] and [ʊ]. The short vowel approaches [ɑ] or [æ]. Arabic has two diphthongs: /(aj / and /aw/. Thus, several GAE vowels are not present in Arabic, for example, [ɪ, e, ɛ, æ, o, ʊ] and the central vowels with and without r-coloring.

Standard Arabic Consonants	Consonant Differences: Arabic and GAE
[p, t, tˤ, d, dˤ, k, q, ʔ, ʕˤ]	■ [t] is a dentalized production in Arabic; the [ˤ] indicates a pharyngealized production.[1] [b] or [g] productions are inconsistent in Arabic but are a portion of the GAE stop-plosive inventory.
[f, θ, ð, ðˤ, s, sˤ, z, ʃ, x, ɣ, ħ, h]	■ [v and ʒ] are inconsistent in Arabic but are a portion of the inventory of GAE. The voiceless and voiced [x, ɣ] have also been labeled as [χ, ʁ], uvular fricatives.
[ʤ]	■ The voiceless affricate [tʃ] is not a consistent realization in Arabic but is a portion of the GAE system.
[m, n]	■ In Arabic, the [n] is a dentalized production, and [ŋ] is an allophonic variation of [n]. This is not the case in GAE in which [n] and [ŋ] are two separate phonemes.
[r]	■ In Arabic, this [r] sound is described as an alveolar trill or as a dental tap or postvelar fricative depending on the dialect. This is a different type of production than the GAE "r".

Standard Arabic Vowels	Vowel Differences: Arabic and GAE
[l], [lˤ], [j, w]	■ The pharyngealized /l/ is noted in Classical Arabic only in the word /alˤlˤah/. ■ All Arabic consonants can occur syllable-initiating, intersyllabically, and in syllable-final positions. Syllables cannot begin with vowels in Arabic. This is not the case in GAE. ■ Consonant clusters can occur at the beginning and end of words in Arabic. There is some restriction on the types of clusters and final clusters in Arabic are often simplified with epenthesis [bint] becomes [binit] ("girl").

[1]*Pharyngealization* involves a secondary approximation of the back and root of the tongue into the pharyngeal area. Based on direct laryngeal observation techniques, Ladefoged and Maddieson (1996) state that there is epiglottal activity.

Sources: Summarized from Dyson and Amayreh (2007), Ladefoged & Maddieson (1996), Thelwall & Akram Sa'Adeddin (1999), and Watson (2002).

CLINICAL APPLICATION

Phonological Changes—Arabic

The following pronunciation difficulties have been noted for Arabic speaker of GAE (Altaha, 1995; Kharma & Hajjaj, 1989; Power, 2003; Val Barros, 2003; Watson, 2002):

1. Arabic typically has a one-to-one correspondence between sounds and letters. Therefore, given written GAE words to pronounce, Arabic speakers could be confused by the lack of sound-letter correspondence in GAE. Also, the influence of the written form can lead to several pronunciation difficulties with both vowels and consonants.

2. The central vowels with and without r-coloring do not exist in Arabic. Therefore, a variation of /a/ - /æ/ or /u/ are substituted for /ʌ/ in GAE. The Arabic r-sound probably replaces the central vowels with r-coloring, which might lead to some acceptable differences in quality of the GAE r-sounds.

3. The distinctions between specific vowels such as /ɪ/, /ɛ/, and /ʊ/ are problematic for Arabic speakers. As the Arabic speaker learns GAE the /ɪ/ may become lengthened and lowered to /e/, whereas /ɛ/ could be produced as /i/ or /æ/.

4. The following consonant distinctions seem to be problematic for Arabic speakers learning GAE: /p/ – /b/, /f/ – /v/, /tʃ/ – /dʒ/ – /ʃ/. This results from the absence of these oppositions in Arabic. For example, /p/ does not exist in Arabic, and /v/ and /dʒ/ are inconsistent.

5. Although /n/ and /ŋ/ exist in Arabic, both are allophones of the same phoneme /n/. On the other hand, in GAE, they are distinct phonemes. In addition, /ŋ/ never occurs at the end of a word in Arabic; therefore, Arabic speakers tend to add /k/ to the end of GAE words that end in /ŋ/. This results in pronunciations such as [duɪŋk] for "doing" or [sɪŋk] for "sing." The GAE phonotactics of /l/ are quite different in Arabic; speakers tend to use the light /l/ in all word positions in GAE. In Arabic, the /d/ is always unreleased and voiceless in word-final positions. GAE words such as "bad," "rod," and "mad" are often pronounced as "bat," "rot," and "mat." Although the phoneme /r/ exists in Arabic, it is pronounced as a trill. There is a strong tendency to transfer this trilled /r/ to GAE. Although this probably does not cause misinterpretations, it does contribute to the speaker's noted foreign accent. Speakers from Egypt also evidence difficulties with /dʒ/ and /ð/. In modern spoken varieties of Egyptian Arabic, /dʒ/ is replaced by /ʒ/ and /ð/ by /h/.

6. Arabic has far fewer consonant clusters in both the word-initial and word-final positions and has no three-segment consonant clusters. In contrast to GAE, which has 78 three-segment clusters and 14 four-segment clusters occurring at the end of words, Arabic has none. GAE clusters are often pronounced with a short vowel inserted to aid in pronunciation.

7. In Arabic, word stress is regular and predictable. Arabic speakers often have problems grasping the unpredictable nature of GAE word stress and the concept that stress can alter meaning, as in con vict' (a verb) versus con' vict (a noun). Thus, word stress could be a problem for Arabic speakers learning GAE.

Implications for Appraisal

A native language can impact a client's acquisition of GAE to varying degrees. Therefore, it is quite possible that a client's irregular pronunciations are a consequence of native language interference. If so, the differences between the sound inventory, phonemic values, and phonotactic constraints of the native language, on the one hand, and of GAE, on the other, provide guidelines for accent reduction. A second possibility is that a client could evidence a phonemic-based disorder in both the native and GAE languages. To determine whether this is so, tests that assess the phonological systems of both languages should be used. For many languages, however, such standardized assessment tools are not available, or the clinician's knowledge of the foreign language is not adequate enough to administer the tests. In these cases, other professionals with knowledge of the language and/or family members could provide valuable information for the appraisal process.

SUMMARY

This chapter considered several aspects of GAE dialect and GAE as a second language. The first section defined dialects and differentiated among what is considered Standard English (including Formal and Informal Standard English) and vernacular dialects. It gave examples of each group. The next section defined and summarized regional, ethnic, and social dialects. The dialects of regions outlined were North, South, Midland, and West. Specific vowel patterns were given for each regional area. The next sections on ethnic and social dialects included definitions of *race, culture,* and *ethnicity* to provide a background for distinguishing this classification of dialects. A summary of features of Appalachian, Ozark, and African-American Vernacular English were discussed with vowel and consonant changes that occur. This section listed phonological variations that appear to be distinctive to Appalachian as opposed to Ozark English as well as those specific phonological characteristics differentiating African-American Vernacular English. The last section of this chapter presented detailed information about speakers of English as a second language. The term *limited English proficient student* was defined and a discussion about the large number of different languages spoken as the first language in the United States followed. For the most prevalent languages that exist in the United States (Spanish, Vietnamese, Filipino/Tagalog, Cantonese, Korean, Hmong, and Arabic), the phonemic inventories were provided as well as specific pronunciation problems that might occur for each GAE language learner speaking these languages. Implications for appraisal were outlined.

CASE STUDY

According to Table 8.4 (pages 219–220), which of the following productions would be indicative of African-American Vernacular English?

house	[haᵘs̞]	matches	[mætʃəs]	thumb	[tʌm]
telephone	[tɛfoᵘn]	lamp	[wæmp]	finger	[fɪŋgə]
cup	[tʌp]	shovel	[ʃʌvə]	ring	[rī]

gun	[gʌ̃]	car	[kɑə]	jumping	[djʌmpən]
knife	[nɑˈt]	rabbit	[wæbət]	pajamas	[djæməs]
window	[wɪnoᵁ]	fishing	[fɪʃĩ]	plane	[pweˈn]
wagon	[wædən]	church	[tʃɜtʃ]	blue	[bwu]
wheel	[wiə]	brush	[bwʌʃ]	bath	[bæf]
chicken	[tʃɪkə̃]	pencils	[pɪnsəz]	drum	[dwʌm]
zipper	[zɪpə]	scissors	[sɪzəz]	Santa	[sænə]
duck	[dʌ]	bathtub	[bæftʌb]	street	[skrit]
vacuum	[vækum]				

Answers: thumb (see item 7), telephone (item 2), finger (item 12), shovel (item 4), ring (item 19), gun (item 19), car (item 11), fishing (item 19), church (item 10), wheel (item 4), bath (item 6), chicken (item 19), pencils (item 4), zipper (item 12), scissors (item 12), duck (item 20), bathtub (item 6), street (item 24), vacuum (item 23)

THINK CRITICALLY

1. Based on the data in Table 8.12, which of the words in the preceding case study might be produced differently according to Standard Arabic American English? What might be the characteristic production?
2. Select one of the phonological inventories of Spanish, Vietnamese, Cantonese, Filipino/Tagalog, Mong Leng Hmong, Korean, or Arabic (Tables 8.6–8.12). Based on these inventories, hypothesize which difficulties children speaking one of these languages might encounter with the GAE words in the preceding case study.

TEST YOURSELF

1. If you are giving an important speech in front of your classroom, which form of Standard English are you probably using?
   a. Informal Standard English
   b. Formal Standard English
   c. vernacular dialect
   d. social dialect
2. Which of the following is true about vernacular dialects?
   a. they are based on geographical regions
   b. all people who use a particular vernacular dialect produce the same set of speech and language features
   c. a wide range of pronunciation features of a vernacular dialect is more accepted than a wide range of grammatical structures
   d. a vernacular dialect and Informal Standard English are the same
3. Regional dialects are
   a. static and do not change
   b. marked by very clear-cut boundaries
   c. not present in the United States
   d. marked by vowel variations
4. African-American Vernacular English is
   a. spoken by all African-American individuals
   b. a systematic, rule-governed dialect

c. only marked by changes in the phonology

d. only used by adolescents

5. Limited English proficient students are
   a. those who have a learning disability and are limited in their language skills
   b. typically students who have not been born in the United States and whose native language is a language other than English
   c. limited in their abilities to learn English
   d. not enrolled in public schools because of their limited abilities in English

6. In second language learning, *transfer* refers to
   a. the ability to process or transfer acoustic data into English
   b. a specific type of technique used to teach second language learners
   c. the language features that occur in the native language that shift to the features of the second language
   d. the carryover of nonnative vowels and consonants to the native language

7. If a child whose native language is Hispanic Spanish says [su] for "zoo," this could be explained as
   a. the fact that there are no voiced fricatives in Spanish
   b. a type of code switching
   c. an acceptable variation of the word "zoo"; most children say it that way

d. a problem with transfer because Hispanic Spanish has no z-sounds

8. How might a child with Vietnamese as their native language say "slide"?
   a. [slaʼɪd]
   b. [θlaʼɪθ]
   c. [slad]
   d. [səlat]

9. Which one of the following statements is *incorrect* about the transfer of sounds from Korean to General American English?
   a. there is no distinction between [r] and [l]
   b. all General American English fricatives are present in Korean with the exception of [z]
   c. because of the realizations of word-final stops, Koreans learning English can have difficulties with [p]-[b], [t]-[d], and [k]-[g] realizations
   d. vowels are often inserted at the end of every word that ends with a consonant

10. Which one of the fricatives is not present in Filipino/Tagalog and could cause difficulties with English pronunciation?
    a. [s]
    b. [ʃ]
    c. [v]
    d. [h]

FURTHER READINGS

Bliatout, B. T., Downing, B. T., Lewis, J., & Yang, D. (1988). *Handbook for teaching Hmong-speaking students*. Los Angeles: Evaluation, Dissemination, and Assessment Center, California State University. The center also has handbooks about Vietnamese-speaking and Korean-speaking students that are excellent sources of the cultural and language issues of these individuals.

Handbooks on Cantonese-speaking, Japanese-speaking, Filipino-speaking, and Portuguese-speaking students.

Sacramento, CA: Bureau of Publications Sales, California State Department of Education.

McLeod, S. (Ed.). (2007). *The international guide to speech acquisition*. Clifton Park, NY: Thomson Delmar Learning.

Roseberry-McKibbon, C. (2007). *Language disorders in children: A multicultural and case perspective*. Boston: Pearson.

Wolfram, W., & Schilling-Estes, N. (2006). *American English: Dialects and variation* (2nd ed.). Malden/Oxford: Blackwell.

Therapy for Articulation-Based Speech Sound Errors

LEARNING OBJECTIVES

When you have finished this chapter, you should be able to:

- Define the traditional-motor approach and be able to structure therapy according to this approach.
- Identify the different phases of sensory-perceptual training.
- Differentiate between phonetic placement, sound modification, and facilitating contexts.

- Describe the phonetic placement and sound modification techniques for the most frequently misarticulated sounds.
- Explain the importance of coarticulatory contexts and identify the easy-to-hard coarticulatory conditions for the most frequently misarticulated sounds.
- Understand the dynamics and interaction when doing group therapy with the traditional motor-approach.

THIS chapter describes techniques that can be used to treat articulation-based errors in the speech of children and adults. As previously defined, these types of speech sound error are motor production problems or an inability to produce certain speech sounds. This chapter emphasizes a *phonetic approach,* which has also been referred to in the literature as a *traditional* or *motor approach* (e.g., Bernthal, Bankson, & Flipsen, 2009; Klein, 1996; Lowe, 1994; Pena-Brooks & Hegde, 2000; Van Riper, 1978). Using this approach, a clinician instructs a client in how to position the articulators in such a way to produce a speech sound that is considered to be within normal limits. Therapy progresses from one error sound to the next. In addition, several of the treatment protocols cited in the literature identify tasks used to improve auditory discrimination skills (e.g., Van Riper & Emerick, 1984; Weiner, 1979; Winitz, 1989).

The goal of this chapter is to provide an information base for clinicians to use in their efforts to help their clients achieve a norm production of specific speech sounds. This foundation requires an understanding of how the sound is normally produced and knowledge of a client's specific misarticulation. In a continuing attempt to unite articulation- and phonemic-based treatment principles, the linguistic function (exemplified by sound frequency, phonotactics, and examples of minimal pairs) is provided for several of the sounds.

The sounds chosen for inclusion in this chapter represent the most frequently misarticulated sounds noted by McDonald (1964). When applicable, the voiced or voiceless cognates are also treated. Not all possible misarticulations for each individual sound are addressed. Only the most frequent misarticulations referenced in the research or as a result of personal clinical experience are included. Therefore, for some sounds, [s] for example, most of the misarticulations treated are distortions. For other sounds, such as [l], the majority of the errors are sound substitutions.

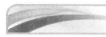

Decision Making: When to Use a Phonetic Approach

Historically, phonetic approaches were first described in Europe around the turn of the twentieth century (Gutzmann, 1895; Kussmaul, 1885). Their first documentation in the United States is attributed to Scripture (1902), Ward (1923), and Scripture and Jackson (1919). Through the years, many authors—including Mosher (1929); Nemoy (1954); Nemoy and Davis (1937); West, Kennedy, and Carr (1937); Van Riper (1939a, 1939b); Young and Hawk (1955); Mysak (1959); West and Ansberry (1968); and Winitz (1969), to mention just a few—have added to and modified these early methods. Van Riper's (1939b) *Speech Correction* is often cited as the text that popularized these techniques that clinicians have used for decades.

Any contemporary view of treatment needs to stress what is new. Thus, noncontemporary roots might cause clinicians to hesitate to take traditional motor approaches seriously. In addition, after so much emphasis has been placed on analyzing our clients' phonemic systems, clinicians wonder whether a traditional phonetic approach should still be used. It should be; there is definitely a place for these methods in our contemporary understanding of speech sound disorders and their remediation.

Articulation-Based Errors

Phonetic or **traditional motor approaches** treat each error sound individually, one after the other. This treatment principle stands in contrast to a **multiple-sound approach**, which attempts to influence several error sounds simultaneously. Traditional motor approaches should not be used automatically with all clients who exhibit a single-sound error. A client with a single-sound error who has problems with the *function* of the sound in the language system, that is, with the underlying system that governs the use of that particular sound, is probably demonstrating a phonemic-based disorder. Omissions and substitutions of an isolated speech sound can be phonemic-based disorders, and other therapy options could be more suitable. The question is never how many sounds are involved but whether the errors, single or multiple, are articulatory or phonological in nature. If they are articulation-based, the best treatment option could be a traditional-motor, phonetic approach.

Decision Making: A Phonetic Approach with a Phonemic-Based Disorder?

As previously discussed, a phonetic approach is probably chosen for a client who demonstrates an articulation-based disorder. This does not necessarily mean that it is unsuitable for a client with phonemic difficulties. Certain portions of these techniques can prove helpful with children who demonstrate phonemic disorders.

Phonological approaches emphasize the function of sounds in a specific language system. Consequently, the internalization of phonemic rules and contrasts is the main goal of these therapies. If, however, the sound is not in a child's repertoire and remains elusive in spite of phonemic-based treatment, the phonetic approach could be implemented to establish the speech sound's norm articulation. This does not mean that clinicians need to go through all steps of the phonetic approach but that certain ideas and procedures of this approach can prove useful. Thus, one of the treatment goals could be to help a child produce the appropriate articulatory features of the speech sound. This in turn could facilitate the primary goal: increasing the child's ability to understand and use phonemic rules and contrasts with that particular sound.

Bernthal, Bankson, and Flipsen (2009) report that the traditional-motor or phonetic approach can also be incorporated into treatment programs for clients who demonstrate linguistic or pattern-based errors, especially if the patterns reflect motor constraints (e.g., prevocalic voicing or certain cluster simplifications). Based on these authors' recommendation, if motor constraints can be identified in the patterns of clients with phonological disorders, the traditional, phonetic approach constitutes a viable option.

Therapy Sequence

This section outlines possibilities for sequencing therapy when working with clients who have phonetic disorders. These sequences have been described by numerous authors (e.g., Secord, 1989; Van Riper, 1978; Van Riper & Emerick, 1984; Waengler & Bauman-Waengler, 1984) and have been used by clinicians for many years. Although the following sequencing is presented, clinicians find that certain training items are necessary for some clients, whereas they might prove unnecessary for others. A specific client's needs and capabilities cause changes in the sequencing of every therapy program.

Each of the treatment phases assumes that a client enters that particular stage with minimal competency and moves to the next stage when a certain level of accuracy has been achieved. The necessary level of accuracy before proceeding to the next stage of treatment is usually relatively high. Paul (2007) notes that correct usage is typically set at 80–90% in structured intervention contexts. Therefore, during structured activities in a therapy setting, 80%–90% accuracy is needed before proceeding to the next stage. However, is this high accuracy necessary in spontaneous speech before a client is dismissed from therapy? As dismissal criteria, Lee, Koenigsknecht, and Mulhern (1975) have suggested a much lower level of accuracy for spontaneous, natural contexts. They argue that termination criteria in spontaneous contexts should be set at 50% accuracy. It appears that once children use targeted behaviors in spontaneous speech the majority of the time, it is probable that they will continue to progress toward more consistent usage. These percentages appear reasonable but, again, can vary according to the individual clinician's expectations and client's capabilities.

General Overview of Therapy Progression

As this therapy was originally outlined, sensory-perceptual or ear training was considered the first step in the treatment process. At least two factors should be considered before implementing sensory-perceptual training: the age of the client and whether specific auditory discrimination difficulties are noted for that client. Age becomes a factor because many of the tasks used to achieve the goals of the training are metalinguistic skills that require the child to think and talk about language. Identifying the position of a sound in a word is a metalinguistic skill, for example. A child must first understand the concept that a "word" is made up of individual "sounds" and their relative relationship to one another. The ability to segment words into sounds develops during the later preschool years. Therefore, for very young children, certain aspects of sensory-perceptual training might not be appropriate. Second, clinicians should carefully evaluate the specific auditory perceptual skills of their clients. The term *specific auditory perceptual skills* refers to clients' abilities to differentiate between their error production and the target sound. If testing reveals no difficulties with specific discrimination tasks, sensory-perceptual training does not seem warranted.

Figure 9.1 is a schematic of the sensory-perceptual training that Van Riper and Emerick (1984) outlined. Few clinicians implement this type of training with this amount of depth. Figure 9.1 can serve as a reference for those clinicians who might think this phase is important or necessary.

The next section outlines the general progression of therapy from producing the sound in isolation to finally using it in spontaneous speech. Although sensory-perceptual training might not be used, it is important to remember that each client must develop specific auditory perceptual abilities in the form of self-monitoring skills. Clinicians constantly need to help their clients develop discrimination of "correct" versus "incorrect" productions. This type of self-monitoring is not an optional portion of therapy.

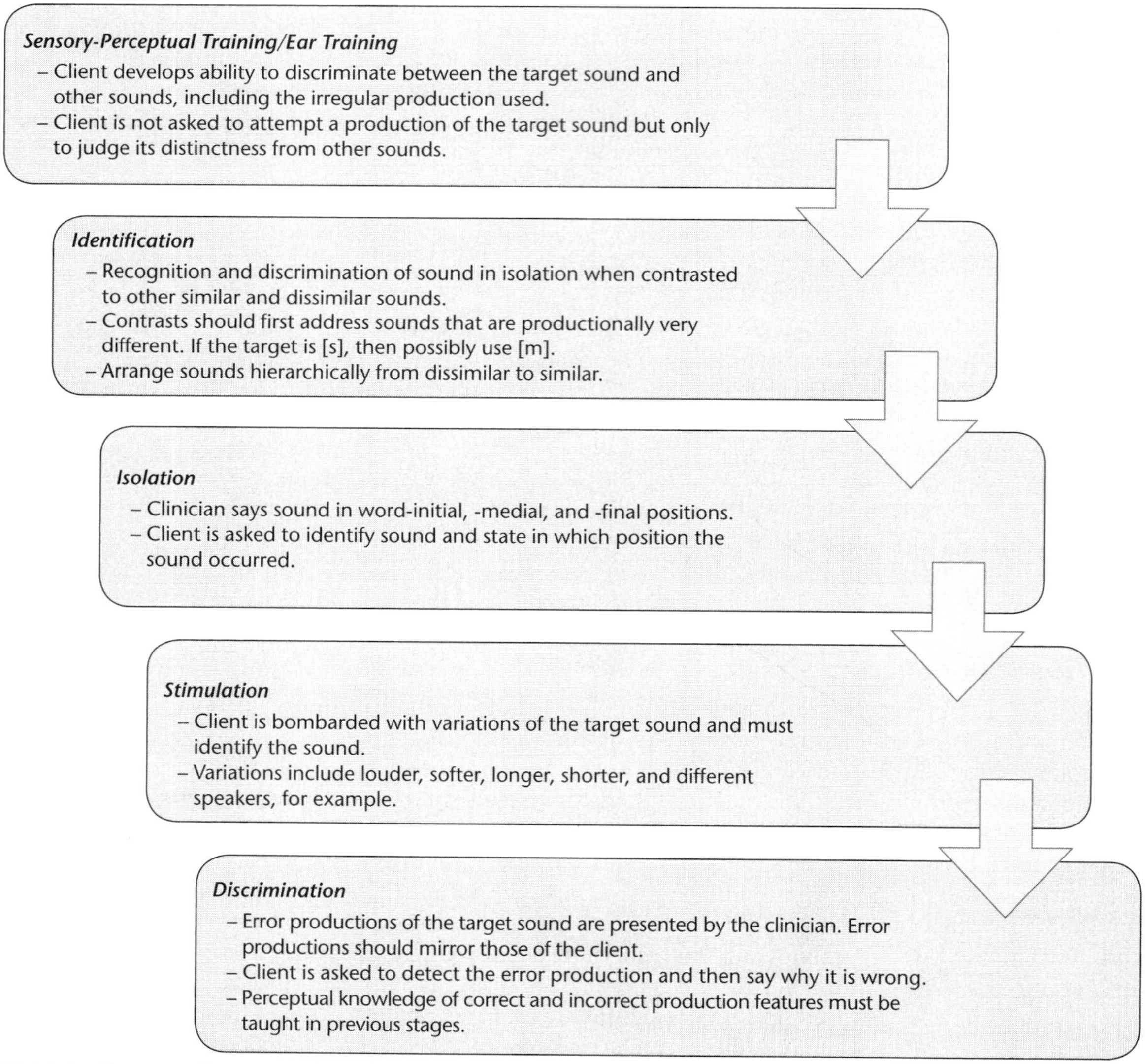

Sensory-Perceptual Training/Ear Training

- Client develops ability to discriminate between the target sound and other sounds, including the irregular production used.
- Client is not asked to attempt a production of the target sound but only to judge its distinctness from other sounds.

Identification

- Recognition and discrimination of sound in isolation when contrasted to other similar and dissimilar sounds.
- Contrasts should first address sounds that are productionally very different. If the target is [s], then possibly use [m].
- Arrange sounds hierarchically from dissimilar to similar.

Isolation

- Clinician says sound in word-initial, -medial, and -final positions.
- Client is asked to identify sound and state in which position the sound occurred.

Stimulation

- Client is bombarded with variations of the target sound and must identify the sound.
- Variations include louder, softer, longer, shorter, and different speakers, for example.

Discrimination

- Error productions of the target sound are presented by the clinician. Error productions should mirror those of the client.
- Client is asked to detect the error production and then say why it is wrong.
- Perceptual knowledge of correct and incorrect production features must be taught in previous stages.

FIGURE 9.1 Sensory-Perceptual Training Progression

Production of the Sound in Isolation. The goal of this phase of therapy is to elicit a norm production of the target sound alone, not in combination with other sounds. This can easily be achieved with fricatives, glides, and liquids, for example—sounds that are continuants. For stop-plosives, young children might find it easier to articulate the target sound with a central vowel, for example [kʌ], or with a noticeable aspiration, [kʰʌ].

There are several possibilities for eliciting the target sound. Beginning clinicians often have the idea that this is a task that can be achieved in a very short time, and this is indeed often the case. However, if norm or near-norm articulation is not obtained in a reasonable time frame (5 to 10 minutes), persisting with the procedure will probably frustrate both the client and the clinician. In this case, either the technique should be changed or other exercises should be initiated to prepare the client for the correct articulation. The following possibilities are offered for eliciting the target sound in isolation.

What Happens When You Cannot Get a Norm Production?

It can often take several therapy sessions to achieve a "correct" production of a specific sound. Which activities can be done to aid this progress? The author offers these as suggestions from clinical experience. First, clinicians should make sure that the client can perceptually distinguish between his or her error sound and the misarticulations. If the client has a dentalized [s], then contrast that to a norm production in words with [s] in various word positions and of varying lengths and complexities. Second, examine the client's articulation test and see whether you noted any words/contexts that were closer approximations than others. For example, the word "tree" provided a context in which a correct or near-correct [r] production was obtained. Use these words to find whether similar words could aid in a norm production. Third, work on stages toward approximating the norm production. For example, have children with a lateral lisp watch their production (the author uses the iPad camera), noting the characteristic lateral movement of the lips and jaw. Try to get the children to produce some type of [s]-like fricative without this movement. Fourth, if the sound in question is a sound substitution, for example a [t] for [k], use minimal pairs to contrast the target to the substitution.

Auditory Stimulation/Imitation. With this procedure, the clinician provides examples of the target sound and asks the client to imitate the sound. A similar procedure is implemented for stimulability testing (see Chapter 6). The clinician instructs the client to "watch me and do exactly what I do." If this works, it is perhaps the easiest and quickest way to achieve the target sound. Unfortunately, though, it does not always succeed.

Phonetic Placement Method. In the **phonetic placement method**, the clinician instructs the client how to position the articulators in order to produce a typical sound production. The phonetic production features of the target sound and the error production are analyzed to determine which articulatory changes need to be initiated so that an accurate production results. In the section Individual Sound Errors, these methods are described in detail for the most common misarticulations.

Sound Modification Method. The **sound modification method** is based on deriving the target sound from a phonetically similar sound that the client can accurately produce. This sound is used as a starting point to achieve the target production. The clinician suggests specific adjustments to the articulators that should result in the target sound.

Once the client has produced the target sound acceptably in isolation, the next task is to stabilize it. This is typically achieved by having the client repeat it immediately.

At first, this probably needs to be carried out with careful monitoring and feedback by the clinician. When the production is more stable, the client should articulate the sound a number of times successively with a softer or louder voice, for example, and when possible, with different durations. This does not need to develop into a tedious drill for client and clinician but can easily be achieved in activities that are fun and motivating. For example, the clinician could hide colored cards or favorite objects around the room. Every time the client finds the object, the target sound could be repeated. The clinician constantly provides feedback as to the acceptability of the productions, also asking the client to attempt judgments about the accuracy of his or her own productions.

Use of Facilitating Contexts: Is an Isolated Production Necessary?

Some clients can produce the target sound quite accurately in some word contexts but not in others. These coarticulatory context conditions seem to aid the client's production of a target sound. Supporting contexts have been called *facilitating contexts* (McDonald, 1964). Van Riper (1978) introduced the term *key words* for words in which the target sound was correctly produced.

Facilitating contexts or key words are often found in the analysis of the client's articulation test or a conversational speech sample. Additional materials examining facilitating contexts include McDonald's (1964) deep testing and Secord's (1981a) probes of articulatory consistency. Van Riper (1978) describes how these key words can be used to move directly to the production of the target sound in isolation. In this case, the target sound is isolated by prolonging the sound in the word or by using its natural syllable structure. In one case, results of an evaluation demonstrated a d/g substitution. However, the word *finger* was found with a correct production of [g]. The facilitating context of a postdorsal-velar nasal [ŋ] aided the client in producing a postdorsal-velar stop. To take advantage of this situation for the purpose of producing an isolated [g], the client first says *fin-ger,* separating the word between [ŋ] and [g]. The *ger* is then reduced to [gʌ].

Facilitating contexts can also be used to begin therapy at the word level. For example, if a small core of words with an acceptable production of the target sound is found, they can be employed to stabilize the production. As Van Riper (1978) pointed out, key words can be used as a model for the client. The clinician should then point out acoustic and articulatory differences between the articulation of these key words and aberrant target sound productions in other words. When the client can feel and hear the target sound, a transition to other words should be attempted. For this transition, it is important that the clinician understand the facilitating context(s) in which the sound occurs. For example, is the target sound always preceded or followed by certain vowels or consonants? Are the key words one- or two-syllable words? Does the target sound occur in a stressed or unstressed syllable? If the clinician can predict the facilitating context, words can be added with similar coarticulatory conditions.

CLINICAL EXERCISES

Tyler, age 4;3 can say "blue" with an accurate [l] but says [bwæk] for "black" and [bwɪŋk] for "blink." Can you suggest two or three words that might be attempted to facilitate [bl]?

The Goldman-Fristoe Test of Articulation noted that Braydon, age 6;4, could produce the word "tree" with an acceptable r-sound. All other words with [r] were in error. Suggest other words that could be practiced to promote a correct [r].

CLINICAL APPLICATION

Using Facilitating Contexts

Using the earlier example of the word *finger,* an analysis suggests that the abutting [ŋ] had a facilitating effect on a norm [g] production; both active and passive articulators are the same for both sounds. Additional words satisfying this coarticulatory context condition include *singer, linger, hunger,* and *longer.* After these words are accurately articulated, a logical sequence might be to proceed to [ŋ] + [k]: *monkey, stinky, thinker.*

Facilitative contexts can be very effective in therapy. If appropriate words can be found, it is relatively easy to isolate the sound in question, which is an excellent start for the isolation phase of production. If the use of meaningful words in a given situation is especially important, facilitative contexts can also be employed for work at the word level. As always, the final clinical choice depends on an individual client's circumstances and capabilities.

Nonsense Syllables. The goal of this therapy phase is to maintain accuracy in producing the target consonant when it is embedded in varying vowel contexts. The therapeutic efficacy of this phase can be greatly increased by ordering the nonsense syllables from those that are easiest for the client to produce to those that are more difficult. The typical sequencing is target sound + vowel (CV), vowel + target sound (VC), and vowel + target sound + vowel (VCV). However, this sequence could change based on the difficulty an individual client demonstrates with each type of nonsense syllable. Vowels can be arranged in a hierarchical order from those that provide favorable coarticulatory conditions to those that do not. Suitable vowel sequences are suggested for each of the misarticulations noted in the following section "Individual Sound Errors." However, the individual client's articulatory ease and production accuracy ultimately determine the sequencing of vowels.

Many clinicians skip the nonsense syllable phase of treatment and move directly to the target sound produced in words. One reason is that words are more meaningful and interesting to clients than is drill work with nonsense syllables. However, work with nonsense syllables does not need to be a tedious exercise. Coming up with motivating and enjoyable activities that incorporate nonsense syllables requires only clinical imagination. In addition, whereas words are more meaningful to children than nonsense syllables, the word material should always be carefully evaluated. Some of the small "articulation cards" with black-and-white line drawings depicting words, for example, are not easily recognizable to the clinician or the client. Such material stretches the concept of meaningfulness. Finally, and probably most importantly, some clients need work with nonsense syllables before they can produce words with any acceptable level of accuracy. If the client produces less than 50% accuracy in two to three practice sessions, the word level is probably still too difficult. The clinician could then work with nonsense syllables or use consonant–vowel words such as *see, sow,* and *saw* until the production has stabilized. In addition, working with nonsense syllables eliminates the interference of the "old" error with the "new" production of the target sound that is inherent in meaningful word material. Years of practice with the old aberrant articulation of the target sound often override the new articulation, especially in familiar words. For example, a child might be quite able to produce the nonsense syllable [ki] accurately in the context of other nonsense syllables. However, when attempting the word *key,* the child might suddenly revert back to the "old" substitution and produce [ti].

Words. The goal of this therapy phase is to maintain productional accuracy of the target sound in the context of words. A large variation in this category exists from one-syllable CV structures to multisyllabic words in which the target sound appears several times, often in consonant clusters. Organizing words from relatively easy to more difficult to produce can prove helpful. This should be done in a systematic manner using the articulatory complexity of the word as a guideline. Several factors affect the articulatory complexity of words. These include the length of the word, the target sound's position in the word, the word's syllable structure, where the syllable stress occurs relative to the target sound, coarticulatory factors within the word, and the client's familiarity with the word.

The Length of the Word. Typically, the fewer the number of syllables, the easier a word is to produce. This would indicate that one-syllable words should be attempted before two- and three-syllable words (Secord, 1989).

The Position of the Sound in the Word. A sound in the initial position of a word or syllable appears to be the easiest. Word- and syllable-final sounds are typically more difficult. Thus, target sounds should generally be placed at the beginning of a word before attempting to realize the target sound at the end (Secord, 1989).

The Syllable Structure. Open syllables (CV) are generally easier than closed syllables (CVC) to articulate. Considering the ease of production, syllable structure can on occasion have precedence over a word's length. Two-syllable words with a reduplicated CVCV structure, such as *Daddy* or *teddy,* can be easier than CVC words such as *bed* or *mad* (Bernthal, Bankson, & Flipsen, 2009).

The Syllable Stress. A target sound is easier to produce in a stressed syllable than when the target is in an unstressed one. Therefore, when choosing two-syllable words, the target sound should first appear in the stressed syllable (McDonald, 1964).

Coarticulation Factors. Certain words might be easier to articulate than others because of the influence of neighboring sounds. This relates not only to preceding and following vowels but also to the neighboring consonants in the word. Knowledge of the vowel and consonant articulations can aid in developing a list of words ordered from relatively easy to produce to more difficult ones. However, the final decision as to ease and difficulty of production depends on the client. Clinicians could find that certain words are "too difficult"; that is, the target sound is consistently misarticulated in that word. These words should then be attempted at a later time when the regular articulation of the target sound is more stabilized.

Coarticulatory factors also include the number of times the target sound appears in a word and whether it appears as a singleton or as a part of a consonant cluster. Words that contain the target sound only once are normally easier to articulate than those that have the target sound more than once. Thus, for [k], *cape* is easier than *cake*. Also, words that contain the target sound as a singleton are typically easier than when the target sound is a portion of a consonant cluster. Thus, *tea* is easier to produce than *tree*.

Familiarity. Familiar words are usually articulated more accurately than unfamiliar words (Secord, 1989). Therefore, clinicians should begin with words that a client knows well or that are high-frequency words. With some clients, however, familiar words might also be more difficult. The impact of years of practicing the misarticulation of a familiar word in a multitude of settings can prove difficult to overcome. These words might need to be targeted later when the client's production and self-monitoring skills have improved.

Structured Contexts—Phrases and Sentences.

The goal of this therapy phase is to maintain the production accuracy of the target sound as words are placed into short phrases and sentences. However, at this point, phrases and sentences should not yet be spontaneous but structured and elicited. If spontaneous sentences are used, the client could choose words containing combinations with the target sound that are still too difficult. This presupposes that clinicians begin work at this phase while still continuing the work at the word level. This is a logical supposition because clinicians typically select a core set of words that can be accurately produced and then put these words into short phrases and sentences.

A *carrier phrase* with a target word at the end is one of the easiest ways to elicit a short phrase. At the beginning, the carrier phrase should probably not contain any other words with the target sound. Another relatively simple way to elicit an utterance is to embed one target word in the carrier phrase, which can be modified to create some degree of spontaneity. For example, if a child is working on [s], the carrier phrase could be "I see a _____." The clinician could have objects or pictures prepared (at first without any s-sounds) that the client identifies to complete the phrase.

During this therapy phase, the clinician moves from highly structured to less structured tasks and might begin to implement target words with more syllables and consonant clusters.

Spontaneous Speech.

The goal of this phase is to maintain accuracy of production when the target sound appears spontaneously in conversation. This goal is first addressed in the therapy setting; however, the client needs to transfer this production accuracy to more and more situations outside therapy. This transfer of behavior to conversational speech in various settings is often referred to as *carryover*.

Both inside and outside the therapy setting, this therapy phase should proceed in a systematic manner. One way of accomplishing this is to vary the length of conversation time. Clinicians could start with 1 to 2 minutes of conversation, increasing the time interval as the client's accuracy increases. Initially, before the conversation begins, the client should be aware that the clinician is "listening for our sound." Later, the time interval can be extended and can include specific contexts that trigger the production of the target sound in many different words. For example, pictures containing words with the target sound could serve as the basis for conversation. Also, certain topics might lend themselves to the production of specific sounds. For example, a topic that includes racing, race cars, and race car drivers would probably trigger [r] in a variety of contexts.

After a relatively high level of accuracy is achieved in the therapy setting, the next decisive step is correct production of the sound outside, in the real world. Parents and teachers can serve as valuable assistants during this phase of therapy. When working outside the therapy setting, the amount of time implemented and the specific tasks should be discussed with the assisting helper. This phase can become overwhelming to both the helper and the client if both suddenly think that the sound needs to be produced accurately all the time in every outside setting. (See following Clinical Application.)

Even when an assistant is employed, the clinician should also monitor a client's level of accuracy in situations outside the immediate therapy setting. This can be accomplished in a variety of ways. For example, to check on the accuracy of sound production outside the therapy setting, the client could bring tape recordings from home, the clinician and child could go out to buy an ice cream, or could go window shopping at a toy store. The clinician could also drop by the child's classroom or telephone home.

Dismissal and Reevaluation Criteria.

The last phase of therapy examines dismissal and reevaluation criteria. Fifty percent accuracy during natural spontaneous speech was mentioned earlier as criterion for dismissal. This relatively low percentage was suggested under the assumption that the client's competency would continue to increase on its own. Such a supposition needs to be checked by some type of reevaluation process. It can be as simple as stopping by the child's classroom and listening to conversation, or it can be more

---

CLINICAL APPLICATION

Structuring a Home Program

When structuring a home program, clinicians need to make sure that a speech assistant (caregiver, teacher, relative, etc.) is informed of several variables:

1. When? Which portion of the day should be set aside for the program?
2. How long? How many minutes should be spent on this program?
3. How often? How many times per week should this program be implemented? Should it be a daily occurrence?

4. What should be done? In detail, what should the assistant do? Does the assistant have written instructions as well as words, phrases, and topics that should be used in the home program?

5. How should accuracy be judged? How should the assistant determine which productions are acceptable and which are not?

6. What should be done if a production is considered unacceptable? How should the assistant react to an aberrant production?

7. How should the assistant motivate and reward the client? What type of reward system should be implemented so that the client stays motivated and continues to work in the home program?

One important question that clinicians need to ask is: How can I be sure that the assistant understands what is to be done? If the assistant does not really understand in detail what has to be accomplished, this can often lead to frustration for both the client and the assistant. (The author had a caregiver assistant who, rather than implement two 5-minute sessions during the day, thought that one 30-minute session twice a week would be better. After two long sessions, the child refused to work at home.) Bringing the assistant into therapy can partially solve this problem. The assistant can see and hear which productions are considered accurate and which are not. After a period of observation, the clinician has the assistant take an active role in the therapy session. The clinician can then give the assistant helpful advice to guide in making decisions about correct and incorrect productions as well as implementation of activities.

Bringing parents into the therapy session is often impractical, especially in a public school setting. Words that a clinician knows that a client can say accurately can be jotted down in a spiral notebook. This notebook can go back and forth between the parents and the clinician. The parents should be instructed to have the child say the word, maybe three to five times, possibly putting the word in a short carrier phrase that you have provided. At home, words that are not produced accurately can be crossed off the list by the parents. This method gives you a fairly easy communication link with the parents.

Katie, who was in second grade, was working on [s] in structured conversation. Katie's mother expressed her willingness to work at home with her.

1. When? After discussing this with the mother, a quiet one-on-one time after dinner was considered the best way to begin.

2. How long? Three to 5 minutes was a good time frame to begin.

3. How often? Every weekday.

4. What should be done? Written instructions were put into a small spiral notebook that the mother could transport in her purse between therapy and home. The clinician described in some detail what the topic of the conversation should be. These topics had been practiced in therapy, and Katie was able to reach a fairly high degree of success with them.

5. How should accuracy be judged? After participating in two therapy sessions, the mother knew what to listen for, and she was given written reminders in the notebook. Katie originally had a θ/s substitution. The mother was aware that [s] should have a clear, sharp quality but not sound like [θ].

6. What should be done if a production is considered unacceptable? It was decided that a small stop sign that was constructed in therapy would be used to signal any unacceptable [s]-productions. The mother would simply hold up the sign when she heard [θ]. Katie knew that when the sign went up, she should repeat the whole sentence and try to monitor her [s]-production.

7. How should the assistant motivate and reward the client? It was decided that if Katie participated for the specified minutes of therapy, she could play on the computer, uninterrupted by her two brothers, for 15 minutes. Also, at the end of each week of therapy, Katie could pick out one of the movies that the family would watch on the weekend.

structured such as administering an articulation test or obtaining a conversational speech sample. Before dismissal, a child who has official school-based documentation for speech/language services (Individualized Family Service Plan or Individualized Education Plan) should be reevaluated typically with a standardized test to determine whether the child is within normal limits with those particular speech sound skills. A spontaneous speech sample is again a necessity as is a consultation with the teacher and parents to be sure that the norm production carries over to other contexts outside the therapy room. Whichever means is employed, *reevaluation* is a portion of the clinician's clinical responsibility. It is the only way to ensure that therapy was indeed successful and the client has continued to generalize across situations. The ultimate therapeutic goal is norm production in all natural, conversational settings. A reevaluation is a way of documenting this.

Individual Sound Errors

This section does not revisit the multitude of traditional-motor approaches that have been suggested throughout the years but focuses on those based on the phonetic features of the target sound in relationship to the error production. Knowledge of the correct phonetic placement and the existing differences between the norm production and the misarticulation is instrumental in facilitating these techniques. Other traditional-motor approaches that might not be quite as "phonetically" oriented are referenced in numerous sources. For example, a compilation of phonetic placement, moto-kinesthetic, and sound approximation techniques can be found in Secord's *Eliciting Sounds* (Secord, 1981b).

This section contains both phonetic placement and sound modification techniques for s-sounds ([s] and [z]); sh-sounds ([ʃ] and [ʒ]); k-g sounds; l-sounds; r-sounds (including [r] and the central vowels with r-coloring, [ɝ] and [ɚ]); th-sounds ([θ] and [ð]); f-v sounds; affricates; voicing problems (e.g., [p] for [b] substitution); and consonant clusters. The discussion should be seen as a reference. It contains a considerable amount of detail that becomes necessary when a clinician is actually working with a client and encountering difficulties achieving an accurate production. The proposed methods also allow the clinician several possibilities for establishing a norm realization for each of the previously noted sounds. To make reading this chapter somewhat less tiresome, several of these techniques have been placed in tables. The word lists with minimal pairs have been placed in Appendix 9.1 at the end of this chapter.

Misarticulations of [s] and [z]

One of the most common speech sound errors is the aberrant production of [s] (Smit, 1993b). Most children at some point in their development have difficulty with [s] realizations. Because [s] and [z] are counted among the latest developing speech sounds, they can pose difficulties into the first school year for some children. This common difficulty can sometimes be heard in the speech of adults. Whether at the grocery store or on television, adults with irregular [s] articulations can be detected.

The productions of [s] and [z] consist of several related physiological factors that make their articulation somewhat complicated: (1) [s] and [z] are both fricatives that are physiologically complex because a rather narrow opening between the articulators must be maintained over a longer period, (2) the fricatives are also the longest sounds in duration

(Bauman & Waengler, 1977; Lehiste, 1970), and production requirements necessitate not only a narrow opening between the articulators but also the maintenance of the right amount of expiratory airflow. (3) There is a precise balance between the articulatory effort required to create the narrow opening and the expiratory air pressure; if this balance is off, even to a small degree, it becomes perceptually noticeable, and (4) aberrant productions can easily cross phonemic boundaries. Thus, if the tongue is too far forward, [s] might sound like [θ]. The same relationship exists between [z] and [ð]. In addition, the voiceless [s] occurs frequently in words in General American English. In summary, [s] and [z] are physiologically difficult, perceptually sensitive, and produced in practically every utterance.

An interesting note: German has no th-sound. The author was surprised at the wide degree of variability that was acceptable for the [s] and [z] sounds in German children. Because there were no distinctive phonemic boundaries between s- and th-sounds, this production variability was generally accepted.

Phonetic Description

Norm productions of [s] and [z] are articulated in essentially two different ways: as an apico-alveolar or as a predorsal-alveolar fricative. These differences are delineated in Table 9.1. The apico-alveolar variation is produced with the tongue tip up, whereas the predorsal-alveolar [s] is realized with the tongue tip down behind the lower incisors. Sagittal grooving of the tongue, which directs the airstream toward the opening between the articulators, is essential for both types of productions. To achieve this, the lateral edges of the tongue must be elevated and touch the first molars to avoid lateral air escape. Although the apico-alveolar articulation is probably the most common, many speakers produce predorsal-alveolar [s] and [z]. Each type of s-production has its therapeutic advantages and disadvantages, which are discussed in "Phonetic Placement. Decision Making: Apico- or Predorsal Placement" on page 257.

Linguistic Function

Frequency of Occurrence. [s] ranks among the top five sounds in frequency of occurrence. Although not as frequent as [s], [z] ranks 11th in the 24 consonants of General American English. The most frequent word-initial clusters include [st], [str], and [sp]; the most frequently encountered word-final clusters are [st], [ns], [nz], [ks], [ts], [rz], and [nts] (Dewey, 1923; Roberts, 1965).

TABLE 9.1 Production Differences: Apico-Alveolar versus Predorsal-Alveolar [s] and [z]

	Phonetic Description	
	Apico-Alveolar Fricative	*Predorsal-Alveolar Fricative*
	[s] voiceless [z] voiced	[s] voiceless [z] voiced
Notable differences	Tongue tip up	Tongue tip down behind lower incisors
Active articulator	Apex (tip of tongue)	Predorsal (front portion of tongue)
Passive articulator	Alveolar ridge	Alveolar ridge
Productional notes	Narrow opening between tongue tip and alveolar ridge	Tongue arches toward alveolar ridge, narrow opening between predorsal section of tongue and alveolar ridge
	Sagittal grooving of tongue Lateral edges of tongue elevated	Sagittal grooving of tongue Lateral edges of tongue elevated

TABLE 9.2 Consonant Clusters with [s]

Word Initiating		Word Terminating			
[sf]	sphere (very infrequent)	[fs]	coughs, roofs		
[sk]	school, skate	[sk]	mask, desk	[ks]	blocks, books
[sl]	sled, sleep	[ls]	false, pulse		
[sm]	small, smile				
[sn]	snow, snack	[ns]	dance, bounce		
[sp]	speed, spin	[sp]	wasp, crisp	[ps]	mops, tips
[st]	stop, stove	[st]	ghost, fast	[ts]	kites, cats
[sw]	sweet, sweater				
[skr]	scratch, scrub	[rs][1]	horse, nurse		
[skw]	square, squash	[lts]	melts, belts		
[spl]	splash, splurge	[mps]	lamps, jumps		
[spr]	spring, spray	[nts]	ants, presents		
[str]	street, string	[rst]	first, worst	[rts]	hearts, skirts
		[sks]	desks, masks		
		[sts]	nests, tastes		

[1]Consonant clusters with [r] are considered centering diphthongs. Therefore, these examples do not really represent consonant clusters. However, because they are included in most consonant cluster lists, they have been included in this one as well.

Phonotactics Both [s] and [z] can occur initiating and terminating a syllable. However, in spontaneous speech, the frequency of their occurrence in initial, medial, and final word positions is not comparable. In the speech of first-, second-, and third-grade children, half of the [s]-sounds occurred initiating a word; the other half were divided fairly equally between medial and final positions. In contrast, more than 90% of the [z] sounds were found in word-final position (Carterette and Jones, 1974).

See Tables 9.2 and 9.3 for the more frequent consonant clusters with [s] and [z] and word examples. All consonant clusters are based on the lists provided by Blockcolsky, Frazer, and Frazer (1987).

Morphophonemic Function. Word-final clusters ending in [s] or [z] can be used, for example, to signal (1) plurality, as in boo<u>ks</u>, goa<u>ts</u>, nes<u>ts</u>; (2) third-person singular, as in he ju<u>mps</u>, she bui<u>lds</u>; and (3) possessives, as in Mom<u>'s</u>, Dad<u>'s</u>. Within phrases, contractible auxiliaries and copulas with the verb *to be* also demonstrate consonant clusters with [s] and [z]. Examples include "the ma<u>n's</u> happy" and "the ca<u>t's</u> running."

Minimal Pairs. Minimal pairs are often used to test the perceptual accuracy of the error production versus the norm production of clients. Several authors (e.g., Grunwell, 1987; Locke, 1980b; Winitz, 1984) have devised protocols to test these types of auditory perceptual skills. In addition, minimal pair contrast therapy (discussed in Chapter 10) employs pairs of words that differ by only a single phoneme. Sounds

TABLE 9.3 Consonant Clusters with [z]

Word Terminating			

Word- or syllable-initiating clusters with [z] do not exist in GAE.

[bz]	ribs, tubs	[vz]	gives, waves
[dz]	adds, toads	[zd]	closed, sneezed
[gz]	bags, bugs	[ldz]	builds, folds
[lz]	bells, shells	[lvz]	wolves, elves
[mz]	teams, games	[rdz]	birds, cards
[nz]	cans, rains	[rlz]	girls, curls
[ŋz]	wings, rings	[rvz]	curves, dwarves
[rz][1]	bears, ears		
[ðz]	bathes, breathes		

[1]Consonant clusters with [r] are considered centering diphthongs. Therefore, these examples do not really represent consonant clusters. However, because they are included in most consonant cluster lists, they have been included in this one as well.

that are frequently contrasted to [s] and [z] include [θ] and [ð], [ʃ] and [ʒ], and [t] and [d]. Appendix 9.1 has examples of minimal pair words and sentences incorporating sound oppositions with [s] and [z]. The section "Types of Misarticulations" contains sound oppositions contrasting [s] and [z] to [ʃ] and [ʒ].

Initial Remarks

Several important variables must first be considered when a clinician sees a child or adult displaying an [s] problem. First, the disorder could be the result of a hearing loss, specifically a high-frequency hearing loss. Acoustically, both [s] and [z] have high-frequency components (6,000 to 11,000 Hz). Because all sound productions are monitored auditorily, even a moderate loss in these frequency areas might impair intensity relationships between formant regions and, therefore, lead to a distorted production. This makes a hearing evaluation prior to conventional diagnostic testing indispensable. If a high-frequency hearing loss is present, a diagnostic evaluation and the subsequent therapy planning need to be organized quite differently.

Second, certain minor structural changes can affect [s] as well. This might include missing teeth in a school-age child or new dentures in an adult. Although circumstances such as these might not cause [s] problems per se, an individual's inability to compensate for such structural deviations can result in unusual production characteristics.

Third, such diagnoses as "tongue thrust" or "tongue thrust swallow" also need to be considered. The term *tongue thrust* refers to excessive anterior tongue movement during swallowing and a more anterior tongue position during rest (Christensen & Hanson, 1981). Hanson (1988) suggests that a more appropriate term would be *oral muscle pattern disorders;* this would avoid the misconception that clients forcefully push their tongues forward. Controversy continues to surround these disorders and their impact on articulation, especially the articulation of [s] and [z]. Not everyone with a tongue thrust develops [s] problems. On the other hand, there is a higher incidence of children with s-distortions who do demonstrate an oral muscle pattern disorder (Fletcher, Casteel, & Bradley, 1961; Hanson, 1988). Although an interdisciplinary approach is strongly urged, it is within the scope of practice of speech-language pathologists to diagnose and treat oral muscle pattern disorders (American Speech-Language-Hearing Association, 1991). Prior to ASHA's 1991 position statement, an ad hoc committee report (American Speech-Language-Hearing Association, 1989) suggested, as do several clinicians (Hanson, 1988, 1994; Hanson & Barrett, 1988; Hilton, 1984), that treatment, often called *oral myofunctional therapy,* might facilitate the correction of [s] difficulties. Knowledge of the diagnostic and treatment procedures of oral muscle pattern disorders at times is necessary to complement work with [s] and [z] misarticulations. Refer to Box 9.1 for literature citations that refer to tongue thrust.

Finally, a client's auditory discrimination abilities should be carefully evaluated. One portion of a clinician's assessment battery should include specific auditory perceptual testing (see Chapter 6). If the client demonstrates auditory discrimination problems between norm productions of [s] and [z] and the client's specific error realization, auditory discrimination training should probably be implemented.

Types of Misarticulations

As with all treatment plans, a solid diagnostic foundation needs to be established before treating misarticulations of [s] and [z]. It is important to find out exactly what the articulation characteristics of the client are during the sound realization—that is, how the client produces the error sound. Although the term *distortion* is often used to label abnormal sound changes, this seldom provides enough diagnostic information. Figure 9.2 is presented to help distinguish between different [s] and [z] "distortions."

The last item in Figure 9.2 refers to the production of a nasalized [s] and [z]. As mentioned, there are two types of nasalized productions: an organic and a functional.

BOX 9.1   Examples of Tongue Thrust Literature

Bigenzahn, W., Fischman, L., & Mayrhofer-Krammel, U. (1992). Myofunctional therapy in patients with orofacial dysfunctions affecting speech. *Folia Phoniatrica, 44*(5), 235–242.

Cayley, A., Tindall, A., Sampson, W., & Butcher, A. (2000). Electropalatographic and cephalometric assessment of myofunctional therapy in open-bite subjects. *Australian Orthodontic Journal, 16,* 23–33.

Christensen, M., & Hanson, M. (1981). An investigation of the efficacy of oral myofunctional therapy as a precursor to articulation therapy for pre-first-grade children. *Journal of Speech and Hearing Disorders, 46,* 160–167.

Forrest, K. (2002). Are oral-motor exercises useful in the treatment of phonological/articulatory disorders? *Seminar in Speech and Language, 23,* 15–26.

Gommerman, S., & Hodge, M. (1995). Effects of oral myofunctional therapy on swallowing and sibilant production. *International Journal of Orofacial Myology, 21,* 9–22.

Hanson, M. L. (1994). Oral myofunctional disorders and articulatory patterns. In J. E. Bernthal & N. W. Bankson (Eds.), *Child phonology: Characteristics, assessment, and intervention with special populations* (pp. 29–53). New York: Thieme.

Hanson, M. L., & Barrett, R. H. (1988). *Fundamentals of orofacial myology.* Springfield, IL: Charles C. Thomas.

Distinguishing functional from organic velopharyngeal competency is the work of a team of professionals. Although an in-depth account of these procedures is not within the scope of this chapter, a few guidelines are given. First, there is a higher degree of probability that a functional problem exists if the nasality is restricted to [s] and [z]. Organic problems usually have an effect on *all* speech sounds, particularly those consonants that require a high degree of intraoral occlusion and the buildup of air pressure (stops, fricatives, affricates). Nasal airflow and its influence on [s]-productions can be verified by pinching the nostrils closed. The nasal resonance immediately disappears during the occlusion of the nasal passageway and is audible again if the nostrils are released. Third, functional nasal productions are usually accompanied by a normal tongue placement for [s] and [z].

For a discussion of nasality because of organic problems and its impact on articulation, see the "Cleft Palate" section of Chapter 11.

Therapeutic Suggestions

Two approaches seem viable when working with a child or an adult displaying an isolated [s] misarticulation: the phonetic placement method and the sound modification method. Simply stated, phonetic placement amounts to describing to the client the positioning of the active and passive articulators as well as the manner of production of the sound in question. Systematic work toward realizing that goal is then implemented in an attempt to change the aberrant production characteristics. Naturally, with children, this needs to be accomplished in an age-appropriate manner. A mirror or a larger portable device with a camera, such as an iPad, not a small cell phone, might be used as visual feedback while the clinician serves as an auditory feedback system. Although this approach is widely used, it is often not easy to describe what exactly needs to be done in a manner that the child can easily understand and follow. The sound modification method, on the other hand, uses another sound or sounds that the child can produce in a regular manner as a point of departure for achieving the target sound. Therefore, [t], which the child can produce, might be used to achieve [s], which the child misarticulates. The sound modification method is

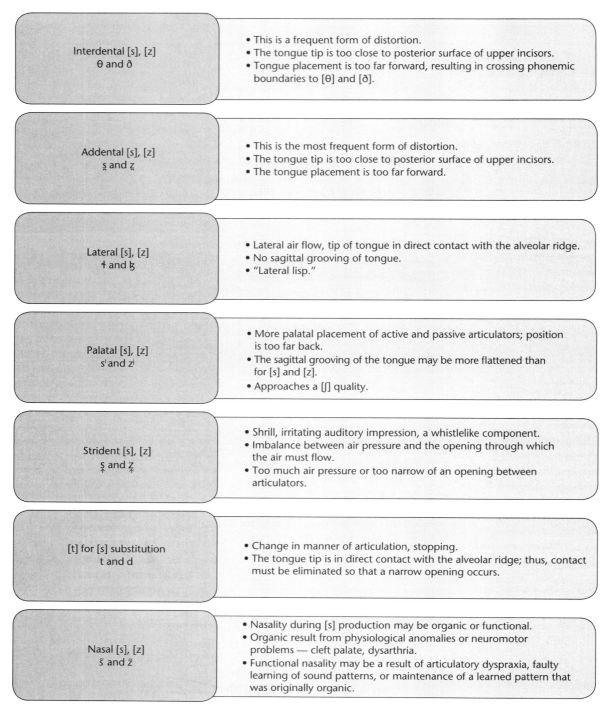

Interdental [s], [z] θ and ð	• This is a frequent form of distortion. • The tongue tip is too close to posterior surface of upper incisors. • Tongue placement is too far forward, resulting in crossing phonemic boundaries to [θ] and [ð].
Addental [s], [z] s̪ and z̪	• This is the most frequent form of distortion. • The tongue tip is too close to posterior surface of upper incisors. • The tongue placement is too far forward.
Lateral [s], [z] ɬ and ɮ	• Lateral air flow, tip of tongue in direct contact with the alveolar ridge. • No sagittal grooving of tongue. • "Lateral lisp."
Palatal [s], [z] sʲ and zʲ	• More palatal placement of active and passive articulators; position is too far back. • The sagittal grooving of the tongue may be more flattened than for [s] and [z]. • Approaches a [ʃ] quality.
Strident [s], [z] s̝ and z̝	• Shrill, irritating auditory impression, a whistlelike component. • Imbalance between air pressure and the opening through which the air must flow. • Too much air pressure or too narrow of an opening between articulators.
[t] for [s] substitution t and d	• Change in manner of articulation, stopping. • The tongue tip is in direct contact with the alveolar ridge; thus, contact must be eliminated so that a narrow opening occurs.
Nasal [s], [z] s̃ and z̃	• Nasality during [s] production may be organic or functional. • Organic result from physiological anomalies or neuromotor problems — cleft palate, dysarthria. • Functional nasality may be a result of articulatory dyspraxia, faulty learning of sound patterns, or maintenance of a learned pattern that was originally organic.

FIGURE 9.2 Frequent Misarticulations of [s] and [z]

easier to apply if the speech sound chosen as a starting point has certain phonetic similarities to the misarticulated sound. This way, a bridge is built between the similar sound that can be correctly articulated by the child and the target sound that is in error. Both methods are discussed for problems encountered with [s] and [z].

Phonetic Placement

Decision Making: Apico- or Predorsal Placement. Although most people produce [s] and [z] as apico-alveolar productions, a predorsal articulation is not without merit. For the apico-alveolar [s], the tongue tip is hovering, so to speak, near the alveolar ridge. This precarious position must be precisely maintained over the entire duration of the sound. In contrast, for the predorsal [s], the tongue tip is resting behind the lower incisors. This provides an easily identifiable spot for the tongue tip, which does not waver or fluctuate; it is something definite to "hold on to." For this reason, the predorsal [s] is noted as being a more stable production. Such relative stability is often especially important for children whose motor capabilities are not yet fully developed. In addition, a large percentage of [s] and [z] misarticulations are interdental or addental in nature; that is, the tongue tip is elevated but too far forward. To move the tongue tip down for

the predorsal-alveolar version provides a solution that is quite different from the child's previous attempts. The natural tendency to return to the previous incorrect [s] is diminished. It is often easier for a child to accomplish a different, new production task than to attempt minor adjustments of a previous one. The final decision of apico-alveolar or predorsal-alveolar [s] production depends on the client's motor abilities or restrictions and on the type and degree of [s] misarticulation. The following two charts outline the procedures for achieving apico-alveolar and predorsal-alveolar productions based on the various misarticulations.

Sound Modification Methods.

Sound modification methods are based on the concept of using a similar, appropriately articulated sound to aid in the production of the misarticulated sound. A similar sound refers to one that is comparable in some of its phonetic production features. This method is easiest to implement when several direct phonetic similarities exist between the sound to be modified and the target sound. However, some successful techniques have evolved out of very limited articulatory similarities.

> Watch the following video and transcribe Mark's [s] difficulty. What type of [s] is the clinician trying to achieve, an apico-alveolar or a predorsal-alveolar? youtube.com/watch?v=nB3D-wi-FSQ

1. *[t]-[s] method.*
   A. Begin with a series of rapid [t] repetitions, which typically produce intermittent [s]-like fricatives. This effect is increased if the child is asked to produce [t] with

PHONETIC PLACEMENT: APICO-ALVEOLAR [s]

Interdental or Addental Misarticulations

- The tongue tip must be moved back, the client must glide the tongue back to the alveolar ridge.
- Lateral edges of tongue must be elevated, edges of the tongue must touch first molars, and the tongue is grooved.
- Visual and auditory feedback is necessary.

Lateral [s] Misarticulation: Apico-Alveolar Production

- Raise the lateral edges of tongue so the edges of tongue touch the first upper molars.
- Direct airstream over the tip of the tongue thus releasing the contact of the tongue with the alveolar ridge.
- Eliminate the lateral jaw and lip movement using visual feedback. The child can produce an overexaggerated "smile" to help in eliminating these lateral movements.

- If the child has difficulty with tongue grooving, place a straw or small cylindrical object (bamboo stick) lengthwise along the center of the tongue and have the child curl the edges of the tongue around the object, raising the edges of the tongue and creating central airflow.

Palatal [s] Production

- Tongue is too far back.
- The client glides the tongue forward until an acceptable sound is achieved.
- Grooving of tongue must be maintained and possibly increased.

Strident [s] Misarticulation

- Balance between expiratory airflow and degree of opening between articulators is crucial.
- The client experiments with reducing the air flow (say the sound softly) or increasing the opening (slight lowering of the tongue).

PHONETIC PLACEMENT: PREDORSAL-ALVEOLAR [s] PRODUCTION

- The tongue tip should be behind the lower teeth.
- The front portion of the tongue is directed toward the alveolar ridge.
- Grooving of the tongue is necessary, and sides of tongue should touch the first upper molars.
- Visual and auditory feedback is important.

Lateral [s] Misarticulation: Predorsal-Alveolar Production

- The tongue tip behind lower teeth eliminates the problem of the contact of the tongue tip and the alveolar ridge.

- The grooving of the tongue is important.
- Eliminate lateral jaw and lip movement using visual feedback.

Palatal [s] Misarticulation

- Predorsal-alveolar production should automatically move the tongue placement forward.
- The grooving of the tongue must be maintained.

lots of air pressure. Have the child listen for the sound in between the [t] repetitions; then ask the child to try to prolong this intermittent [s].

B. Begin with a [t]-production in which the stop phase is prolonged, building up air pressure behind the occlusion. The client is then instructed to release the [t] very slowly. The result should approximate [s].

2. *[ʃ]-[s] method.* Three steps are necessary to change [ʃ] to a normal [s]-production:
   A. Eliminate the lip rounding associated with the production of [ʃ]. Have the client smile while saying [ʃ].
   B. Have the client move the tongue slightly forward to change the place where the friction occurs.
   C. Increase the sagittal grooving of the tongue. Have the client raise the lateral edges of the tongue touching the upper molars.

3. *[f]-[s] method.* This method assumes that the tongue tip for [f] is already situated behind the lower incisors; therefore, a predorsal [s] is the goal.
   A. Pull the middle of the lower lip away from contact with the upper incisors during the production of [f].
   B. Raise the front portion of the tongue slightly as the upper and lower incisors come closer together.

For this modification, the client must be aware that a friction sound should be maintained during the entire attempt.

4. *[i]-[s] method.* Phonetic similarities between [i] and [s] consist of the lip spreading and the high, anterior tongue placement for both sounds. For [i], the tongue tip is typically in a lowered position, whereas the anterior portion of the body of the tongue is elevated toward the palate. Thus, this modification normally results in a predorsal (tongue tip down) [s].
   A. Instruct the client to bring the teeth slightly closer together during the [i] production.
   B. Elevate the front portion of the tongue until a friction-type sound is heard.
   C. Raise the lateral edges of the tongue touching the upper molars.

The [i] could easily be modified to a voiced [z] if a decision has been made to initiate work with that sound. In addition, the [i]-[z] method has the advantage of maintaining voicing throughout the modification, which is not the case with the [i]-[s] method. See the section "Where to Begin: [s] or [z]."

Functional Nasal [s] and [z] Problems. Therapy for functional nasal [s] and [z] problems does not fit readily into the categorizations of phonetic placement or sound modification methods. The reason for the aberrant nasal [s] is not a deviant tongue placement but rather the inadequate velopharyngeal closure leading to nasal emission. Specific consonants can be used as a bridge to promote sufficient velar closure.

1. [t]-[s]. If [t] can be produced without hypernasality, instruct the client to hold the stop phase of the [t], building up pressure during the occlusion. [t] is then *slowly* released, producing [s]. Complete velopharyngeal closure is normally necessary when producing [t]. By increasing the air pressure, the occlusion is strengthened because of the higher degree of production effort. This heightened effort might promote more velopharyngeal closure for the following [s] approximation as well. Visual and auditory feedback should also be implemented to increase the client's awareness of nasal emission versus no nasal emission.

2. Using consonant clusters [t] + [s] and [s] + [t]. This method is a slight variation of #1. It uses the build-up of intraoral air pressure of [t] to facilitate a non-nasal [s] production. The [t] is paired with [s] in a consonant cluster such as

---

CLINICAL EXERCISES

Tommy, age 7;2, has an addental s-production. Outline the steps you would take—in age-appropriate terms—to achieve an apico-alveolar [s] production.

You have decided to attempt a sound modification approach with Tommy for his dentalized production. However, Tommy's [ʃ] is also in error. Which sound modification method would you use? Why?

"hits" or "bats." If the nasality is eliminated with these phonetic contexts, try [s] + [t] as in "stop" or "stick." At first do not include any nasal sounds in the word. Therefore, such words as "mats" or "nuts" would be avoided.

Where to Begin: [s] or [z]? When attempting to achieve an isolated sound production, most clinicians automatically begin with voiceless [s]. The reasoning seems to be that the fricative, although complicated enough for the client, should not be further burdened with the addition of voicing. However, beginning with [z] could be advantageous under certain conditions.

First, voiced consonants normally are produced with less air pressure than the voiceless ones. Increased air pressure can at times be counterproductive to establishing norm articulations. Especially with an apico (tongue tip up) [s], this increased air pressure could lead to the client's "losing" the precariously new approximation between active and passive articulators.

A second factor that supports a choice of [z] is the ability of the voicing component to mask minor productional differences. Listeners seem to be more critical of even slight deviations of the voiceless [s]. The same articulatory features used for the production of [z] are not as noticeable. Naturally, we do not want the client to acquire an [s] that is somehow not acceptable.

The following scenario can serve as an example. We have begun work on [s]; however, even with our best efforts and those of the child, the production is still slightly off target. We have tried several times to correct for the minor mispositionings, but the articulation is still not quite accurate. We are becoming somewhat frustrated; the child, we feel, is already frustrated. This could be a good time to attempt a voiced [z]. If the articulatory variation is minor enough, the voicing should provide an acceptable sound. While giving the child success (finally), it also allows practice time for the new sound. This practice with [z] is often all the child needs to achieve an acceptable [s] articulation.

A third consideration in favor of [z] is a coarticulatory consideration. If the voiceless [s] is placed in a consonant–vowel (or vowel–consonant) context, the client must change the voicing halfway through the utterance. This sudden change in voicing could strain an already difficult articulatory-motor task. By using [z], voicing can be maintained throughout the production. To attain [s] once [z] is acceptable is relatively easy. If the child whispers [z], [s] results. The next task is to put the isolated sound production into specific contexts.

Coarticulatory Conditions

The phonetic context in which a target sound is placed can have a considerable impact on the production of that sound. Certain contexts can support the production features of the target sound and others might undermine them. Phonetic contexts that support the production of a target sound can be used effectively by clinicians in certain phases of therapy. On the other hand, ignoring coarticulatory contexts could lead to endangering a "new" sound production that is still relatively unstable. Facilitative coarticulatory conditions rely on knowledge of, and comparison between, phonetic features.

If the newly acquired [s] is practiced in syllables or words, the vowels that precede or follow it should be considered. Recall that [s] is articulated with the tongue in a relatively anterior position and with some degree of lip spreading; [i] seems phonetically comparable. Both [s] and [i] require unrounding of the lips while the anterior portion of the tongue is elevated toward the palate. This is not the case with [u]. This vowel is produced with the back of the tongue elevated and requires lip rounding. The coarticulatory effects of the lip rounding on [s] can be demonstrated by saying the word *Sue*. The lip rounding for [u] is already present as one begins to say the initial [s]. This lip rounding and the additional posterior tongue placement could actually work against a newly acquired [s] articulation.

By examining phonetic comparability, it would seem that the front vowels are better suited for initial context work with [s]. The front vowels [i], [ɪ], [eɪ], [ɛ], and [æ] support the relatively forward tongue placement and the lack of lip rounding. The back vowels have

---

CLINICAL APPLICATION

Analyzing Coarticulatory Conditions

When analyzing words according to coarticulatory conditions, several factors should be kept in mind:

1. *The vowel following or preceding the target sound.* Consider the comparability of production features of certain vowels relative to the target sound. Some vowels have production features that are phonetically similar to the target sound, whereas others are clearly different. For example, the lip rounding of the high-back vowels and the lip spreading of [s] are dissimilar articulatory conditions.
2. *The syllable structure of the word.* Consider the articulatory gesture as a whole. A word that contains a consonant followed by a vowel (CV) is a less complex articulatory unit than one with a CVC structure. CVCC words are relatively more complex than either CV or CVC structures. Single syllable words are far simpler to produce than two or three syllable words.
3. *The phonetic features of the surrounding consonants.* Consider the movement of the articulators for the production. The target sound's production features can be compared to the other consonants in the word. Again, these similarities can be used to create favorable coarticulatory conditions. For example, the active and passive articulators and the voicing of [s] and [t] are phonetically the same. This is not the case for [s] and [k].

   Other consonants may provide supportive coarticulatory conditions based on their relative neutral tongue positions. For example, the tongue is not directly involved in the articulation of the bilabials and [h]. Within an articulatory unit, if [s] precedes or follows a sound that does not require tongue activity, then the coarticulatory effects on [s] are minimal. Therefore, [m], [p], [b], and [h] can provide supportive coarticulatory conditions for those consonants in which the tongue is the active articulator.
4. *The misarticulation of the client.* Consider the type of misarticulation the client demonstrates. She or he is accustomed to this motor pattern and has practiced it for a long period. The new motor task, the norm articulation of the target sound, is relatively new. If the new motor task is put into a phonetic environment similar to the misarticulation, the newly established articulation could be jeopardized. For example, a child's misarticulation of [s] involves a tongue position that is too anterior, an addental or interdental [s] problem. If this [s] is in a word together with [θ], this could trigger the original misarticulation. Or if the child has a lateral [s], it is probably not a good idea to begin practice words that contain [l], a lateral sound that might trigger the lateral [s] misarticulation.

---

specific features that lack support for [s] and [z]. First, a more posterior tongue placement is associated with all back vowels. In addition, the degree of lip rounding increases from [ɔ] to [oᵘ] and from [ʊ] to [u]. The [ɑ] is considered to be an unrounded vowel. Thus, if lip rounding presents a problem for [s], the low-back vowel [ɑ] should demonstrate more favorable coarticulatory conditions than the mid- and high-back vowels.

The speech-language specialist should keep in mind the phonetic context when moving through every stage of therapy. By contrasting the phonetic features of the target sound and the surrounding consonants and vowels, a hierarchy of contexts can be established that move step-by-step from more to less supportive coarticulatory conditions. Not every client needs such small steps. However, for those who do, this hierarchy can prove invaluable. On the other hand, some clients might demonstrate phonetic contexts that could be more facilitating

CLINICAL EXERCISES

The following words are from a published card set that is available to work on s-sounds.

Word-Initially: Santa, sailboat, cereal, sunflower, soccer player, sock, seal, sand, sandwich, cell phone

Word-Finally: cups, paints, mouse, dice, horse, blocks, jacks, grapes, nurse

How would you rank order these words for a child just beginning with s-words? Several of the words should not be used at the beginning of therapy. Which ones should be eliminated until a later date?

for them than those previously mentioned. The clinician should then use those specific contexts. The suggested sequence should not be seen as part of a "therapy cookbook" approach to be followed with every client but as one possibility that incorporates phonetic comparability.

Word Examples. The following one-syllable words are ordered from relatively easy to more difficult coarticulatory conditions:

[s] Words	[z] Words
see - seep - seam - seat - seed - seen	zee - zeal - Zeke
sip - sit - sin - sing	zip - zing - zipped - zinc
say - same - save - sail	Zane
set - said - sell	Zeb - Zed - Zen
sap - Sam - sat - sash - sang	zap - zag - zapped - zagged
sum - sun - suck - sung	
sob - sod - sock - song	czar
sow - soap - sewed - soak	zone - zoned
soot	
Sue - soup - suit - soon	zoo - zoom - zoomed

Misarticulations of [ʃ] and [ʒ]

This section describes typical norm and aberrant productions of [ʃ] and [ʒ]. It then addresses specific phonetic placement and sound modification methods. Because [s] and [ʃ] show many similarities in error productions as well as in the diagnostic procedures that would be implemented, the reader is referred back to the section on [s] misarticulations at several points.

Phonetic Description

Phonetically, [s] and [ʃ] are closely related. However, the sagittal groove is considerably wider for [ʃ] than it is for [s]; the tongue is flatter for [ʃ]. This is one reason that the friction noise for [ʃ] is not as "sharp" as that for [s]. In addition, the place of articulation is not the alveolar ridge as with the [s]; it is located slightly posterior to it at the anterior part of the palate, the postalveolar or prepalatal area. Finally, [ʃ] has lip rounding rather than the lip spreading common for [s]-productions. Putting this all together, the phonetic description of [ʃ] is a voiceless coronal-postalveolar or coronal-prepalatal fricative with lip rounding. The voiced counterpart of [ʃ] is [ʒ].

Linguistic Function

Frequency of Occurrence. The voiceless [ʃ] is an infrequent sound ranking 20 of the 24 General American English consonants. The voiced [ʒ] is the most infrequent sound in General American English, occurring only in words of foreign origin, such as *beige* or *rouge* (Dewey, 1923; Roberts, 1965).

Phonotactics. Both [ʃ] and [ʒ] can occur initiating and terminating a syllable. There are very few consonant clusters with [ʃ] and [ʒ]. See the more frequent consonant clusters and word examples in Table 9.4.

Morphophonemic Function. Word-final clusters that end in [ʃ] or [ʒ] can be used to signal past tense in regular verbs that end in these sounds, such as *splashed* and *massaged*.

TABLE 9.4 Consonant Clusters with [ʃ] and [ʒ]

Word-Initiating [ʃ]	Word-Terminating [ʃ]	Word-Terminating [ʒ]
[ʃr] shrimp, shrub	[rʃ] marsh, harsh	[ʒd] rouged, massaged
	[ʃt] washed, wished	

Minimal Pairs. Frequent sounds that are substituted for [ʃ] and [ʒ] include [s] and [z] and [t] and [d]. See Appendix 9.1 for examples of minimal word pairs and sentences

Initial Remarks

Preliminary considerations are similar to those presented for [s]. Thus, the client's hearing acuity, minor structural or functional deviations, and the auditory discrimination abilities should be assessed before beginning work on the isolated articulation of [ʃ] and [ʒ].

Types of Misarticulation

The most common forms of [ʃ] and [ʒ] misarticulations are outlined in Figure 9.3.

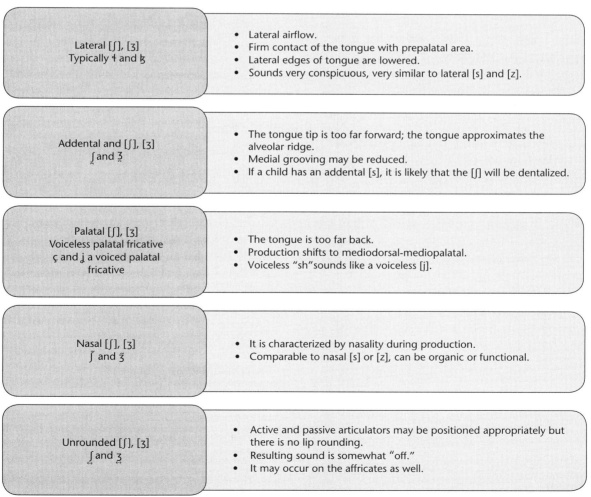

FIGURE 9.3 Frequent Misarticulations of [ʃ] and [ʒ]

Therapeutic Suggestions

Phonetic Placement. Although most [ʃ] and [ʒ] realizations are produced with the tongue tip up, approximating the area directly behind the alveolar ridge, [ʃ] can also be produced with the tongue tip down behind the lower incisors. As with the tongue tip down [s], the tongue arches upward with the front portion of the tongue approximating the postalveolar or prepalatal area. The accompanying chart outlines both productions, the tongue tip up (coronal-postalveolar or prepalatal) and tongue tip down (predorsal-prepalatal) [ʃ] and [ʒ].

Sound Modification Methods

1. *[s]-[ʃ] method.* Because [s] and [ʃ] sounds are phonetically similar, clients who have difficulty with [ʃ] often demonstrate [s] problems as well. If that is the case, this method cannot be used. If [s] is intact, the [s]-[ʃ] method would certainly be a good choice. Only lip rounding and a slight retraction of the tongue are initially required. Fortunately, both requirements are often fulfilled simultaneously. If the lips are clearly protruded, the tongue tip has a tendency to retract a bit (Weinert, 1974). If this natural retraction is still not enough, the client should be instructed to glide the

PHONETIC PLACEMENT: [ʃ] AND [ʒ]

Placement: Coronal-Postalveolar or Prepalatal Articulation (Tongue Tip Up Production)

- Frontal portions of the tongue approximate the anterior area of the palate either posterior to the highest point of the alveolar ridge (postalveolar) or the anterior area of the palate (prepalatal).
- Sagittal grooving of tongue is present but is wider and flatter than for [s].
- Lips are rounded.

Lateral [ʃ] Misarticulations

- Raise the lateral edges of tongue.
- Release the contact of the tongue with the alveolar ridge.
- Use similar techniques outlined for lateral [s].

Addental [ʃ] Misarticulation

- The tongue must be retracted.
- The client should glide the tongue slowly backward until an acceptable sound is achieved.

- The tongue can be pushed back with a tongue depressor.

Palatal [ʃ] Misarticulation

- The tongue is too far back.
- During production of [ʃ], instruct the client to slowly glide the tongue forward.

Not Enough Lip Rounding

- Lip protrusion is needed.
- The client should place both hands on cheeks and push lips forward; clinician can say to the child "Look like a fish."

Placement: Predorsal-Prepalatal Production

- The tip of tongue should be down, touching inside of lower incisors.
- The front portion of the tongue arches upward toward the alveolar ridge.
- A narrow opening is created between the predorsal portion of tongue and slightly behind the alveolar ridge.
- A slight medial groove is necessary.
- Lips are slightly protruded and rounded.

tongue back slightly. If the [ʃ] still sounds somewhat off, slight adjustments might need to be made.

2. *[t]-[ʃ] method.* The main phonetic dissimilarity between [t] and [ʃ] pertains to the manner of articulation, stop versus sibilant fricative. The positioning of the active and passive articulators are close enough to be usable.

   A. Begin with a prolonged [t] production (prolonging the implosion phase) with lip protrusion.
   B. Maintaining the lip protrusion, instruct the client to slowly release the [t] while gliding the tongue back slightly.

3. *[tʃ]-[ʃ] method.* The goal of this method is to isolate the friction portion of the affricate. This can be done in the following manner:

   A. Begin with a very slow production of [tʃ], making sure that lip protrusion is realized.
   B. Instruct the client to lengthen the final fricative portion of the affricate.

Functional Nasal [ʃ] Problems. Each of the following methods must first be evaluated to find whether adequate velopharyngeal closure is achieved. Therefore, no hypernasal resonance should be noted for the sounds coupled with [ʃ].

1. *[t]-[ʃ].* This is similar to the technique described in functional nasal [s] problems. The addition of lip rounding will be necessary for [ʃ] realizations.

2. *[tʃ]-[ʃ].* First, a forceful [tʃ] is produced with an increased buildup of air pressure behind the point of closure. The [t] portion is then slowly released. The client should be instructed that this release should be only minimal. The goal is a slightly narrower opening between the articulators than is normally the case with [ʃ]-productions. This narrow opening with its increased air pressure should help support the velopharyngeal closure necessary for [ʃ].

> ## CLINICAL EXERCISES
>
> You are seeing Erin, age 7;3, in speech therapy. She has both lateral [s] and [ʃ] misarticulations, which are also evident in her affricate productions. Which sound would you start with first, or would you work on both simultaneously? Why?
>
> You have chosen to use a sound modification technique for Erin's misarticulations. Which one would you choose for [s] and for [ʃ]? Why?

Coarticulatory Conditions

When describing context conditions that support regular [ʃ]-productions, two questions must be considered:(1) Is the problem based on difficulties with the tongue placement? (2) Is the problem primarily the result of not enough lip rounding? The answer plays a role in the selection of coarticulatory conditions.

(1) If the problem is a result of faulty tongue placement—that is, if addental, palatal, or lateral [ʃ]-realizations result—the sequence of supportive vowel coarticulations follows those described for [s]. Thus, the front vowels [i], [ɪ], [eɪ], [ɛ], and [æ], particularly the high-front vowels [i] and [ɪ], support the relatively high anterior position of the tongue during regular [ʃ]-productions.

(2) If the [ʃ] misarticulation is primarily the result of a lack of lip rounding, a different coarticulatory sequence should be considered. The natural lip rounding of the back vowels would support the articulatory necessities for [ʃ]. The high-back vowels [u] and [ʊ] with the most lip rounding would be especially helpful, followed by [oʊ] and [ɔ]. Even the central vowels [ɜ] and [ɚ], which are produced with some degree of lip rounding, could support the lip protrusion necessary for [ʃ]. The unrounded features of the low-back vowel [ɑ] and the front vowels would initially not be indicated.

Word Examples. The following one-syllable words are ordered from relatively easy to more difficult coarticulatory conditions:

[ʃ] Words	
Primary Problem: Tongue Placement	Primary Problem: Lip Rounding
she - sheep - sheet - she'd - shield	shoe - shoot
ship - shin - shipped - shift	should - shook
shape - shame - shade - shave - shake	show - showed - shown - shore
shed - chef - shell - shelf	sure - shirt
shack - shag - shaft	shot - shawl - shock - shocked - shop
shut - shove	shack - shag - shaft
shop - shot - shawl - shock - shocked	shed - shell - chef - shelf
show - showed - shown - shore	shade - shave - shake - shape - shame
should - shook	shin - shift - ship - shipped
shoe - shoot	she - sheet - she'd - shield - sheep

Misarticulations of [k] and [g]

Many children go through a phase of substituting [t] for [k] and [d] for [g]. For example, Preisser, Hodson, and Paden (1988) reported that this is the most common deviation involving the [k] and [g] sounds in children from 18–29 months of age. Some children seem to "get stuck" in this usually short transient period. In spite of a normal progression in other aspects of their speech-language development, they might retain the [t/k] [d/g] substitution into their preschool or even beginning school years. This poses obvious dangers because the child's enormous increase in vocabulary during this time necessitates the understanding and observation of the phoneme oppositions /t/ versus /k/ and /d/ versus /g/. Many minimal pairs exemplify these contrasts in General American English—*tea* versus *key,* for instance.

Phonetic Description

[k] and [g] are voiceless or voiced postdorsal-velar stops: The back of the tongue is raised, creating a complete blockage of the expiratory airflow at the anterior portion of the velum. A buildup of air pressure occurs until the tongue suddenly moves away from the velum, releasing the air into the oral cavity. Typically, [k] is produced with higher pressure and more tension than [g]. That makes [k] in most cases aspirated and [g] unaspirated. However, the [k] is not usually aspirated in certain context conditions, for example, in word-medial position and as a component of a consonant cluster.

Linguistic Function

Frequency of Occurrence. [k] and [g] occur fairly frequently in General American English. Of 24 consonants, [k] is ranked in the top 10 most frequent, whereas [g] ranks approximately 15 (Carterette & Jones, 1974; Mines, Hanson, & Shoup, 1978). Frequent word-initiating consonant clusters include [gr], [kw], [kl], and [kr]. Frequent word-final clusters with these sounds are [ks] and [kt].

Phonotactics. Both [k] and [g] can occur initiating and terminating a syllable. Most [g] sounds occur initiating words, whereas [k] sounds are fairly equally distributed across initial, medial, and final word positions. A list of the more frequent [k] and [g] consonant clusters with word examples are in Tables 9.5 and 9.6.

Morphophonemic Function. Word-final clusters that end in [ks] or [gz] can be used to signal plurality, as in boo<u>ks</u>, le<u>gs</u>, or do<u>gs</u>. In number and tense marking, [k] occurs with [t] or [s] to produce words such as p<u>icked</u> and p<u>icks</u>. The [g] preceding either [d] or [z] can also mark number and tense in verbs such as lo<u>gged</u> or wa<u>gs</u>. In phrases, contractible auxiliaries and copulas with the verb *to be* also demonstrate clusters with [k] and [g]. Examples include the du<u>ck's</u> waddling and the do<u>g's</u> barking.

Minimal Pairs. The most common substitutions for [k] and [g] are [t] and [d]. At the end of the chapter in Appendix 9.1, examples of minimal pairs and sentences contrast these sounds.

Initial Remarks

Because [k] and [g] misarticulations are often substitutions of one speech sound for another, it is especially important that the client be evaluated for a phonemic disorder.

TABLE 9.5 Consonant Clusters with [k]

Word Initiating		Word Terminating	
[kl]	clown, clean	[kl]	uncle, tickle
[kr]	cry, crumb	[ks]	box, six
[sk]	school, sky	[kt]	backed, looked
[skr]	scream, scrape	[lk]	milk, silk, elk
[skw]	squeak, squirt	[rk]	dark, work
		[rkt]	worked, parked
		[sk]	ask, desk
		[sks]	asks, disks

TABLE 9.6 Consonant Clusters with [g]

Word Initiating		Word Terminating	
[gl]	glad, glue	[gz]	pigs, bugs
[gr]	grape, grouch	[gd]	wagged, flagged
[gw]	Gwen, very infrequent cluster		

Types of Misarticulation

The most frequent forms of [k] and [g] substitutions are noted in Figure 9.4.

Substitution of [t] and [d]	• This is most frequent form of substitution. • The manner is maintained (stop-plosive) but point of articulation is moved anteriorly. • Velar fronting occurs.
Substitution of postdorsal-velar fricative [x] and [ɣ]	• Stop-plosive production is replaced by a fricative. • The place of articulation remains the same. • Back of tongue is raised, but there is no contact between the articulators.
Substitution of a postdorsal-uvular stop-plosive [q] and [G]	• Stop-plosive production but the place of articulation is too far back. • The resulting production can sound "guttural."

FIGURE 9.4 Most Frequent Substitutions for [k] and [g]

PHONETIC PLACEMENT: [k] AND [g]

[t] and [d] Substitutions

- Prevent the tip of the tongue from touching the alveolar ridge; the tip of the tongue must remain down behind the lower incisors.
- Place the client's clean finger or clinician's gloved finger sagitally (or a tongue depressor can be used if the client can tolerate it), holding down the front half of the tongue (not just the tip). If the frontal portion of the tongue cannot be raised, an appropriate [k] can result.
- A similar procedure can be attempted with a tongue depressor placed flat and transversely across the client's tongue, keeping the front portion of the tongue down.
- The client tips his or her head back and tries to "gargle". This demonstrates the posterior positioning of the tongue. The client then attempts [g] maintaining this position.

Postdorsal-Velar Fricative Substitution

- A fricative is produced instead of a stop, therefore, the tongue needs to be elevated to achieve contact between the articulators.
- Demonstrate with [t] or [d] to emphasize the stop phase and the release aspiration.
- It might be helpful to apply slight pressure under the chin at the throat (do not push too hard, the client can gag).

Postdorsal-Uvular Stop-Plosive Substitution

- The place of articulation must be moved more anteriorly.
- The client repeats a rapid sequence of [i] - [k], [i] - [k], [i] - [k], trying to keep the tongue in the [i] position while saying [k]; the front vowel has a tendency to create a more forward positioning of the tongue.

Therapeutic Suggestions

The chart "Phonetic Placement: [k] and [g]" represents various ways to treat the misarticulations of [k] and [g].

Sound Modification Methods

1. *[ŋ]-[g] method.* These two speech sounds are phonetically very similar: Active and passive articulators are directly comparable; however, [ŋ] is a nasal whereas [g] is a stop. The easiest way to use this modification method is to have the client:

   A. Prolong the [ŋ] sound while holding the nostrils closed.
   B. Release the buildup of air pressure into the oral cavity; [g] should result. If [k] is the goal, have the child whisper [ŋ] with the same procedure but with an increase in air pressure.

2. *[u]-[k] method.* This is based on using the high-back vowel [u] to facilitate the tongue positioning for [k]. Have the client:

   A. Prolong [u] and then elevate the back of the tongue.
   B. Suggest that the client try to "stop" the sound by blocking it with the back portion of the tongue. The goal is to obtain complete closure between the posterior portion of the tongue and the soft palate.
   C. Release the sound. If the tongue positioning for [u] is maintained, an acceptable [k] or [g] should result.

Coarticulatory Conditions

[k] and [g] also demonstrate context-dependent modifications during their productions. In the context of back vowels such as [u] or [ɑ], the articulation is typically made farther back in the mouth. In the context of front vowels, such as in the word *key,* the point of contact is more frontally located. These modifications can be used to structure coarticulatory conditions that support specific production goals.

If the goal is to move the positioning of the articulators posteriorly—for example, when a [t] for [k] substitution is realized—combining [k] with the back vowels [u], [ʊ], [oᵘ], [ɔ], and [ɑ] is advantageous. During the production of back vowels, the posterior part of the tongue is elevated, supporting the placement necessary for [k]. The front vowels do not provide this coarticulatory support. In fact, the high-front vowels pose an additional danger in this respect. Because of the influence of the high-frontal tongue placement for these vowels, a client might be tempted to revert back to the [t] substitution. With a t/k substitution, the phonetically supportive vowel sequence follows the order high back, mid back, low back, central, low front, mid front, and high front.

If the goal is a more anterior tongue position, as in the substitution of a postdorsal-uvular stop for [k] and [g], the opposite vowel sequence is indicated. In this case, the front vowels aid a more anterior placement with the sequence high front, mid front, low front, central, low back, and mid back followed by high-back vowels.

It seems advisable to let [g] follow [k] in the sequencing of therapy; the lower degree of the overall muscular effort with the voicing component make [g] usually more difficult to achieve. According to personal clinical experience, a coarticulatory condition that seems to support [g] articulation is not a vowel context but an abutting consonant. Often in the context of [ŋ], as in the word *finger,* clients have produced a standard [g] that was not evidenced in other g-words. It is always worth a trial period to search for individually based starting points.

Word Examples. The following one-syllable words are ordered from relatively easy to more difficult coarticulatory conditions for a child with a t/k substitution.

[k] Words	[g] Words
coo - coop - cool - cooed[1] - cooled[1]	goof - goose - goofs
could[1]	good[1] - goods[1]
cope - comb - cove - coal - coach - coat[1]	go - goal - goes - ghost[1] - gold[1]
cop - cob - cough - call - caught[1] - cart[1]	gong - gob - gone - gauze - got[1]
cup - cub - come - cuff - cut[1]	gum - gull - Gus - gush - gulp
curb - curve - curl - Kurt[1]	girl
cap - cab - can - calf - cash - cat[1]	gang - gap - gab - gas - gash
Ken - kept[1] - Kent[1]	guess - get[1] - guest[1]
Kay - cape - came - cane - cave - cage	gay - game - gave - gain - gate[1]
king - Kim - kiss - kit[1] - kid[1]	give - gill - gift[1] - guilt[1]
key - keep - keen - keel	geese

[1]These words contain [t] and [d] and probably need to be evaluated to determine whether the coarticulatory influence of [t] and [d] has a negative impact on the newly acquired [k] and [g].

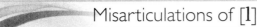

Misarticulations of [l]

Problems with [l]-productions are common in the speech of 3- and 4-year-old children (Prather, Hedrick, and Kern, 1975; Vihman & Greenlee, 1987). By age 4;6 to 5, normally developing children demonstrate a decrease in [l] misarticulations (Haelsig & Madison, 1986). Aberrant articulations include substitutions of [w] and [j] for [l]. Because of the relatively high frequency of occurrence of [l] in General American English, misarticulations are also fairly conspicuous errors.

Phonetic Description

[l] sounds are phonetically described as voiced apico-alveolar laterals. During most [l] realizations, the tip of the tongue touches the alveolar ridge. The neighboring coronal areas are relaxed, allowing air to escape laterally. Whereas some articulatory modifications do occur—for example, typical changes take place when [l] is in word-initial versus word-final positions—the main feature for [l], which is a laterally free passage for the expiratory airway, remains constant.

Common descriptions of [l] realizations note that the free lateral passage exists on both sides (bilaterally). However, Faircloth and Faircloth (1973) confirm that during spontaneous speech and under certain articulatory conditions, [l] can be realized unilaterally. Heffner (1975) describes the unilateral production as a common [l] realization. Because very little air actually escapes through the lateral openings, a unilaterally free passage usually results in a perfectly acceptable auditory [l] impression. Quite in contrast to the escape of air during lateral [s] misarticulations, the lateral airflow during [l] realizations is very minimal and not actually detectable.

General American English has two [l] varieties: the "light" (or "clear") and the "dark" [l]. Different authors have categorized the production features of the two types in various ways. Some distinguished between them by using the location of the tongue tip (Wise, 1958), whereas others have discussed the qualitative differences (Heffner, 1975). The "light" [l] has an [ɪ] quality that results from a convex shape of the tongue, especially its frontal portion near the palatal or prepalatal area (Heffner). The "dark" [l] has an [ʊ] or [o] quality caused by the elevation of the tongue's posterior portion. This high-back elevation produces a concave upper surface of the tongue behind the alveolar occlusion. Light l-sounds are transcribed [l], whereas dark l-sounds are symbolized [ɫ] or [lˠ].

Although both [l] varieties represent one single phoneme in General American English, /l/, their usage is nevertheless regulated: Light [l] is typically realized in the initial word position when /l/ precedes a vowel or follows an initial consonant—for example, in the words *like, leap, play,* and *sleep.* Dark [ɫ] is found in word-final positions as syllabics and when it precedes a consonant—for example in the words *full, kettle,* and *cold* (Heffner, 1975). Occasional lack of tongue tip contact has also been noted in [l] following a vowel in word-final position. This becomes important to clinicians when evaluating children. If the tongue tip contact is not established—for example, in the word *wheel*—the final [l] might assume an [o] or [ʊ] quality. It is a good idea to test /l/ production in more than one word position before ascribing the /o/-like sound to an articulatory error.

Linguistic Function

Frequency of Occurrence. [l] is a frequent sound in General American English; it ranks eighth in children's speech and fifth in adult's speech (Carterette & Jones, 1974). Frequent word-initial clusters include [pl], [kl], and [bl], whereas [ld] and [lz] are commonly occurring word-final clusters (Dewey, 1923; Roberts, 1965).

Phonotactics. [l] is realized in all word positions, although, as previously noted, allophonic variations that in part depend on the sound's position in the word exist. It appears that [l] occurs more frequently in medial and final word positions than when initiating a word. See Table 9.7 for lists the most frequent consonant clusters with [l].

Morphophonemic Function. Consonant clusters with [l] are used to signal plurality (do<u>lls</u>, ha<u>lls</u>), possessive (Ji<u>ll's</u>, Bi<u>ll's</u>), third-person singular (he sai<u>ls</u>, she ro<u>lls</u>), and contractible auxiliaries and copulas (the ba<u>ll's</u> rolling, the doll's little). The consonant clusters [ld] and [lvd] signal past tense, as in sai<u>led</u> or so<u>lved</u>.

Minimal Pairs. Common substitutions for [l] are [r], [w], and [j]. Minimal pair words and sentences exemplifying these substitutions are in Appendix 9.1 at the end of the chapter.

Initial Remarks

Distortions and substitutions are common [l] errors. Typical substitutions include w/l, j/l, and r/l. Because these substitutions are phonemically relevant, it is important to establish whether they represent phonemic difficulties. This information should be the basis for any therapeutic decision. Also, knowing the articulatory features of the misarticulated [l] is required. Determining these features should include probes into contexts that would promote light and dark [l] realizations. Because their articulation is different, one type could be closer to norm production than the other.

TABLE 9.7 Consonant Clusters with [l]

Word Initiating		Word Terminating	
[bl]	black, blue	[lb]	bulb
[fl]	flower, flake	[ld]	mild, gold
[gl]	glue, glad	[lf]	Ralph, golf
[kl]	clean, clown	[lk]	milk, elk
[pl]	play, plane	[lm]	film, elm
[sl]	sled, slide	[lp]	help, gulp
[spl]	splash, splinter	[ls]	false, pulse
		[lt]	belt, salt
		[lθ]	health, filth
		[lv]	shelve, twelve
		[lz]	bells, dolls
		[ldz]	folds, worlds
		[lts]	belts, adults
		[lvd]	solved, shelved
		[lvz]	shelves, wolves

Types of Misarticulation

The most common types of [l] misarticulations are outlined in Figure 9.5.

[w] for [l] Substitution	• This substitution occurs in word- or syllable-initial position. • Because of the phonotactics of GAE (no [w] word-finally) at the end of a word, the [l] substitution has more of a back vowel quality. • There is a high back position of tongue for [w]; the frontal area of the tongue is dropped and not in contact with the alveolar ridge. • Lip rounding is present.
[j] for [l] Substitution	• This is heard in word-initial position because [j] does not exist at the end of a word in GAE. • The tongue tip does not make contact with the alveolar ridge. • The tongue body is dropped to a mediodorsal-mediopalatal position. • The distance between articulators is widened somewhat.
[r] for [l] Substitution	• The entire tongue is lowered for the mediodorsal-mediopalatal [r] production. • The tongue tip does not touch the alveolar ridge; it is lowered. • If the retroflexed [r] is used as a substitution, the tongue has been slightly lowered from the alveolar ridge and is curled back.
[l] Distortion possibly [ɮ]	• The lateral openings for the l-production are too small and narrow. • This can cause a friction noise quality that sounds like a voiced lateral [z].

FIGURE 9.5 Frequent Misarticulations of [l]

Therapeutic Suggestions

Phonetic Placement. For norm productions of [l], the apex and coronal edges of the tongue are in direct contact with the alveolar ridge. The lateral edges of the tongue are not elevated but rather relaxed, allowing free passage of the air to the right and left of the contact at the alveolar ridge. Visibility of the articulation is often very helpful when establishing the placement of an isolated sound. Because visibility for most [l]-productions is limited, a wide-open mouth posture can enhance it. Under this condition, the tip of the tongue should touch the alveolar ridge in such a way that a good portion of the tongue's underside becomes visible. The chart in the accompanying box outlines the phonetic placement for the various substitutions of [l].

Sound Modification Methods

1. *[d]-[l] method.* Active and passive articulators for these two sounds are very similar; the manner of articulation, though, is different.

    A. Use the passive method mentioned below of pulling the lateral edges of the tongue down during [d]-production.

PHONETIC PLACEMENT: [l]

[w] for [l] Substitutions

- The lip protrusion on [w] needs to be eliminated (use [u] - [i] as a contrast of lip protrusion–no lip protrusion).
- The contact with the alveolar ridge needs to be established.
- The edges of the tongue are relaxed; instruct the client to use a "flat tongue" and then raise it to the alveolar ridge.
- If the back of the tongue is still elevated for [w], the result might sound like a dark [l]; put a front vowel after this production and see if it improves qualitatively.

[j] for [l] Substitutions

- The tongue tip must be elevated to the alveolar ridge; this could be the only adjustment necessary.
- If a frictionlike sound occurs, the lateral edges of the tongue need to be lowered to allow more airflow.
- A straw or small cylindrical object (bamboo stick) placed the length of the tongue and pushed down slightly can be used to aid in raising the edges of the tongue if the lateral airflow is too excessive.

[r] for [l] Substitutions

- Contact of the front part of tongue with the alveolar ridge is needed.
- The body of the tongue needs to be moved forward; see the "Sound Modification Methods" for using the [i] - [l] sound modification method.

[l] Distortions—[l] Produced as a Lateral Fricative

- If [l] is being produced as a fricative, the opening between the active and passive articulators is too narrow. Thus, the edges of the tongue need to be lowered.
- Contrast a flattened tongue versus a rolled tongue, and then place the tongue tip on the alveolar ridge with a more flattened tongue.

Passive Method of Lowering Lateral Edges of the Tongue

- Place a narrow ribbon (1/2 inch wide) flat across the front of the tongue so that the ends hang down on either side to the client's chin.
- Have the client pull down gently on both sides of the ribbon during [l] production.

B. A second possibility during the stop phase of [d] is to have the client release the air without losing the tongue tip–alveolar contact.

2. *[i]-[l] method.* This method is based on similarities between the [i] and the light [l] productions.
   A. Prolong [i] ([ɪ] can also be used) while moving the tongue tip to the alveolar ridge. Although production similarities exist between [i] or [ɪ] and the light [l], this method does not offer much visual feedback for the client. If visibility is important, the [ɑ]-[l] method might be a better choice.

3. *[ɑ]-[l] method.*
   A. Prolong the [ɑ] with a wide-open mouth posture.
   B. Elevate the tongue tip to the alveolar ridge and provide visual feedback. Not only is visibility good with this open-mouth posture but also it helps to lower the lateral edges. Often a child can say la-la-la, which is a slight variation of this method. If the [l] is correct, try [lɑ]—a pause—and then possibly [t] or [d] at the end of the new words ([lɑt], [lɑd].

CLINICAL EXERCISES

Usually the initial-word position for [l] is the easiest. Make a list of 10 two-syllable words that could be used for [l] in the medial-word position with the light [l] such as "jelly" or "silly." Try to make your list without using consonant clusters with [l].

What advantages does the [d]-[l] sound modification method have?

Coarticulatory Conditions

Favorable coarticulatory conditions, specifically the sequence of vowels that support regular [l] articulations, depend on the goal to be achieved. If visibility is important, low vowels might be the choice. Low vowels provide a client with a means of visual control that can be continued until [l] is somewhat stabilized. A desirable sequence of context exercises might begin with the low-back [ɑ] and continue with the low-front [æ]. Mid-front vowels [ɛ] and [eɪ] and mid-back [ɔ] and [oʊ] still offer some visibility if produced with a relatively open-mouth posture. Because of the possible coarticulatory influence of the lip rounding, the mid- and high-back vowels probably should be the last in the sequence for a client who demonstrates a [w/l] substitution.

In the case of [l] distortions based on an opening that is too narrow, creating a lateral fricative sound, the back vowels probably should be the choice. The slightly concave shape of the tongue supports the relaxing of the lateral edges. Here, the dark [l] in word-final position could be easier for a client to achieve.

If a later goal is to produce both light *and* dark /l/ sounds, two coarticulatory conditions need to be considered; first, the position of /l/ in the word, and second, the tendency for certain vowels to promote light versus dark [l] sounds. Back vowels, especially high-back ones, support the dark [l], whereas front vowels, especially high-front ones, aid the production of light [l]. Depending on the momentary goal—light [l] or dark [ɫ]—the sequence of vowels must vary. For the coarticulatory support of light [l] articulations, the sequence could be [l] +: high-front, mid-front, low-front, central, low-back, mid-back, and high-back vowels. The opposite sequence is suggested preceding dark [ɫ] realizations: high-back, mid-back, low-back, central, low-front, mid-front, and high-front vowels.

CLINICAL EXERCISES

There are several published word cards available for working on many types of misarticulations. The following are presented for [l] in the final-word position.

Word-final position [l] words: seal, pinwheel, whale, pencil, doll, beach ball, squirrel, windmill, apple

How could you rank order these words from easiest to more difficult? Are there any words that you might not use or wait until a much later time to attempt?

Several supportive coarticulatory possibilities have been suggested. Based on the momentary goal, different vowel sequences should be considered. However, the order of supporting coarticulatory circumstances for the new sound achievement must be determined by whatever is easiest for a client to attain.

Word Examples. The following one-syllable words are ordered from relatively easy to more difficult coarticulatory conditions for a client with an [l] problem. Word examples are given for both light and dark /l/.

Words with Light l-Sounds	Words with Dark l-Sounds
Lee - leap - leaf - leave - leak - leash	pool - tool - fool - cool - school - spool
limb - lip - lid - lit - lick - live	wool[1] - bull - pull - full
lay - lame - late - laid - lake - lace	bowl - pole - foal - goal - coal
led - let - leg - ledge - left - lend	all - hall - ball - mall - doll - fall - call
lamb - lad - laugh - lag - lamp	hull - dull - gull - skull
lug - luck - love - lump - lunch	bell - tell - fell - sale - shell
law - lot - loss - log - long - lock	mail - bale - pail - Dale - nail - sale - jail
low - load - loan - loaf - loaves	ill - hill - will[1] - Bill - pill - fill - gill
look - looked	eel - heel - meal - deal - kneel - feel
Lou - loom - loop - loon - loot - Luke	

[1]If a client has a [w/l] substitution, these words would need to be evaluated to determine whether the initial [w] might negatively impact [l] articulations.

Misarticulations of [r] and the Central Vowels With r-Coloring

The misarticulations in this section include those occurring with the consonantal r-sound, as in *rabbit* or *red,* and/or the central vowels with r-coloring, [ɝ] and [ɚ] as in *bird* or *father.* A client who has difficulty producing "r-qualities" typically demonstrates problems with both consonantal [r] and central vowels with r-coloring.

Consonantal [r] develops relatively late; it is frequently still in error during the preschool years. Smit (1993b) reported that only by age 7 were 75% of the children in her study able to produce [r] at the word level.

The central vowels with r-coloring appear to be the last vowels to be mastered. Data from the Smit (1993b) study demonstrated that only approximately 80% of the children from 6–7 years of age correctly used the vocalic [r] in the middle of the word (as in "earring").

Although it is expected that r-sounds (both consonantal and central vowels with r-coloring) are "mastered" by school age, some children continue to have difficulties with these sounds. Typical problems include sound substitutions of the consonantal [r] in word- or syllable-initial positions and derhotacization or vowelization of the central vowels with r-coloring.

Phonetic Description

Consonantal [r]. The articulation of [r] in General American English is extremely variable. In fact, the production of [r] might well be the most inconsistent consonant of our language. In different contexts, the same speaker might use various tongue and lip positions when producing this sound. The different types of [r]-productions are usually placed into two broad categories: the bunched and the retroflexed [r] (Shriberg & Kent, 2013).

The bunched [r] is phonetically classified as a voiced mediodorsal-mediopalatal central approximant. For this production, the corpus of the tongue is elevated toward the palate while the tongue tip points slightly downward. The voiced expiratory air passes sagittally through this fairly wide passage. The sides of the tongue touch the bicuspids and molars. This tongue position can vary with the vowel context, and lip rounding could be present.

The retroflexed [r] is phonetically classified as a voiced apico-prepalatal central approximant. The tip of the tongue points to the alveolar ridge or its neighboring prepalatal areas. Because the lateral edges of the tongue are raised, preventing lateral air escape, the voiced expiratory air is again channeled sagittally out of the oral cavity. During this action, the dorsum of the tongue is somewhat depressed. This makes the elevation of the tip of the tongue appear even more pronounced. Often the tip of the tongue might even be slightly bent backward or curled up. Such an articulatory position gave these [r] realizations their characteristic name: retroflexed.

Although [r] is extremely variable in its production features, recognizing some frequent allophonic variations that occur in General American English is therapeutically helpful. After [θ], the [r] can be produced as a trill. The term **trill** depicts a sound produced by the vibratory action of the active articulator tapping rapidly against a place of articulation, in this case the tongue tip against the alveolar ridge. After [t], [r] could have a fricativelike quality caused by the preceding [t], which in its release phase creates a closer approximation between the articulators than is normally the case. Also, following voiceless consonants, such as in the words *try, cry,* and *fry,* [r] could be partially devoiced.

Central Vowels with r-Coloring.   [ɝ] and [ɚ] have been called *rhotic* or *rhotacized vowels* and *retroflexed vowels.* The term *r-colored* or *rhotacized vowels* describes their perceptual quality; they appear to contain r-features. The second term, *retroflexed,* refers to a possible tongue position during their production. Because these vowels are not always produced with a retroflexed tongue articulation, this label is somewhat imprecise.

The central vowel [ɝ] is stressed and is usually produced with some degree of lip rounding; [ɚ] is the unstressed counterpart of [ɝ]. Both vowels show similar articulations, although lip rounding could be lacking when [ɚ] is produced. Based on the results of palatography, Fletcher (1992) noted that tongue actions for the rhotic vowels are similar to those for the rhotic approximants. The r-like vowels can be produced in two ways. First, the tongue can be curled upward and backward in a retroflexed position. Second, the tip can be dropped slightly, the body of the tongue bunched and moved posteriorly in the mouth. These articulations are comparable to the "retroflexed" and "bunched" consonantal [r]-productions previously discussed.

Linguistic Function

Frequency of Occurrence.   Both consonantal [r] and the central vowels with r-coloring are frequent sounds in General American English. According to Carterette and Jones (1974), these sounds are the second most frequently occurring sound category. There are many consonant clusters with [r] that are also prevalent. These include [pr], [tr], [fr], and [gr] in the word-initial

There is some disagreement as to the exact nature of the r-substitutions in children. Very often the misarticulation is simply called a *w/r substitution.* Shriberg and Kent (2013) argue that most [w/r] substitutions are actually derhotacized r-productions. Based on extensive clinical experience, Gibbon (2002) states (based on intuition, not clinical data) that most typically developing children acquiring [r] pass through a stage in which they produce [w] substitutions, and some seem to go through another stage in which they progress from [w] to [ʋ], a labiodental approximant, before reaching [r]. Children with speech disorders seem to follow the same path, but more slowly, and some continue with [ʋ] into adulthood. However, Gibbon believes that [r] realized as [w] could be more common in children with speech sound disorders.

TABLE 9.8 Word-Initiating Consonant Clusters with [r] and Final Consonants Following Rhotic Vowels

Word Initiating		Word Terminating	
[br]	bread, broom	[rb]	Herb, curb
[dr]	dream, drink	[rd]	bird, card
[fr]	frog, friend	[rg]	iceberg, Pittsburgh
[gr]	grass, green	[rk]	fork, Mark
[kr]	Craig, cry	[rl]	Karl, girl
[pr]	prune, prince	[rm]	arm, worm
[ʃr]	shrimp, shrub	[rn]	barn, learn
[tr]	train, truck	[rp]	burp, chirp
		[rs]	nurse, horse
[skr]	scream, scratch	[rʃ]	harsh, marsh
[spr]	spring, sprite	[rt]	dirt, short
[str]	straw, strong	[rv]	serve, starve
		[rz]	doors, ears
		[rdʒ]	large, George
		[rkt]	worked, parked
		[rlz]	girls, Charles
		[rst]	first, pierced
		[rts]	shirts, sports
		[rtʃ]	March, birch

position. The central vowels with r-coloring also occur with final consonants exemplified by [rd], [rt], [rn], and [rz] (Dewey, 1923; Roberts, 1965).

Phonotactics. Whereas the consonantal [r] occurs in initiating syllables or in specific clusters, the central vowels with r-coloring function as syllable nuclei. The noted word-final [r] "clusters," such as [rn] and [rt], contain [ɝ] (e.g., *turn, hurt*) or centering diphthongs preceding a consonant (e.g., *barn, farm*); they are, therefore, technically not consonant clusters. They are, however, included in Table 9.8.

Minimal Pairs. The most frequent substitutions for [r] include [w], [j], and [l]. See Appendix 9.1 at the end of the chapter for a list of examples of minimal pair words and sentences with these phonemic oppositions.

Initial Remarks

Because several misarticulations of the consonantal [r] include substitutions of one phoneme for another, it is important that a client's phonemic system be evaluated. Dialectal variations should also be examined. Dialects that characteristically lose r-coloring on central vowels include Southern, South Midland, Eastern New England, and African American Vernacular English (e.g., Iglesias & Anderson, 1995; Pollock and Berni, 2001).

Types of Misarticulation

Figure 9.6 is an outline of the most common substitutions for [r] and the central vowels with r-coloring.

Therapeutic Suggestions

Phonetic Placement: [r]. Two possibilities can be used for phonetic placement therapy with [r]: (1) the apical-alveolar "retroflexed" [r] articulation and (2) the mediodorsal-mediopalatal "bunched" [r] articulation. The retroflexed [r] is often easier to implement because its features can be explained more easily. The choice of retroflexed or bunched [r] depends on the client and the type of aberrant production presented.

CLINICAL APPLICATION

Dialect and r-Problems

The dialect of the family should always be considered when evaluating young clients. For example, in the Midwest, a diagnostic situation in which the client demonstrated a lack of r-coloring on all rhotic vowels occurred. The clinician was first convinced that the child had "r problems" until she met the mother and father. Both parents, who had lived most of their lives in Boston, spoke in a similar manner. Derhotacization was a characteristic of their Eastern New England dialect.

Apico-Prepalatal Retroflexed Articulation. The client is instructed to elevate the front of the tongue so that the tongue tip is pointing behind the alveolar ridge. The tongue tip should come close to the area behind the alveolar ridge but should not touch it. The posterior edges of the tongue should be in contact with the upper molars. First, instruct the client to glide the tongue, which is touching the alveolar ridge, forward and backward, "sweeping" the palatal area. Next instruct the client to execute, with a

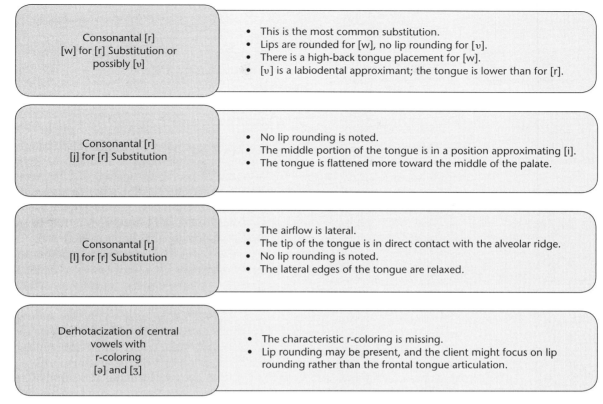

FIGURE 9.6 Common Substitutions for [r], [ɝ], and [ɚ]

slightly open-mouth posture, the same action but this time *without* touching the palatal area. If, at the same time, the back edges of the tongue are raised and voicing is added, an r-like quality might be heard. If the [r]-production seems close but is not quite on target, it is important to remember the tension of the tongue. Clinicians often have a child try to "tense" the tongue by pushing on the desk or pretending that he or she is lifting something heavy. This slight tongue tension could be enough to change the quality to an acceptable-sounding [r].

> Watch the following video of Hope who is 5 years old. Listen and try to transcribe her [r] errors. Is she having difficulty with the consonantal and vocalic r-sounds? Also note the [ʃ] in "fishing" and the [f] in "finger."

Mediodorsal-Mediopalatal Bunched Placement. The bunched [r] is produced with the tongue tip down while central portions of the tongue's body are elevated. The characteristic rhotic resonance is created by a voiced medial-sagittal airflow over the relatively broad surface of the tongue. The client should be instructed to lower the tongue tip so that it rests close to the top of the lower incisors. The client must also be aware that the lateral edges of the tongue need to touch the upper molars. A practice progression might start with the client articulating [d], noting how the back portions of the tongue touch the molars. Next, the tongue tip should be lowered, leaving the back of the tongue in the same position. Finally, the whole body of the tongue, including the tongue tip, must be moved posteriorly. The necessary change could be aided by gently pushing back the tip of the tongue with a tongue depressor so that the mediodorsal portion of the dorsum becomes more elevated. Ehren (2010) suggests that the tongue depressor be placed horizontally

PHONETIC PLACEMENT: [r], [ɝ] AND [ɚ]

[w] for [r] Substitutions

- The lip protrusion on [w] needs to be eliminated/reduced (use [u]-[i] as a contrast of lip protrusion-no lip protrusion).
- The back portion of the tongue should not be as elevated as for the production of [w]; the tongue body needs to be moved slightly anterior.
- Retroflexed [r]: The tongue tip must be elevated to approximating (but not touching) the prepalatal area for the retroflexed [r].
- Bunched [r]: The lips should be somewhat retracted, and the front portion of the tongue needs to be elevated slightly.

[j] for [r] Substitutions

- Elevation of the tongue or tongue tip is an important factor.
- Retroflexed [r]: This is marked by a concave shape (= ˘), and the tongue tip points in the direction of the prepalatal area; [j] is characterized by a slightly convex shape (=ˆ).
- Bunched [r]: The dorsum of the tongue must be lowered slightly (lower jaw).

[l] for [r] Substitutions

- Retroflexed [r] and bunched [r]: The contact between tongue tip and alveolar ridge should be released; the lateral edges of the tongue should be raised so airflow is directed medially.

Addition of r-coloring to [ɝ] and [ɚ]

- Only r-coloring needs to be added if the client produces [ɜ] and [ə].
- Two possibilities are (1) to point the tongue tip in the direction of the prepalatal area and (2) to push the tongue posteriorly, creating more of a bulge in the middle of the tongue

---

CLINICAL EXERCISES

A child has a [w] for [r] substitution but the central vowels with r-coloring are correctly articulated in the words "bird" and "turn." Construct a list of words that account for these contexts to expand the correct productions of the central vowels with r-coloring to the consonantal [r].

in the mouth, pushing the flattened surface back to the corners of the mouth., The child places the tongue against the posterior edge of the tongue depressor inside the mouth and then attempts the [r] production. The chart in "Phonetic Placement: [r], [ɝ] and [ɚ]" lists the steps that need to be taken for the other substitutions.

Sound Modification Methods: [r] and Central Vowels with r-Coloring. Several of the following modification methods use sounds that were noted as substitutions for [r]. For example, a client could have a [j/r] substitution; [j] is one of the sounds that can be modified to an [r]. The [l]-[r] *and* [j]-[r] *methods* are included in the section "Phonetic Placement: [r], [ɝ] and [ɚ]." The following methods can also be used.

1. *[d]-[r] method.* With this sound modification method, the goal is a retroflexed r-sound. The client is instructed to:
   A. Produce [d] and note where the tongue placement is.
   B. Attempt to produce [dr] by gliding the tongue tip back, pointing into the direction of the prepalatal area. The tongue tip should not touch the palate, but the movement should follow the release of the [d]; that is, the tongue tip should drop and then move back. The [d]-production as a point of departure for [r] also underlines the necessary contact of the posterior edges of the tongue with the mo-

lars. This in turn aids the elevation of the lateral edges of the tongue, reinforcing the [r] resonance.

2. *[ɝ] or [ɚ]-[r] method.* Clients who have difficulty with [r] usually show problems with the r-colored central vowels as well. However, if a clinician decides to work on the consonantal [r] and the client has acceptable productions of the central vowels with r-coloring, a transfer of this r-coloring would be the method of choice. If the client has [ɝ] and [ɚ] but not [r], a word could be specifically divided to elicit the [r] sound. For example, the client could begin with the word *purr*. Then the client tries *purring*. Next a pause is made in the word: *pu-rring*. Finally, the last syllable is isolated as *ring:* a consonantal [r] is achieved.

Where to Begin Therapy? Certain clinical decisions need to be made in respect to therapy. First, should therapy begin with the consonantal [r] or the central vowels with r-coloring? This choice should be based on stimulability probes and the perceptual sali-

ency of the error sound. Perceptual saliency refers to the conspicuousness, or noticeability, of the error sound to listeners. If one client has substitutions such as [w/r] or a [j/r] and a second client produces derhotacization of central vowels, the substitutions are probably more prominent perceptually. Dialect might also play a role in clinicians' decision making. If dialect features include derhotacization of central vowels, the consonantal [r] would be the only therapy choice. Second, which type of [r]-production, the bunched or the retroflexed [r], should be the goal of phonetic placement or sound modification techniques? Again, the client's stimulability plays a role. Placement techniques for both therapies can be implemented, and the resulting [r] can be evaluated. If an acceptable [r]-production is achieved in isolation, probes can determine which vowels or words promote the accurate use of the newly acquired sound. The therapeutic goal is to appraise the client's individual possibilities and determine the most efficient means of changing aberrant productions to acceptable articulations. Every client presents a different set of challenges.

Coarticulatory Conditions

The retroflexed [r] sound offers a challenge when clinicians try to determine which vowel sounds might present coarticulatory conditions that assist its production. There are no vowels in General American English with a tongue placement similar to the retroflexed [r] position. If the retroflexed [r] follows front vowels, especially high-front vowels, at least elevated frontal portions of the tongue are promoted. But combinations with these vowels would necessitate a quick movement from a concave retroflexed [r] to a convex "bunched" tongue shape for the front vowels. On the other hand, the back vowels, with their characteristic posterior elevation of the tongue, clearly do not support any retroflexed articulation. The central vowels without r-coloring, especially those produced with an elevated mandibular position, offer perhaps the best possibility. The front vowels would clearly be better in supporting retroflexed [r] than the back vowels.

Similar coarticulatory conditions would exist for the central vowels and the bunched r-production with its relative centralized elevation of the tongue's dorsum. However, the secondary feature of lip rounding, which often characterizes the bunched [r], is also characteristic of the back vowels. Therefore, if the goal is the bunched [r], the sequence of vowels might be central vowels, back vowels, and, finally, front vowels.

As noted previously, the articulatory features of [r] can change with individuals and with the context in which the sound occurs. Because of this, clinicians need to concentrate on the possibilities of each individual client and on the coarticulatory conditions that seem to foster the norm production of these sounds.

Word Examples. Keep in mind that individual and contextual variations often dramatically alter the production of [r]. The following one-syllable words exemplify one possible vowel sequence that could be used for a child with an [r] problem. This order is based on the retroflexed [r] as target. The vowel sequence is the one suggested at the beginning of this section. Word examples are given for both the consonantal [r] and central vowels with r-coloring.

Consonantal [r] Words

rub - rough - run - rut - rush - rug - rung

ram - rap - ran - rat - rag - rack - rang

red - wren - rent - wrench - wreck

Ray - rain - rail - raid - race - rake

rim - rib - rip - ridge - rig - Rick - ring

real - read - reach

raw - Ron - rod - rot - rock - wrong

row - robe - rope - roll - road - wrote

room - roof - rude - rule - root

Central Vowels with r-Coloring

Words with the central vowel with r-coloring - [ɝ]	Words with centering diphthongs
her - burr - purr - fur - sir - spur - stir	air - hair - mare - bear - pear[1]
earn - earth - urge	ear - fear - deer - near - cheer - gear
worm - burn - turn - word - hurt - learn	are - bar - far - jar - car - star
slurp - skirt	oar - more - bore - pour - door
	blur
	lure - tour

[1]Pronunciation of the words with centering diphthongs can vary from speaker to speaker. Thus, the word *hair* might be pronounced [hɛɚ] or [heˈɚ]. These differences could have an influence on the sequencing of the words.

Misarticulations of [θ] and [ð]

[θ] and [ð] are among the latest sounds to develop in the speech of children. Difficulties in articulating them often extend into the beginning school year. Common errors are the substitution of [t/θ] and [d/ð]. Other misarticulations include the substitution of the labiodental fricatives [f] and [v] for [θ] and [ð]. Clinicians should also be aware that variations in [θ] and [ð] productions can be a feature of African American Vernacular English. The realization of these features is conditioned by the position of [θ] and [ð] in the word. These dialectal features are not considered articulation errors.

See the "Dialects" section of Chapter 8 for more information on the influence of word position on [θ] and [ð] variations.

Phonetic Description

[θ] and [ð] can be produced as interdental or as addental fricatives. For the interdental realization, the tongue tip is protruded slightly between the front incisors. For the addental articulation, which is phonetically described as apico-dental, the tongue tip approaches the inner surface of the front incisors. The friction that characterizes these sounds as fricatives is created by restricting the breath stream between the apex of the tongue and the backside of the upper front teeth. For the interdental productions, this friction occurs between the apex and the cutting edge of the front incisors. For both productions, the tongue remains relatively flat.

Linguistic Function

Frequency of Occurrence. On a frequency of occurrence list for General American English speech sounds, [θ] and [ð] are not neighbors. Whereas [ð] is slightly above the middle, occupying a rank order of approximately 10 among 24 consonants, [θ] is among the last on the list, ranking 21 of a total of 24 (Carterette & Jones, 1974). Only word-initial [θr] is considered a fairly frequent cluster in General American English.

Phonotactics. Both [θ] and [ð] are found in word-initial and word-final positions. [ð] occurs primarily in word-initial positions, whereas [θ] occurs approximately half the time in word-initial positions; the other half is fairly evenly split between word-medial and word-final positions. See Table 9.9 for examples of consonant clusters with [θ] and [ð].

Morphophonemic Function. Word-final clusters that end in [θ] and [ð] can signal (1) plurality, as in mo*nths* and mou*ths*; (2) third-person singular, as in ba*thes* and brea*thes*; and (3) past tense, as in ba*thed* and brea*thed*.

Minimal Pairs. Frequent sounds substituted for [θ] and [ð] include [s]-[z], [t]-[d], and [f]-[v]. See Appendix 9.1.

Types of Misarticulations
See Figure 9.7 for the most common substitutions for [θ] and [ð].

Therapeutic Suggestions
Phonetic Placement
Interdental Productions. [θ] and [ð] are articulated as follows:

1. The tongue tip is *slightly* protruded between the upper and lower incisors.
2. The top of the tongue lightly touches the lower edges of the front teeth.

TABLE 9.9 Consonant Clusters with [θ] and [ð]

Word Initiating		Word Terminating	
[θr]	thread, three	[tθ]	width, hundredth
		[lθ]	health, wealth
		[nθ]	ninth, month
		[ŋθ]	length, strength
		[ðd]	bathed, breathed
		[ðz]	bathes, breathes

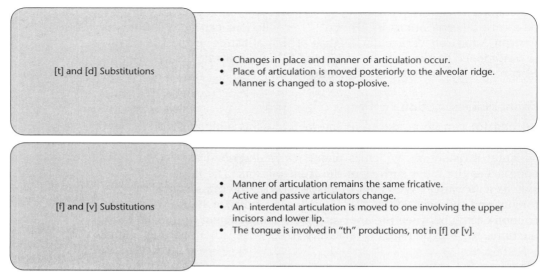

FIGURE 9.7 Frequent Misarticulations of [θ] and [ð]

3. The underside of the tongue rests on the top edges of the lower incisors.
4. The body of the tongue is relatively flat.

The expiratory airflow should be directed over the surface of the tongue between the tongue tip and the bottom edge of the front incisors. Specific tongue activities could be implemented before this placement. For example, a client could move the tip of the tongue forward and backward over the bottom edge of the front incisors. Next, with the tip of the tongue placed lightly on the bottom edge of the front incisors, the client lowers the tongue tip minimally during expiration. The goal is to create awareness of the airflow over the surface and tip of the tongue. Because the tip of the tongue is visible during the interdental production, visual feedback can be helpful. Care should be taken that this placement is not established with excessive tongue protrusion. The tongue tip should barely be visible between the teeth.

Apico-Dental Productions. The tongue tip is placed touching the posterior surface of the front incisors. The body of the tongue should be relatively flat. During expiration, a client should glide the tongue back slightly until a friction noise is heard. The required posterior movement is minimal. For the client with a [t/θ] substitution, care must be taken that the posterior movement does not result in the tongue tip coming into contact with the alveolar ridge.

The substitutions [t/θ] and [f/θ] can be effectively influenced by employing sound modification methods. The following list describes how to change the articulation from [t] and [f] to an interdental or addental [θ] and [ð].

Sound Modification Methods

1. *[t]-[θ] method.* These two sounds are distinguished by their place and manner of articulation. To move from [t] to [θ], the place of articulation must be moved

anteriorly. Also, the manner of articulation changes from a stop to a fricative. The client should be instructed to:

A. *Slowly* release [t]. This should result in a frictionlike sound.
B. Maintain this frictionlike quality while moving the tongue forward until its tip comes very close to the back of the front incisors. If this constriction is continued, the client should feel the air flowing over the tip of the tongue, forcing its way between the tongue and the back of the upper front teeth.

2. *[f]-[θ] method.* For this method, both active and passive articulators must be modified; the manner of articulation remains the same. The easiest articulation to achieve when modifying [f] to [θ] is the interdental one. Two different methods can be used:

A. During the production of [f], the client pulls the bottom lip away from the upper incisors.
B. The friction sound must continue during the placement of the tongue tip between the upper and lower incisors.

Or during the production of [f], the client is instructed to:

A. "Split the /f/ in half with his tongue by sticking his tongue between his teeth" (Secord, 1981b, p. 32). The goal is the release of the labiodental placement when the client places the tongue between the incisors.
B. The friction sound must continue during the placement of the tongue.

3. *[s]-[θ] method.* If the client has an acceptable [s], this could be an easy sound modification method to use because the place of articulation is the only feature distinguishing the two sounds. The goal is an apico-dental [θ]. During the [s]-production, the client should:

A. Glide the tongue forward until the tip almost touches the back of the upper incisors.
B. Feel the air flowing between the tongue tip and the back of the teeth.

Coarticulatory Conditions

Because of the high-front position of the tongue during [θ] and [ð] realizations, high-front vowels offer perhaps the best coarticulatory conditions following these sounds. The back vowels with the positioning of the tongue toward the back of the mouth would not aid the production. Therefore, a possible vowel sequence is high front, mid front, low front, followed by central vowels and finally the back vowels moving from low- to mid- to the high-back vowels.

Compared to the voiceless [θ], the voiced [ð] has a much higher frequency of occurrence in General American English. This would suggest that practice with [ð] is an important aspect of therapy.

Word Examples. The following one-syllable words are ordered from relatively easy to more difficult coarticulatory conditions for a child with [θ] and [ð] problems.

[θ] Words	[ð] Words
theme	thee - these
thin - thick - thing - think	this
theft	they
thank - thanks	them - then - their - there
thumb - thud - thug - thump	that - than - that's - the
third - thirst	though - those
thaw - thought - thawed - thong	

The following sections describe phonetic errors that clinicians encounter less frequently. These errors include voicing problems and difficulties with f-sounds, affricates, and consonant clusters.

Misarticulations of [f] and [v]

One of the earliest fricatives to emerge in the speech of children is [f], and it is usually mastered between 3 and 4 years of age. However, if sound mastery data are examined (see Chapter 5), the voiced [v] is consistently noted as being later in acquisition than its voiceless cognate. When Sander (1972) reinterpreted the data from Wellman, Case, Mengert, and Bradbury (1931) and Templin (1957), he reported that 90% of the children had mastered [f] by age 4 but only 51% had mastered [v]. It was not until age 8 that 90% of the children had mastered the voiced [v]. Therefore, approximately 4 years separate similar levels of competency for [f] versus [v].

What could account for this large difference in the age of acquisition? Although differences between the mastery ages of other consonant cognates exist as well, such large age variations are noted only for [f] and [v]. Perhaps the later acquisition of [v] reflects a much lower frequency of occurrence in General American English when compared to [f]. If it is not a frequent sound, children might simply not be using it, seemingly extending the mastery age. However, frequency of occurrence data for children (Carterette & Jones, 1974) do not support this hypothesis. The frequency of occurrence for [f] and [v] is relatively similar. A second possibility is that it is not the quantity of different words but a limited number of highly frequent words with [v] that raise the frequency count. (A similar case can be made for the voiced [ð]. Its relative high frequency of occurrence can be attributed to a small number of very frequently used words, such as *the.*) Two studies (Denes & Pinson, 1973; Dewey, 1923) might support this hypothesis. These investigators found that *of* [ʌv] was among the 10 most frequently used words in General American English. Such words as *have* and *give* also seem to be fairly common words. If the frequency of occurrence according to the position in the word is examined for first-, second-, and third-grade children, the majority of the [v]-sounds occur in word-final positions. These are merely possibilities for explaining the differences between the reported ages of acquisition for [f] and [v]. Whatever the reason, the later age of acquisition for [v] could have clinical implications.

The previous therapeutic discussion of phonetic errors has assumed that clinicians would proceed clinically from one consonant cognate to the other. Thus, therapy with [s] would closely coincide with [z] work. The acquisition information might cause clinicians to question the validity of this procedure for [f] and [v]. Acquisition data suggest that therapy for [f] should be initiated prior to [v]. Depending on the age of the child, it might not be realistic to expect the same level of accuracy for [v]. One of the predictions established by Elbert and Gierut (1986) is that if one member of a cognate pair is achieved in therapy, improvement occurs with the other member. Interpreted in regard to the acquisition data, therapy would most often begin with [f]. However, clinicians might want to wait and watch to see whether [v] would develop on its own. For many children, [v] acquisition appears to take place much later than the mastery of the voiceless [f].

CLINICAL EXERCISES

In the case of [f] and [v], how could you monitor whether [v] becomes established in a child's inventory?

Children with phonemic-based disorders often substitute [p] for [f]. Although [f] is an early developing sound, what might you do if you find that a child uses stop-plosives for all fricatives? In this case, would it be a good idea to go sound by sound through all the fricatives?

Phonetic Description

[f] and [v] are labiodental fricatives. A constriction is created by bringing the inner edge of the lower lip into close contact with the edges of the upper incisors. If this contact is very light, the breath stream can pass between the inner edge of the lower lip and the cutting edge of the upper incisors. Firmer contact between the lower lip and upper teeth might cause the breath stream to flow around the incisors, some of the air being forced out in the region of the canine and premolar teeth. The upper lip remains inactive during [f] and [v] articulation.

Types of Misarticulations

1. *[p/f] and [b/v] substitutions.* Examples of these substitutions include [pɪŋɡɚ] for *finger* or [ʃʌbəl] for *shovel.* Place and manner of articulation have been modified for this substitution. The labiodental articulation is replaced by a bilabial one, and the fricative is changed to a stop-plosive.

    Phonetic transcription of the error: [p] or [b].

2. *Bilabial fricative substitution.* For this substitution, only the place of articulation has been altered from a labiodental to a bilabial production. The symbols [ɸ] and [β] are used to denote voiceless and voiced bilabial fricatives.

    Phonetic transcription of the error: [ɸ] or [β].

Therapeutic Suggestions

Phonetic Placement. To develop an awareness of the labiodental articulation, the client should "bite down" on the lower lip with the upper teeth. This probably results in the client's touching the outside edges of the lower lip. However, [f] is produced with the inside of the lower lip approximating the upper incisors. Therefore, the client should then glide the lower lip along the cutting edges of the upper teeth toward the inside of the lip, letting the lip "pop out" of the bite. When the upper incisors are lightly positioned on the inner edge of the lower lip, the client should blow, allowing air to escape between this narrow slit. If the labiodental contact is too firm, the jaw can be lowered *slightly*.

If the client realizes a [p/f] substitution, the presence of airflow should be targeted. Although the airflow for [f] is relatively weak, a light feather or a small piece of tissue placed in front of the mouth should show some movement during the entire [f] production. This could then be contrasted to the lack of movement during the stop phase of the [p] articulation. In isolation, producing [p] causes movement of the feather only at the very end during the plosive part of the articulation.

The labiodental contact is also an important aspect of the phonetic placement for the client who demonstrates a bilabial fricative ([ɸ] or [β]) substitution. Because the substitution and the target sound are both fricatives, if the labiodental positioning can be established, an acceptable [f] results. A passive method might assist in this placement. During the bilabial fricative production, the bottom lip is pushed inward with the tip of the index finger. This should position the bottom lip approximately in the right spot for [f]. When a mirror is used, this passive method offers the client visual feedback regarding the relative positioning of the lower lip and the upper incisors. In addition, auditory feedback is provided when the two different sound qualities are compared.

Watch the following video as a speech/language therapist demonstrates one way to achieve an [f] with 3-year-old Aiden. As you listen, do you notice any other speech sounds Aiden still has difficulty with? youtube.com/watch?v=9xAoIxsyj38

Sound Modification Methods

[p]-[f] method. During the stop phase of the [p]-production, the bottom lip is pushed inward with the tip of the index finger so that air can escape. The lower lip should be positioned in such a manner that its inner edge approximates the upper incisors. Initially, maintaining the position of the index finger can serve as an aid until the client is aware of the necessary articulatory placement.

Coarticulatory Conditions. Vowels with lip rounding, such as the back vowels (with the exception of [ɑ]), should be avoided when beginning syllable or word practice with a newly acquired [f]. Lip rounding is clearly an unfavorable coarticulatory condition. The central vowels with r-coloring, which are often produced with lip rounding, would not provide a beneficial coarticulatory condition either. When comparing the tongue placement and the relatively closed position of the jaw during normal [f] realizations, the sequence of vowels to be considered might be high front, mid front, and low front followed by the central vowels without r-coloring. The final vowel sequence would start with the low-back vowels followed by the mid- and high-back as well as central vowels with r-coloring.

Word Examples. The following one-syllable words are ordered from relatively easy to more difficult coarticulatory conditions for a child with [f] difficulties. One-syllable words beginning with [v] are also included. However, it should be kept in mind that a large percentage of [v] sounds occurs in the medial and final word positions.

[f] Words	[v] Words
feet - feed - feel - field	
fit - fill - fin - fig - fish - fist	Vic - Vince
fade - fail - face - fake - faint	veil - vein - vase
fed - fell - fence	vet - vest
fat - fan - fast - fact	van - Val - vamp
fun - fudge	
fought - fall - fog - false	vault
phone - phones - fold	vote
foot - full	
food - fool	
fur - fern	Vern - verb

Affricate Problems

The affricates [tʃ] and [dʒ] develop relatively late in children's speech. The reason for this could be the complexity of their production or their low frequency of occurrence in General American English. Several investigations (e.g., by Carterette & Jones, 1974; Shriberg & Kwiatkowski, 1982a) analyzed the utterances of children and adults consistently ranking both [tʃ] and [dʒ] as two of the least frequently used consonants. This is further exemplified in Olmsted's (1971) study. In spontaneous speech, only 1 of the 48 children ranging from 36 to 54 months of age in the study attempted [dʒ], and that child produced it in an aberrant manner. Although several of the acquisition studies did not test both [tʃ] and [dʒ], others (Arlt & Goodban, 1976; Prather et al., 1975; Smit, 1993b) reported that there is a somewhat later age of acquisition for [tʃ] compared to [dʒ].

Phonetic Description

Although some descriptions of affricates give the reader the idea that they are merely the stops [t] and [d] followed by the fricatives [ʃ] and [ʒ], this is not entirely accurate. Based on palatograms, Kantner and West (1960) reported two factors that differentiate isolated consonant sequences from affricate productions: (1) the initial position of the stop portion and (2) the nature of the movement from the stop to the fricative portion of the affricates. First, the initial stop portion of [tʃ] is articulated closer to the articulatory position for [ʃ]; therefore, it is produced more posteriorly than is normally the case with an isolated [t]. Second, movement from the stop to the fricative portion of the affricate is characterized by the front of the tongue dropping relatively slowly, momentarily creating a constriction that is typical for the [ʃ]-sound. This is different from the release of an isolated [t] in which the tongue drops suddenly to a neutral position. The degree of lip rounding during the production of these affricates depends primarily on the speaker and the phonetic context.

An affricate is not merely a stop followed by a fricative production. Its realization varies in characteristic ways from the articulation of an isolated stop followed by a fricative. However, in an attempt to simplify the directions for children, it often seems that the goal is merely to fuse the stop with the fricative. In addition, the previously reported differences between affricates versus stop plus fricative productions might prove helpful to clinicians if the resulting sound quality is perceptually still not acceptable.

Types of Misarticulations

1. *[t/tʃ] and [d/dʒ] substitutions.* These misarticulations are characterized by the substitution of a stop for the affricate production. Examples include [tɜt] for the word *church* or [pədaməz] for *pajamas.* Because the substituted stop and the stop part of the affricate are the same, only the slow release of the stop to [ʃ] distinguishes these two speech sounds.
   Phonetic transcription of the error: [t] or [d].

2. *[ʃ/tʃ] and [ʒ/dʒ] substitutions.* A substitution of a fricative for the affricate is exemplified by [waʃ] for *watch* and [ʒʌmp] for *jump.* The lack of the initial stop portion of the affricate distinguishes this substitution from the affricate production.
   Phonetic transcription of the error: [ʃ] or [ʒ].

3. *[s/tʃ] and [z/dʒ] substitutions.* Examples for these substitutions include [pis] for *peach* and [zæm] for *jam.* This realization does not have any initial stop portion, only a fricative element. In addition, the fricative segment is articulated more anteriorly than the normal fricative portion of the affricates.
   Phonetic transcription of the error: [s] or [z].

4. *[ts/tʃ] and [dz/dʒ] substitutions.* Examples for these substitutions include [tsɪp] for "chip" and [dzip] for "jeep." The fricative element of these substitutions is too far forward.
   Phonetic transcription of the error: [ts] or [dz].

Therapeutic Suggestions

Phonetic Placement. The tongue tip is placed on the posterior edge of the alveolar ridge in a manner similar to [t]. This [t] realization should be released *slowly.* It is important that the client be aware that during the release, the lateral edges of the tongue need to remain in contact with the premolars and molars, similar to a [ʃ]-production. In addition, the tongue glides slightly back during the release. The posterior movement of the tongue can be aided by pushing the tongue back with a tongue depressor during the slow release of [t].

Sound Modification Method

1. *[t]-[tʃ] method.* The description for employing this method is similar to the one explained in the previous paragraph "Phonetic Placement." To achieve success with this method, it is important that the lateral edges of the tongue remain in contact with the premolars and first molars during the slow release of the [t]. If this is not the case, a [tʰʌ] quality can result rather than [tʃ].

Secord (1981b) suggests telling "the client to practice saying /t/-/ʃ/ slowly at first, then rapidly until they blend and become one sound" (p. 41).

CLINICAL EXERCISES

The following examples are from word cards which can be purchased for use in therapy. These are the words for "ch":

Initial: chair, chalkboard, chocolate, cherry pie, chicken, Chinese food, cheerleaders, children, cheese, chimpanzee

Medial: highchair, poncho, beach ball, wheelchair, nachos, teacher, enchilada, peaches, pitcher

Final: beach, coach, wrench, ostrich, sandwich, witch, watch, bench, lunch

Which one of the words would you want to eliminate at the beginning of therapy work on [tʃ] because the target sound is in a consonant cluster? Rank order the remaining words from easiest to more difficult coarticulatory conditions.

Coarticulatory Conditions

Because of the anterior placement of the tongue for both the stop and the fricative portions of the affricate, the front vowels seem to offer more coarticulatory support than the back vowels. Consequently, a possible vowel sequence would be high-, mid-, and low-front vowels followed by the central vowels and the back vowels. The back vowels, however, offer two advantages: (1) the lip rounding, especially of the high-back vowels, might provide coarticulatory support for the lip rounding noted in the [tʃ]-production, and (2) the back positioning of the tongue for the back vowels might enhance the backward gliding movement of the tongue in its transition from stop-plosive to the fricative portion of the affricate. If this proves to aid the production of [tʃ] in a given case, the vowel sequence might be the high-, mid-, and low-back vowels followed by the central and the front vowels. Clinicians should use probes to determine which vowel sequence would be more beneficial for their particular client.

Word Examples. The following one-syllable words are ordered from relatively easy to more difficult coarticulatory conditions for a child with an affricate problem. In this case, affricate-vowel probes demonstrate that the series of back vowels offers better coarticulatory conditions than the front vowels.

[tʃ] Words	[dʒ] Words
chew - choose	June - juice
choke - chore - chose	Joe - joke - Joan
chalk - chop - chopped - chops	jaw - jog - jar - job - John - jaws
chirp - churn	jerk - germ
Chuck - chug - chum - chunk	jug - junk - jump - jumped
chat - champ - chance	Jack - jam - jab
check - Chet	gem - jet - Jeff
chain - chase	jay - Jane
chick - chin - chill - chips	Jim - Jill
cheek - cheep - cheese - cheat - chief	gee - jeep - Gene - jeans

Voicing Problems

Voicing problems manifest themselves in the substitution of a voiced for a voiceless cognate, such as [du] for *two,* or a voiceless for a voiced cognate, such as when *ball* is pronounced as [pɑl]. Voicing has phonemic value in General American English. Different word meanings are established by the presence or absence of a voicing component. This can be exemplified by the minimal pairs *face* and *vase* and *tot* and *dot.* Because of its phonemic relevance, a voicing problem should trigger evaluation to determine whether a phonemic disorder exists.

Several authors (e.g., Grunwell, 1987; Smit & Bernthal, 1983; Smith, 1979) have noted that children at age 4 still show difficulties with certain aspects of voicing. The most common pattern is the voiced production of normally voiceless stops, fricatives, and affricates initiating a syllable or word (prevocalic voicing). Thus, *toe* and *soup* might be pronounced as [doᵘ] and [zup]. In addition, voiceless cognates are substituted for their voiced counterparts terminating a word or syllable (postvocalic devoicing); that is, *cub* becomes [kʌp] and *dog* [dɑk]. *Context-sensitive voicing* is a term used to refer to these types of voicing errors. According to Grunwell, context-sensitive voicing, especially postvocalic devoicing, continues in some children beyond 3 years of age.

Specific factors that need to be appraised before implementing therapy for difficulties with consonant voicing–devoicing include the frequency of occurrence in the client's speech and the contexts in which the voicing–devoicing occurs. First, the voicing–devoicing difficulties should occur at a relatively high frequency before therapy is implemented. Second, some specific contextual modifications resulting in devoicing are commonly heard in General American English; these modifications would not be considered misarticulations. For example, devoicing final consonants and assimilations of voicelessness are common (Abercrombie, 1967). Devoicing final consonants can be found most often before a pause. Therefore, devoicing final consonants could be realized during an articulation test as well as in spontaneous speech samples. Personal clinical experience has shown that final devoicing often occurs on plurals that end in [əz]: *matches* is pronounced as [mætʃəs] and *dishes* as [dɪʃəs]. Assimilations of voicelessness can be either progressive or regressive. During an utterance, these assimilations can often be heard if a voiceless consonant precedes or follows a voiced stop, fricative, or affricate. For example, we pronounce *news* as [nuz]. However, *news* is typically pronounced [nus] in the word *newspaper.* This devoicing of [z] is a regressive assimilation influenced by the following voiceless [p]. Although these types of sound change in context are common, they must be evaluated in relationship to their frequency of occurrence for a particular client. If the frequency is so high that intelligibility is somehow affected, even these "normal" modifications might warrant therapy.

Therapeutic Suggestions

Probably all children use some voicing distinctions in their speech. The task is to create an awareness of voicing versus lack of voicing for a particular cognate pair. The following guidelines can be supplemented with auditory discrimination exercises to enhance the general awareness of voicing versus devoicing. Minimal pair words that target the particular voicing–devoicing cognate difficulty can also be employed.

The following sequencing of auditory discrimination exercises is suggested:

1. Aid a client's general awareness of the presence or absence of voicing by having her or him listen to two sounds—[s] and [z], for example—and identify which one is

voiced. This could be combined with the tactile feedback method, which is explained in the "Tactile Feedback Method" next section.

2. Place the cognates in minimally paired words and ask the client to identify voiced versus voiceless sounds at the beginning or end of a word. Word pair discrimination exercises would use the particular consonant cognates and the position of these sounds in words that are problematic for the client. If a client has trouble with devoicing the final stops, word pairs such as *cap* versus *cab* and *lock* versus *log* could be identified.

Tactile Feedback Method. This method develops a client's awareness of the vibratory sensation associated with voicing. This is then contrasted to the lack of vibration present during voiceless sounds. Clients place their fingers on or slightly above the thyroid cartilage during the production of a voiced sound. Attention should be directed to the vibration that is felt. For children, this vibration can be compared to a motor being "on" during voiced versus "off" during unvoiced consonants. This method works well with fricatives and affricates but is difficult to implement with stop-plosives. The natural tendency to add a vowel after the production of stop sounds can trigger the feeling of vibration on unvoiced stop sounds. Actually, the vibration for the vowel *follows* the stop production, but many children will not be able to discern this. A clinician who decides to implement the tactile feedback method for establishing an awareness of voiced versus voiceless stop-plosives should instruct a child to whisper the stop to attain a voiceless realization while saying the voiced cognate with a "big (loud) voice." This should eliminate the voicing influence of the following vowel on the voiceless stop.

Auditory Enhancement Method. This method enhances the humming effect heard during the production of voiced consonants. The client's hands are cupped and placed over the ears. During the production of voiced consonants, the client should hear a humming not present during the production of voiceless consonants. A similar effect can be achieved by plugging each ear with an index finger. Difficulties could arise when using this method to discriminate between voiced and voiceless stops; the instructions noted in the tactile feedback method should be followed here as well.

Whispering Method. If a child produces a voiced consonant and its voiceless cognate is the goal, the clinician can have the child whisper the sound. As with all the previously noted methods, this one is implemented only until the client understands the distinction between voiced and voiceless productions.

Singing Method. This method is implemented for clients who can produce a voiceless consonant but the goal is its voiced cognate. Here, the client "sings" the voiceless consonant. A familiar melody such as "Happy Birthday" is sung with the voiceless consonant combined with the [ʌ] vowel replacing the words: [pʌpʌpʌpʌpʌpʌ]. If the client actually continues to sing—that is, to produce continuous voicing—the voiceless consonant becomes voiced. If this is accomplished, the client is made aware of the voiced production, which can then be isolated from the tune.

Developing Voiced Stop Productions. This technique is actually a sound modification method. It modifies the voiced stop-plosives from the nasals [m], [n], and [ŋ]. Personal clinical experience has shown that this technique is often surprisingly effective if one of the previously mentioned methods has failed. During the nasal production, the nostrils are pinched closed. The client releases the air orally. If the voicing of the nasal continues, [b] should result from [m], [d] from [n], and [g] from [ŋ]. The success of this technique depends on the continuation of the voicing component of the nasal sounds.

Consonant Cluster Problems

For some children, the acquisition of consonant clusters can extend into the beginning school years. Smit (1993a) reported that it was not until children were 9 years of age that all consonant clusters were realized in a regular manner. Children also seem to go through certain stages in acquiring consonant clusters (see Chapter 5). Consonant cluster reduction and substitution are two processes that describe these stages. One of the earliest stages in a child's attempt to produce consonant clusters is consonant cluster reduction. This is exemplifed by the production of [dʌm] for *drum*. Typically, though not always, the marked member of the cluster is the one that is deleted (Ingram, 1989b). The next phase in acquiring clusters is a consonant cluster substitution, which is demonstrated when [dwʌm] is realized for *drum*. The last phase is the norm articulation of the consonant cluster.

According to the phonotactics of General American English, most consonants can be members of a consonant cluster. Consonant clusters at the end of a word are often used to signal certain linguistic functions such as plurality (exemplified by the word *dogs*), third-person singular tense (as in *kicks*), past tense (as in *kicked*), and possessives (as in *Jack's*). At the spontaneous speech level, any consonant cluster can occur. Therefore, the treatment of consonant clusters often is one stage of a therapy program. In addition, children who can produce the individual sounds of a cluster but have difficulty with clusters containing those sounds might be referred for therapy. Depending on the number and type of consonant clusters affected, this problem could reduce the intelligibility of a child's speech considerably. The following guidelines are given to aid in the treatment of consonant clusters.

Therapeutic Suggestions

In General American English, consonant clusters consist of either two or three consonants in word-initial position and from two to four consonants in word-final position. Consonant clusters with only two consonants are typically easier to produce than those with three or four. In addition, before therapy with consonant clusters begins, all members of the consonant cluster should be sounds that the child can produce accurately. For example, if a clinician is working on [k] clusters but the child cannot produce [r], [kr] clusters should be avoided.

Production of Word-Initial Clusters

Epenthesis. During the acquisition of clusters, children often insert a schwa between the two consonants. This is a process referred to as *epenthesis*. Epenthesis can also be used to aid a client's production of a cluster. If the cluster is [sk], as in the word *skate,* the client starts with [səkeˈt]. At first, the word should be slowly pronounced so that the schwa is somewhat prolonged. After a period of practice, the client attempts to shorten the schwa vowel gradually. This can often be achieved by increasing the tempo of the entire word. The end result should be a smooth transition from the first to the second consonant.

Pausing. For this method, a pause is inserted between the first and second member of the consonant cluster. Using the previous example, [sk] becomes [s] (pause) [keˈt]. After a period of practice, the client again shortens the pause between the two consonants.

Personal clinical experience has shown that visual feedback in the form of a drawn line or gestures can often aid children in shortening this pause. For example, a long line is drawn that can be successively shortened, or the clinician can start with hands out-spread moving them closer and closer together to indicate a shorter pause. Because of the natural pause that occurs between two syllables, this method is especially effective for consonant clusters that could occur across syllable boundaries, such as [ns] in *answer* or *pencil.*

Production of Word-Final Clusters

Prolonging the First Sound. This method is best suited for clusters whose first element can be easily prolonged, such as the fricatives, affricates, nasals, or liquids. The first sound is prolonged for about 2 seconds and is then followed by the second element of the cluster, as in the word *nest,* "sssssssssss-t" for [st]. With repeated practice, the prolongation of the first sound is then successively shortened.

Pausing. This technique presents itself as a possibility if the first element of the consonant cluster is a stop-plosive. The instructions are similar to those described for initial consonant clusters.

Production of Word-Medial Clusters.

Many word-medial clusters, especially two-consonant clusters, occur across syllable boundaries, as in *base-ball* or *an-swer.* Other clusters can be found initiating a syllable, as in *ze-bra* or *A-pril.* Although common pronunciations do not syllabify these clusters between the two elements, for therapeutic purposes, they could be artificially divided into *zeb-ra* or *Ap-ril.* The previously mentioned pausing method could be easily implemented by inserting a pause between the two syllables. This pause could first be lengthened and then shortened as the client gains stability of production.

Coarticulatory Conditions

Three variables should be considered when working on consonant clusters: (1) the length of the cluster, (2) the position of the cluster in the word, and (3) the coarticulation between the specific elements of the cluster.

The *length of the cluster* refers to how many individual consonants form the cluster. Typically, the fewer the consonants, the easier the cluster is for the client. Therefore, consonant clusters with two elements should be attempted prior to three-element clusters.

The *position of the cluster* in the word refers to whether the cluster initiates the word, terminates it, or occurs somewhere in the middle. Although most clinicians probably begin with clusters initiating the word, medial clusters offer some positive features. The "natural" pause between two syllables can be used to separate the cluster into two discrete elements: For example, the [ns] cluster in *pencil* is divided into *pen-cil.* Again, this pause is at first prolonged and later shortened. This procedure gives the client time in a relatively natural word situation to produce the transition between the elements of the cluster. Inserting a pause can also be used for clusters that typically are not syllabified between the two elements. If the consonant cluster [st] is selected, practice could include *Eas-ter, toas-ter,* and *roos-ter,* for example. If the client can produce the cluster without a pause between the syllables, it can then be transferred to the word-initiating position. The client would be instructed to whisper the first part of the word, saying the last *ster* portion in a louder voice. This necessitates changing the syllable boundary from between the cluster, s-t, to initiating the cluster, st-. However, if the client can make this transition, the consonant cluster now stands at the beginning of a word, *stir.* A similar technique can be used to gain word-final consonant clusters. In this case, the last *er* portion of the word is whispered, which results in *east (from Easter) toast (from toaster),* and *roost (from rooster).*

A disadvantage to using the clusters medially is that the client must deal with a two-syllable rather than a one-syllable word. If more difficulty is noted when the client has to articulate a two-syllable word, this technique loses its appeal. Both word-initiating and word-terminating consonant clusters should then be practiced in one-syllable word contexts. Words for [st] practice could include *star* and *stone* or *nest* and *lost.* Here, word-initiating clusters would probably be easier than word-terminating clusters. As with all stages of therapy, the clinician needs to establish which sequence offers more favorable effects for each individual client.

The third factor to be considered is the coarticulation between the elements of the cluster. Given a specific target sound in the cluster, certain sound combinations could be easier to produce than others. For example, if the target sound is [s], consider the consonant cluster [sk], as in *skate,* versus [sp], as in *spot.* For [sk], the tongue must move quickly from a front approximation of the articulators to a stop closure involving the back of the tongue. With [sp], on the other hand, the [p] element can be articulated with very little or no tongue movement from the [s] position. When the coarticulation features are considered, [sp] appears easier to articulate than [sk].

CLINICAL EXERCISES

You have been working with Anna who had a lateral s-problem. You are now ready to work on consonant clusters. Based on the principles mentioned previously, rank order the following clusters from easy to hard: [sp, st, str, sl, sw, sk, skr, str, sm, sn].

[k] clusters in both the word-initial and word-final positions are on page 267. Rank order the clusters from easy to hard.

Certain consonant clusters might also need to be carefully evaluated based on the original misarticulation. For a child who originally demonstrated a lateral [s], clusters with [l], a lateral sound, might trigger the old misarticulation, for example. Or for the child who originally had a [t] for [k] substitution, the word-final cluster [kt], as in *kicked* or *locked,* might prove troublesome.

In addition, specific techniques used to elicit the norm production can be reinforced by selecting specific consonant clusters. If the [t]-[s] method was used to establish [s], the cluster [ts] used at the beginning of therapy might reinforce the [s]-production. Similarly, a clinician who has established an acceptable [r] realization by means of the [d]-[r] method might use the consonant cluster [dr] to aid in stabilizing [r] during the initial stages of therapy.

The preceding guidelines have been provided to suggest, not dictate, clinical decision making. The choice of the cluster and the sequencing of clusters in the therapy program depend on the needs and the articulatory possibilities of an individual client. However, one of the tasks of a clinician is to understand and consider the factors that could have a positive or negative influence on the production of a specific target sound. This understanding increases the efficacy of therapy.

Group Therapy with the Traditional-Motor Approach

In many speech/language therapy positions, the clinician has the possibility to work one-on-one with a client. University clinics, hospitals, and private practice, for example, usually offer these opportunities. However, clinicians working in the public school—and more than 50% of the speech/language therapists do (American Speech-Language-Hearing Association, 2013)—there is a necessity to incorporate group therapy in your sessions. The following are a few suggestions for clinicians working with speech sound disorders in a group setting.

First, it is a good idea to group the clients according to grade levels. Even if a child in kindergarten and one in first grade have similar goals, the difference at this young age is large. With older children, fifth grade and middle school, it might be possible to group them from similar grades. For example, a group of sixth and seventh graders would probably be functional, whereas a group of sixth- and eighth-graders would be problematic. Occasionally, you have a student who is mature or immature for the particular grade level, and the grouping could be adjusted accordingly. However, students enjoy being with other members of their grade, and activities can be at the same level.

Second, limit the number of children in each group. Groups of two students are the best; a group of three is still doable. When four or more students are in one group, the author has found that, even with middle schoolers, problems occur. When you have larger groups, it is very easy for the students to be unruly. Remember that the reason students typically really enjoy speech therapy is that it is fun. They get to interact and do interesting activities. When it becomes a continual issue with discipline, the fun is gone, and students withdraw from therapy. They make up excuses for not going to therapy, they sit in therapy and not talk, and they complain. This is not a conducive atmosphere for speech services. Also keep in mind that from about fifth grade on, speech therapy becomes a chore. Students are often teased about going to "speech" (although bullying is supposed to be totally unacceptable) or they feel "different," singled out. At fifth-grade age, being part of the group is very important. This is another reason why it is essential to address those speech sound disorders as early as possible and dismiss the child from services. As a last note, most speech/language therapy sessions in the public schools are 25–30 minutes in length. If you have four students in a group and alternate between each, a student has a total of 6–7 minutes of individual time per session. That is certainly not very much time for changing speech behavior.

Third, if possible, put students with similar speech sound disorders in one group. If you have two or three second graders who are still working on r-sounds, they would make a great group. Again, that might not be possible. However, a group can function if all members have different speech sound disorders. It is important that students know what sound they are working on. A therapy session can begin quickly by all telling the sound that is their goal. It is often surprising that after months, some children still might not know why they are in speech services. And if they do not know "their" sound, a clinician cannot expect that there be any conscious carryover to the classroom. You can have a group with one student working on some language goals; this just takes a bit more planning. However, it is difficult to put students with fluency problems and children who are autistic in a group of students with speech sound disorders. Children who are autistic should be put into a group of students who are not autistic if possible. Social interaction with other nonautistic children is often very beneficial.

During the course of a school year, a clinician will continually be evaluating new students and some children, especially those in kindergarten and first-grade, come to speech services with articulation-based speech sound disorders. It is perhaps a good idea to see a child who cannot produce a target sound individually until the goal sound can at least be produced in some type of syllable, either a nonsense syllable or simple CV words such as "see" for [s] or "ray" for [r]. There are two reasons for this. The child who is trying to acquire a new sound needs a clinician's constant and undivided attention to try to position the articulators, the clinician is possibly trying to find facilitating contexts, and give feedback as to the correct and incorrect sound productions. This is very hard to do in a group. Second, a child might be very self-conscious about the speech sound error, and therapy is a hard task to complete in front of a group of fellow students. If the clinician's time is restricted due to a very large caseload, the clinician might say, "I really don't have time for individual therapy." One possibility for dealing with a child individually would be to take the child out of class, sit anywhere close to the classroom (speech therapy rooms are often way off the beaten track on the outskirts of the campus, and the walk back and forth could take more than 5 minutes), and try to get the sound in isolation for 5 minutes. If a clinician attempts this procedure for just a very limited amount of time every day for a week, this is often enough time to be able to move the student into a group after that week. Clinicians should continue to look for facilitating contexts. Those contexts are true shortcuts to word production with a particular sound. For example, a child pronounced the [r] in the word *tree* correctly on the articulation test. That facilitating context was used as a starting point to expand: "tree" (which was repeated several times) moved to "treat" and then "trees," and then [tr] + [ɪ] words were explored. The possibilities to move from "tree" are numerous; one could try [t] pause [ri], then just [ri], then "reef," "reel," and so on.

It is the clinician's task to know in each group the exact level at which each child is working. Is it the CV, CVC level, or has the child progressed to short carrier sentences or even short spontaneous sentences? **It is critically important to keep notes on every therapy session.** You could have a list of words that seem to be good possibilities and then jot down the word with a + or − depending on the student's production accuracy. From personal experience, the best possibility seems to be to have a sheet with lines for each child. The date can be written at the margin and the words written in with a + or − for each therapy session. This log can easily be used later to document progress when speech "report cards" are the task. In the public schools, this is usually the same time that classroom report cards/progress reports are given to the parents. If you have no notes, these progress reports become guesswork and meaningless.

What type of activities lend themselves to group work? One possibility is a set of games that one of the children of the group picks each therapy session. (Some of the favorites for even second graders are Chutes and Ladders, Candyland, and Monkeying Around). These have to be games that do not involve time setting up or lots of time taking a turn. The students really enjoy choosing a game and often keep very close track of whose turn it is to pick. Turns move from one child to the next. The goal is to get as many productions from a student as possible in one 30-minute session. One possibility is to have the student repeat each word at least 10 times before taking a turn or make up four sentences with a specific word or use "his or her" sound in spontaneous sentences for 30 seconds. The possibilities for activities are really only as limited as your imagination. Although tempting, clinicians should very carefully use published packs of word cards. This is boring, and students tire quickly of just looking at a picture and saying the word. And as noted earlier, these word cards range from coarticulatory conditions that are easy to very difficult. This is also true for workbooks for particular sounds that have pages and pages that can be copied and distributed. These also are boring and do not have the words ordered according to any type of phonetic principles.

Again, clinicians should try to keep speech therapy services fun. Students should be praised and rewarded when they are doing a good job. One idea is to give each child a small colorful sheet of paper with his or her name on it. Staple it to the bulletin board and stamp it at the end of every therapy session (stickers take too much time). A child who accumulates a certain number of stamps can choose a prize from a treasure chest. This has proven to be a real incentive for children up to fourth grade.

SUMMARY

This chapter has dealt with the phonetic (traditional-motor) approach to the treatment of articulation-based disorders, which focuses on placement of the articulators in such a manner as to achieve an acceptable articulation of the sound in question. First, a sequence for therapy was outlined, beginning at the sound level and systematically moving to more complex articulatory conditions. Dismissal criteria were also suggested in the first portion of this chapter.

Misarticulations of several consonants were discussed in detail in the second part of this chapter. These consonants represented the most frequently misarticulated speech sounds: [s] and [z], [ʃ] and [ʒ], [k] and [g], [l], [r], the central vowels with r-coloring, and [θ] and [ð]. Other sound problems included misarticulations of [f] and [v], the affricates [tʃ] and [dʒ], voiced and voiceless substitutions, and consonant clusters. When applicable, phonetic placement as well as sound modification techniques were described. In addition, effects of coarticulation were examined for each noted problem.

Therapy with a group of students is often a necessity. The final section of this chapter examined some possibilities for group therapy. Suggestions of how to structure the groups were given and examples of some activities provided.

Any successful application of the traditional-motor approach to articulation therapy presupposes a firm knowledge base not only of the phonetic characteristics of the sound's norm realization but also of the misarticulated sound. An attempt has been made to provide both in this chapter.

CASE STUDY

The following are results from the Arizona Articulatory Proficiency Scale for Lori, age 7;6.

1. horse	[hoɚθ]	20. car	[kɑɚ]
2. wagon	[wægən]	21. ear	[ɪɚ]
3. red	[rɛd]	22. swing	[θwɪŋ]
4. comb	[koᵘm]	23. table	[teɪbəl]
5. fork	[foɚk]	24. cat	[kæt]
6. knife	[naˈf]	25. ladder	[lærɚ]
7. cow	[kaᵘ]	26. ball	[bɑl]
8. cake	[keˈk]	27. airplane	[ɛɚpleˈn]
9. baby	[beˈbi]	28. cold	[koᵘld]
10. bathtub	[bæθtəb]	29. jumping	[dʌmpɪŋ]
11. nine	[naˈn]	30. television	[tɛləvɪzən]
12. train	[treˈn]	31. stove	[s̩toᵘv]
13. gun	[gʌn]	32. ring	[rɪŋ]
14. dog	[dɑg]	33. tree	[tri]
15. yellow	[jɛloᵘ]	34. green	[grin]
16. doll	[dɑl]	35. this	[ðɪθ]
17. bird	[bɝd]	36. whistle	[wɪθəl]
18. pig	[pɪg]	37. chair	[tɛɚ]
19. cup	[kʌp]	38. watch	[wɑt]

39. thumb	[θʌm]	45. sun	[θʌn]
40. mouth	[maᵘθ]	46. house	[haᵘθ]
41. shoe	[ʃu]	47. steps	[stɛpθ]
42. fish	[fɪʃ]	48. nest	[nɛst]
43. zipper	[ðɪpɚ]	49. carrots	[kɛɚəts]
44. nose	[noᵘð]	50. books	[bʊkθ]

Lori demonstrates difficulties with [s], [tʃ], and [ʤ]. If you analyze the patterns for [s]-production, you find that she substitutes [θ] for [s] and [ð] for [z] in most words. However, she dentalizes [s] when it occurs at the beginning of a word with [t] (see *steps* and *stove*). Facilitating contexts can be noted at the end of a word in which [s] is produced correctly in [s] + [t] or [t] + [s] blends in words such as *nest* and *carrots*. It seems as if the combination with [t] produces coarticulatory conditions that are favorable for [s]. Although [s] is a later developing sound than [tʃ] or [ʤ], these facilitating contexts could be used initially to begin work on [s]. In addition, [s] is a sound that occurs frequently in General American English.

THINK CRITICALLY

1. You are working with a 7-year-old child, Larry, who has a [θ] for [s] substitution (as well as a [ð] for [z] substitution). He seems unable to distinguish between [s] and [z] when used in minimal pairs with voiced and voiceless "th." Based on his errors and his lack of discrimination abilities, construct a sensory-perceptual training program using identification, isolation, stimulation, and discrimination. Try to be as specific as possible about the targets you would use for each of the phases.

2. Maureen, a 7;6-year-old child, shows evidence of consistent dentalized [s̪] and [z̪] productions for [s] and [z] in all contexts. You cannot find facilitating contexts and have decided to do phonetic placement with the child. Describe the advantages and disadvantages of using an apico-alveolar (tongue tip up) versus a predorsal-alveolar (tongue tip down) production. Select one of the phonetic placement techniques and describe step-by-step how you would explain the tongue placement and what the child would need to do to achieve a correct [s]-production.

3. Molly has a [w] for [r] substitution. Describe in detail the steps you would complete to achieve an [r]-production using the phonetic placement technique for the apico-predorsal [r]. If you now have [r] in isolation, what CV nonsense syllables and simple words would you use to stabilize the [r]?

TEST YOURSELF

1. Which of the following is *not* a phase of sensory-perceptual training?
   a. identification
   b. production
   c. isolation
   d. stimulation
   e. discrimination

2. Instructing the client how to position the articulators in order to produce a norm production describes the
   a. auditory stimulation/imitation procedure
   b. phonetic placement method
   c. sound modification method
   d. facilitating context of a sound

3. In the word phase of the traditional-motor approach, all of the following contribute to the articulatory complexity of a word *except* the
   a. length of the word
   b. position of the target sound in the word
   c. type of word (nouns are more concrete and should be used first)
   d. syllable structure

4. The transfer of behavior to conversational speech in various settings is referred to as
   a. coarticulatory assistance
   b. facilitating context
   c. home program
   d. carryover

5. What percentage of accuracy during natural spontaneous speech was mentioned as a possible criterion for dismissal?
   a. 100%
   b. 80%
   c. 50%
   d. 60%

6. Which would be an appropriate progression of a therapy sequence?
   a. phrases/sentences, words, spontaneous speech, sensory-perceptual training
   b. words, nonsense syllables, sounds in isolation, spontaneous speech
   c. sounds in isolation, nonsense syllables, words, phrases/sentences
   d. sensory-perceptual training, sounds in isolation, phrases/sentences, nonsense syllables

7. Which of the following is part of a clinical responsibility that helps ensure that therapy was successful and the client has generalized sound productions across situations?
   a. reevaluation
   b. dismissal
   c. screening
   d. intervention

8. All of the following are therapeutic suggestions for problems with voicing *except*
   a. phonetic placement method
   b. tactile feedback method
   c. auditory enhancement method
   d. whispering method

9. A child has a [t] for [k] substitution. Which one of the following words might be problematic when working at the simple word stage?
   a. *king*
   b. *comb*
   c. *coop*
   d. *coat*

10. If you are working primarily on lip rounding for a correct [ʃ] production, which of the following words would be a good coarticulatory context?
    a. *shop*
    b. *shook*
    c. *shed*
    d. *sheep*

FURTHER READINGS

Bleile, K. M. (1996). *Articulation and phonological disorders: A book of exercises for students* (2nd ed.). San Diego, CA: Singular.

Bowen, C. (2014). Children's speech sound disorders (2nd ed.). Hoboken, NJ: John Wiley & Sons.

Dodd, B. (2013). Differential diagnosis and treatment of children with speech disorder (2nd ed.). Hoboken, NJ: John Wiley & Sons.

Passy, J. (2003). *A handful of sounds: Cued articulation in practice.* Camberwell, Melbourne, Victoria: Australian Council for Educational Research (ACER) Press.

Williams, A. L. (2006). *Sound contrasts in phonology (SCIP).* Eau Claire, WI: Thinking Publications.

APPENDIX 9.1

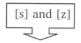

Minimal. Pair Words and Sentences Contrasting [s] and [z] to [θ] and [ð]

[s] versus [θ]		[z] versus [ð]		[s] versus [θ]		[z] versus [ð]	
sank	thank	Zen	then	bass	bath	breeze	breathe
sick	thick			Bess	Beth	close	clothe
sink	think			face	faith	seize	seethe
sing	thing			mass	math	she's	sheathe
saw	thaw			miss	myth	Sue's	soothe
sigh	thigh			moss	moth	tease	teethe
sin	thin			mouse	mouth		
song	thong			pass	path		
sought	thought						
sum	thumb						

He was *sicker* after dinner.
He was *thicker* after dinner.

Did he *breeze* close by her?
Did he *breathe* close by her?

He had to *saw* the pipes.
He had to *thaw* the pipes.

They walked by the *closing* store.
They walked by the *clothing* store.

The captain was *sinking*.
The captain was *thinking*.

There's a strange-looking *moss* on the tree.
There's a strange-looking *moth* on the tree.

Something was wrong with his *sum*.
Something was wrong with his *thumb*.

The boy had a big *mouse*.
The boy had a big *mouth*.

Minimal Pair Words and Sentences Contrasting [s] and [z] to [t] and [d]

[s] versus [t]		[s] versus [t]		[z] versus [d]		[z] versus [d]	
sell	tell	ace	ate	Z	D	as	add
cent	tent	base	bait	zing	ding	bees	bead
sack	tack	brass	brat	zip	dip	buzz	bud
sag	tag	case	Kate	zoo	do	cries	cried
sail	tail	kiss	kit	zoom	doom	dries	dried
sank	tank	hiss	hit	zipper	dipper	knees	need
sea	tea	lice	light			rose	rode
seam	team	mice	might			size	side
sew	toe	nice	night			toes	towed
sip	tip	peace	Pete			ways	wade
sock	talk	rice	write			trays	trade

(Continued)

Minimal Pair Words and Sentences Contrasting [s] and [z] to [t] and [d] (Continued)

He wanted to *sell* his story. He wanted to *tell* his story.		He looked at the big *zipper*. He looked at the big *dipper*.	
The *seam* was split. The *team* was split.		The airplane *zipped* through the clouds. The airplane *dipped* through the clouds.	
He thought it was *nice*. He thought it was *night*.		It wasn't the right *size*. It wasn't the right *side*.	
She gave him a large *kiss*. She gave him a large *kit*.		The *bees* can't be lost. The *bead* can't be lost.	

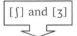

[ʃ] and [ʒ]

Minimal Pair Words and Sentences Contrasting [ʃ] and [ʒ] to [s] and [z]

[ʃ] versus [s]		[ʒ] versus [z]	[ʃ] versus [s]		[ʒ] versus [z]
shack	sack	No words found	bash	bass	no words found
shag	sag		clash	class	
shame	same		gash	gas	
shave	save		leash	lease	
she	see		mesh	mess	
shed	said		plush	plus	
sheep	seep				
sheet	seat				
shell	cell				
shine	sign				
ship	sip				
shock	sock				
shoe	Sue				
shoot	suit				
show	sew				
shy	sigh				

What a *shine*! What a *sign*!	It was a big *bash*. It was a big *bass*.
The *shell* was very small. The *cell* was very small.	He broke the *leash*. He broke the *lease*.
It was a large *shock*. It was a large *sock*.	The *clash* was over. The *class* was over.

Minimal Pair Words and Sentences Contrasting [ʃ] and [ʒ] to [t] and [d]

[ʃ] versus [t]		[ʒ] versus [d]	[ʃ] versus [t]		[ʒ] versus [d]	
shack	tack	No words found	bash	bat	rouge	rude
shag	tag		cash	cat	beige	bade
shake	take		fish	fit		
shape	tape		flash	flat		
sharp	tarp		hash	hat		
she	tea		mash	mat		
shed	ted		rash	rat		
shell	tell		rush	rut		
ship	tip		wish	wit		
shop	top					
shoe	two					
shoot	toot					

He found a larg *shack* in the woods.
He found a large *tack* in the woods.

The *ship* was broken.
The *tip* was broken.

He tried to *shake* it.
He tried to *take* it.

It was a long *shape*.
It was a long *tape*.

She had a funny *wish*.
She had a funny *wit*.

He couldn't find his *cash*.
He couldn't find his *cat*.

What a *fish* he had!
What a *fit* he had!

It was a large *flash*.
It was a large *flat*.

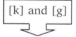

[k] and [g]

Minimal Pair Words and Sentences Contrasting [k] and [g] to [t] and [d]

[k] versus [t]		[k] versus [t]		[g] versus [d]		[g] versus [d]	
cake	take	ache	ate	gate	date	bag	bad
cop	top	back	bat	gown	down	beg	bed
cape	tape	bake	bait	go	doe	bug	bud
cub	tub	beak	beat	got	dot	leg	led
key	tea	bike	bite	gull	dull	sag	sad
kite	tight	knock	knot				
cool	tool	lake	late				
car	tar	like	light				
corn	torn	neck	net				

(Continued)

They didn't like the cold *coast*.	The *cub* was small.	They had a *bake* sale.
They didn't like the cold *toast*.	The *tub* was small.	They had a *bait* sale.
The teacher *caught* the boy.	The *gate* was fixed.	He twisted his *neck*.
The teacher *taught* the boy.	The *date* was fixed.	He twisted his *net*.
He was stuck in the *car*.	There is a scratch on her *back*.	He *likes* it.
He was stuck in the *tar*.	There is a scratch on her *bat*.	He *lights* it.
Hand me the *key*.	The *lock* was big.	Her big brother made her *beg*.
Hand me the *tea*.	The *lot* was big.	Her big brother made her *bed*.

Minimal Pair Words and Sentences Contrasting [l] to [r], [w], and [j]

[l] versus [r]		[l] versus [ɚ]		[l] versus [w]		[l] versus [j]	
lace	race	bowl	boar	lag	wag	lung	young
lane	rain	Dale	dare	life	wife	loose	use
led	red	feel	fear	lake	wake	lard	yard
lick	Rick	male	mare	leave	weave	Lou	you
long	wrong	mole	more	leap	weep	less	yes
lie	rye	owl	our	leak	weak	let	yet
light	right	tile	tire	light	white		
lead	read			let	wet		
lock	rock						

She knew it was the *long* way home. She knew it was the *wrong* way home.	She didn't want to *leave*. She didn't want to *weave*.
He stumbled on the *lock*. He stumbled on the *rock*.	*Lou* cannot come to the party. *You* cannot come to the party.
What a *deal*! What a *dear*!	It was a *light* coat. It was a *white* coat.
The *tile* needed to be replaced. The *tire* needed to be replaced.	The *lung* fish swam in the aquarium. The *young* fish swam in the aquarium.

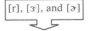

Minimal Pair Words and Sentences Contrasting [r] with [l], [w], and [j]

[r] versus [l]		[ɚ] versus [l]		[r] versus [w]		[r] versus [j]	
race	lace	boar	bowl	rag	wag	rung	young
rain	lane	dare	Dale	rail	whale	ram	yam
red	led	fear	feel	rake	wake	rank	yank

[r] versus [l]		[ɚ] versus [l]		[r] versus [w]		[r] versus [j]	
Rick	lick	mare	male	rate	wait	rot	yacht
wrong	long	more	mole	red	wed	rear	year
rye	lie	our	owl	ray	way	roar	you're
right	light	tire	tile	right	white		
read	lead			rent	went		
rock	lock			ring	wing		
				ripe	wipe		
				ride	wide		
				raced	waste		
				rest	west		
				round	wound		
				rake	wake		
				run	won		

It was a long *rain*.
It was a long *lane*.

She won the *race* at the county fair.
She won the *lace* at the county fair.

He walked to the *right*.
He walked to the *light*.

He *feels* the earthquake.
He *fears* the earthquake.

Across the field ran a large *mare*.
Across the field ran a large *male*.

The *ring* was broken.
The *wing* was broken.

The athletes always *run*.
The athletes always *won*.

She didn't want to *rake* it up.
She didn't want to *wake* it up.

The *rot* was moldy and damp.
The *yacht* was moldy and damp.

Roar loud, he said.
You're loud, he said.

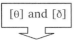

Minimal Pair Words and Sentences Contrasting [θ] and [ð] to [s] and [z], [t] and [d], and [f] and [v]

[θ] versus [s]		[θ] versus [s]		[ð] versus [z]		[ð] versus [z]	
thank	sank	Beth	Bess	then	Zen	clothe	close
thick	sick	faith	face			teethe	tease
thin	sin	path	pass			breathe	breeze
think	sink	mouth	mouse				
thinner	sinner	myth	miss				

[θ] versus [t]		[θ] versus [t]		[ð] versus [d]		[θ] versus [d]	
thank	tank	bath	bat	than	Dan	breathe	breed
thick	tick	Beth	bet	then	den	loathe	load
thin	tin	math	mat	though	dough		

| thought | taught | tooth | toot | thine | dine | |
| | | path | pat | | | |

[θ] versus [f]		[ð] versus [v]				
thin	fin	than	van			
		that	vat			
		thine	vine			

The fog was *thickening*.	They walked by the *clothing* store.
The fog was *sickening*.	They walked by the *closing* store.
It hurts when children *teethe*.	She couldn't *breathe* through the testing, so she left.
It hurts when children *tease*.	She couldn't *breeze* through the testing, so she left.

Treatment of Phonemic-Based Speech Sound Disorders

LEARNING OBJECTIVES

When you have finished this chapter, you should be able to:

- Define minimal pair contrast therapy and be able to explain how these contrasts can be used in the intervention process.
- Differentiate between minimal, maximal (including complexity approaches), and multiple oppositions approaches and know how to select treatment targets for each.
- Apply a generalization matrix for predicting phonological generalization, which can be used when selecting treatment targets.
- Establish a treatment protocol using phonological processes and minimal pairs.

- Explain the "cycles training," its goals, and therapeutic progression.
- Describe metaphon therapy as a phonological awareness approach to treating phonemic errors.
- Describe how to treat a child with an emerging phonological system.
- Identify ways to connect the treatment of phonemic-based disorders to language, specifically morphosyntax intervention and core vocabulary.
- Analyze vowel errors and prepare an intervention program.

T HIS CHAPTER focuses on phonemic-based approaches to treatment. Fey (1992) lists three basic principles underlying most of these approaches:

1. *Groups of sounds with similar patterns of errors are targeted.* In direct contrast to treating individual sounds in a sequential order, patterns of errors are noted, and selected targets are chosen for therapy.
2. *Phonemic contrasts that were previously neutralized are established.* Many of the phonemic-based treatment methods use minimal pairs to contrast phonemic oppositions. If these distinctions can be made, the assumption is that

the child will generalize this knowledge to other contrasts.
3. *A naturalistic communicative context is emphasized.* Work on individual sounds or nonsense syllables is, strictly speaking, not a part of phonemic-based therapy techniques.

Several of these treatment approaches are described in this chapter. Although each uses a somewhat different analysis system to describe the patterns of errors, most of them employ minimal pairs in their remediation program. These *minimal pair contrast therapies* have been grouped together; however, their differences are discussed. Other treatment techniques, such as *cycles training* and *metaphon therapy,* which incorporate different concepts into their methodology, are also addressed. The last portion of this chapter contains some guidelines for combining phonemic-based approaches with other treatment necessities. This includes their integration with language therapy exemplified by a child with co-occurring phonemic and language disorders and a child with an emerging phonological system. Finally, phonemic-based approaches are discussed in relationship to *vowel therapy* in children with multiple vowel errors.

As discussed earlier, the production of speech sounds—the phonetic form—and the contrastive use of phonemes within the phonological system—the phoneme function—are closely related. In addition, the phonological system interacts with other language areas. Although phonemic-based approaches emphasize the function of phonemes, both the production of speech sounds and the relationship of phonology to other language areas should not be overlooked. This chapter integrates these factors with a discussion of intervention techniques for phonemic-based speech sound disorders.

Treatment Principles

Several principles underlie the treatment of phonemic errors in the following approaches. First, the phoneme as a basic unit differentiating between word meanings is at the core of these phonemic-based therapies. Consequently, intervention begins at the word level. This differs considerably from the traditional or motor approach, which typically begins with the production of the respective sound(s) in isolation. In addition, word materials used to treat phonemic errors are structured in a very specific manner. Phonemes are usually arranged contrastively between words, resulting in "minimal pairs"—two distinct words that differ by only one phoneme value.

Second, treatment focuses on a child's phonological system. An analysis of the child's phonology as an integrated system results in knowledge of (1) the inventory and distribution of speech sounds, (2) the syllable shapes and phonemic contrasts used, and (3) the error patterns displayed. All of these factors become important when the child's phonological system, not the individual speech sound, is at the center of the remediation process.

Third, very often groups of sounds or sound classes rather than only individual speech sounds, are targeted. Children with these speech sound disorders often have difficulties with several phonemes. Their aberrant realizations might extend to whole classes of sounds making it impossible for the children to establish phonemic contrasts; neutralization of phonemic oppositions, therefore, occurs. Phoneme-based remediation focuses on more than one sound or perhaps on an entire class of sounds at the same time. Several sounds can be targeted simultaneously, as in the cycles training approach (Hodson & Paden, 1991), or two sounds can be used to demonstrate phonemic oppositions as in minimal contrast therapy (e.g., Blache, 1982; Lowe, Mount-Weitz, & Schmidt, 1992). With phonologically based therapies, generalization is assumed to occur to other sounds or sound classes.

Important differences exist between the traditional-motor approach (which is often used to treat articulation errors) and phonemic-based remediation methods (which targets phonemes). Traditional-motor approaches represent therapy for *speech form,* the production of speech sounds. In contrast, phonemic-based remediation methods target *phonemic function,* the contrastive use of phonemes to establish meaning differences. However, in the actual therapy situation, separating these two different approaches entirely is often impossible. Form and function constitute an interactive unity that work together in our treatment of children with phonemic difficulties.

Minimal Pair Contrast Therapy

The term **minimal pair contrast therapy** refers to the therapeutic use of pairs of words that differ by only one phoneme. These minimal pairs are used to establish contrasts not present in the child's phonological system. For example, an analysis reveals that a child does not differentiate between stops and fricatives; that is, all fricatives are produced as homorganic stops (e.g., [s] → [t], [f] → [p]). One type of minimal pair therapy might use [f], representing the fricatives, and [p], exemplifying stops in word pairs such as *fin* and *pin* to establish this opposition. The underlying principle is that by establishing the contrast between [f] and [p], generalization will occur to other stops and fricatives.

Minimal Opposition Contrast Therapy

What Is Minimal Opposition Contrast Therapy?   Minimal opposition contrast therapy is a method in which minimal pairs are employed as the beginning unit of therapy. The selection of the sounds for the minimal pairs was originally based on the principle that two sounds are selected with as many articulation similarities as possible. Articulatory similarities are typically measured according to the phonetic production features of place, manner, and voicing. In minimal opposition contrast therapy, the sounds chosen differ in only one or two of these production features.

Although minimal opposition contrast is considered a phonemic-based approach, the parameters for establishing these contrasts are phonetic in nature: Differences between phonetic production features are employed to determine the minimal contrast. Both speech "form," exemplified by the phonetic production features, and "function," the use of phonemic contrasts, are united for this therapy approach.

When to Use Minimal Opposition Contrast Therapy.   Which clients seem to be good candidates for this remediation plan? The minimal opposition contrast procedure targets the substitution of one phoneme for another. Sound distortions and assimilations cannot be adequately addressed using phonemic contrasts. Clients who display a large number of these types of errors would probably not benefit from this therapy. Beginning with Weiner's (1981) study, more than 40 peer-reviewed published investigations of the minimal pair approach have documented its use with children (see Baker, 2010, for a summary). Children participating in these studies had moderate, moderate-to-severe, or even severe phonological impairments. All children had normal hearing, age-appropriate receptive language skills, and no evidence of oral-motor difficulties.

In addition, Lowe (1994) states that "the minimal opposition procedure is most appropriate for clients who are stimulable for the target sound" (p. 190). Hodson (1992) supports this view and adds that it appears inappropriate to set up a potentially frustrating situation by requiring differential productions of word pairs until a child can spontaneously and effortlessly say the target sounds in the pairs.

Before considering the minimal opposition contrast approach, clinicians need to know whether any data document its successful therapeutic use. Saben and Costello-Ingham (1991) found that therapy based on minimal opposition contrasts alone produced little progress in two clients. However, these clients improved when a traditional-motor approach was implemented with the minimal opposition contrasts. So, then, does minimal opposition contrast seem a viable therapy method? Baker (2010) points out in her summary of the research literature, "Together the majority of the research suggests that the minimal pair approach is effective for children with consistent phonological speech errors" (p. 57).

Place-voice-manner analysis for the various consonants can be found on pages 188-189.

How to Select Target Sounds for Minimal Opposition Contrast Therapy.
When establishing the target sounds for minimal pairs, the following principles should be kept in mind (Lowe, 1994):

1. Phonemic substitutions form the basis for target selection. The norm production and the substitution(s) should first be seen as possibilities for minimal pairs.

2. The place-manner-voicing features for both the target sound and the substitution should be considered and the differences counted. For example, if a child demonstrates an [f/v] and a [d/v] substitution, the number of differences between the two substitutions should be listed. The production features that primarily distinguish [f] from [v] are voicing; those that differentiate between [d] and [v] are manner and place.

3. The sound substitutions chosen should reflect the least number of differences in production features. Therefore, [f] and [v] should be selected because they demonstrate only one production feature difference; [d] and [v] differ in two production features.

4. A child's age and the developmental level of the child's phonemic system should be evaluated. Earlier sounds have priority. For example, when place, manner, and voicing characteristics are analyzed, both [t/s] and [p/b] substitutions represent differences of one production feature. However, [b] is earlier than [s]. Therefore, the [p]-[b] contrast is probably the better choice. See Table 10.1 (next page) for an overview of early and later developing sounds.

5. Sound substitutions that affect a child's intelligibility the most should have priority over those with little negative effect on intelligibility. This choice is primarily related to the frequency of occurrence of the two sounds. Therefore, if two sound substitutions demonstrate an equal number of differences in production features, priority should be given to the sound that impacts the child's intelligibility the most.

6. Stimulable sounds have priority over those that are not stimulable.

This procedure can be exemplified in the following manner. A 7;7-year-old child demonstrates the following substitutions: [w/r], [θ/s], [ð/z], [d/dʒ], [t/tʃ], and [w/ʃ]. The production differences are as follows:

Substitution		Main Production Differences	
	Place	Manner	Voicing
w/r	w = labial	glide	voiced
	r = palatal	liquid	voiced
θ/s	θ = dental	fricative	voiceless
	s = alveolar	fricative	voiceless
ð/z	ð = dental	fricative	voiced
	z = alveolar	fricative	voiced
d/dʒ	d = alveolar	stop	voiced
	dʒ = postalveolar	affricate	voiced
t/tʃ	t = alveolar	stop	voiceless
	tʃ = postalveolar	affricate	voiceless
w/ʃ	w = labial	glide	voiced
	ʃ = postalveolar	fricative	voiceless

TABLE 10.1 Early to Late Sounds: Approximate Development

Early Sounds	
Nasals	Typically, [m] and [n] develop before [ŋ].
Stops and [h]	[p], [b], [t], and [d] are early stops; [k] and [g] later ones. The appearance of [k] and [g] can extend into the development of early fricatives. [h] appears around the time of early stop development.
Glides	[w] is usually earlier than [j].
Liquids	[l] develops earlier than [r]. For some children, [r] may be among the later developing sounds.
Fricatives	[f] is an early fricative, often appearing much earlier than [v].
Later Sounds	
Fricatives	The sibilants [s], [z], [ʃ], are late, whereas [ʒ], [θ], and [ð] often belong to the latest developing sounds.
Affricates	Typically [tʃ] and [dʒ] develop after, or approximately at the same time, the fricatives [ʃ] and [ʒ] appear.

Source: Summarized from Bauman-Waengler, (1994).

Based on the number of production differences, two possibilities exist for target sounds: [θ-s] or [ð-z]. Both sound pairs are acquired at about the same time. Given that both sounds are stimulable, the best target sound selections are probably [θ] and [s] because [s] has a higher frequency of occurrence and, therefore, has more of an impact on the child's intelligibility.

How Is Minimal Opposition Contrast Therapy Used? The two target sounds selected are placed in minimal pair words with the chosen sounds at the beginning: *think-sink, thing-sing,* or *thick-sick,* for example. However, often few words are appropriate for children. Therefore, it has been suggested that if meaningful minimal pairs cannot be found for contrastive phonemes, near-minimal pairs should be used (Elbert & Gierut, 1986). **Near-minimal pairs** are pairs of words that differ by more than one phoneme; however, the vowel preceding or following the target sound remains constant in both words. For example, *sir-third* or *thorn-sore* would be considered near-minimal pairs. These near-minimal pair words can be very helpful in establishing more practice material for the client.

Many of the treatment protocols of minimal opposition contrast therapy include discrimination, imitation, and spontaneous production of the word pairs. After minimal pairs are chosen, the following steps are suggested (Blache, 1989).

STEP 1: *Discussion of words.* The therapist must be certain that the child knows the concepts portrayed. To confirm this, the child can be asked to point to the picture named, and the clinician could ask questions about it. For example, for the chosen word pair *fig-pig,* ask, "Which one is a fruit?" or "Which one is an animal?"

STEP 2: *Discrimination testing and training.* In this phase, the client's discrimination between the two sounds is tested. The therapist repeats the two words in random order while the child is instructed to point to the respective picture. If the response is correct seven consecutive times, the therapist can be reasonably certain that the client is differentiating between the two sounds.

It is advised that if the criterion level of seven correct discriminations in a row cannot be reached, poor auditory discrimination or memory skills may be the cause. These skills need to be addressed before continuing the program.

You are setting up a program using minimal oppositions contrast therapy. Leo, age 4;0, has the following substitutions: t/s, d/z, t/ʃ, w/l, w/r, t/k, d/g, and w/j. Based on the outlined principles (and the child's age), which two phonemes would you target?

Make a list of minimal pairs that you could use with this child.

Watch the following demonstration of minimal opposition contrast therapy. Can you think of concepts and words you could use for a child working on the minimal pair /s/ versus/t/? youtube .com/watch?v=06DGe83dNpI& index=93&list=PLXpt2SP7467n TqEDHqTE3ExWes-zwvlyCh

STEP 3: *Production training.* This phase is directed toward the elicitation of the minimal pair words. The child is instructed to be the teacher, saying the words while the therapist points to the correct picture. In the selection of the target sound for the minimal pairs, the child can produce one of the sounds chosen while the other is not in the child's inventory. If the target sound is stimulable, the child is probably able to contrast the minimal pair. If the target sound is not stimulable, which is typically the case, the child says one word of the pair incorrectly. For example, in the previous example, [f] and [p] were selected. The child could produce [p] but not [f]. If the child says [pɪn] for *pin* and [pɪn] for *fin,* the therapist points to *pin* both times; that is, the therapist points to a word not intended by the child. Blache (1989) states, "The therapist then uses traditional cues to elicit the distinctive feature property" (p. 368). If the child cannot articulate the sound correctly, a traditional or motor approach could be implemented to achieve the sound at the *word level.* The word level is emphasized as the minimal unit. Immediate reinforcement should follow the correct sound production.

STEP 4: *Carryover training.* Once the target word can be accurately articulated, the following sequence is suggested:

Model	Example
"a" + word	a pig, a fig
"the" + word	the pig, the fig
"Touch the" + word	Touch the pig, Touch the fig
"Point to the" + word	Point to the pig, Point to the fig
longer expressions + word	That is a big pig, That is a big fig

Maximal Oppositions Approach

What Is the Maximal Oppositions Approach? This treatment method is similar to minimal opposition contrasts in that minimal word pairs are used as the beginning unit of training. However, in direct contrast to minimal opposition contrasts in which target sounds that are similar in production are selected, the maximal oppositions approach chooses sounds that are very different. Differences in production were originally defined according to the number of variations in place, manner, or voicing between the two sounds (Elbert & Gierut, 1986; Gierut, 1989). If possible, sounds that demonstrated differences in all three production features were then selected.

In the meantime, the conceptual framework for this therapy has changed somewhat. As this concept evolved, the term *maximal oppositions* referred to differences in distinctive features. These differences vary along two dimensions: (1) the number of unique features that differentiate between the two phonemes and (2) the nature of the features—that is, if differences are major or nonmajor class features. The Chomsky and Halle (1968) system, which defines major class features as consonantal, sonorant, and vocalic, is used.

Elbert and Gierut (1986) first introduced the concept of maximal oppositions training in response to their continuum of productive phonological knowledge (see Chapter 7). A series of investigations (Dinnsen & Elbert, 1984; Elbert, Dinnsen, & Powell, 1984; Gierut, 1985) examined the relationship between "most" and "least" phonological knowledge and

CHAPTER 10 *Treatment of Phonemic-Based Speech Sound Disorders* **311**

the amount of generalization that occurred in the phonological system of children. The findings of one of these studies indicated that children treated in the order of least to most phonological knowledge showed generalization across the overall sound system (Gierut, 1985). In other words, if treatment focused first on sounds that the child could not produce (consistent "error" productions) and only later targeted sounds that appeared in some contexts (inconsistent "error" productions), the most generalization occurred. On the other hand, if the order of treatment proceeded from most to least phonological knowledge, generalization was very limited. These findings led to the development of the maximal oppositions approach.

When to Use the Maximal Oppositions Approach. Which clients benefit most from maximal oppositions training? By examining the children in the series of investigations conducted to demonstrate this method (Gierut, 1990, 1992), most subjects had at least six sounds that were missing from their phonetic and phonemic inventories. This suggests that clients who would benefit the most from this intervention strategy would be those with moderate to severe phonemic-based disorders.

CLINICAL APPLICATION

Selecting a Target for Minimal Opposition Contrast Therapy

The following substitutions are noted in the speech of the child H. H.

Substitution	Main Production Differences
[tʃ] → [t]	place, manner
[dʒ] → [d]	place, manner
[k] → [t]	place
[g] → [d]	place
[f] → [b]	manner, voicing
[θ] → [b]	place, manner, voicing
[ð] → [d]	place, manner
[ʃ] → [d]	place, manner, voicing
[ʃ] → [s]	place
[s] → [t]	manner
[z] → [t]	manner, voicing
[r] → [w]	place, manner
[l] → [w]	place, manner

Four substitutions are candidates for this approach: [k-t], [g-d], [ʃ-s], and [s-t]. Stimulability of the sounds would need to be ascertained before target sounds could be selected. If all are stimulable, [k] and [t] would be a good choice because they are early developing sounds.

The maximal oppositions technique has been described in several research investigations in which its efficacy has been tested on several children. Gierut (1989) reported that after 3 different word pairs contrasting maximal oppositions had been presented, the child learned 16 word-initial consonants and restructured his phonological system. Other studies (Gierut, 1990, 1991, 1992; Gierut & Neumann, 1992) supported these findings. When minimal versus maximal oppositions approaches were therapeutically contrasted, more generalization was noted using maximal contrasts (Gierut, 1990). Other studies challenged one of the basic principles of minimal pair therapy, the selection of sounds based on the concept of "substitution" and "error" sounds (Gierut, 1991, 1992; Gierut & Neumann). If both sounds used to establish word pairs were *not* in the child's inventory, this proved to be as effective as, or at times even more effective than, teaching one sound versus its substitution. In the last of the series of investigations, word pairs comparing two previously unknown phonemes that differed by maximal and major class features were found to be the preferred way to change the phonological system of the child (Gierut, 1992). Research findings seem to support the efficacy of maximal oppositions therapy.

How to Select Target Sounds for the Maximal Oppositions Approach. Between the earlier and the later versions of maximal oppositions therapy, the procedure for target selection changed (Elbert & Gierut, 1986; Gierut, 1989, 1992). Only the later selection procedures are outlined here.

The therapist selects two sounds not in the child's inventory (i.e., two unknown sounds). In addition, these two sounds should be maximally different according to their distinctive features. Two parameters are used to determine the maximum distinctive feature differences: (1) the number of unique distinctive features that differentiate the two sounds (more distinctive feature differences = maximum feature distinction) and (2) the nature of the feature—that is, whether it is a major or nonmajor feature class (major class features = maximum feature distinction) (see Box 10.1). Major class features are:

[+ vocalic]	differentiates vowels and liquids
	from
	stops, fricatives, affricates, nasals, and [h]
[+ consonantal]	differentiates stops, fricatives, affricates, nasals, and liquids
	from
	vowels, glides, and [h]
[+ sonorant]	differentiates nasals, liquids, glides, and [h]
	from
	stops, fricatives, and affricates

How Is the Maximal Oppositions Contrast Approach Used?   The perception of or discrimination between the phonological contrast is not directly trained; rather, treatment includes two phases, *imitation* and *spontaneous production,* for each sound pair. However, it should be noted in this context that this treatment protocol originated from a research project comparing different word pairs and their impact on changes in the phonological systems

---

BOX 10.1   Major Class Features

Sonorants	Consonantal	Vocalic
vowels +	stops +	vowels +
glides +	fricatives +	liquids +
nasals +	affricates +	stops −
liquids +	nasals +	fricatives −
[h] +	liquids +	affricates −
stops −	vowels −	nasals −
fricatives −	glides −	[h] −
affricates −	[h] −	

Distinctive Feature Differences

Number of Features Excluding Major Class Features

	p	b	t	d	k	g	f	v	s	z	ʃ	ʒ	θ	ð	tʃ	dʒ
r	4	3	3	2	5	4	4	3	3	2	3	2	2	1	5	4
l	4	3	3	2	7	6	4	3	3	2	5	4	2	1	7	6
w	6	5	7	6	3	2	6	5	7	6	5	4	6	5	7	6
j	4	3	5	4	3	2	4	3	5	4	3	2	4	3	5	4
h	3	4	4	5	4	5	3	4	4	5	4	5	3	4	6	7

CLINICAL APPLICATION

The following example (Subject 11 from Gierut, 1992) is given to illustrate the selection process used in maximum feature distinctions:

Inventory	Sounds Not in Inventory	Major Class Difference
m, n, ŋ,		
w, j, h,	r, l	
p, b, t, d,	k, g	yes, between r, l versus k, g
f, v, tʃ, ʤ	s, z, ʃ, ʒ, θ, ð	yes, between r, l versus s, z, ʃ, ʒ, θ, ð

Major class differences are evidenced between /r/ and /l/ and several other phonemes. Because both /r/ and /l/ are [+ voice], the voiceless consonants [– voice] demonstrate one more distinctive feature difference than the voiced consonants. When feature differences for the noted voiceless consonants and /r/ and /l/ are counted, the following number of distinctive feature differences emerges[1]:

[r] and [k] = 5	[l] and [k] = 7
[r] and [s] = 3	[l] and [s] = 3
[r] and [ʃ] = 3	[l] and [ʃ] = 5
[r] and [θ] = 2	[l] and [θ] = 2

Therefore, considering both major class distinctions and the differences in distinctive features, according to maximal oppositions the target phonemes are /l/ and /k/. These phonemes are then used to form minimal pairs such as *lane-cane, leg-keg,* and *lamp-camp.*

---

[1]The categories sonorant, consonantal, and vocalic are not counted again when figuring the number of distinctive features.

of children. For clinical purposes, practitioners may want to implement additional activities to serve the needs of individual clients.

1. *Imitation phase.* Minimal pair picture cards are presented to the client who is asked to repeat the clinician's model of the pictures. Several activities can be used to maintain interest, such as matching or sorting pictures during imitative production, moving a car around one space on a track each time the word is imitated, playing various card games with the pictures, and so on. This phase of treatment continues until the child achieves 75% imitative accuracy over two to maximally seven consecutive sessions.
2. *Spontaneous phase.* Word pairs are now produced by the client without the clinician's model. Again, various activities can be found to keep the child's interest. This phase continues until 90% accurate production without a model for at least 3 (maximally 12) consecutive sessions is achieved.

Evolution of Maximal Oppositions — The Complexity Approach
What Is the Complexity Approach? The complexity approach emerged from a series of studies that examined the pretreatment knowledge of the phonological system and its

CLINICAL APPLICATION

Selecting Target Sounds with the Maximal Oppositions Approach

The following results are provided for H. H.

Inventory	Sounds Not in Inventory	Major Class Difference
m, n, ŋ w, j, h p, b, t, d f, v, s[1]	r, l k, g tʃ, dʒ, z, ʃ, θ, ð	yes, between r, l versus k, g yes, between r, l versus z, ʃ, ʒ, tʃ, dʒ, θ, ð

[1][f] and [v] were each produced correctly one time during the articulation test; [s] was used as a substitution for [ʃ].

Major class differences are evidenced between /r/ and /l/ and several other phonemes. Because both /r/ and /l/ are [+ voice], the voiceless consonants [– voice] render more distinctive feature differences. When feature differences are counted between the noted voiceless consonants and /r/ and /l/, the highest number of feature differences exists between /l/–/k/ and /l/–/tʃ/ (seven different features). Therefore, previously noted word pairs for /l/ and /k/ or word pairs such as *lane* versus *chain* and *Lynn* versus *chin* could be used in this maximal oppositions approach.

impact on generalization in a child's phonological system (e.g., Elbert et al., 1984; Gierut, 1985; Williams, 1991). These findings suggested that more complex linguistic input promotes more change on untreated related targets in a child's phonological system. Contrast approaches to intervention, such as the maximal oppositions approach, were a product of this concept. The complexity approach focuses on *what* is targeted in intervention as opposed to *how* it is targeted. Target selection becomes very important and is based on analyzing a child's productive phonological knowledge.(See "Assessment of Productive Phonological Knowledge" in Chapter 7, pages 194–195.) To specifically test the productive phonological knowledge, an extensive list of words was used. These words tested almost all of the phonemes of General American English in at least five contexts. When appropriate, word-initial, -medial, and -final positions were examined. Minimal pairs were also included ("face" versus "vase") as well as morphophonemic alterations ("soup" versus "soupy"). This list was used to assess a child's understanding of his or her phonemic system and of the underlying lexical representation of morphemes. This list is included in Gierut, Elbert, and Dinnsen (1987, p. 477).

When to Use the Complexity Approach Which clients seem to be good candidates for the complexity approach? It was designed for children with phonemic-based speech sound disorders. This disorder cannot be attributed to physical difficulty of the oral structure or musculature. Based on several research investigations, children's' ages ranged from 2;8 to 7;11 with most being around 4;0 years of age. The children were monolingual speakers of General American English with normal hearing, intelligence, and oral-motor abilities. Most of the children had receptive and expressive language skills in what is considered the average range. All children typically excluded six or more sounds from their phonetic and/or phonemic inventory across three manner classes (e.g., Gierut, 1999). The children also scored one or more standard deviations below the mean on a standardized articulation assessment and therefore could be described as having a moderate or severe phonological impairment of unknown origin.

The complexity approach is appropriate for children who primarily have limited phonemic inventories rather than limited word length or stress pattern inventories. Extensive word lists such as the Phonological Knowledge Protocol (Gierut, 1999) or a shorter list Onset Cluster Probe (Gierut, 1998) were used to assess the child's productive phonological knowledge.

Does the complexity approach seem a viable option for creating therapeutic change? Several studies have documented that the use of consonant clusters in treatment demonstrated more widespread change when compared to children for which only singletons were targeted (e.g., Gierut, 1998; Powell and Elbert, 1984). When sonority level differences were targeted (see the section "How to Select Target Sounds for the Complexity Approach" on how to calculate sonority level differences), Gierut (1999) reported that smaller sonority differences in consonant clusters brought about more widespread change in the phonological system. On the other hand, Williams (1991) noted that partial productive phonological knowledge of one of the consonants of the cluster was more advantageous to widespread generalization than no productive phonological knowledge. To summarize, it appears that most of the literature supports prioritizing consonant clusters although this concept requires further investigation.

How to Select Target Sounds for the Complexity Approach. In the complexity approach, sonority, stimulability, markedness, and complexity guide the selection of target sounds.

Sonority, (which was discussed in Chapter 2, page 17) refers to a sound's loudness relative to other sounds of the same length, stress, and pitch. Sounds were ranked according to a numerical sonority hierarchy (Steriade, 1990). Vowels are considered to be the most sonorous with a rank of 0, the other consonant classes demonstrating the following hierarchy: glides = 1, liquids = 2, nasals = 3, voiced fricatives = 4, voiceless fricatives = 5, voiced stops = 6, and voiceless stops = 7. Gierut (1999) examined the difference in the ranked score between consonant clusters; "clue" [kl] would have a sonority difference of 7 (voiceless stop) – 2 (glide) = 5. She reported that intervention targeting clusters with small sonority differences, such as [fl] (a score of 5 – 2 = 3), facilitated greater widespread generalization when compared to other clusters with larger sonority differences such as [kl]. The clusters with [s], such as [sp], [st], and [sk], are exceptions to this sonority principle and were not included in these relationships (see Chapter 2, page 33).

Stimulability testing is also an important aspect of this approach. A stimulable sound was considered one in which the sound could be produced accurately in isolation or in CV, VCV, VC syllables with at least 20% accuracy. If a child is stimulable for a specific sound, the child is thought to have some degree of phonological knowledge of that sound versus a child who is not stimulable at all. Studies on the role of stimulability and intervention progress suggest that nonstimulable sounds promote greater widespread change when compared to stimulable ones (Powell, Elbert, and Dinnsen, 1991). Thus, stimulability testing is important for potential intervention targets that are complex in nature.

In respect to markedness, marked sounds have been reported to be later developing and have been described as being more complex. According to this construct, sound classes are hierarchically structured where the existence of a more marked feature at a higher level implies the existence of a less marked feature at a lower level. Thus, the existence of a more marked (higher-level feature) implies the existence of a lower level one, but not vice versa. For example, consonants imply vowels. The following is the hierarchically based complexity structure for consonants from *more* to *less* complex:

True consonant clusters imply affricates
⇩
Affricates imply fricatives
⇩
Fricatives imply stops
⇩
Liquids imply nasals
⇩
Voiced obstruents imply
voiceless obstruents

> **CLINICAL EXERCISES**
>
> Consonant clusters appear to be the most complex. Based on the complexity approach, order the clusters [tr], [kl], [bl], [gl], [fl], and [tw] based on their sonority.

CLINICAL APPLICATION

Selecting Targets According to the Complexity Approach

The following results are provided for H. H.

In Inventory	Sounds Not in Inventory
m, n, ŋ	
w, j, h	r, l
p, b, t, d	k, g
f, v, s[1]	tʃ, dʒ, z, ʒ, ʃ, θ, ð

[1]Both [f] and [v] were produced one time correctly during the articulation test. H. H. is stimulable for these sounds. In addition, [s] was used as a substitution for [ʃ]. H. H. is stimulable for this sound. Stimulability probes documented that H. H. was not stimulable for the other noted sounds.

According to complexity, affricates would be the most complex sound class not in H. H.'s inventory which are nonstimulable. If consonant clusters were to be targeted, there are several possibilities: [θr], [kr], [kl], [gl], and [ʃr]. The sonority ranking reveals the following: [θr] (5 − 2 = 3), [kr] (7 − 2 = 5), [kl] (7 − 2 = 5), [gl] (6 − 2 = 4), and [ʃr] (5 − 2 = 3). The most complex (those with the lowest sonority ranks are [θr] and [ʃr].)

CLINICAL EXERCISES

Based on the concept that nonwords create a quicker system wide change, make a list of minimal pair nonwords you could use in therapy for [dʒ] and [tʃ]. Also make a list using [θr] and [ʃr].

What advantage do you see in using nonwords in therapy as opposed to real words? What disadvantages?

Thus, the higher the consonant type is, the more complex are its traits. Voiceless obstruents have the least complexity, whereas true consonant clusters (those without [s]) are the most complex.

The perspective of complexity underlies the other principles of sonority, stimulability, and markedness. As can be noted in previous sections, target selection is always based on the more complex features of the sounds in question. Intervention targeting more complex traits or features is thought to facilitate widespread change in a child's phonological system. The concept is that the existence of more complex features implies the existence of less complex ones.

One additional factor should be noted: When nonwords were targeted, as opposed to real words, more rapid system wide generalization was found as a function of treatment. Children exposed to nonwords sustained those levels of performance even after treatment had been concluded. Children exposed to real words eventually reached comparable levels of phonological generalization, but not until 55 days after the cessation of treatment (Gierut, Morrissette, & Ziemer, 2010). However, these results are based on a small number of children and may not generalize to all children seen in therapy.

How Is the Complexity Approach Used? Based on a review of the literature, the complexity approaches were typically delivered in one-on-one therapy sessions in university speech and hearing clinics. Sessions were approximately 30–60 minutes three times per week. However, other research has been conducted for 30-minute sessions once per week noting that most speech/language therapists cannot provide 1-hour sessions three times per week (Dodd, Crosbie, McIntosh, Holm, Harvey, et al., 2008). More research is necessary to determine a realistically optimal time frame for therapy.

Therapy guidelines were as follows:

1. When *nonword* minimal pairs were used, they were structured according to the phonotactics of General American English and had the targeted phonemes in the word-initial position. Examples might be [lib] versus [mib] or [lænu] versus [mænu]. These words were introduced as characters of a story or unusual objects in the story.

2. Intervention was conducted in two phases, *imitation* and *spontaneous production.* These guidelines were provided on page 312 under How Is the Maximal Oppositions Contrast Approach Used? These two phases were used in the same manner with the complexity approach.

Further Evolution of the Complexity Approach: A Matrix for Predicting Phonological Generalization. This matrix described by Gierut and Hulse (2010) is another possibility for selecting targets to induce generalization with the complexity model. The matrix is based on four factors and is somewhat similar to what has already been described. These factors are error patterns, implication universals, developmental norms, and stimulability. Error patterns suggest that those sounds excluded from the child's phonemic inventory could be optimal targets for treatment (e.g., Gierut, Elbert, and Dinnsen, 1987). *Implication universals* refer to the co-occurrence of specific sound properties in language in which one property is predictive of another. This is stated as X implies Y, but not vice versa. This was introduced on page 315 but changed somewhat in the Gierut and Hulse (2010) matrix. The following implicational universals are incorporated into their matrix:

Fricatives are predicted to change *stops*

Affricates are predicted to change *fricatives*

Voiced obstruents are predicted to change *voiceless obstruents*

Liquids are predicted to change *nasals*

Pairs /s θ/, /z ð /, /l r/ are predicted to change *all phonetic manner categories*

CLINICAL APPLICATION

Using the Gierut and Hulse (2010) principles, which sounds would we target for H. H.? The following is the noted inventory:

Sounds in Inventory	Sounds Not in Inventory
m, n, ŋ	
w, j, h	r, l
p, b, t, d	k, g
f, v, s	tʃ, dʒ, z, ʒ, ʃ, θ, ð

It appears that H. H. is stimulable for one of the consonant pairs /sθ/ but is not stimulable for /zð/. In addition, the /lr/ pair is not stimulable. The affricates /tʃ/ and /dʒ/ and the fricatives /ʃ/ and /ʒ/ are not one of the later developing sounds, so they would probably not be potential targets. Because the pair /lr/ is predicted to change all phonetic manner categories, this might be a good target possibility. On the other hand, affricates are predicted to change fricatives, which would impact several sounds that are not in H. H.'s inventory. Trial therapy might demonstrate which would support more system-wide change.

The third factor in this matrix, developmental norms, is based on research that has shown that treatment of *later* acquired sounds results in system-wide phonological changes (e.g., Gierut, Morrissette, Hughes, and Rowland, 1996). Therefore, what has been termed the late-8 sounds—/θ, ð, s, z, ʃ, ʒ, l, r/—are weighted as being more efficient treatment targets. The final factor, stimulability, is similar to that noted previously. Treating nonstimulable sounds demonstrates more generalization to other sounds than does treating stimulable sounds. Gierut and Hulse (2010) offer a complex matrix chart that a clinician could use to actually calculate which treatment targets are the best. It is rather detailed and the reader is referred to the National Institutes of Health website where the Gierut and Hulse matrix can be obtained.

Multiple Oppositions Approach

What Is the Multiple Oppositions Approach? This treatment method, developed by Williams (1992, 2000a, 2000b), is an alternative approach to contrastive minimal pairs. The approach directly addresses the collapse of multiple phonemes. For the child with extensive phoneme collapses, homonymy, in which two or more words are pronounced alike but have different meanings, results. This has a negative effect on the intelligibility, and, thus, communication breakdowns result. In the multiple oppositions approach, the child is presented with several sounds simultaneously that address the collapse of several phonemes into one phoneme. The supposition is that by treating more contrasts, several phonemic oppositions could be added to the child's system. This should result in a shortened length of treatment, improved intelligibility, and more efficient intervention.

When to Use the Multiple Oppositions Approach.

According to Williams (2000a), the multiple oppositions approach is used to treat severe speech disorders in children. When evaluating the method in an efficacy study, the children included for treatment exhibited moderate to profound phonological impairments. This was defined as the exclusion of at least six sounds across three manner categories. The children in these studies were between 36 and 72 months of age, and their hearing and intelligence were considered to be typical as were the structure and function of the speech mechanism. Because this treatment protocol is specifically designed to treat the collapse of multiple phonemic contrasts, the children should definitely demonstrate a collapse of phonemic contrasts that incorporates several sounds.

Children who were treated using this method all demonstrated documented improvement. Although children who had more severe disorders required a longer time to reach the generalization stage, system-wide changes were especially noted in the children with the most severe disorders.

How to Select Target Sounds for the Multiple Oppositions Approach.

Selection of treatment targets is based on phonemic factors. Both maximal distinctions and maximal classifications are used to guide target selection. Maximal distinctions, similar to the maximal oppositions method, are those that are maximally different from a child's error. Maximal classifications indicate that those targets selected differ maximally in respect to place, voice, and manner. In addition, a child's unique organizational structure is considered. Sounds that have the potential for the greatest impact on the child's phonological reorganization should be targeted.

For example, the following demonstrates one phonemic collapse noted in our case study child H. H.:

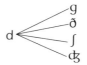

In this case, [d] would be contrasted with [g], [ð], [ʃ], and [dʒ] in minimal pair sets. These sounds would then be used to form minimal pairs such as *doe–go–though–show–Joe*.

How Is the Multiple Oppositions Approach Used?

Multiple oppositions has been used primarily in one-on-one therapy sessions of 30–45 minutes. However, it appears that this approach can be implemented in a small group. Parents have been engaged to help promote change in naturalistic play activities. The frequency of the therapy sessions was typically twice per week. The number of sessions varied, ranging from 21 to 42 sessions in the research studies. However, when Williams (2000b) followed 10 children longitudinally; other treatment options were included in later phases, making the average number of intervention sessions 60. The more severe the problem was, a longer time frame of intervention was needed. Bauman-Waengler and Garcia (2011) documented a case study with one child in which progress had plateaued after 8 months of using the cycles approach. The multiple oppositions approach was then implemented and in 14 weeks very rapid progress was noted. This may be the result of several factors, however, this case study adds to the growing body of knowledge that supports multiple oppositions as being a viable treatment protocol.

Treatment has been structured in several different ways using multiple oppositions. One paradigm using minimal contrast therapy demonstrated positive results (Williams, 2000a). A second study used a specific treatment procedure (Williams, Epperly, Rodgers, & Feltes, 1999) that consisted of four treatment phases:

1. *Imitative phase* until 70% accuracy across two consecutive treatment sets was obtained.
2. *Spontaneous phase* until accuracy reached 90% across two consecutive treatment sets.
3. *Spontaneous contrasts or generalization* based on 90% accuracy of the target sound in untrained words.
4. *Conversation* based on naturalistic intervention procedures.

Williams (2003) provided a slightly different treatment paradigm.

1. *Familiarization* and *production* of the contrasts.
2. *Production of the contrasts* through focused practice and interactive play (naturalistic activities).

These first two phases emphasize familiarization of the contrast rule, of the target sounds, and of the pictured stimuli and vocabulary. Imitative responses are numerous.

3. *Production of contrasts* with communicative contexts.
4. *Conversational recasts.*

These last two phases place more emphasis on the contrastive function of the target sounds in conversational contexts.

Phonological Process Therapy

What Is Phonological Process Therapy?   Phonological processes are often used to assess error patterns in the speech of children. As an assessment tool, its practical application is often traced to David Ingram's (1976, 1989b) *Phonological Disability in Children*. Since that time, several assessment protocols and tests founded on the concept of phonological processes have been developed (e.g., Bankson & Bernthal, 1990; Dean, Howell, Hill, & Waters, 1990; Hodson, 2004; Khan & Lewis, 2002; Lowe, 1996). Although some therapy methods, such as cycles training and metaphon therapy, use phonological process *assessment* to determine training goals, a phonological process *therapy* as such does not exist. Typically, a phonological process is selected, and then minimal pair contrasts are employed. If the child can produce the minimal pair distinctions, the phonological process has been suppressed (i.e., it has been eliminated).

To bridge the gap between the assessment of phonological errors (see Chapter 7) and their treatment, the following section describes how minimal contrasts can be established when specific phonological processes have been selected as intervention targets.

When to Use Phonological Process Therapy   Which clients would benefit the most from specific phonological process therapies using minimal contrasts? For the young client

---

CLINICAL EXERCISES

H. H. demonstrates other phonemic contrasts that are not being realized. Pick one other collapse of phonemic contrasts and demonstrate it using the type of multiple oppositions diagram that is outlined for H. H. on page 318.

Make a list of words that could be used for this specific collapse of phonemic contrasts. Did you have any difficulty making this list of minimal paired words? If you considered using nonwords, make a list of single-syllable words with the targets at the beginning of the word.

It is fairly easy to construct minimal pairs with the substitution processes. For example, when treating velar fronting, minimal pairs contrasting /t/ and /k/ could be used. However, syllable structure processes are a bit more difficult. Final consonant deletion could be treated by contrasting words that contain a final consonant versus those that do not, for example, *bow* versus *boat*. Minimal pairs could also be constructed for consonant cluster reduction—*street* versus *treat*—and for unstressed syllable deletion—*before* versus *four*. On the other hand, reduplication does not seem to lend itself effectively to the use of minimal pairs.

whose phonological system is characterized primarily by the persistence of only a limited number of phonological processes, the phonological process therapy approach is probably a viable option. However, for the child who is unintelligible or who demonstrates a wide variety of phonological processes, other approaches (cycles training, maximal oppositions, and metaphon therapy) might offer better possibilities.

As mentioned earlier, phonological processes are frequently used to assess patterns of phonemic errors. However, would minimal contrast therapy targeting specific phonological processes also influence their reduction? Weiner (1981) tested this hypothesis with two children by using minimal contrast therapy in game activities. Accurate production was required or a breakdown in communication would occur. For example, in attempting to reduce the frequency of occurrence of final consonant deletion, *bow* and *boat* were contrasted. The child had to gather a certain number of pictures of *boat* from the clinician. If the child said *bow* although *boat* was intended, the clinician would pick up the picture of *bow*. A communicative breakdown had occurred. This intervention method achieved a reduction of specific phonological processes that generalized to nontrained words as well. Based on the results of this one study, phonological process therapy seems to enhance suppression of phonological processes. However, far more research is needed, especially in consideration of the newer developments that multiple and maximal feature distinctions seem to offer.

How to Select Target Sounds with Phonological Process Therapy.

Which phonological processes should be chosen for therapy, and how does this choice impact target selection? Phonological processes should be chosen based on

- Their relative frequency of occurrence
- The effect these processes have on a client's intelligibility
- A child's age and phonological development

For a list of the most common processes and the approximate age of suppression, see Chapters 4 and 5.

Good candidates for process selection are those processes that occur most often in the speech of the child because they will probably affect intelligibility to a higher degree. However, certain phonological processes have more impact on intelligibility than others. For example, the process final consonant deletion affects many different sounds, whereas velar fronting is typically limited to a t/k substitution. Therefore, if a decision must be made between final consonant deletion versus velar fronting, final consonant deletion is probably the process to work on first. Finally, the child's age must be considered. Some phonological processes are normally suppressed at an early age, such as reduplication, and others continue to operate until the end of the preschool years, such as stopping of /θ/ and /ð/. Therefore, earlier processes are typically targeted before later processes.

Consider an example: A 4;6-year-old child demonstrates a high frequency of final consonant deletion, consonant cluster reduction, gliding (/r/ → /w/), and stopping of /θ/ and /ð/. Based on the age and the impact on intelligibility, final consonant deletion is a good choice for beginning therapy. The others are "late" processes that would probably not affect the intelligibility of a 4-year-old as much as deletion of many final consonants would.

After an appropriate phonological process is selected, word pairs must be found for the beginning phase of minimal contrast training. The child's phonetic inventory and the stimulability of specific sounds often guide the selection. See Table 10.2 for examples of numerous phonological processes.

How Are Minimal Pairs Used with Phonological Processes?

These minimal pairs can be used in many ways in a therapy situation. Several of them are discussed on pages 309–310 and 313. These activities can be as varied as the clinician's imagination but should always incorporate the client's interest and level of ability. Communicative function should stand at the forefront of any activity. See Appendix 10.1 for some concrete ideas to construct minimal pairs with phonological processes.

Table 10.2 provides an overview of the different types of therapy using minimal pairs.

Cycles Training

What Is Cycles Training? This approach was developed by Hodson and Paden (1983, 1991). It is referred to as cycles training because the phonological patterns that are to be remediated are trained successively during specific time periods known as cycles. For example, certain patterns are trained for a given period in Cycle 1, others in Cycle 2.

TABLE 10.2 Comparisons of Minimal Pair Therapy Methods

Type of Therapy	Minimal Opposition	Maximal Oppositions	Complexity Approach	Multiple Oppositions	Phonological Process
Age range	2;1–10;5 Children were usually between 4;0 and 5;0 years old.	2;8–7;11 The majority of children were around 4 years old.	2;8–7;11 Most children were around 4 years old. This is an extension of maximal oppositions.	Children were between 36–72 months old.	Age has not been determined. A child around 4–5 years old would likely benefit the most.
Severity of disorder	Moderate, moderate to severe, or severe phonological disorders.	Moderate to severe phonological disorders. At least 6 sounds were missing from phonemic inventory.	Moderate to severe phonological disorders. At least 6 sounds were excluded across 3 manner categories.	Moderate to severe level of phonological disorders. Six sounds were in error across 3 manner categories.	This has not been evaluated. The child should demonstrate only a limited number of phonological processes.
Targets phonetically similar sounds	Yes Minimal pair words have place, manner, and voicing similarities with ideally only 1 production difference.	No Targets should be maximally different based on distinctive features.	No Targets should be as complex as possible based on sonority, stimulability, markedness, and complexity.	No Ideally, targets have maximal distinctions and differ maximally in respect to place, manner, and voicing characteristics.	No Based on phonological processes that occur most often in children's speech.
Targets based on	A sound that the child can make versus one that is a substitution.	Sounds that demonstrate major class distinctions and as many distinctive feature differences as possible.	Small sonority differences in consonant clusters, marked later developing consonants, and more complex features. Nonwords are advantageous.	Based on collapse of phonemic contrasts. One sound is used as a substitution for several different sounds. Up to 4 target sounds can be selected.	Relative frequency of occurrence of phonological process, the effect the process has on a child's intelligibility, and the child's age and phonological development.
Necessary stimulability of sound	Yes Stimulable sounds have priority as targets.	No Nonstimulable sounds are preferred targets.	No Nonstimulable sounds are preferred targets.	This is not a deciding variable. The collapse of phonemic contrasts relative to the sound system has high priority.	It is assumed that sounds are stimulable.

CLINICAL APPLICATION

Selection of a Phonological Process

In H. H.'s speech consonant cluster reduction, final consonant deletion and stopping are the most prevalent processes. Consonant cluster reduction is a relatively late process and would not, therefore, be a good therapy selection. Final consonant deletion would probably impact the intelligibility of H. H.'s speech the most. Using a sound that H. H. can produce, minimal pairs would contrast a word with a final consonant versus no final consonant. For example, [b] and [t] can be articulated in an acceptable manner but are deleted in word-final position. Selected minimal pairs would be exemplified by *meat* versus *me, boat* versus *bow,* or *tube* versus *two.*

This approach is distinctive for several reasons. First, each cycle has no predetermined level of mastery for phonemes or phoneme patterns. Therefore, clients are not required to reach 75% or 90% accuracy of any phoneme or pattern realization to move to the next cycle. The targeted patterns in the cycle are used to stimulate the *emergence* of a specific sound or pattern, not the *mastery* of it. The underlying premise for this procedure is based on the known observation that phonological acquisition is gradual. The cycles approach is an attempt to approximate closely the way phonological development normally occurs as a gradual process. Second, several sounds are targeted within one cycle. Although some of the patterns from Cycle 1 might be "recycled" in the next phase, new sound patterns are also introduced. Third, this approach targets very specific clients: It is explicitly designed for highly unintelligible children. The goal of cycles training is to increase intelligibility in a relatively short time. A by-product is the acquisition of certain sounds and patterns.

When to Use Cycles Training. Which clients benefit most from cycles training? This therapy targets highly unintelligible children. "This approach was *not* designed for children with mild speech disorders" (Hodson, 1989, p. 331). Although *highly unintelligible* is not explicitly defined, these children seem to be in the profound-to-severe range on the Hodson Assessment of Phonological Processes—Revised (Hodson, 2004). Utterances of the children in the profound category were characterized by extensive omissions, some phoneme substitutions, and a very restricted repertoire of consonants. Utterances of the children in the severe category had fewer omissions, but more substitutions and consonant classes were limited (Hodson & Paden, 1991).

Is cycles training a viable therapy? According to the authors, it was developed, tested, and refined at experimental clinics in which this approach was used with more than 200 clients (Hodson & Paden, 1991). Hodson (1992) states that "most clients have been dismissed from our clinic as essentially intelligible in less than 1 year" (p. 252). This seems to indicate that the cycles approach is an effective treatment method. Whereas numerous case studies have been published using it (e.g., Gordon-Brannan, Hodson, and Wynne, 1992; Hodson, 2007), there appears to be only one randomized controlled intervention study with a larger number of children (Almost and Rosenbaum, 1998). Twenty-six children were assigned to two groups with either immediate or delayed therapy for similar intervals. After 4 months, the immediate therapy group had larger gains than the delayed therapy group. However, even after therapy had been discontinued, the group of children with immediate therapy continued to make progress.

How to Select Target Sounds with Cycles Training. The following are guidelines for potential target patterns or phonemes for Cycle 1 training.

1. *Early developing phonological patterns.* These patterns are typically present in very young normally developing children. Highly unintelligible children should be assessed to determine their individual abilities in the following categories. Deficiencies in these categories would be potential targets for Cycle 1 training:

- *Syllableness.* This refers to two- and three-syllable equal stress word combinations such as *cowboy* or *cowboy hat.* This category is evaluated according to whether the vowel nuclei exist, not in respect to the accurate production of all sounds.
- *Word-initial singleton consonants.* These include CV structures with the following phonemes: /m, n, p, b, t, d, w/.
- *Word-final singleton consonants.* These are VC structures with the phonemes /p, t/ and/or /k, m, n/.
- *Other word structures.* Both CVC and VCV words are found in the child's speech.

2. *Posterior/anterior contrasts.* The child's speech is examined to see whether either alveolar or velar sounds are absent.

3. */s/ clusters.* The child's speech is examined to see whether /s/ clusters are produced. Based on clinical experience, Hodson and Paden (1991) have found that word-final /s/ clusters are the most facilitating for these children. Singleton /s/ is not targeted until a later cycle.

4. *Liquids.* The child's speech is examined to see whether /l/ and /r/ are produced. If absent, these phonemes should be stimulated during each cycle.

If a child does not have one or more of these patterns or phonemes, any of them would be acceptable targets for Cycle 1. Target selection of specific phonemes also depends on the child's stimulability. The clinician should select the child's most stimulable sounds or patterns so that he or she can experience immediate success. Unacceptable targets include /ŋ/, /θ/, /ð/, the syllabic /l/, and weak syllable deletion.

Consider this example: A child demonstrates a high frequency of occurrence of the following processes: final consonant deletion, consonant cluster reduction, velar fronting, gliding (w/l and w/r substitutions), and stridency ([s]) deletion. The list of potential primary targets includes the following:

1. Word-final singleton consonants
2. CVC structures
3. s-clusters
4. Liquids
5. Velars

Patterns Eliminated

1. Word-final singleton consonants were not considered a Cycle 1 target because the child did produce [p], [t], [m], and [n] in the word-final position.
2. The child was not stimulable for stridents.

Patterns Targeted

1. CVC structures to stimulate the understanding of final consonants
2. Liquids
3. Velars

Because the child was not stimulable for stridents, /s/ clusters, which would normally be a primary target, were delayed until a later cycle.

CLINICAL APPLICATION

Selecting Targets According to the Cycles Approach

These results are provided for H. H.

In Inventory	Sounds Not in Inventory
m, n, ŋ	
w, j, h	r, l
p, b, t, d	k, g
f, v, s1	tʃ, dʒ, z, ʒ, ʃ, θ, ð

[1]Both [f] and [v] were produced once correctly during the articulation test, so H. H. is stimulable for these sounds. In addition, [s] was used as a substitution for [ʃ]. H. H. is stimulable for this sound.

Which patterns would you target with H. H.? Posterior–anterior contrasts are important for differentiating [t] and [d] from [k] and [g]. Liquids offer another possibility. In addition, s-clusters might be good because H. H. does seem to be able to produce this sound; however, it is used as a substitution for [ʃ].

How Is Cycles Training Used?

Establishing a Cycle. Each phoneme in a pattern should be targeted for *60 minutes per cycle.* If therapy is 30 minutes per session twice a week, the first phoneme would be targeted for 1 week of therapy. After completion of the first phoneme, a second one is initiated for the next 60 minutes. All remaining phonemes are presented consecutively for 60 minutes each. If the goal is a specific phonological pattern rather than an individual phoneme, at least two exemplars of the pattern should be presented in two consecutive 60-minute time intervals before moving to the next phoneme or pattern. If the pattern targeted is CVC structures, two different CVC word types should be used, for example, CVCs with final voiced stops versus final nasals. Only one phonological pattern or phoneme should be targeted during any *one* session. In Cycle 1, all the patterns determined from the assessment should be presented consecutively. Typically, this cycle has between three and six different patterns or phonemes.

Preparing Word Cards for Therapy. Words are used as the minimal unit of production practice, so word cards that picture each of the chosen concepts are developed. Chosen words should be monosyllabic and incorporate facilitative phonetic environments. For example, words with sounds produced at the same place of articulation as the substitute sound should be avoided. Thus, *cat, can, kite*, and *goat* should not be used if the child has a t/k substitution (Hodson, 1989). Object and action words are preferred. Obviously, the words should also be appropriate for the child's vocabulary level.

Structuring the Remediation Session. Each therapy session should follow these steps:

1. *Review.* The child reviews the preceding session's word cards.
2. *Auditory bombardment.* Amplified auditory stimulation is provided for 1 to 2 minutes while the clinician reads approximately 12 words that contain the target pattern for this session.
3. *Target word cards.* The child draws, colors, or pastes pictures of three to five target words on large index cards while repeating the words modeled by the clinician.
4. *Production practice through experiential play.* During experiential play (e.g., fishing, bowling), the clinician and the child take turns naming the pictures. The clinician provides models and/or tactile cues (such as touching the child's upper lip to indicate an alveolar sound or the throat to indicate a velar production) so that she or he achieves 100% success on the target patterns. (This is why it is essential that target words are carefully selected.) The clinician also provides opportunities to engage in conversation to determine whether the pattern is beginning to emerge spontaneously.
5. *Stimulability probes.* The clinicians assesses the child's stimulability for the next session's potential targets. For example, if /s/ clusters are prospects for the next session, the child is asked to model several words that contain different /s/ clusters. The most stimulable /s/ cluster is then targeted for the next session.
6. *Auditory bombardment.* Step 2 is repeated.
7. *Home program.* The parent or school aide participates in a home program that is 2 minutes per day. This program consists of reading the week's listening list (Step 2) and having the child name picture cards of the production practice words.

CLINICAL EXERCISES

The cycles approach targets for the next cycle only those words that are stimulable. How is this different from maximal opposition therapy and the complexity approach?

Prepare a word list for /k/ in the word-initial position that has the following characteristics: is a single syllable, has no other /k/ or /g/ sounds, does not contain the substitutions /t/ or /d/ or sounds that occur at this place of articulation, and contains only singletons, not consonant clusters.

Metaphon Therapy: One Type of Phonological Awareness Approach

What Is Metaphon Therapy? Metaphon therapy orginated in the 1980s as a result of dissatisfaction with minimal pair management strategies for phonologically disordered children. In the experience of its developers, Janet Howell and Elizabeth Dean, the use of minimal pair contrasts was often not causing the necessary changes in the child's phonological system. This led to questioning the metaphonological skills of these children. In other words, what do children with phonological disorders know about sounds?

Similar to cycles training, metaphon therapy has evolved out of clinical experience and incorporates different approaches that are merged into two therapy phases. However, the framework established to guide therapy is obviously different from that proposed by cycles training. Metaphon therapy is based on metalinguistic awareness. **Metalinguistic awareness** is the ability to think about and reflect on the nature of language and the way it functions. Specifically, metaphon therapy is structured to develop children's metaphonological skills. *Metaphonology* is defined as the ability to pay attention to and reflect on the phonological structure of language (Howell & Dean, 1991, 1994).

Is there evidence that supports the notion that children with phonological disorders have problems with metaphonological skills? Using different metaphonological tasks, several investigations have demonstrated that children with phonological disorders generally do not perform as well as normally developing children of a similar age (e.g., Bird & Bishop, 1992; Gillon, 2005; Hesketh, Dima, & Nelson, 2007; Magnusson, 1991).

Metaphon therapy also assumes that phonologically disordered children fail to realize the communicative significance of the phonological rule system. Their difficulties do not pertain to producing speech sounds in a normal manner but to their failure to acquire the rules of the phonological system. Howell and Dean (1991, 1994) postulate that the best way to help these children change their rule systems is to provide them with information that will encourage them to make their own changes and thus impact their speech output. The phases of metaphon therapy are constructed in an attempt to provide this knowledge.

When to Use Metaphon Therapy. Which children can benefit the most from metaphon therapy? Howell and Dean (1991, 1994) target preschool children because it is at this age that metaphonological knowledge is developing. In the existing case studies cited by Howell and Dean (1994), several common features can be noted: Most of the children presented had very restricted phonetic inventories; all the children had unusual or idiosyncratic processes, such as initial consonant deletion; and all the children had a wide variety of phonological processes operating in their speech. These results might indicate that metaphon therapy would be a good match for children who have moderate to severe phonological disorders and who have at least two or three processes that predominate their speech patterns.

Does metaphon therapy work? Both the first and second editions of Howell and Dean's book (1991, 1994) provide the results of an efficacy study that evaluated several aspects of metaphon therapy. Originally, 13 children participated in the study; in the second edition, the number of subjects increased to 50. Preliminary results indicate that metaphon therapy does indeed work. First, they indicate a reduction in the use of specific phonological processes pre- and post-treatment. Second, changes in the phonological system were accelerated beyond the expected level according to chronological development. Because the children in this study were not divided into treatment versus no-treatment groups, two different measures of language were used to verify whether treatment, not development, was actually responsible for the changes. Pre- and post-treatment scores for phonological processes were compared to those obtained from a second nontreated language area that was measured by the British Picture Vocabulary Scale (Dunn, Dunn,

Whetton, & Pintilie, 1982). Although significant differences could be verified with pre- and post-treatment phonological process scores, the scores from the British Picture Vocabulary Scale remained the same, verifying that treatment, not development, had caused the noted changes. Third, some subjects demonstrated a reduction in the targeted phonological processes, but for others the change generalized, causing a reduction in processes that were unrelated to those specifically targeted in treatment. Based on these results, metaphon therapy appears to be a viable therapeutic option, but more controlled studies are needed.

How to Select Target Sounds for Metaphon Therapy. Howell and Dean (1991, 1994) use the *Metaphon Resource Pack* (Dean et al., 1990) as the basis for their assessment procedure. Seventy words (44 monosyllabic and 26 multisyllabic) are elicited and 13 different phonological processes are identified.

Howell and Dean (1991, 1994) provide the following general considerations that influence the choice among the processes to be treated:

1. Those selected should not be the same as the ones that are seen in normally developing children of the same age.
2. Variable use of a simplifying process, which might be evidence of spontaneous development in the child's phonological system, should be given priority in the selection process.
3. The effect the phonological process has on the intelligibility of the child is important. Processes that cause an increased loss of intelligibility, such as stopping of fricatives or atypical processes, should be given priority.
4. The sounds available to the child, both spontaneously and on an imitative basis, play a role in the selection process; sounds that are not in the inventory but can be imitated are usually given priority.

An example is a child, age 4;4, who demonstrates the following processes with an occurrence of more than 50%:

Velar fronting	Word-initial and -final positions
Stopping of fricatives	All positions
Stopping of affricates	All positions
Initial consonant deletion	Limited to fricatives
Initial consonant cluster reduction/deletion	All contexts
Phonetic inventory	[m, n, ŋ]
	[p, b, t, d, k, g]
	[w, j]
	[l]

Based on the child's age, the velar fronting, stopping of fricatives, and initial fricative deletion were all potential target processes. Consonant cluster reduction could be seen as a consequence of the child's lack of fricatives and of the limited phonetic inventory. Velar fronting was chosen as the first target because the child showed evidence of suppression of this process in some contexts. Initial fricative deletion was selected as the second target because the introduction of fricatives might generalize, eliminating the stopping of fricatives as well.

How Is Metaphon Therapy Used? This therapy has two phases. Phase 1 is designed to develop an awareness of the properties of sounds. This is accomplished in a motivating setting where success is facilitated. Phase 1 is the most important phase because it forms the basis for the application to more realistic communicative settings emphasized in Phase 2.

Phase 1 Therapy: Developing Phonological Awareness. The primary aim of Phase 1 is to capture the child's interest in sounds and the entire sound system. Although this is a natural activity of normally develop-ing preschoolers, Howell and Dean (1991, 1994) believe that such awareness has not been possible for a child with a phonological disorder. The child and the clinician explore the properties of sounds together, how sounds differ from each other (i.e., place, manner, and voicing distinctions), and the importance of realizing these distinctions.

> ### CLINICAL EXERCISES
>
> Refer to the child who was described on page 326 and whose velar fronting was targeted. Can you identify some concrete ideas of how you could develop phonological awareness of the differences in these sounds (front–back) at the concept and sound levels? Remember, the child is 4;4.

Phase 1 therapy is divided into four levels: concept level, sound level, phoneme level, and word level. Although the emphasis is somewhat different depending on whether the target selection is a substitution or a syllable structure process, every client moves through each of the levels with each process. Throughout Phase 1, the child remains a listener only.

Therapy for Substitution Processes

1. *Concept level.* During the discussion and exploration of sounds with a child, it is essential that there be a shared understanding of the vocabulary and concepts used. At the concept level, the child and the clinician play games that involve this vocabu-lary when talking about different classes of sounds. At this level, individual speech sounds are not contrasted; rather, some of their characteristics—such as long versus short, front versus back, and noisy versus whisper—are considered. The child plays games such as matching long and short socks, ribbons, or strings; putting bricks at the front or back of the house; and growling noisily and in a whisper. These activities are used to identify the respective characteristics as preparation for later place-man-ner-voicing comparisons of actual speech sounds. At this level, 100% success should be achieved. Therapy at this level may be brief, depending on the child's success.

2. *Sound level.* In this phase, the previous achievements are transferred to the description of sounds in general. Games might involve musical instruments, noisemaking rattles, shakers, and vocalizations made by the therapist and child, such as lions "roaring," (supporting the "noisy" concept), people "singing," (supporting the "noisy", voicing concept) and girls "whispering." (supporting the "whisper", voiceless concept), The aim is to show that all sounds can be classified according to the dimensions specified in the concept level, that is, long–short, front–back, and noisy–whisper.

3. *Phoneme level.* After having achieved success at the first two levels, the child is now ready to move on to activities involving speech sounds. The child and clinician take turns producing a range of sounds that varies along the three dimensions previously indicated. Individual sounds are not yet the focus; rather, all sounds from one class are contrasted with sounds from another (e.g., different stops are con-trasted with various fricatives). The respective speech sounds may be produced spontaneously or in response to a visual referent (a card with a mnemonic of the property in question). At this level, speech sound activities can also be paired with those introduced at the con-cept level—for example, first the matching of long and short strings and then the identification of long and short sounds.

> Watch the following video of a short demonstration of metaphon therapy using the examples of long versus short. Can you think of ways you could construct something for noisy (voiced) versus whispered (voiceless) sounds? youtube .com/watch?v=r7j4fKTlmWg

4. *Word level.* After the phoneme level, minimal pairs of words contain-ing the targeted contrast are introduced. A child is asked to make a

judgment about whether the sound is, for example, long or short, front or back, or noisy or whispered. Although the child is only a listener at this level, some discussion about the sound properties are included. For example, a noisy (voiced) sound is identified and then knowledge of other "noisy" sounds is questioned. Later, other minimal pair words can be introduced. In addition, visual referents used in previous levels can be placed on the back of the card to provide additional feedback about the target item.

Therapy for Syllable Structure Processes

1. *Concept level.* For syllable structure processes, such as initial or final consonant deletion, other concepts are introduced, such as "beginning" and "end." These concepts could be exemplified by the engine at the beginning of a train and the caboose at the end or the nose of the alligator at the beginning and the tail at the end. If cluster simplification is the target, suitable contrasts could consist of the concepts of one horse in front of the wagon, two engines pulling the train, or three dogs pulling the sled.

2. *Syllable level/Word level.* At this stage, syllables representing the targeted contrast are used. For initial consonant deletion, for example, V and CV structures with nonsense syllables could be introduced with the analogy of a train with no engine versus one with an engine. Because therapy may not be motivating if the clinician stays with nonsense syllables, some words might be selected as well.

Phase 2 Therapy: Developing Phonological and Communicative Awareness. The link between Phases 1 and 2 is established by incorporating Phase 1 activities into Phase 2. Phonological awareness needs to be well developed before Phase 2 can be successful. Both Phase 1 and Phase 2 activities are essential for the core activity.

The core activity is structured so that the clinician and the child take turns in producing minimal pair words. If the child says the word pictured on the card accurately, the clinician provides positive feedback and this feedback is expanded into a relevant discussion. For example: "Right, that was a noisy sound. I bet you know lots of other noisy sounds." If, however, the child produces one of the minimal pair words incorrectly, intending the other word, the clinician picks the word that was said, not the intended one. This might stimulate the child to produce a spontaneous repair. The clinician never comments directly on the child's inappropriate production of a particular word but draws the child's attention to the salient features of the contrast: "That was a noisy sound. Should it have been a whisper sound?" Phase 1 activities can be used prior to or after the core activity.

There are no instructions regarding a child who repeatedly does not produce the sound or sound pattern in question correctly. The assumption is that the child goes back to Phase 1 activities. Therefore, for children who are not stimulable for a particular sound and remain unstimulable throughout Phase 1, Phase 2 could prove to be frustrating. In a later portion of the text, Howell and Dean suggest that based on the child's increased metalinguistic awareness, a discussion of the reasons for the loss of contrast should be explored. "Referring to sounds in a way which allows children to discuss them allows specific exploration of the reasons why a child has failed to convey meaning" (Howell & Dean, 1994, p. 110).

The last phase moves the minimal word pairs into sentences such as "Put the picture of the pea/key in the box," and "Draw a picture of the pea/key on the board." Situations that facilitate communication and promote repairing communicative breakdowns are important variables. It is stressed that a supportive environment is an essential ingredient of this therapy.

The following is a short video of Phase 2, metaphon therapy. Again, try to think of ways you could use this format to represent noisy versus whispered and front versus back contrasts. youtube.com/watch?v=DwlprCqdPkA

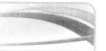

Speech Sound Disorders with Concurrent Language Problems: Therapeutic Suggestions

Speech sound disorders often co-occur with language disorders. Based on a variety of studies, the estimated co-occurrence rate was 35–60% (e.g., Botting and Conti-Ramsden, 2004; Shriberg, 2004). Thus, many children seen clinically for a speech sound disorder also demonstrate other language problems.

In an attempt to deal with this co-occurrence of language and speech sound disorders, several approaches have attempted to link speech sound intervention to other language components. For example, Hoffman and Norris (2010) have supported a whole language approach in which phonological development is targeted at the same time as development of discourse structure, semantic, morphosyntactic and letter-sound knowledge. In addition, the morphosyntax intervention approach (Haskill, Tyler, & Tolbert, 2001; Tyler & Haskill, 2011) focuses on structures that interface with phonology and are significant for language development. This approach targets as many as four grammatical morphemes in a cycle for approximately a week. This cycle can be repeated or alternated with direct speech intervention every other cycle. Singleton or final consonant clusters can be targeted in past tense (row<u>ed</u>, wal<u>ked</u>), third person singular (he go<u>es</u>, she dri<u>nks</u>), or in a copula sentence (He <u>is a</u>way, He <u>is m</u>ad). Specific studies have suggested that participants made significant gains in speech and morphosyntax (Tyler, Lewis, Haskill, & Tolbert, 2002, 2003). Although more research is needed on the interaction of phonology with other language areas, it is currently safe to say that (1) many children with phonemic-based disorders also demonstrate language difficulties and (2) intervention needs to target both phonology and any additional deficient language areas. To achieve this, a specified amount of time could be allotted to each deficient area: phonology, morphosyntax, semantics, or pragmatics. It would, of course, be more time efficient if some language therapy goals could be unified. The following section on "Connecting Phonology to Morphosyntax: Morphosyntax Intervention" offers some suggestions on how specific phonological remediation goals could be combined with noted morphosyntactic problems.

Connecting Phonology to Morphosyntax: Morphosyntax Intervention

Various morphological problems in children with specific language impairment (SLI) have often been observed (e.g., Bishop, 1994; Eyer & Leonard, 1994; Leonard, 1994; Leonard, McGregor, & Allen, 1992; Oetting & Horohov, 1997; Oetting & Rice, 1993; Rice & Oetting, 1993; Rice, Wexler, & Cleave, 1995). Based on findings of several of these investigations, Leonard and colleagues (1992) summarized the grammatical morphemes that were used less frequently by children with SLI: among others, these grammatical morphemes include plurals, regular and irregular past tense, possessives, third person singular, and copula/auxiliary sentence forms.

Based on production difficulties, it becomes clear that speech sound disordered children might have problems actually producing some of these grammatical morphemes. Plurality, past tense -ed, possessive, and third-person singular, for example, very often result in word-final consonant clusters. If a child deletes final consonants or reduces consonant clusters, the grammatical function of these morphemes will be lost. Even for a child displaying primarily substitution processes, these morphemes might not be realized accurately. In order to preserve morphemic contrasts, attention must be given to final consonants and consonant clusters when working with a child with a speech sound disorder.

Remediation Suggestions

1. If a therapy goal is the elimination of final-consonant deletion, words that incorporate specific grammatical morphemes in contrasting word pairs could be targeted. The use of such pairs depends on the sounds in the client's inventory and

the targeted sound(s), but could include, whenever possible, aspects of morphology, especially grammatical morphemes. The following are given as examples of words/ phrases incorporating grammatical morphemes which end in VC structures:

Grammatical Morpheme	Examples
Plurality	toe-toes, key-keys, shoe-shoes
Possessive	Joe-Joe's, Ray-Ray's
Regular past tense	row-rowed, lay-laid, show-showed
Third-person singular	I go–he goes, I do–he does

2. If a therapy goal pertains to reducing consonant cluster reduction or deletion, contrastive word pairs such as these incorporate grammatical morphemes in a word-final VCC structure:

Grammatical Morpheme	Examples
Plurality	boat-boats, cup-cups, wheel-wheels
Possessive	cat-cat's, Dad-Dad's, dog-dog's
Regular past tense	walk-walked, kiss-kissed
Third-person singular	I walk–he walks, I sip–he sips
Irregular past tense	drink-drank, hold-held

3. In sentences, minimal pair words could be used systematically to represent other grammatical morphemes:

Grammatical Morpheme	Examples
Copula	She is sad versus She is mad
	He is tall versus He is small
Auxiliary	He is shopping versus
	He is hopping
	She is kissing versus
	She is hissing

4. Subject and object pronouns could also be used in sentences:

	Examples
Subject pronouns	She is here versus He is here
	She opened the door versus
	Lee opened the door
	She has the tea versus She has the key
	He helped the man versus
	We helped the man
Object pronouns	Give it to Jim versus Give it to him
	The tea belongs to her versus
	The key belongs to her

5. Length and complexity of the utterance also need to be considered because syntactical complexity affects productional accuracy. The more complex the syntax is, the more likely a child is to demonstrate a breakdown in articulatory accuracy. Although one therapeutic goal could be to increase the length and complexity of a

child's utterances, this should always be evaluated with respect to the interaction between production accuracy and syntactic complexity.

Connecting Phonology to Semantics: Vocabulary Intervention

The majority of research on the semantic limitations of children with language impairments has focused on their use of nouns (Leonard, 1988; Rice, 1991). Such studies have found that language-impaired children are slow in using their first words, and subsequent vocabulary development occurs at a slower rate than in normally developing children. Other literature has examined the use of verbs in language-impaired children (Conti-Ramsden & Jones, 1997; King & Fletcher, 1993; Paul, 1993; Rice, 1994; Rice & Bode, 1993; Rice et al., 1995; Watkins, Rice, & Moltz, 1993). These studies suggest that verbs and verb-related grammatical properties can be a particular problem for children with language impairments.

Lizbeth, age 4;0, has a /t/ for /k/ substitution. She is also delayed in language and has difficulty with subject-object pronouns. Can you suggest five sentences in which you could target /k/ versus /t/ and work on subject pronouns (he, she, it) and object pronouns (him, her)?

Marcus, age 5;11, is working on [s] and [z]. He also deletes the "s" ending of third-person singular forms (He walks, She thinks). Create eight sentences, four that work with [z] in word-final position as a singleton (for example "He goes") and four that are in word-final position as clusters with [s] or [z] that address third-person singular forms (for example "She hops").

Remediation Suggestions

1. Although minimal pair words typically incorporate nouns ("things" are easier to picture), various verbs could also be targeted. These could be selected in accordance with the child's targeted sound or process. Some examples follow:

Velar Fronting	[t/k] Substitution
taught-caught, knot-knock, bait-bake	
Stopping of fricatives	[t/s]
tell-sell, , tip-sip, talk-sock	
Final consonant deletion	
pay-paid, , say-sail, show-shown	
Initial consonant deletion	
eat-beat, aid-made, earn-burn	

2. When targeted sounds emerge in the child's speech, expand vocabulary with new words containing the target. Children appear to learn more new words easier and quicker that begin with consonants that they have used previously in other words. Therefore, if a targeted sound is emerging in the child's speech, the clinician could try to use new practice words that also expand the child's vocabulary.

The Child with an Emerging Phonological System: Therapeutic Suggestions

As previously noted, the term *emerging phonological system* refers to a time period when sounds are beginning to be used to form conventional words—in other words, the emergence of expressive language. At approximately age 2, normally developing toddlers begin to combine single words into two-word utterances. However, this communicative development seems to lag behind in some 2-year-olds. Children whose comprehension abilities are considered normal but who fail to achieve a 50-word vocabulary and 2-word combinations by age 2 are referred to as "late talkers," toddlers with "slow expressive language development or delay" (Paul & Jennings, 1992; Reed, 1994; Rescorla & Schwartz, 1990), or as children with "specific expressive language impairment" (Rescorla & Ratner, 1996). It has been estimated that approximately 10–15% percent of the total 2-year-old population meets these criteria (Rescorla, 1989). Half of them seem to outgrow this delay; the other half continues to demonstrate language problems at age 3 and beyond.

When children with slow expressive language development are compared to norm children of similar ages, their vocalizations occur less often. In addition, the phonetic profiles of these children show a reduced repertoire of consonants and syllable shapes. Inventory constraints are especially notable in word-final positions (Paul & Jennings, 1992; Rescorla & Ratner, 1996).

To evaluate a child's emerging phonological system, an independent analysis was suggestedin Chapter 6. Such an analysis examines the child's productions of individual sounds, however, the sound productions are not compared to the adult model. At this point in the child's development, it is far more important to note her or his actual usage of specific sounds in words. To this end, two types of data need to be collected: (1) the inventory of speech sounds and (2) the syllable shapes used.

General remediation strategies for children with slowly emerging language development include developing expressive language skills; specifically expanding the number of vocabulary items, the consonant inventory, and syllable shapes; and finally the use of two-word utterances (Paul, 2007). At this stage of a child's development, therapy must represent a unified package. Therapy to promote phonological skills needs to be combined with increasing the child's lexicon. The use of specific syllable shapes is also a consideration when selecting which words to target. Remediation for the child with an emerging language system must account for the interdependencies that exist among all language areas.

The following suggestions provide some points to consider when choosing the first words for children with small expressive vocabularies. The consonant inventory and the syllable shapes the child uses are especially important variables in this selection process.

Combining Phonology with Semantics: Developing a Lexicon

1. First, children's consonant inventory needs to be considered. Early vocabularies are influenced by the phonological composition of the word. Words that are easier for children to produce are more likely to be included in their early vocabularies. In addition, children appear to learn more easily and quickly new words that begin with consonants that they have used previously in other words. Therefore, new words that contain sounds already in a child's inventory should be targeted.

   An example: The child's inventory contains the following sounds:

   [m, n]

   [p, b, t, d]

   [h, j]

   Depending on the child's present lexicon, the following might be good word choices:

   me, no-no

   puppy, baby, bye-bye, teddy, toe

   happy, yeah

2. The child's present use of syllable shapes needs to be considered. Early syllable shapes include V, CV, CVCV, and CVC. The therapist selects words with syllable shapes the child already uses, possibly including other early syllable shapes. In doing so, it should be kept in mind that the therapy goal is to *expand* the child's use of syllable shapes; therefore, early syllable shapes not in the child's repertoire should also be stimulated.

   An example: If the child primarily realizes V, CV, and CVCV syllable shapes:

   mama might be easier than *mom*

   papa might be easier than *dad*

   puppy or *doggie* might be easier than *dog*

   kittie might be easier than *cat*

   baby might be easier than *doll*

3. When expanding a child's consonant inventory, the normal developmental sequence should be the guiding principle. Children with slow emerging language seem to acquire consonants in the same order as normally developing children, only at a slower rate (Paul & Jennings, 1992). Therefore, early sounds that are not yet in the child's inventory should be targeted. For the child with only a few expressive words, Paul (2007) suggests introducing the sound by first using a babbling game activity rather than by putting it directly into words. The clinician begins by imitating the child's vocalizations. Once a reciprocal babbling exchange is established, the clinician introduces the new consonant into the babbling activity. The goal of this activity is not to get the child to produce that particular sound but to increase the consonant inventory. Therefore, any new consonant, even if it is not the one modeled by the clinician, should be rewarded.

4. New words should be similar to those used first by normally developing children. These include, for example, names of important people in the child's environment, names for objects the child directly acts on, labels for objects that move and change, actions, games, and routines in which the child is an active participant (Owens, 2008, Berko Gleason & Bernstein Ratner, 2009). Table 10.3 provides some examples of children's earliest words.

5. After having evaluated the child's inventory and use of syllable structures, words from a wide variety of grammatical classes should be selected. Although nouns dominate young children's early speech, children's vocabularies include words from a variety of grammatical classes from the beginning (Berko Gleason & Bernstein Ratner, 2009). Therefore, not only nouns should be targeted but also words that can be used to talk about the *relations* between objects. These relational words express more communicative functions and can be readily combined with other words into two-word utterances. Refer to Table 10.4 for some of the words that Lahey and Bloom (1977) and Lahey (1988) proposed for a first lexicon. These one- or two-syllable words include both nouns and relational words as well as early syllable shapes.

At this stage in the child's development, articulation patterns very seldom mirror adult pronunciation. However, the therapy focus for these children is on expanding the use of consonants, syllable shapes, and words, not on norm production. Therefore, any word approximations produced by the child should be rewarded, not corrected. For example, if the word is *down* and the child says [da] or [ta], the clinician should reward this word approximation. Even if the child produces the final [n] in another word, that does not mean the child can produce [n] under different coarticulatory conditions in a new word. The goal during this phase of therapy is to stimulate word production, not articulatory "correctness."

CLINICAL EXERCISES

Melody, age 2;2, is just beginning to say first words. She says [mɑmi], [dæ.i] for "daddy," [ta] for "cat," [mi], [nono], [beᵗbi], [dɑ] for "there," and [up] for "oops."

Can you make a list of additional words that you might target using these sounds?

Which sound(s) might you target for stimulation?

TABLE 10.3 Children's Earliest Words: Examples from the Vocabularies of Children Younger Than 20 Months

Sound effects
baa baa, meow, moo, ouch, uh-oh, woof, yum-yum
Food and drink
apple, banana, cookie, cheese, cracker, juice, milk, water
Animals
bear, bird, bunny, cat, cow, dog, duck, fish, kitty, horse, pig, piggy
Body parts and clothing
diaper, ear, eye, foot, hair, hand, hat, mouth, nose, shoe, toe, tooth
House and outdoors
blanket, chair, cup, door, flower, keys, outside, spoon, tree, TV
People
baby, daddy, gramma, grampa, mommy, [child's own name]
Toys and vehicles
ball, balloon, bike, boat, book, bubbles, plane, toy, truck
Actions
down, eat, go, sit, up
Games and routines
bath, bye, hi, night-night, no, peekaboo, please, shhh, thank you, yes
Adjectives and descriptive
allgone, cold, dirty, hot

Source: Berko Gleason, Jean, *The development of language*, 4th Edition, © 1997. Reprinted by permission of Pearson Education, Inc., Upper Saddle River, NJ.

Treatment of Multiple Vowel Errors

An abundance of information about children's difficulties with consonant articulation and their remediation is available. In contrast, vowel problems have not received the same degree of attention. This has been generally justified by the fact that vowels are mastered at an early age in the child's development. Therefore, children with speech sound disorders probably show few vowel errors. However, this assumption stands in contrast to the documented vowel errors that have been noted in many case studies and in the literature (e.g., Ball & Gibbon, 2002; Clark & Goldstein, 1996; Khan, 1988; Pollock & Keiser, 1990; Renfrew, 1966; Reynolds, 1990; Stoel-Gammon & Herrington, 1990).

Although vowels are normally among the earliest sounds acquired, it appears that some speech sound disordered children demonstrate difficulties with regular vowel realizations. Using the Pollock and Keiser (1990) data as an estimate for the frequency of occurrence, 1 of their 15 children with phonemic-based problems (6.7%) had distinct difficulties with vowel productions. This child's speech showed that approximately half of the vowels were in error. Vowel difficulties could well belong to the clinical profile of some children with speech sound disorders.

A review of several studies containing vowel data from children with speech sound disorders seems to indicate that two patterns emerge (Stoel-Gammon & Herrington, 1990). First, there are children with extremely limited vowel inventories. These children's vowel productions seem to resemble those of the babbling period with lax, non-high vowels

TABLE 10.4 Words for a First Lexicon

Content Category	Relational Words		Substantive Words
	Relational words that are not object specific	Relational words that are more specific to objects but still relate to many objects	
Rejection	no		
Nonexistence or disappearance	no, all gone, away		
Cessation of action	stop, no		
Prohibition of action	no		
Recurrence of objects and actions on objects	more, again, another		
Noting the existence of or identifying objects	this, there, that		
Actions on objects		give, do, make, get, throw, eat, wash, kiss	
Actions involved in locating objects or self		put, up, down, sit, fall, go	
Attributes or descriptions of objects		big, hot, dirty, heavy	
Persons associated with objects (as in possession)			person names

Source: © American Speech-Language-Hearing Association. Reprinted by permission.

predominating. A second group demonstrates relatively large vowel inventories but a high incidence of vowel errors—that is, a large number of vowel substitutions. The sequence of vowel acquisition in this group of children appeared to be similar to the one for younger normally developing children. In both groups of children with vowel problems, the vowels represented by the corners of the vowel quadrilateral were mastered earlier.

Very little information on deviant vowel systems is available. Although several authors state that some children with phonological disorders do have deviant vowel systems (e.g., Ball & Gibbon, 2002; Grunwell, 1987; Hodson & Paden, 1991; Lowe, 1994), neither assessment nor remediation procedures are described in these texts. However, Pollock (1991) described an assessment procedure for identifying vowel errors. Klein (1996) appears to be one of the first to describe therapy for vowel problems in some detail. If a child's vowel inventory is severely restricted or if the child's speech contains a high proportion of vowel substitutions, remediation focusing on vowel distinctions should be implemented.

How disordered should a vowel system be to warrant therapy? Three types of diagnostic information for vowel analysis are suggested: (1) the vowel inventory, (2) the accuracy of production, and (3) error patterns. Examination of the vowel inventory can determine whether the child has a limited or near normal inventory. Data on the accuracy of vowel production are important when assessing children with a fairly complete vowel inventory but a high proportion of vowel substitutions. The third diagnostic information, error patterns, is especially valuable when planning therapy. Figure 10.1 is a matrix that can be used to record the child's vowel inventory. The use of this matrix is similar to that of the consonant matrix presented in Chapter 7. Accurate and irregular vowel realizations can be recorded directly on the matrix. This provides the inventory and the number of occurrences of accurate productions. Error patterns can also be identified by comparing the substitutions to the norm productions.

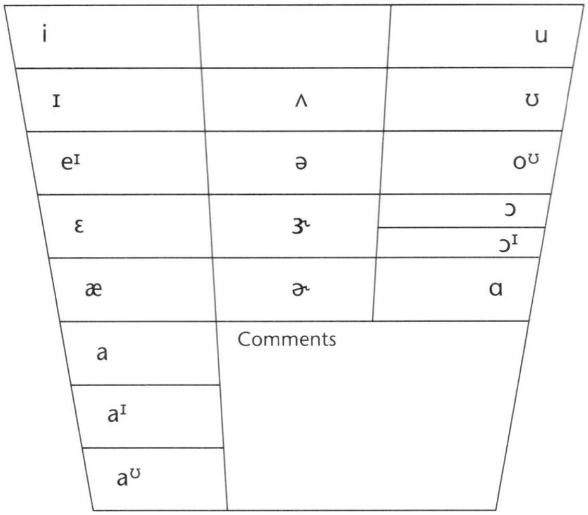

FIGURE 10.1   Vowel Matrix

The Child with a Very Limited Vowel Inventory: Therapeutic Suggestions

According to the rather limited data available, it appears that the vowel system of these children is characterized by only two or three vowels. These vowels are lax and non-high vowels such as [ɑ], [ɛ], [æ], or [ʌ]. Such lax, non-high vowels are typical for the babbling period. Stoel-Gammon and Herrington (1990) group vowel acquisition into three categories:

Group 1	
Vowels that are mastered relatively early	i, ɑ, u, o, ʌ
Group 2	
Vowels acquired somewhere between early and late (some investigations reported early acquisition, others later)	æ, ʊ, ɔ, ə
Group 3	
Vowels that are mastered relatively late	e, ɛ, ɪ, ɝ, ɚ

Using One Known and One Unknown Vowel in Minimal Pairs

1. *The child's vowel inventory needs to be compared to those vowels that are mastered relatively early.* A vowel from Group 1 that is productionally very different from one of the child's vowels is selected. For example, if the child has [ɑ], a lax, low-back vowel, the tense high-front vowel [i] would be a good candidate.

2. *The two vowels should be contrasted in minimal pairs.* Whenever possible, consonants from the child's inventory should be used. Examples follow:

Not in Inventory	In Inventory
me	ma
beet	bought
team	Tom
hee	haw

CLINICAL EXERCISES

Refer to Melody (page 333). Based on her limited vocabulary, what is her vowel inventory?

Are there "early" vowels that she does not have in her inventory? Can you identify four words that you could use in therapy to stimulate these vowels? Make sure that you also consider her consonant inventory.

3. *Other early vowels in minimal contrasts with the original vowel are introduced.* Using the example with [ɑ], another productionally distinct vowel is [u]. Examples are:

Not in Inventory	In Inventory
moo	me, ma
boo	bee
moon	mean
new	knee

Using Two Unknown Vowels in Minimal Pairs

1. *This variation of the complexity approach uses two unknown vowels in minimal pairs.* Two vowels that are not in the child's inventory should be chosen from Group 3 if possible. The vowels should again be as productionally different as possible. If the child's inventory includes [ɑ] and [ʌ], [ɪ] and [ɝ] might be selected. These sounds are placed in minimal pairs. Examples follow:

bit-Burt
bid-bird
ill-Earl
gill-girl

2. *Two different unknown vowels are then targeted.* The selection process should consider the complexity of the vowel and its lack of stimulability.

The Child with a High Proportion of Vowel Substitutions: Therapeutic Suggestions

Children with a high proportion of vowel substitutions usually show a relatively intact vowel inventory. An error pattern analysis can be helpful in selecting the target vowels.

This analysis procedure contrasts the target vowel to the substituted vowel. A list of all vowel substitutions with their relative percentage of occurrence is generated. One possible target could be inconsistent vowel substitutions, i.e., those vowels that are sometimes produced correctly but also have different substitutions. For example, the following are noted for /æ/:

ɛ/æ, frequency of occurrence = 30%

ɪ/æ, frequency of occurrence = 35%

correct production of [æ], frequency of occurrence = 35%

One of the substitutions for [æ] would be selected as the second vowel. In addition, the substitution chosen should be as productionally different as possible from the target. These two vowels would then be used as the vowel nuclei of minimally paired words. Using these criteria, [æ] and [ɪ] would be a good choice. These two vowels are then placed in minimal word pairs. Examples are:

mat-mitt

bag-big

pan-pin

ham-him

A second possibility is to target a vowel that is used as a substitution for several vowels. The following exemplifies this scenario:

Target Vowel	Substitution
i	ɪ
eᴵ	ɑ
ɛ	ɑ
æ	ɑ
ʊ	u

In this case, [ɑ] is used as a substitution for [eᴵ], [ɛ], and [æ]. Therefore, [ɑ] would be contrasted with either [eᴵ], [ɛ], or [æ]. Clear production differences should be given priority when selecting the targeted vowel. Contrasting [ɑ], a lax, low-back vowel to [eᴵ], a diphthong with a mid-high tense onglide, would provide such distinct differences. These two vowels would then be placed in minimal pairs. Examples are:

tall-tail

cop-cape

top-tape

Therapy proceeds from vowels with dissimilar to more similar production features. In this example, [ɑ] and [ɛ] would be the next vowels targeted as the nuclei for minimal pairs.

Using a multiple oppositions approach several different minimal pairs could be contrasted using the three substitutions of [eᴵ], [ɛ], and [æ]. The following words would then be targeted simultaneously : bought – bait – bet – bat.

SUMMARY

This chapter described several intervention approaches for the treatment of children with phonemic-based disorders. Some of these remediation programs use minimal pair contrasts as the beginning unit of remediation—for example, minimal opposition contrasts, maximum oppositions, complexity approaches, multiple oppositions, and therapy designed to reduce the use of phonological processes. Other remediation techniques are unique, such as cycles training and metaphon therapy. These two therapy protocols, which have been developed and refined through actual clinical experience, forge together a combination of methods that can be effectively used to treat speech sound disorders in children.

Discussion of the treatment approaches has been designed to answer specific questions. First, when should this therapy be chosen? Which clients could best be treated with this approach? Guidelines that broadly separate clients who might be better versus poorer candidates for each particular approach were explored. The chapter also discussed selections of beginning targets and clinical applications that exemplify the transition from assessment to intervention. Intervention methods were outlined in some detail to indicate the use of each approach in a therapy setting.

The last part of this chapter explored and suggested some special applications of phonological therapy. Phonological remediation principles with children displaying concurrent language difficulties and those with emerging phonological systems exemplified the merging of phonological intervention strategies with other language areas such as morphology and semantics. Finally, treatment principles for children with disordered vowel systems were presented to demonstrate how minimal pair contrasts can be structured in a remediation program.

This chapter emphasized assessment results and their connection to therapy goals. Whenever possible, the assessment results outlined in Chapter 7 and the therapy procedures in this chapter were directly linked. Several clinical applications were provided to demonstrate the assessment–treatment connection, which is essential for professional speech-language services.

CASE STUDY

The following results are from the *Hodson Assessment of Phonological Patterns* (HAPP-3) (Hodson, 2004) for Andrew, age 5;6.

1. basket	[bætə]	26. shoe	[du]
2. boats	[boᵘ]	27. slide	[jaˈd]
3. candle	[tænə]	28. smoke	[boᵘt]
4. chair	[teˀ]	29. snake	[deˈt]
5. clouds	[jaᵘd]	30. soap	[doᵘp]
6. cowboy hat	[taᵘbo æt]	31. spoon	[pun]
7. feather	[pɛdə]	32. square	[twɛˀ]
8. fish	[pɪd]	33. star	[tɑˀ]
9. flower	[taᵘə]	34. string	[twɪn]
10. fork	[pot]	35. swimming	[twɪmɪn]
11. glasses	[jætət]	36. television	[tɛdəbɪdən]
12. glove	[dʌb]	37. toothbrush	[tubət]
13. gum	[dʌm]	38. truck	[twʌt]
14. hanger	[hændə]	39. vase	[beˈd]
15. horse	[hoˀt]	40. watch	[wɑt]
16. ice cubes	[aˈt jub]	41. yoyo	[jʌjoᵘ]
17. jumping	[dʌmp]	42. zip	[jɪp]
18. leaf	[jif]	43. crayons	[tweˈən]
19. mask	[mæt]	44. black	[bæt]
20. music box	[mu ɪt bɑt]	45. green	[dwin]
21. page	[peˈd]	46. yellow	[jɛjoᵘ]
22. plane	[peˈn]	47. three	[twi]
23. queen	[twin]	48. thumb	[tʌm]
24. rock	[wɑt]	49. nose	[noᵘd]
25. screwdriver	[dwu dwaˈvə]	50. mouth	[maᵘf]

We have decided to use the cycles approach. The following process is used to determine which patterns to target.

1. *Early developing phonological patterns:*
    Syllableness. The child seems to demonstrate evidence of this in words such as *cowboy hat* and *ice cubes.*
    Word-initial singleton consonants. The child uses [m] *mouth,* [n] *nose,* [p] *page,* [b] *boats,* [t] *television,* [d] *snake* (although the pronunciation is incorrect, Andrew did use [d] initially), and [w] *watch.*
    Word-final singleton consonants. Andrew uses [p] *soap,* [t] *truck* (he substitutes [t] for [k], but [t] is in word-final position), [m] *thumb,* and [n] *spoon.* No [k] is found in the word-final position.
    Other word structures. Andrew can produce CVC structures (e.g., *mouth*) and CVCV structures (e.g., *yoyo, feather*).
2. *Posterior/anterior contrasts.* Although alveolar sounds are present, velar sounds are absent in Andrew's speech.
3. *[s] clusters.* Andrew does not seem to be able to produce [s] as a singleton nor in clusters.
4. *Liquids.* Andrew does not demonstrate that he can produce the liquids [l] and [r].
    Patterns targeted: Based on stimulability, the following patterns could be targeted.

1. *Anterior–posterior contrasts.* Andrew has [t]; therefore, the velar [k] would be a target for the first cycle.
2. *[s] clusters.* Hodson and Paden (1991) recommend that word-final [s] clusters be targeted. The clinician should determine which one(s) might be stimulable.
3. *Liquids.* Andrew does not produce any liquids. Stimulability should be probed on both [l] and [r]. One or both of these could be used in the first cycle.

THINK CRITICALLY

1. Based on the earlier case study from Andrew, age 5;6, we note that the following consonants are not in his inventory: [k], [g], [s], [z], [ʃ], [z], [θ], [ð], [ŋ], [l], and [r]. If you were going to use maximal oppositions, which two sounds would you target? First, find the sounds that have major class feature differences. Second, find the two sounds that have the most distinctive feature differences.
2. Based on the earlier case study from Andrew, age 5;6, note the collapse of phonemic contrasts. For example, the consonants [k], [s], [f] (one time in *flowers*), [ʃ], [tʃ], and [θ] are all collapsed to [t]. What other neutralization of phonemic contrasts can be noted in Andrew's articulation test results? Use this information to establish treatment targets with the multiple oppositions approach.

TEST YOURSELF

1. Intervention using phonemic-based approaches begins
   a. by teaching sounds in isolation
   b. by teaching sounds in syllables
   c. at the word level using any type of one-syllable words
   d. at the word level using minimal pairs

2. Which one of the following pairs would be considered near minimal pairs?
   a. *bird-bad*
   b. *look-lake*
   c. *bird-sir*
   d. *rip-ship*

3. If meaningful minimal pairs cannot be found for contrastive phonemes, what should be used as the alternative?
   a. oral motor exercises
   b. near-minimal pairs
   c. a new set of contrastive phonemes
   d. cycles training

4. Cycles therapy was designed for a specific group of clients—those with
   a. highly unintelligible speech
   b. mild to moderate speech disorders
   c. articulation-based errors
   d. [s] and [r] problems

5. In the cycles approach, each phoneme in a pattern is targeted
   a. for four sessions
   b. for 30 minutes
   c. for 60 minutes
   d. until 50% accuracy is achieved

6. The ability to think about and reflect on the nature of language and how it functions refers to
   a. cognition
   b. intelligence
   c. pragmatics
   d. metalinguistic awareness

7. Which of the following therapy approaches uses metalinguistic awareness?
   a. cycles training
   b. metaphon therapy
   c. maximal oppositions
   d. multiple oppositions

8. Of the following therapy approaches, which contrasts two very different phonemes, neither of which is in the child's inventory?
   a. cycles training
   b. metaphon therapy
   c. maximal oppositions
   d. multiple oppositions

9. Which of the following therapy approaches attempts to mirror the normal developmental process of a child's phonological system?
   a. cycles training
   b. metaphon therapy
   c. maximal oppositions
   d. multiple oppositions

10. If you are working at the word level on [s], which of the following would represent combining work on phonology and morphology?
    a. working on third-person singular forms
    b. working on expanding sentence structures
    c. working on new vocabulary words with [s] in the final position
    d. working on subject versus object pronouns *she* and *her*

FURTHER READINGS

Ball, M. J, & Gibbon, F. (Eds.) (2012) *Handbook of vowels and vowel disorders*. New York: Taylor & Francis.

Hodson, B., & Paden, E. (1991). *Targeting intelligible speech: A phonological approach to remediation*. San Diego, CA: College-Hill Press.

Howell, J., & Dean, E. (1998). *Treating phonological disorders in children: Metaphon—theory to practice* (2nd ed.). London: Whurr.

McLeod, S. & Baker, E. (2015). *Children's speech: An evidence-based approach to assessment and intervention*. Boston, MA: Pearson.

Williams, A. L., McLeod, S., & McCauley, R. J. (2011). *Interventions for speech sound disorders in children*. Baltimore: Paul H. Brooke.

APPENDIX 10.1   Examples for Constructing Minimal Pairs Using Phonological Processes

Substitution Processes	
Underlying principle	Construct word pairs with the target sound and the substitution. If the target sound is not stimulable, a traditional approach might be necessary to achieve correct production of the sound in a specific word context.
Velar fronting	For t/k and d/g substitutions, find word pairs contrasting /t/ and /k/ and /d/ and /g/. Examples: *tea* versus *key, tape* versus *cape. Dumb* versus *gum, dull* versus *gull.*
Palatal fronting	For s/ʃ substitution, find word pairs contrasting /s/ and /ʃ/. Examples: *sip* versus *ship, sell* versus *shell.*
Stopping of /s/ and /z/	For t/s and d/z substitutions, find word pairs contrasting /t/ and /s/ and /d/ and /z/. Examples: *toe* versus *sew, tee* versus *sea. D* versus *Z, do* versus *zoo.*
Gliding /r/ → /w/	For w/r substitution, find word pairs contrasting /w/ and /r/. Examples: *wed* versus *red, weed* versus *read.*

Unusual Processes	
Stops replacing glides /j/ → /d/	For d/j substitution, find word pairs contrasting /d/ and /j/. Examples: *yacht* versus *dot, yarn* versus *darn.*
Denasalization of /n/ → /d/	For d/n substitution, find word pairs contrasting /n/ and /d/. Examples: *knot* versus *dot, near* versus *deer.*

Processes Affecting Groups or Classes of Phonemes	
Underlying principle	Select contrast pairs containing sounds that the child can produce or are stimulable.
Final consonant deletion	Start with word pairs with and without final consonants, such as *bow* versus *boat.* If generalization does not occur, present word pairs contrasting another final consonant against no final consonant. Example: Child can produce [m, n, t, d, l, f, v, p, b] but not in word-final position. First, present contrasts such as *toe* versus *toad, low* versus *load.*
Consonant cluster reduction	Use singletons in the child's inventory to structure reduced consonant clusters contrasted to standard consonant clusters. Example: Cluster reductions are noted on several consonant blends. Child can produce [b], [p], [k], and [l] but says [kaʊn] for *clown,* [peⁱ] for *play,* [bu] for *blue.* Begin with [pl] and contrast word pairs such as *plan* versus *pan, peas* versus *please.*
Stopping of fricatives	Select a stimulable fricative, which is then contrasted with the homorganic stop. Example: Child is stimulable for [f] but uses p/f substitution in most contexts. Use word pairs such as *fig* versus *pig, fin* versus *pin.*

Unusual Processes	
Initial consonant deletion	Start with word pairs contrasting one initial consonant versus no initial consonant. If generalization does not occur, present word pairs with another initial consonant. Example: Child can produce [p, b, t, d, h, w, m, n] but inconsistently deletes these sounds at the beginning of a word. Use word pairs such as *beet* versus *eat, bee* versus *E.*
Sound preference substitutions	Select a stimulable sound and use it in a contrasting word pair with the sound preference. Child produces [s], [z], [ʃ], [tʃ], and [dʒ] as [t]. The child is stimulable for [ʃ]. Contrast word pairs such as *two* versus *shoe, top* versus *shop.*

Speech Sound Disorders in Selected Populations

LEARNING OBJECTIVES

When you have finished this chapter, you should be able to:

- Understand the definitions and general characteristics of childhood apraxia of speech, cerebral palsy, children with cleft palates, intellectual disabilities, hearing loss, acquired apraxia of speech in adults, and adults with dysarthrias.
- Describe the speech sound characteristics of the previously mentioned disorders.

- Identify the specific tasks that can be used to assess the speech sound disorders of previously identified populations.
- Explain specific speech sound treatment goals for each of the given disorders.
- Access general and specific materials for assessing and treating the mentioned disorders.

THIS CHAPTER provides an overview of the speech characteristics of selected populations in which speech sound problems are among their primary difficulties. Many comprehensive books have been written on each of these disorders. Therefore, the following synopsis represents only selected aspects of the main characteristics and the diagnostic-treatment principles for each of these relative to their speech sound disorder. Each individual discussion is organized into four sections: (1) definition and general features, (2) speech sound characteristics, (3) clinical diagnostics, and (4) therapeutic implications.

This chapter is not organized to reflect all the disorders that speech-language specialists assess and treat in clinical practice. It is also not within the scope of this book to examine all the techniques that are available when working with individuals who have these disorders. Instead, it is an overview of the disorders, assessment possibilities, and treatment options that are directly related to the individual's speech sound difficulties.

Childhood Apraxia of Speech: A Disorder of Speech Motor Control

Definition and General Features

The term *developmental articulatory dyspraxia* was first used by Morley, Court, and Miller (1954) to describe a small subset of children with speech sound disorders that seemed to be very different from those of other children with speech problems.

These children have subsequently been categorized as having developmental apraxia of speech, congenital articulatory apraxia, and developmental verbal apraxia, to mention a few labels. Currently, the preferred term is *childhood apraxia of speech (CAS)* as opposed to other terms such as developmental apraxia of speech or developmental verbal dyspraxia (American Speech-Language-Hearing Association, 2007a). The preferred use of *childhood apraxia of speech* distinguishes this disorder from merely a "developmental" disorder that the child under normal circumstances could outgrow.

After surveying the literature, The Ad Hoc Committee on Childhood Apraxia of Speech (American Speech-Language-Hearing Association, 2007b) found that childhood apraxia of speech occurs in children in three clinical contexts: known neurological etiologies (e.g., intrauterine stroke, infections, trauma), as a result of complex neurobehavioral disorders (e.g., genetic, metabolic), and as an idiopathic neurogenic disorder with no known neurological or complex behavioral disorders. To paraphrase the Ad Hoc Committee on Childhood Apraxia of Speech (American Speech-Language-Hearing Association, 2007b) definition, it could be stated that childhood apraxia of speech (CAS) is a neurological childhood (pediatric) speech sound disorder in which the precision and consistency of movements underlying speech are impaired in the absence of neuromuscular deficits (e.g., abnormal reflexes, abnormal tone). The main difficulty appears to be the planning and/or programming of spatiotemporal parameters of movement sequences that results in errors in speech sound production and prosody. The term *childhood apraxia of speech* implies a shared core of features (both speech and prosodic) regardless of the time of onset and whether it is congenital or acquired or has a specific etiology. Definitions of childhood apraxia of speech have universally described it as being based on a neurological deficit (as the American Speech-Language-Hearing Association, 2007b, definition indicates); there is also clear agreement that whatever neuroanatomical sites/circuits are involved, they are clearly different than those underlying the dysarthrias.

An exact delineation of symptoms of childhood apraxia of speech is problematic. Early reports delineating the symptoms were based on acquired apraxia of speech in adults. Similarities and differences between the specific articulatory problems noted in adults with acquired apraxia of speech and children with so-called developmental apraxia of speech were compared. The most important similarity between these two groups of clients pertains to the lack of sequential volitional control of the oral mechanism. However, initial studies could never verify a neurological basis for comparable speech symptoms in children with developmental apraxia of speech. Although verifiable neurological impairment can cause childhood apraxia of speech, by far the most children who are diagnosed are in the group of children with no known neurological or behavioral disorders.

There remains a clinical necessity to delineate the speech characteristics of CAS children from those evidenced by children with developmental speech sound disorders. Both groups of children have certain characteristics in common: The onset is early in the developmental period, and the course is long term, often extending into adulthood (Shriberg, Aram, & Kwiatkowski, 1997a). Review of the research literature indicates that, at present, there is no validated list of diagnostic features of CAS that differentiates this symptom complex from other types of childhood speech sound disorders, including those primarily caused by phonological delay or neuromuscular disorder (dysarthria) (American Speech-Language-Hearing Association, 2007b). Its estimated prevalence of occurrence is approximately 1 to 2 children per 1,000 or 0.1–0.2% (Shriberg et al.). However, in a study by Delaney and Kent (2004), the prevalence noted for 12,000–15,000 children was much higher, or between 3.4–4.3%. See Box 11.1 for additional information on the demographics of childhood apraxia of speech.

> **BOX 11.1**   Childhood Apraxia of Speech: Demographics
>
> • More than 80% of children with CAS have at least one family member with reported speech and/or language disorders (Velleman, 2003).
>
> • CAS demonstrates higher rates of family history than other speech sound disorders, which suggests a genetic basis in at least some cases (Lewis et al., 2003).
>
> • Up to 3% to 4% of children with speech delay are given the diagnosis of CAS (Delaney & Kent, 2004).
>
> • CAS symptoms are common among children with Down syndrome (Kumin & Adams, 2000).
>
> • Approximately 60% of children with autism spectrum disorder have speech problems; about 13% report primarily symptoms of apraxia of speech (Marili, Andrianopoulos, Velleman, & Foreman, 2004).

Articulatory/Phonological Characteristics

Several studies have reported speech characteristics of children with suspected CAS. However, some of these reports refer to case studies describing only one or two children. Other investigations cannot be compared because uniform criteria were not used when selecting the subjects. Therefore, when interpreting the data of these reports, it should be remembered that methodological differences exist between the studies. With this in mind, the following speech characteristics are offered for children with CAS (American Speech-Language-Hearing Association, 2007a, 2007b; Hall, Jordan, & Robin, 1993).

According to the American Speech-Language-Hearing Association's (2007a, 2007b) technical report and position statement, three segmental and suprasegmental features of apraxia of speech in children are consistent and have gained some consensus among investigators:

1. *Inconsistent errors on consonants and vowels in repeated productions of syllables or words.* Therefore, if a child says a specific word or syllable in different contexts, variability of performance is noted. Whereas the child might say [fit] the first time, this could be [pit], [vit], or [fɪt] in a repeated performance.

2. *Lengthened and disrupted coarticulatory transitions between sounds and syllables.* The relatively smooth transitions between speech sounds that are noted in children with normally developing speech sound systems are problematic for children with CAS. These transitions could be slow, broken, or appear difficult to achieve.

3. *Inappropriate prosody, especially in the realization of lexical or phrasal stress.* Both word and sentence stress could be noticeably different. In a series of studies by Shriberg, Aram, and Kwiatkowski (1997a, 1997b, 1997c), inappropriate stress was found to be the only linguistic domain that differentiated CAS children from those with delayed speech development.

The diagnostic challenge is to differentiate childhood apraxia of speech from speech delay, a dysarthria, and a speech sound disorder that might be moderate to severe in nature. The following general areas of behaviors have been studied: nonspeech motor, speech production, speech perception, prosody, language, and metalinguistic/literacy variables. See the following list for each of these areas.

Nonspeech Motor

1. *Impaired nonspeech oral volitional movements.* This behavior includes imitated or elicited postures and sequences such as making the movements of "smile" versus "kiss" (e.g., Shriberg et. al, 1997b).

2. *Groping behavior and silent posturing.* **Groping behavior** is an ongoing series of movements of the articulators in an attempt to find the desired articulatory position. **Silent posturing** refers to the positioning of the articulators for a specific articulation without sound production. Both groping behaviors and silent posturing have been noted in the speech of children with CAS (e.g., Davis, Jakielski, & Marquardt, 1998).

Speech Motor

3. *Difficulty sequencing speech sounds and syllables.* According to Hall and colleagues (1993), sequencing problems are central to this disorder. Difficulty with sequencing seems to increase as the complexity and/or length of the utterance increases (e.g., Davis et al., 1998). Also included in this category are poor performance on the maximum repetition of syllables and slow diadochokinetic rates (e.g., Nijland et al., 2002).

4. *More errors made in the sound classes involving more complex oral gestures.* Consonant clusters, fricatives, and affricates evidence a larger percentage of difficulty (e.g., Davis et al., 1998). These same sound classes are also troublesome for children with developmental phonological disorders.

5. *Unusual errors not typically found in children with speech sound disorders.* These include sound additions, prolongations of vowels and consonants, repetitions of sounds and syllables, and unusual substitutions, such as glottal plosives and bilabial fricatives (e.g., Lewis et al. 2003: McCabe, Rosenthal, & McLeod, 1998).

6. *A large percentage of omission errors.* Several investigators (e.g., Lewis et al., 2003) have found that sound and syllable omissions are the most frequent type of errors noted in children with CAS. This could be related to the complexity of the speech tasks. Polysyllabic words demonstrated more syllable omissions whereas spontaneous speech included more sound omissions.

7. *Difficulty producing and maintaining appropriate voicing.* Children with CAS might voice unvoiced sounds and devoice voiced sounds (e.g., Lewis et al., 2004). These errors have also been verified by acoustic analyses (e.g., Nijland et al., 2002).

8. *Vowel and diphthong errors.* Several studies have identified these errors in children with CAS (e.g., Nijland et al., 2002). Pollock and Hall (1991) specifically describe the vowel errors of five school-age children with CAS. All of these children had difficulty with tense-lax vowel contrasts, and four of the five evidenced diphthong reduction.

Prosodic Characteristics

9. *Variable nasal resonance, pitch, loudness, and stress.* These have been reported in children with CAS. It appears that this group of children has a tendency to use excessive equal stress (Shriberg et al., 1997a, b, c). Their inability to fully contrast stressed versus unstressed syllables gives the impression of inappropriate stress patterns.

10. *Prosodic impairment.* General and more specific difficulties with prosody have often been reported in the speech of children with CAS (e.g., Boutsen & Christman, 2002; Davis et al., 1998).

Speech Perception

11. *Difficulty in discriminating sound sequences in nonsense words.* This was noted by Bridgeman and Snowling (1988) as was poor discrimination of vowels (Maassen, Groenen, & Crul, 2003).

Language Difficulties

12. *Significant language delays.* These have been reported in children with CAS (e.g., Velleman & Strand, 1994). Lewis et al. (2004) reported that language impairments were more significant and persistent in these children. They found that gains in articulation did not eliminate the language deficits; both receptive and expressive language deficits were noted as was a strong family history of language impairment in the families of children with CAS.

Metalinguistic/Literacy Characteristics

13. *Difficulty identifying rhymes and syllables.* Investigators (Marion, Sussman, & Marquardt, 1993; Marquardt, Sussman, Snow, & Jacks, 2002) have found that children with suspected CAS demonstrate problems with rhyming and syllabification. These disorders could be evidence of a more broad-based phonological or linguistic problem as opposed to motor-based difficulties alone (Velleman, 2003).

CLINICAL EXERCISES

Childhood apraxia of speech is marked by an increase in errors on sound classes involving more complex oral gestures. Based on simple to complex oral gestures (for example, number of syllables, presence of consonant clusters) rank order the following words: street, butterfly, big, spreads, fig, caterpillar, no, baseball.

Children with CAS could have difficulty identifying rhymes and syllables. Which area of development do these tasks represent? Based on difficulties with rhyming and syllabification, are there other problems for which these children might be at risk?

Although all of these error patterns have been reported in the speech of children with CAS, not all of them occur in all these children. Inconsistency and variability of errors is probably the most frequent pattern characterizing this disorder. Children with CAS are often highly unintelligible. Another common feature is the lack of progress these children make in spite of a considerable amount of therapy over a long period.

> Watch this video of Jewel who is 4 years 9 months old with childhood apraxia of speech. Note the difficulties that she has with her speech. youtube.com/watch?v=tYmm23EPXjU&list=PL122A3871DE5687FA

Clinical Implications: Diagnostics

Generally, a broad cluster of symptoms is assumed to represent CAS, including speech, nonspeech, and language deficits. However, not all symptoms must be present, nor is there one characteristic or symptom that must be present. In addition, the typically reported symptoms are not exclusive to childhood apraxia of speech. Compounding the problem is the observation that children change over time. Assessment, therefore, must be organized in a way that allows us to look at a wide range of symptoms.

In respect to assessing a child with CAS, the American Speech-Language-Hearing Association technical report (2007b) adopted the position that referrals to other professionals, including neurologists, occupational therapists, and physical therapists, are often appropriate for associated, nonspeech issues. It is the speech-language pathologist, however, who is responsible for making the primary diagnosis of CAS and for designing, implementing, and monitoring the appropriate individualized speech-language treatment program.

The following assessment procedures are recommended for the child who is suspected of demonstrating CAS:

- Hearing screening
- Language testing
- Thorough speech-motor assessment, including diadochokinetic rates

- Articulation test
- Language sample
- Tests to examine the sequencing of sounds and syllables as well as their consistency.

Hearing screening is a portion of every assessment; however, it should be verified that the child with suspected CAS does not have a hearing loss as the basis for the noted articulatory problems. Language testing is also an important dimension of the assessment process. Although some research studies have used the absence of receptive language problems as one of the criteria for inclusion in the group with suspected CAS, others report both expressive and receptive language difficulties co-occurring with CAS (e.g., Lewis et al., 2004). Formal and informal assessment of language should always be used to gain a more complete understanding of the language proficiency of children suspected to have this disorder.

A speech-motor assessment needs to include sequential volitional movements of the oral mechanism for both speech and nonspeech tasks. Oral diadochokinetic rates in nonspeech and speech activities should be evaluated as well (e.g., Love, 2000). Such information helps document the structural and neuromuscular adequacy of the oral peripheral mechanism. Its functional adequacy for nonspeech and speech tasks should be described and compared. See Chapter 6 for diadochokinetic rates (page 157) and for specific structural and functional measures of the oral peripheral mechanism, Appendix 6.1.

An articulation test and language sample can be used to appraise several speech parameters: types of errors, any unusual errors, voicing problems with consonants, vowel and diphthong errors, difficulties with nasality and nasal emission, and prosodic problems. Differences between productions of one-word responses and those requiring increased articulatory length or complexity need to be ascertained. Groping behavior and/or silent posturing are additional areas that require close observation.

Tests and protocols specifically designed to assess children with CAS are available. A study by McCauley & Strand (2008) reviewed several standardized tests of nonverbal oral and speech motor performance in children according to very specific parameters. Tests published between 1990 and 2006 were selected; only 6 of the 22 tests reviewed met their parameters. These six tests are outlined in Table 11.1.

Clinical Implications: Therapeutics

An established set of therapeutic approaches for the treatment of CAS does not exist. This is not surprising when one considers the limited understanding of the cause, nature, and differential diagnostic markers for this disorder. Even after a careful diagnostic evaluation of the appraisal data, only *suspected* CAS can normally be assumed. Based on this assumption, many different remediation approaches have been suggested. The following is a synopsis of the treatment suggested by Hall and colleagues (1993) and the American Speech-Language-Hearing Association technical report (2007b). It is based on the analysis of outcome measures from many different remediation programs as well as their clinical experience.

1. *Intensive services are needed.* Children with suspected CAS require an extraordinarily high amount of intensive therapy on an individual basis. A child, his or her caregivers, and the clinician must be dedicated to this concept. Hall and associates (1993) recommend a summer program in which the children are in residence for 6 weeks, receiving 4 hours of therapy per day, 5 days a week.

2. *Remediation should progress systematically through hierarchies of task difficulty.* Where to begin with remediation and how to progress depend on the assessment data from each individual child. Hall and associates (1993) evaluate the child's strengths and progress in very small, carefully manipulated steps. They analyze what the child can do successfully and proceed from there. Because of the variability of their developmental progress, therapy goals might need to be changed or modified (Bauman-Waengler &

TABLE 11.1 Description of Standardized Tests for Assessing Nonverbal Oral and Speech Motor Performance in Children

Test	Age Range	Oral Structure Assessed	Approximate Percentage of Items Nonverbal / Speech Oral Motor	Provides Screening Measures	Used for a Complete Diagnosis	Aid in Treatment Planning	Assessment of Change over Time
The Apraxia Profile[1]	3;0 to 13;11	No	Nonverbal = 10% Speech = 90%	No	Yes	Yes	No
Kaufman Speech Praxis Test for Children[2]	2;0 to 6;0	No	Nonverbal = <10% Speech = 90%	No	Yes	Yes	No
Oral Speech Mechanism Screening Examination[3]	5;0 to 78	Yes	Nonverbal = 40% Speech = <10% Oral structure = 50%	Yes	No	No	No
Screening Test for Developmental Apraxia of Speech[4]	4;0 to 7;11	No	Nonverbal = 0% Speech = 100%	Yes	No	No	Yes
Verbal Dyspraxia Profile[5]	Not specified in manual but could be used for children and adults	No	Nonverbal = 75% Speech = 25%	No	Yes	Yes	No
Verbal Motor Production Assessment for Children[6]	3;0 to 12;0	Yes	Nonverbal = < 50% Speech = > 50%	No	Yes	Yes	Yes

[1]*The Apraxia Profile,* by L. A. Hickman, 1997, San Antonio, TX: Psychological Corporation.

[2]Kaufman Speech Praxis Test for Children, by N. Kaufman,1995, Detroit, MI: Wayne State University Press.

[3]*Oral Speech Mechanism Screening Examination* (3rd ed.), by K. O. St. Louis & D. Ruscello, 2000, Austin, TX: Pro-Ed.

[4]Screening Test for Developmental Apraxia of Speech (2nd ed.), by R. W. Blakeley, 2001, Austin, TX: Pro-Ed.

[5]*Verbal Dyspraxia Profile*, by J. M. Jelm, 2001, DeKalb, IL: Janelle.

[6]Verbal Motor Production Assessment for Children, by D. Hayden & P. Square, 1999, San Antonio, TX: Psychological Corporation.

Garcia, 2011). Therefore, the consonant inventory, distribution, and syllable shapes provide important information when evaluating where to begin and continue with therapy. Speech sounds that can be successfully articulated are combined into syllable structures already present in the child's speech. These are then gradually expanded to include a few monosyllabic words of high utility and, possibly, carrier phrases.

3. *Remediation stresses sequences of movements.* Careful incremental increases in sequencing movements and the "memory" for such movements are important. Articulation "memory" should be based on internalized tactile-kinesthetic-proprioceptive information relating sounds that are heard to specific motor patterns.

4. *Many repetitions of speech movements are required in drill-oriented sessions.* Hall and colleagues (1993) use 3 to 10 repetitions of each stimulus. Stimuli range from CV utterances to multisyllabic words. Pausing is used between each set of repetitions so that the client can return to a neutral or resting position to reduce perseverative behavior.

5. *The clinician must determine the need for auditory discrimination tasks.* Not all children need enhancement of auditory discrimination skills. Based on assessment data, the clinician should determine whether an individual child needs work in this area.

6. *Remediation should emphasize self-monitoring.* Self-monitoring should be emphasized as early as possible within the remediation program. Some suggest that tactile and kinesthetic self-monitoring be trained (e.g., Square, Martin, & Bose, 2001).

7. *Input from multiple modalities is needed.* Multisensory input appears helpful to many children with suspected CAS. Various types of cueing have been introduced and can be used to meet the specific needs of these children. All of the cueing techniques represent visual and/or tactile cues used to help a child articulate certain sounds or sound sequences (see the following "Clinical Application" for sources).

8. *Remediation should include manipulation of prosodic features as an integral part of the total remedial program.* Whenever possible, rhythm, intonation, stress, and rate manipulation should be integrated into the therapy program from the beginning. The diagnostic data should reveal the areas that specifically need to be targeted. However, some children do not seem capable of manipulating articulatory and prosodic features simultaneously. In this case, an articulatory goal is established first and prosody added later to articulation tasks that are relatively easy for the client.

9. *If necessary, the clinician should teach compensatory strategies.* Compensatory strategies include slowing the overall rate of speech, increasing the use of pauses between words and syllables, vowel prolongation, and the intrusion of a schwa vowel between consonants in a cluster. Hall and associates (1993) state that compensatory strategies could be a necessary portion of therapeutic measures but generally should be seen as only a stage of remediation to facilitate a child's progress. When the compensatory strategies are no longer necessary, productions without them should become the goal.

10. *The clinician must provide successful experiences.* Treatment should begin at a level at which children can succeed. Therefore, it is important that the clinician understand a child's baseline level of articulatory functioning and the strengths that this individual demonstrates. Children with suspected CAS need success with speech goals to keep them motivated throughout the typically long and slow remediation process.

It is perhaps overwhelming for clinicians to read about all the different therapy methods and to choose which one might be best for a client who has been diagnosed with childhood apraxia of speech. A valid concern is which of the many treatment protocols demonstrates verifiable efficacy. Murray, McCabe, and Ballard (2014) evaluated peer-reviewed published articles from 1970 to 2012 to identify treatment methods for CAS that were of good quality; defined the treatment procedures adequately; examined the treatment outcomes, especially maintenance and generalization of the behavior; and established a level of certainty for each treatment approach. Central to this review was treatment efficacy. Demonstration of efficacy extends beyond treatment effects but also requires assessing maintenance and generalization of the treatment effects and hopefully demonstrating increased performance on untrained items that are somehow related to those trained items. A total of 42 articles were reviewed and analyzed according to very specific parameters. Three approaches emerged as having sufficient evidence to be considered for interim clinical practice: (1) integral stimulation/dynamic temporal and tactile cueing, (2) rapid syllable transition treatment, and (3) integrated phonological awareness intervention. These three techniques are explained briefly and references given in the following "Clinical

CLINICAL EXERCISES

Pick one of the therapy techniques noted in the following "Clinical Application." Use the Internet to find information about that technique. List what population it is intended for, how the technique works, what resources you could find (materials or tests, for example), and how you would specifically use the technique in therapy.

Application." It must be kept in mind that this is the beginning of an attempt to evaluate published articles and is based on a limited number of cases. However, it does point to the future need for maintenance and generalization measures to established efficacy.

CLINICAL APPLICATION

Therapy Techniques Which Demonstrated Treatment Efficacy (Murray, McCabe, & Ballard, 2014)

Integral Stimulation/Dynamic Temporal and Tactile Cueing.

Brief Summary: Integral stimulation involves repetition and imitation with visual and auditory models. Visual and tactile inputs, such as touches to the face or adjustments of the jaw and lip postures are used at first. The therapist says the word or syllable with the child and the child looks at the therapist as the word is pronounced and listens carefully. Dynamic Temporal and Tactile Cueing is a variation of integral stimulation that was developed for children who cannot achieve a close approximation of consonants or vowels. The following stages are utilized: (1) imitation (to determine the severity of the disorder), (2) simultaneous production of lengthened vowels with a gradual reduction of lengthening to normal, (3) reduction of therapist's vocal cueing to miming the sound, (4) a clinician's presentation of an auditory model that the child repeats, (5) a delayed response after presenting the model, and (6) spontaneous production. According to Murray and colleagues (2014), this approach works well with clients who have severe CAS.

Sample References: Edeal & Gildersleeve-Neumann, 2011; Maas & Farinella, 2012; Strand & Debertine, 2000; Strand & Skinder, 1999.

Rapid Syllable Transition Treatment (ReST).

Brief Summary: This method is based on principles of motor learning and attempts to address three core problem areas of childhood apraxia of speech: inconsistent sounds, transition between sounds and syllables, and stressing difficulties, specifically lexical stress. The concept is that high-intensity, difficult targets with low frequency knowledge should lead to long-term change in behavior. Items used are nonwords that are three syllables in length such as "baguti" [bəguti]. Targets presented are strong stress SW on the first two syllables (strong stressed first syllable, followed by a weak unstressed second syllable) "'baguti" and weak stress WS (an unstressed weak first syllable followed by a stressed second syllable) "ba'guti" nonwords. Consonants should be minimally stimulable and targets are presented orthographically. The clinician begins by repeating the non-word and the client attempts to say it until the word is recognized and produced correctly. There is immediate feedback on all trials. There are prepractice and practice phases with 10 randomly selected treatment stimuli in the prepractice phase in a carrier phrase such as "He bought a ____." The practice phase consists of 10–12 treatment targets for a total of 100–120 trials. According to Murray and colleagues (2014), this approach seems to work better for children 7–10 years of age with mild-to-moderate CAS.

Sample References: Ballard, Robin, McCabe, & McDonald, 2010; McCabe, Murray, Thomas, Bejjani, & Ballard, 2013.

Integrated Phonological Awareness Intervention.

Brief Summary: This approach targets three areas, speech production, phonological awareness, and printed word decoding skills. Specifically targeted speech sound production practice, developing phonological awareness, and linking graphemes to phonemes are all parts of this approach and are trained in a block design. One speech error pattern was selected based on a phonological process analysis in which the children must demonstrate at least 40% usage of the pattern.

Speech Production: A long "cycle" of intervention was used for each speech error pattern consisting of 12 sessions over 6 weeks.

Phonological Awareness: Different phoneme awareness tasks such as phoneme segmentation or initial phoneme identification were probed to determine whether the tasks were developmentally appropriate. The phoneme segmentation probe used 10 trained and 5 untrained words. For this task, the child was required to segment the probe word into its components using colored blocks. All the stimulus words for this task were taken from the child's target speech production task.

Linking Graphemes to Phonemes: For the initial phoneme identification portion, the child was required to select one of three words with a target sound that corresponded to her or his target error pattern. This approach seems to work best with children from 4–7 years of age.

Sample References: Crosbie, Holm, and Dodd, 2005; Moriarty & Gillon, 2006; McNeill, Gillon, & Dodd, 2009a, b.

Motor Speech Disorders: Cerebral Palsy

Definition and General Features

Cerebral palsy (CP) is a nonprogressive disorder of motor control caused by damage to the developing brain during pre-, peri-, or early postnatal periods (Dillow, Dzienkowski, Smith, & Yucha, 1996; Hardy, 1994; Love, 2000). The condition results in a wide variety of motor disabilities, dysarthria among them. Approximately 400,000 children have cerebral palsy, making this disorder the most common developmental motor impairment (Best, Bigge, & Sirvis, 1994; Love, 2000), occurring about 3 times in every 1,000 births (Bigge, 1991). The lack of volitional speech-motor control is among its central clinical features. However, the cerebral palsy symptom complex, characterized by a host of neurological malfunctions, is far more than disordered articulation. In addition to general movement and coordination problems, primarily caused by spastic conditions of muscles and increased tendon reflexes"these dysfunctions include disturbances in cognition, perception, sensation, language, hearing, emotional behavior, feeding, and seizure control" (Love, 2000, pp. 49–50).

The treatment of cerebral palsy requires a team approach to the problem, which is typically a cooperative effort of a physician specializing in such disorders, a physical and occupational therapist, a psychologist, a social worker, and a speech-language pathologist. Clinical management by the speech-language pathologist requires special considerations that differ considerably from those employed in the treatment of other children with speech sound disorders. Clinical management can be effective only if the complexity of the disabling condition is understood. Among other important factors, this management involves being able to evaluate the intricate interrelationships between respiration, phonation, resonance, and articulation in individuals with cerebral palsy.

Articulatory/Phonological Characteristics

In addition to respiratory, phonatory, and articulatory problems, speech-related dysfunctions in cerebral palsy include prosodic abnormalities and velopharyngeal inadequacies (Bishop, Brown, & Robson, 1990; Dillow et al., 1996; Hardy, 1994; Love, 2000). Cerebral palsy encompasses many different types and degrees of speech-related problems. To facilitate an understanding of the various articulatory/phonatory characteristics, a distinction is usually made between three types of involvement commonly found in individuals with cerebral palsy: (1) spasticity, (2) dyskinesia, and (3) ataxia.

Among clients with cerebral palsy, spastic involvement is the most frequently found. Four major types of spastic involvement are recognized: (1) hemiplegia, (2) paraplegia, (3) diplegia, and (4) quadriplegia. With *spastic hemiplegia,* the arm and leg on one side of the body show signs of spastic paresis. *Spastic paraplegia,* which is relatively uncommon, is characterized by involvement of the legs only. *Spastic diplegia* affects all four limbs, but the lower limbs show more involvement than the upper ones. All four limbs are about equally involved in *spastic quadriplegia.* Individuals with spastic diplegia and quadriplegia are more likely to have speech disorders than are people who have hemiplegia or paraplegia. Respiratory, phonatory, resonatory, and articulatory symptoms of individuals with spasticity include the following:

> *Respiratory difficulties.* Reduced vital capacity resulting in inadequate breath support for phonatory and articulatory purposes
>
> *Laryngeal dysfunction.* Harsh voices and, when coupled with respiratory aberrations, short phrasing and prosodic disturbances

Velopharyngeal inadequacies. Hypernasality

Articulatory deficiencies. Production of fricatives and affricates as well as an overall laborious, slow rate of speech; muscle weakness, articulatory instability, and inaccuracy in finding target articulation points are also noted (Love, 2000)

Dyskinesias in cerebral palsy are best exemplified by athetoid conditions marked by unilateral or bilateral disturbances of posture, tonus, and motion. They have been reported to be far less frequent than spastic involvement within the cerebral palsy population, but their effects on speech performance are often severe. More often than not, the degree of limb dysfunction mirrors the impairments of the speech mechanism. Many clients with athetoid dysarthria show dysfunction of every physiological component contributing to speech:

Respiratory difficulties. Breathing might be rapid and irregular, showing a lack of thoracic respiratory movement or even "reverse breathing" in which the sternum is flattened instead of lifted during inspiration.

Laryngeal dysfunction. General hypertonicity, which can immobilize the phonatory process altogether, can be more pronounced than in spastic involvement. If any voice results, it is commonly marked by an especially strained quality, hard glottal onset, and reduced intensity and prosody realizations.

Velopharyngeal inadequacies. Slow velar activity often results in hypernasal effects.

Articulatory deficiencies. Distortions of consonants are possible as well as vowel productions (positioning of the mandible during speech can somehow establish necessary differences in tongue height but not in anterior-posterior tongue movements for the production of front versus back vowels).

Ataxia is infrequent among clients with cerebral palsy. Its main symptom is lack of coordination of hypotonic muscle action. Based on clinical observation, the speech characteristics of individuals with ataxic cerebral palsy appear to be similar to those of adults with ataxic dysarthria but are more severe than other children with dysarthria (Nordberg, Miniscalco, & Lohmander, 2014). The following characteristics are noted in children and adults with ataxia:

Respiratory difficulties. Shallow inspiration and lack of expiratory control

Laryngeal dysfunction. Harsh voice productions, reduced range of prosodic feature realization.

Velopharyngeal inadequacies. Hypernasality is not typical.

Articulatory deficiencies. Imprecise consonants and vowel distortions, inconsistent sound substitutions and omissions and a general dysrhythmia (Nordberg, Miniscalco, & Lohmander, 2014).

See Table 11.2 for a summary of the three different types of cerebral palsy.

Milloy and Morgan-Barry (1990) describe the following phonological processes that relate to the speech errors of temporal and motor control:

Phonological Processes

Related to temporal coordination. Voicing difficulties, including devoicing initial consonants or voicing unvoiced sounds, variable realizations of voiced-voiceless cognates, prevocalic voicing, consonant cluster reductions, final consonant deletions, stopping of fricatives or frication of stops, and weak syllable deletions predominate.

Related to motor control, errors of phonetic placement. Fronting, backing, stopping, gliding, lateral realization of apical and coronal fricatives, vowelization of [l] and [r], and nasalization have been noted.

TABLE 11.2 Summary of Types of Cerebral Palsy

Type of Cerebral Palsy	Muscular Involvement	Speech Disorder
Spasticity		
1. Hemiplegia	Upper and lower limbs on one side demonstrate hypertonicity.	Speech is acceptable, and a developmental delay is possible.
2. Paraplegia	Lower limbs and possibly torso musculature demonstrate hypertonicity.	Problems with respiration and breath control exist.
3. Diplegia	All four limbs are involved although the lower limbs are more severely affected. Torso and neck muscles could also be involved.	Speech is variable depending on the extent of the neuromotor problem; prosodic and articulation difficulties could be present.
4. Quadriplegia	Spasticity in all four limbs occurs with equal degree.	Dysphonia and articulation difficulties depend on the severity of the disorder.
Athetosis	Impairment of voluntary movements result from extreme hypertonicity or extreme flaccidity; involuntary continuous muscle movements are present.	Speech difficulties can occur, although variable in severity; speech is generally slow with poor articulation; and problems with phonation, stress, and rhythm are possible.
Ataxia	This is characterized by incoordination of movement with the inability to maintain posture and balance.	Speech problems are typically present; articulation and problems with rhythm are evident.

Clinical Implications: Diagnostics

The primary communicative impairment of children with cerebral palsy is clearly motor speech in nature. But these children present a variety of clinical symptoms having to do with both the type and the severity of involvement. On the other hand, all children with cerebral palsy share some common factors that directly relate to basic functions subserving speech, namely, problems with respiration, phonation, resonation, and articulation. It is important to assess the type and degree of interference that each of these systems could have on speech.

Problems with *respiration* could lead to difficulties in initiation of vocalizations, difficulties sustaining vocalizations, variations in loudness that could affect word and sentence stress, inability to sustain vocalization for multisyllabic words or longer sentences, and loss of expiratory support at end of utterance.

Problems with *phonation* could result in interruptions in phonation, breathy voice, harsh voice, pitch and intensity variations, and problems in coordinating voicing and articulation.

Problems with *resonation* could result in various degrees of hypernasality, variations in nasality within an utterance, and lack of intelligibility caused by nasality problems.

Problems with *articulation* could result in difficulties in achieving speech sound productions, sound distortions, and disorganized phonological systems, possibly leading to problems with language and learning to read.

When assessing children with cerebral palsy, it is essential to remember that the smooth integration of all systems subserving speech is a real problem. Therefore, the assessment and treatment of children with this disorder must account for far more than speech sound production difficulties.

The high diversity of possible involvements requires an encompassing evaluation. In addition to respiratory, phonatory, resonatory, and articulatory limitations and possibilities, data regarding the following areas should be obtained:

- Cognitive skills
- Sensory and perceptual abilities beginning with an audiological evaluation
- Emotional behavior
- Feeding/eating characteristics
- Language competence

Odding, Roebroeck, &, Stam (2006) report that about 40% of the population with cerebral palsy shows some degree of cognitive impairment,the rest of these individuals demonstrating intelligence within normal limits. Impaired language development, learning difficulties, and academic problems often occur in children with cerebral palsy (Rosenbaum et al. 2007). An audiological evaluation is a necessity for children with cerebral palsy; those with athetosis in particular have higher auditory detection thresholds, poorer speech reception thresholds, and poorer speech discrimination than do children without cerebral palsy.

Often the speech-language pathologist becomes part of an early intervention team for infants who have been identified with cerebral palsy. As a member of this team, the speech-language pathologist could be asked to assess prespeech skills as prerequisites for the development of articulation skills. These prerequisites include:

1. Head control with stability of the neck and shoulder girdle. Such stability provides later control and mobility of oral structures.
2. A coordinated pattern of respiration and phonation.
3. A variety of feeding experiences to enhance normal feeding patterns.
4. Babbling practice (Levin, 1999).

CLINICAL EXERCISES

Identify two assessment measures of prespeech behavior in your clinic or on the Internet. List their characteristics. For what age population are they intended, how do you get the information (e.g., testing, interview), what type of behaviors do they test, and are they specially designed for cerebral palsied children?

Explain briefly how respiration, phonation, resonance, and articulation work together for an integrated speech system. Pick one of the three main types of dysarthrias (spasticity, dyskinesia, ataxia) and discuss in general terms how a child's speech might sound based on respiratory, phonatory, resonatory, and articulatory difficulties.

Clinical Implications: Therapeutics

As always, the selection of appropriate therapeutic measures to influence the communicative abilities of clients with cerebral palsy is a direct outgrowth of specific diagnostic results. Established methods for the treatment of various "types" of cerebral palsy amount only to guidelines for elementary orientation.

There are, nevertheless, general principles that apply to all remediation efforts with young clients who have cerebral palsy. First, some prespeech prerequisites must be met (the previously mentioned head control and the coordination of respiratory patterns with voice production, for example). The necessity of coordination between breathing and phonation for future articulation work is self-evident, but a certain degree of posture control is equally indispensable. Another, although controversial prerequisite, pertains to the inhibition of certain chewing and swallowing behaviors, specifically the chewing reflex, which might interfere with oral-motor activities for articulatory tasks. Neurodevelopmental therapy—for example, the so-called Bobath approach to the treatment of infants with cerebral palsy—heavily emphasizes the early reduction of abnormal oral reflexes within a prespeech program (Bobath, 1967; Bobath & Bobath, 1972).

The next therapeutic phase with young children who have cerebral palsy pertains to communication and speech-language stimulation. In infants, this might start with vocal play and babbling practice. Chapter 6, pages 162–166, offers some considerations for speech therapy for children with emerging phonology.

For older children with cerebral palsy, a basic consideration is the facilitation of desired movements while inhibiting the abnormal reflex patterns. Before a speech-language clinician can address the coordination of respiration, phonation, resonation, and articulation, the child must be able to maintain some reflex-inhibiting postures that the physical therapist recommends. Because this is usually one of the primary goals of the early intervention team, the children should already have developed some skills in this area. If they can inhibit abnormal reflexes and realize certain movements required for speech, articulation training can be initiated.

Traditionally, therapy began by establishing temporal coordination and motor control of the speech musculature. Goals were to increase the speed, range, and accuracy of movement of the tongue, lips, and jaw (Gibbon & Wood, 2003). These goals were then integrated with the maintenance of body and head tonus as well as respiration, phonation, and resonation (Barlow & Farley, 1989). Oral exercises usually preceded phonetic placement. Selection of the target sound was guided by stimulability, consistency, visibility, and whether the sound developed early or late. Therefore, stimulable, visible sounds that in some contexts were produced accurately and were early to be acquired were normally given priority (Love, 2000).

However, there were those who felt that groups of sounds rather than a single sound should be treated. Guidelines by Hardy (1994) and Crary (1993) include the following procedures:

1. *Consonants that are realized correctly in prevocalic positions but are misarticulated in postvocalic positions should be treated first.* Generally, postvocalic errors are more easily remedied if the child can produce the sound in a prevocalic position.

2. *Distortions should be treated before substitutions.* This includes distortions that fall short of the target because of motor involvement. Prognosis should be better if the child can produce the sound somewhat distorted rather than delete or use a substitute for the sound.

3. *Training articulatory omissions and substitutions that fall short of the target because of motor involvement should be delayed.* Compensatory articulatory efforts for sounds that are difficult to produce should be trained instead. Children usually have already developed some type of compensatory sound realization. The clinician's duty is to refine this production as much as possible.

4. *A multiple auditory-visual stimulation approach should be used.* It is preferred over auditory stimulation alone.

5. *Voice–voiceless distinctions should be trained by slowing the speech process* and then concentrating on the production of the sound's voicelessness. This is important because children with cerebral palsy have a tendency to substitute voiced for voiceless consonants.

6. *It is important to remember that some children with cerebral palsy cannot achieve "normal" articulation.* In these cases, *reasonable compensations* are the goal; they can be very efficient for communicative purposes.

Occasionally, the physical handicap is so severe that effective verbal communication

---

CLINICAL APPLICATION

Augmentative and alternative communication (AAC) refers to an area of research as well as clinical and educational practice. AAC involves attempts to study and when necessary compensate for temporary or permanent impairments, activity limitations, and participation restrictions of individuals with severe disorders of speech-language production and/or comprehension, including spoken and written modes of communication. It is the position of the American Speech-Language-Hearing Association (ASHA) that communication is the essence of human life and that all people have the right to communicate to the fullest extent possible. No individuals should be denied this right, regardless of the type and/or severity of communication, linguistic, social, cognitive, motor, sensory, perceptual, and/or other disability(ies) they might present (American Speech-Language-Hearing Association, 2005).

cannot be achieved at all. If that is the case, *augmentative communication*—the use of other systems (gestural, boards with words or pictures, electronic devices) to promote meaningful communicative exchange—must be implemented.

Cleft Palate

Definition and General Features

Occurring in 1 of about 700 births (Grames, 2008), palatal and (upper) lip clefts are among the most frequent congenital anomalies (American Cleft Palate–Craniofacial Association and Cleft Palate Foundation, 1997). **Clefting** refers to a division of a continuous structure by a cleavage, a split prominently caused by a failure of the palate to fuse during fetal development (Shprintzen, 1995). Examples of clefting are cleft palate and cleft lip. Both the hard and soft palates and the lips form normally uninterrupted structures within their anatomical boundaries. If clefting occurs, a gap severs their unity, dividing the roof of the mouth (which also constitutes the floor of the nasal cavity) and/or the upper lip sagitally into separated left and right portions.

There are several etiologies that cause a failure of the regular median fusion of the embryo's oral-facial structures between the 8th and 12th weeks of gestation. In addition, there is also the possibility of a rupture of already fused oral-facial elements (Kitamura, 1991). Contrary to common understanding, no single cause for clefting exists; "clefting is . . . a clinical outcome of many possible diseases" (Shprintzen, 1995, p. 5).

Although there are many classification systems, the recommendations by the American Cleft Palate–Craniofacial Association have been most frequently adopted (Bzoch, 1997).

1. Clefts of prepalate
   - *Cleft lip:* unilateral, bilateral, median, prolabium (central segment of upper lip), congenital scar
   - *Cleft of alveolar process:* unilateral, bilateral, median, submucous
   - *Cleft of prepalate:* any combination of types, prepalate protrusion, prepalate rotation, prepalate arrest (median cleft)
2. Clefts of the palate
   - *Clefts of soft palate:* extent, palatal shortness, submucous
   - *Clefts of hard palate:* extent, vomer attachment, submucous
3. Clefts of prepalate and palate
4. Facial clefts other than prepalate and palate.

Unilaterality or *bilaterality* of hard palate clefts refers to their presence on one or both sides of the hard palate; *median clefts* refers to their presence at the midline. These clefts are along a line where the lower edge of the nasal septum attaches to the palate. *Submucous clefts,* on the other hand, are characterized by an intact mucous membrane covering a cleft. This cleft could be separating muscular portions of the soft palate and/or a cleavage of the posterior bony portions of the hard palate. A V-shaped indentation in this area might be felt with the finger. Another sign of the probable existence of a submucous cleft is a divided uvula, a *bifid uvula.* Quite in contrast to unilateral and bilateral clefts, submucous clefts seldom cause feeding problems or abnormal speech.

Articulatory/Phonological Characteristics

Children with cleft palate may exhibit developmental and/or compensatory articulatory and phonological disorders (Bzoch, 1997; Pamplona, Ysunza, Gonzalez, Ramirez, & Patino, 2000; Whitehill, Francis, & Ching, 2003). Developmental speech-language delays are similar to those in children without clefts, but they occur more frequently in children with cleft palates (Schonweiler, Schonweiler, Schmelzeisen, & Ptok, 1995; Trost-Cardamone, 1990). Therefore, children with developmental delays are characterized by speech sound skills that resemble those of younger normally developing children. Developmental delays cannot always be said to be completely independent of the underlying condition. Consonant cluster reductions—for example, a frequent occurrence in children with speech-language delays—can often be traced to placement or omission errors that are disorder specific in children with palatal clefts.

Compensatory errors pertain to specific errors in the placement of active and passive articulators that could occur in patients who have inadequate closure of the velopharyngeal valve or a cleft or fistula in the hard palate (Witzel, 1995). They have also been described as "compensatory adjustments." These sound substitutions or distortions are produced more posteriorly and inferior in the vocal tract by posterior positioning of the tongue, associated true and false vocal fold adduction, or abnormal positioning of the arytenoid cartilage and epiglottis. Because of difficulties with velopharyngeal closure, these errors are thought to be a compensatory attempt to modify the airstream below the velopharyngeal valve. But compensatory errors are not always a direct result of velopharyngeal incompetence. They could actually result from compensatory articulation caused by limited movements of the velopharyngeal valve during productions of specific sounds. Refer to Table 11.3 for the types of compensatory articulation errors (Witzel).

Although specific sound production difficulties have often been noted in the speech of children with cleft palate, these may not be entirely phonetic in nature. Children with cleft palate could also evidence difficulties with the organization of phonemes within their language system; that is, they might demonstrate phonemic-based disorders (Broen & Moller, 1993; Chapman, 1993; Chapman & Hardin, 1992; Chapman, Hardin-Jones, & Halter, 2003). Early delays in phonological development include a high frequency of deletion of final consonants, syllable reduction, and backing. However, at the age of 4 to 5 years, these problems were less apparent.

CLINICAL EXERCISES

In the speech of children with a cleft palate, a mid-dorsal palatal stop can be a compensatory articulation for [t], [d], [k], and [g]. Based on the production features between these sounds, what would you want to do in therapy to achieve [t] and [d]? [k] and [g]? (Refer to Table 11.3.)

Pick one of the compensatory articulation errors for fricatives. Explain how you would want to change the production features between that compensatory articulation and [s] and [z]. Be as specific as possible.

Watch this video of a boy who has a repaired cleft palate but still has severe articulation problems. Which errors do you note in his speech? youtube.com/watch?v=-LR_YDBPWIY

Clinical Implications: Diagnostic

Obviously, the initial diagnosis of clefting in a newborn—its nature, site, and extent—is a medical task. So is the beginning of its management, typically involving at least a pediatrician, an orthodontist, and an otolaryngologist. But clefts are a matter of long-term care requiring a team of specialists for successful assessment and management. Speech-language pathologists are important members of this team. Their primary job is to assess the child's communicative status and development, a challenging task. Not only are all clefts different (including their various effects on verbal communication) but also the personalities of the children and their caregivers vary regarding their ability to cope with the situation and its clinical consequences. However, the biggest diagnostic challenge might be the developmental aspects of the disorder, that is, the changing nature of the appraised findings. Today's status can differ from tomorrow's because of natural growth factors, necessary corrective measures of medical intervention, and compensatory prospects. Diagnostics involving children with clefts is a truly ongoing process.

TABLE II.3 Compensatory Articulation Errors

Compensatory Articulation	Production Characteristics	Substitution For
Glottal stop	Adduction of true vocal folds; increased air pressure could even result in false vocal fold adduction.	Stop-plosives
Laryngeal stop	Abnormal positioning of epiglottis; the epiglottis comes in contact with the pharynx.	Stop-plosives, consonants
Laryngeal fricative	Abnormal positioning of epiglottis; it approaches the pharynx.	Fricatives
Laryngeal affricate	Epiglottis briefly contacts pharynx; it then constricts the airstream.	Affricates
Pharyngeal stop	Posterior movement of the dorsum of the tongue; it contacts the pharynx, causing a buildup and release of air.	Stop-plosives
Pharyngeal fricative	Posterior movement of the dorsum of the tongue toward the pharynx; it constricts the airstream, causing frication.	Fricatives
Pharyngeal affricate	Brief contact of the dorsum of the tongue with pharynx; it then constricts the airstream.	Affricates
Posterior nasal fricative	Posterior dorsum of tongue and soft palate positioned to generate friction at velopharyngeal valve; this is always accompanied by nasal air emission.	Fricatives
Posterior nasal affricate	Posterior dorsum of tongue and soft palate are positioned to create both stopping and friction; always accompanied by nasal air emission.	Affricates
Middorsum palatal stop	Middorsum of tongue contacts the hard palate at approximate place for [j].	[t], [d], [k], and [g]
Middorsum palatal fricative	Middorsum of tongue approaches the hard palate to create friction.	Fricatives
Middorsum palatal affricate	Middorsum of tongue contacts the hard palate followed by frication.	Affricates

The areas of diagnostic concern again underline the necessity of a team approach to the clinical management of children with cleft palate. For example, they are all prone to intermittent middle ear infections and their concomitant conductive hearing loss. This means that an otolaryngologist and an audiologist need to be involved to closely monitor the condition and hearing ability of all children with palatal clefts. The findings are important for the speech-language clinician because "evidence indicates that children with recurrent middle ear problems are slower to acquire speech production skills" (Broen & Moller, 1993, p. 230).

The central diagnostic issue pertains to the phonatory, resonatory, and articulatory effects of velopharyngeal port incompetency (VPI) which includes both structural abnormalities and neuromuscular inadequacies. Whereas structural abnormalities largely can be corrected by surgical and/or prosthetic measures, some functional deficits in respect to speech often remain, resulting in hypernasal resonance, nasal air emission, sound distortions, and sound substitutions. The latter two are characterized by *articulatory backing* in children with cleft palate. This is a compensatory measure to produce speech sounds more posteriorly in the oral cavity than is normally the case. Velopharyngeal incompetency impairs the intraoral pressure buildup necessary for the norm production of many speech sounds—primarily stops, sibilants, fricatives, and affricates, the so-called pressure consonants. Nasals and semivowels such as [w] and [j] remain relatively intact.

One of the most striking features characterizing the speech of children with cleft palates with velopharyngeal incompetence is the substitution of glottal stops for stop-plosives. This compensatory articulatory behavior is triggered by the impossibility of accumulating the intraoral pressure required for the regular production of these pressure consonants. During this substitution, the standard positioning of the articulators is sometimes retained. For example, for [p], the lips are closed and suddenly opened simultaneously with the release of the glottal stop. This often results in an impression of a slightly distorted yet acceptable [p]-production. In addition to the articulatory consequences of velopharyngeal incompetency, dental anomalies and problems with occlusion of the mandibular and maxillary arches often contribute to the aberrant articulation of children with cleft palate.

"The primary clinical task for the speech-language pathologist is to assess the child's phonological status and then infer the effects of structural deviations on the phonological behavior observed" (Trost-Cardamone & Bernthal, 1993, p. 317). Such a task differs considerably from child to child, primarily according to age and linguistic/cognitive levels, but it always involves:

1. Speech sampling and analysis, including sound inventory and phonological pattern development
2. Stimulability probes
3. Intelligibility judgments
4. Oral-facial examination

Each of these assessment areas has been discussed previously in some detail (see Chapters 6 and 7), and the procedures do not differ significantly for children with cleft palate.

One important aspect of the diagnosis with these children is to find and distinguish between error patterns that are developmental in nature and those that, as a result of the cleft, have a structural or physiological basis. Some patterns are sometimes seen in children with cleft palate but are not typical for children with structurally and functionally intact oral and pharyngeal mechanisms. Trost-Cardamone and Bernthal (1993) provide the following list:

1. *Consonant distortions associated with nasal emissions.* Three error patterns are associated with nasal emission. It is important to distinguish between them because different interventions could be in order for each.
   - *Nasal emission caused by persistence of velopharyngeal inadequacy.* This is characterized by nasal emission during production of all pressure consonants and pervasive hypernasality accompanying production of vowels and the vocalic consonants [l], [r], [j], and [w].
   - *Nasal emission caused by oronasal fistulae.* An oronasal fistula is an opening between the oral and nasal cavity. Although some can be easily eliminated surgically, others are too large for successful closure. There is a relationship between the location of the fistula and the consonants affected. Posteriorly located fistulae (near the juncture between the hard and soft palate) affect primarily [k] and [g] with little influence on anteriorly produced consonants. When the fistula is anteriorly located, [t], [d], [s], [z], [p], and [b] are likely to be distorted.

- *Nasal emission that is speech sound specific.* This could occur in the absence of clefting or velopharyngeal impairment. It does not affect a class of sounds and is rarely associated with hypernasality. Nasal emission does not require surgical intervention; it is probably caused by faulty learning and can usually be treated with speech therapy if properly diagnosed (see pages 259–260).

2. *Vowel distortions secondary to hypernasality.* It is important for clinicians to differentiate between vowel distortions that could result from deviant articulatory placement and those that are deviations due to hypernasal resonance as the result of deficient velopharyngeal valving.

3. *Compensatory articulations.* Several types of compensatory articulations are noted in Table 11.3. The clinician should differentiate between compensatory articulations that are used as substitutions and those that occur as coarticulations.

4. *Atypical backed articulation.* These articulations include back-velar substitutions for [l], [r], and [n]. The posterior shifts could result from attempting to capture airflow or using the back of the tongue to help seal the velopharyngeal port. Such productions should be analyzed to determine whether they are part of a phonological pattern of backing or represent selective articulatory substitutions.

CLINICAL APPLICATION

Clinical Test Battery for Children with Cleft Palates

Bzoch (1997) recommends the following clinical test battery:

1. *Language testing*
2. *Audiometric evaluation*
3. *Nasal emission test.* A small mirrored surface or a headset listening device is sufficient to enhance the auditory and visual perceptions of nasal airflow. This test uses ten two-syllable words, each containing two [p] or [b] sounds.
4. *Hypernasality test.* This measure uses 10 one-syllable words beginning with [b] and ending with [t]. The subject repeats each word twice. On the second repetition, the examiner pinches the nares closed. A perceptual judgment of hypernasality is indicated if words shift in quality between the first and second repetition.
5. *Hyponasality test.* This measure uses 10 one-syllable words beginning with [m] and ending with [t]. The subject repeats each word twice; on the second repetition, the examiner pinches the nares closed. On this test, there *should be a shift in quality* between the first and second repetition.
6. *Phonation test.* The subject prolongs [i], [ɑ], and [u] for 10 seconds. The examiner notes any aspirate or hoarse phonation. Also, failure of the client to sustain phonation for 10 seconds would indicate a habituated breathy voice. This can be confirmed by the conversational speech sample.
7. *Articulation test.* Special tests examining typical errors noted in the speech of children with cleft palate are available. These include, for example, the Iowa Pressure Test (Morris, Spriestersbach, & Darley, 1961), the Bzoch Error Pattern Diagnostic Articulation Test (Bzoch, 1979), and the Great Ormond Street Speech Assessment (Sell, Harding, & Grunwell, 1994).
8. *Screening nasometer test.* This test is used for children from 2 to 6 years of age. Procedures can be found in many sources. Two examples are found in Dalston (1997) and Dalston, Warren, & Dalston (1991).

Clinical Implications: Therapeutics

Many children with cleft palates undergo palate repair by the age of 18 months. They remain free of compensatory sound production errors such as glottal for oral stops and pharyngeal for oral fricatives. Other children require therapeutic intervention. To implement therapy with clients with cleft palates, four overall goals should be kept in mind:

1. Improve the placement of consonant productions by promoting a more forward place of articulation.
2. Improve velopharyngeal valve function and decrease hypernasal resonance quality.
3. Modify compensatory articulations.
4. If developmental phonological errors exist, improve the child's phonological system (Van Demark & Hardin, 1990).

Improving the placement of consonant productions and modifying compensatory articulations are usually accomplished by direct work on the place of articulation—that is, motor placement techniques. Glottal stops can easily be eliminated by using maneuvers, such as gentle whispering, overaspiration, or the use of a sustained [h] that keeps the vocal folds apart (Golding-Kushner, 1995). Slight overaspiration by using a sustained [h] usually breaks the glottal pattern because it requires an open glottis. Voiceless oral stops are first introduced at the end of a prolonged [h]. In addition, the voiceless stop itself is overaspirated. If the word were *pie,* the production would sound similar to a prolonged [h] + [p] + *high.* Teaching voiceless homorganic oral fricatives before establishing oral stops is a good technique for breaking up compensatory coarticulations. Nasal occlusion and release help to eliminate nasal snorting and to establish stops and fricatives. By occluding the nares, clients quickly learn to direct the airstream orally.

Sometimes even after surgery, the velopharyngeal mechanism is only marginally adequate for articulatory function; hypernasality may still persist to varying degrees. If further surgery and/or prosthodontic intervention is not indicated, improving velopharyngeal valve function and decreasing hypernasal resonance quality might then become a treatment goal. Several ways have been suggested to improve velopharyngeal valve function. The velum is massaged and electrically stimulated; various devices have been used to improve the effectiveness of these exercises (Starr, 1993). Behavioral approaches that provide feedback to clients are attempts to enhance their awareness and control of the velopharyngeal mechanism. Perceptual and acoustic feedback, visual feedback, and airflow and air pressure feedback have been offered with varying degrees of success (see Starr for a review of these techniques). However, due to lack of clinical studies, outcome measures for these techniques remain unclear.

Decreasing hypernasal resonance could be another important therapy goal for these clients. Hypernasal resonance occurs in individuals with adequate and inadequate velopharyngeal competency. The following describes one such technique, increased mouth opening or orality (Boone, McFarlane, Von Berg, & Zraick, 2013), because of its overlap with previously mentioned articulatory principles.

> ## CLINICAL APPLICATION

Case Study JD

This case study is adapted from Albery and Russell (1990). JD was born with a cleft of the soft palate, which was repaired relatively late at age 2;6.

According to the authors, progression through the early speech stages with an open cleft had influenced his articulatory development. His deviant and restricted inventory is not, therefore, typical but does exemplify some of the compensatory articulation errors noted in Table 11.3.

JD's speech was highly unintelligible because the inventory restrictions resulted in the loss of numerous phonemic contrasts.

Phonetic Inventory

[m], [n], [w], [j], [h]	Articulated in a regular manner in the prevocalic, intervocalic, and, where applicable, postvocalic word positions.
[ʔp], [ʔb]	A glottal component accompanied the bilabial productions in the prevocalic word positions.
[p], [b], [t], → [ʔ] [d], [k], [g], → [ʔ] [f], [v], [ʃ], → [ʔ] [ʒ], [θ], [ð], [tʃ], [dʒ],	Stop-plosive productions (including [p] and [b] in intervocalic and postvocalic positions), most fricatives, and affricates were realized as glottal stops.
[s] → [ħ]	[s] was realized as a voiceless pharyngeal fricative [ħ] in all word positions.
[z] → [ʕ]	[z] was realized as a voiced pharyngeal fricative [ʕ] in all word positions.
[l] → [l̃]	[l] was nasalized in the postvocalic word position.
[r] → [w]	[r] was realized as [w].

In the United States, the trend for many years has been toward early closure of palatal clefts, typically between the ages of 6 and 18 months (Marsh & Lehman, 1988).

During sound articulation, varying degrees of velar activity occur. For example, stop-plosives require complete closure of the nasopharyngeal port for the necessary buildup of intraoral air pressure. Productions of [ɑ] or [w], on the other hand, do not demand the same degree of closure to prevent undue nasal resonance. Complete velopharyngeal closure is necessary only during the production of stops and sounds with little articulatory possibility for oral air escape, sibilants, and affricates, for example. With more "open" sounds, the same degree of closure is not required.

If open sounds require less velar activity to keep nasality effects from occurring, increasing the opening of the respective phoneme realizations should at least lessen, and possibly prevent, such consequences. Consider /i/ realizations as an example. They can be achieved in several ways, specifically with a more or less restricted oral passageway and without violating phonemic boundaries. Under otherwise comparable conditions, more open oral productions put less demand on proper velar function than the more restricted oral ones and are, therefore, preferable for the purpose at hand.

Examples such as this illustrate the clinical practicalities of the principle to be applied: The task is to train the hypernasal child to systematically use the widest oral-articulatory posture for the sound in question. This posture should not interfere with the phoneme value the sound represents.

Intellectual Disability (Intellectual Developmental Disorder)

Definition and General Features

The various attempts to define intellectual disability reflect the different understanding of, and attitudes toward, the disorder at different times. At least 10 different "official" definitions of intellectual disability have existed since 1921. Changes from the American Psychiatric Association's *Diagnostic and Statistical Manual DSM-IV* (APA, 2000) to the DSM-5 (APA, 2013) include the use of the term *intellectual disability* (intellectual developmental disorder) to reflect the more common terminology that has been used for decades by professional and lay groups. The definition has stayed relatively the same from DSM-IV (APA, 2000) to DSM-5 (APA, 2013), noting that this mental disorder is characterized by significant limitations both in intellectual functioning and in adaptive behavior as expressed in conceptual, social, and practical adaptive skills.

In such a definition, three criteria stand out:

1. Limitations in adaptive skills
2. Subaverage intellectual functioning
3. Manifestation of a cognitive impairment before 18 years of age

The term *adaptive skills* refers to functioning in three domains or areas of specified everyday living activities: the conceptual domain includes skills in language, reading, writing, math, reasoning, knowledge, and memory; the social domain refers to empathy, social judgment, interpersonal communication skills, the ability to make and retain friendships and similar capacities; the practical domain relates to self-management in areas such as personal care, job responsibilities, money management, recreation and organizing school and work tasks.

The individual must also show significant deficits in adaptive behavior relative to his or her own cultural group. This delineation is used to rule out linguistic and cultural differences that might limit the individual's functioning in a larger setting.

Subaverage intellectual functioning in this definition refers to approximately 2 standard deviations below the mean on suitable standardized intelligence quotient tests, translating into a score of about 70 or below. The *manifestation of a cognitive impairment before age 18* identifies such deficiencies as a developmental disorder beginning somewhere between the time of conception and official adulthood. This would eliminate individuals who in adulthood might show signs of dementia and demonstrate similar problems in adaptive behavior, for example.

Previously, the DSM-IV (APA, 2000), reported 2–3% of people meet the criteria for intellectual disability. This was the result of the diagnostic criterion that required an IQ score of approximately 70 or below. Statistically, 2 standard deviations below average (a score of 70) equal 2.5% of the population, thus the estimates of between 2–3% of the population. However, DSM-5 (APA, 2013) has moved away from relying on specific IQ scores. The estimates in DSM-5 report a prevalence rate of approximately 1 percent.

The DSM-5 defined severity in terms of adaptive functioning, not IQ scores. The level of adaptive functioning determines the levels of support necessary. The manual further states that IQ scores are less valid in the lower end of the IQ range.

Specific associated problems could also impact the communicative behavior of this population. Both sensorineural and conductive hearing losses as well as abnormal middle ear function are prevalent in these individuals. Individuals with intellectual disability are at least 40 times more likely than the general population to have a hearing impairment (Carvill, 2001).

Articulatory/Phonological Characteristics

All subgroups of children with intellectual disabilities demonstrate a higher prevalence of speech problems. They tend to lack articulatory precision and appropriate pauses and phrasing. The phonological characteristics of this population can be summarized as follows (Kumin, 1998; Shriberg & Widder, 1990; Stoel-Gammon, 1998):

1. Speech sound errors are more common than in the normally developing population.
2. Deletion of consonants is the most frequent error.
3. Errors are typically inconsistent.
4. Patterns are similar to those of children who are not cognitively disabled but demonstrate a functional delay.

In general, individuals with cognitive impairments demonstrate the same phonological processes as norm children but with a higher frequency of occurrence. However, children with Down syndrome might show other developmental patterns. In a review of articles from 1950, Kent and Vorperian (2013) found that children with Down syndrome demonstrated both delayed and deviant phonological patterns. The most common phonological processes are the reduction of consonant clusters and final consonant deletion. Variable use of these processes is also noted in this population. It has been hypothesized that individuals with intellectual disabilities might use these processes for other reasons than to simplify their speech. For example, Shriberg and Widder (1990) suggest that consonant deletions might reflect cognitive processing constraints in the motor assembly stage of speech production.

Clinical Implications: Diagnostics

Individuals who are intellectually disabled compose a diverse group of people. Not only are individuals with cognitive disabilities quite different among themselves but also the boundaries between disabled and what is considered to be norm are rather indistinct. That is not to say that individuals with intellectual disabilities are not different from individuals who are considered to be developing in a normal manner; they are. Although the cognitive development of children with intellectual disabilities is said to be generally similar to that of nondisabled children, only slower (Owens, 2009), and their cognitive skills have been proven to keep growing through adulthood. However, organizational and recall problems as well as difficulties in recognizing the significant feature of a given situation distinguish children with intellectual disabilities from their normally developing peers.

With this group diversity in mind, assessment procedures largely depend on the age of the individual and the level of speech and language functioning. Some individuals with intellectual disabilities do not have speech at all and alternative means of communication need to be explored. For the very young child who is beginning to develop first words, an independent analysis can examine the inventory of sounds being used. For older children and adults with more developed speech and language skills, the following assessment procedures could be used:

An independent analysis for children with emerging phonological systems is discussed in Chapter 6.

1. *Articulation test.* This determines the consonant and vowel inventory. Phonological patterns and the intelligibility of speech at the single-word level can also be analyzed.
2. *Spontaneous speech sample.* This determines the consonant and vowel inventory in conversational speech. Phonological patterns can be noted as well as the overall intelligibility in natural communicative situations. Differences in intelligibility between spontaneous speech and the articulation test should be evaluated.
3. *Motor-speech capabilities.* Speech structure and function should be assessed to determine the individual's motor capabilities.
4. *Hearing acuity and middle ear function.* Because of the large percentage of hearing losses and problems with middle ear function, having a complete understanding of the individual's current hearing realities is important .
5. *Language.* The client's language should be assessed to determine the level of linguistic functioning.
6. *Assessment of the environment.* The environment in which the individual lives and works will determine communicative needs. One of the major roles of a clinician is to assess the communicative environment in which the individual resides. This should provide information about the circumstances demanding communication of some type and the way the client is currently communicating to express needs, wants, and desires.

Although the diagnostic assessment of an individual with intellectual disabilities is conducted in a manner essentially similar to that used with normally developing clients, specific factors need to be kept in mind. Individual differences, such as age, level of cognitive functioning, level of speech and language functioning, and learning style, naturally alter the methods used.

Clinical Implications: Therapeutics

Each child with an intellectual disability presents a unique pattern of communicative abilities and difficulties that must be identified. Some guiding principles for clinicians can nevertheless be suggested within an intervention framework. The following principles have been suggested for the treatment of speech sound disorders in the population with intellectual disabilities (Owens, 2009; Swift & Rosin, 1990):

1. Use overlearning and repetition.
2. Train in the natural environment.
3. Begin as early as possible.

4. Follow developmental guidelines.
5. Concentrate more on overall intelligibility than on training individual sounds.
6. Enlist the help of the client's caregivers.
7. Direct all therapeutic activities to communication training serving the daily routine.
8. All intervention efforts should be commensurate with the client's ability to grasp and attend to the respective tasks. This typically translates into short, repetitive, reinforced activities that are meaningful to the situation and result in real, tangible consequences (Owens, 2009).

With very few exceptions, traditional motor approaches with these individuals have been of little value in the treatment of speech production problems. Therefore, a sound-by-sound approach using placement techniques is probably not a good choice. The cycles approach has been adapted for use with children with intellectual disabilities in classroom settings. In these cases, time allotments have been doubled for the children; thus, each phoneme or pattern is targeted for 2 hours rather than for 60 minutes (Hodson & Paden, 1991). A training period of 3 years or more might be required before substantial intelligibility gains are observed.

Many of the treatment programs for children and adults with intellectual disabilities target the increase of overall functional language skills. Although intelligibility often is a noted problem with these individuals, very little information on the treatment of the phonological systems is available. One possibility, developed by Swift and Rosin (1990), presents a remediation sequence for improving intelligibility of children with Down syndrome. Although this program was designed for a specific population of children, it could be adapted for other children with intellectual disabilities (in Swift and Rosin's study, the children were at mild and moderate levels of intellectual disability with little evidence of hypotonicity).

The early linguistic stage emphasizes single words and early two-word utterances. In structured sound play, the clinician selects objects and toys that should elicit intended sounds. For example, if bilabial sounds were targeted, *ball, baby, bye-bye,* and *moo* could be selected. Drill work is then used to increase the target behavior, attention, and syllable sequencing. Swift and Rosin (1990) also use other techniques, such as melodic speech, visual cues, cued speech, auditory bombardment, and an auditory training unit. Overlearned phrases associated with frequently occurring situations (scripts) are trained as well. In addition, augmentative communication is recognized as a valid option within the oral language intervention program.

During the late linguistic stage, drill work and the learning of scripts continue. In addition, repair strategies that could aid overall

CLINICAL APPLICATION

Speech Goals and Activities for Facilitating the Development of Speech and Improving Intelligibility

Miller (1988) offered the following goals and suggestions. Although they were proposed for Down syndrome children, they could be used with other children with intellectual disabilities who are in the beginning stages of speech and language development.

Speech Goals for the Child

1. *Increase the ability to respond to people and objects.* The more this skill can be promoted, the greater the opportunity for enhancing communication.
2. *Increase the frequency of vocal and verbal productions.* The more output, the more opportunity for modifying the quality of speech.
3. *Increase the production of sounds and the variety of sounds made.* This includes not only the actual production of speech sounds but also speaking rate, loudness, and intonation changes. These variables add to the child's intelligibility.
4. *Transition from babbling behavior to using words to represent objects and actions in the environment.* It appears that children who are intellectually disabled are trying to say words earlier than they are recognized by the caregivers in the children's environments. Their speech is often difficult to understand, and the words they use are simply labels but are not descriptive.

speech intelligibility are then taught. Repair strategies include a listener's request for clarification when a message is not understood, for example. Repair strategies from a speaker's point of view include repeating, rewording, and adapting the prosodic features (e.g., slowing the rate, adjusting phrasing, and using stress and inflection to enhance the meaning). Throughout the program, communication should be as functional as possible.

The decision to use an augmentative or alternative system for communication with individuals with intellectual disabilities should be based on the same criteria used with any client. If the cognitive and language comprehension levels allow it, alternative/augmentative communication devices can certainly increase the potential for successful communication. The general advice is to try speech therapy first—for 1 year at least—before nonspeech communicative means are introduced even if all requirements for their use are met (Long & Long, 1994).

Suggestions for Caregivers

1. Identify situations and activities throughout the day in which a child is most vocal. List these situations over a week or two, noting the situation, the length of time they continue, and how many times they occur during the day.
2. Document how much a child responds to people and things by looking, touching, or playing during a particular situation. Communication depends to a large degree on responsiveness.
3. Try to increase the time a child spends in these communication-enhancing situations (noted in speech goal 1).
4. Introduce a child to music at an early age. Children frequently respond enthusiastically to this stimulation. The type of music depends on the child.
5. Speech activities should be a natural part of a child's day. Talk to the child about objects and activities during ordinary caregiving tasks. Introduce interactive games such as "pat-a-cake," "peek-a-boo," and "so big." These activities promote vocalizations and develop responsiveness to turn taking and social interaction.

Based on a thorough assessment, the speech-language clinician can suggest sounds, sound patterns, and words that could be included in activities for a child's day. Suggestions offered in "The Child with an Emerging Phonological System: Therapeutic Suggestions" section of Chapter 10 could also be incorporated here.

CLINICAL EXERCISES

Pick two of the four speech goals for a child (from Miller [1988] on page 366) and give three concrete examples for each of how you could implement this in therapy.

You should treat in a natural environment (page 365), that is, in situations the child encounters on a daily basis or wants and needs that are a portion of his or her daily activities) and follow developmental guidelines. Lucas, age 5;6 with an intellectual disability, has the following sounds: [p, b, t, d, w, h, and f]. According to developmental guidelines, which sound(s) would you target next?

List eight words that you could then target in a natural environment. What types of environments would you target?

Hearing Impairment

Definition and General Features

Hearing loss (or hearing impairment) is a generic term for any diminished ability in normal sound reception. The different etiologies that can result in hearing loss are only indirectly part of this definition. Commonly, hearing loss is described by type and degree of the particular auditory dysfunction (Northern & Downs, 2002). As far as the types of hearing impairment are concerned, conductive, sensorineural, and mixed dysfunctions are distinguished. The degree of hearing loss is categorized by reference to decibel (dB) levels, indicating the increase in intensity needed to make sound audible for the individual in question.

Conductive hearing loss refers to transmission problems affecting the travel of air-conducted sound waves from the external auditory canal to the inner ear. This affects the mechanical transfer of sound waves. A prominent medical condition causing conductive hearing loss is otitis media. **Sensorineural hearing loss** occurs as a consequence of damage to the sensory end organ, the cochlear hair cells, or the auditory nerve. In these cases, air-conduction and bone-conduction thresholds are typically comparable. Mumps, among other medical conditions, can cause a sensorineural auditory dysfunction. If both a conductive and a sensorineural loss can be established, a *mixed hearing loss* exists.

The different degrees of hearing loss indicate the severity of the problem and are calculated according to the (approximate) threshold findings obtained. (*HL* stands for "hearing level.")

26 to 40 dB HL = mild hearing loss

41 to 55 dB HL = moderate hearing loss

56 to 70 dB HL = moderately severe hearing loss

71 to 95 dB HL = severe hearing loss

96 + dB HL = profound loss

Severity levels of hearing loss, which are determined by objective audiometric means, are not necessarily reliable indicators of speech-language function. Individuals deal differently with losses of hearing ability, especially within the context of communication. A loss of 50 dB HL bilaterally in two children, for example, can have a notably different influence on their verbal communication. Such different effects of an objectively established hearing loss can become especially important when dealing with children in various phases of their speech-language development. Even relatively mild auditory dysfunctions with relatively minor communicative consequences for adult speakers/listeners might have lasting detrimental developmental effects in children. Nevertheless, the diminished ability to receive sound for comprehension is normally identified by the degree of hearing loss.

Articulatory/Phonological Characteristics

Speech production in the hearing impaired is affected by the degree of hearing impairment and the frequencies involved. Generally, the greater the hearing loss, the more likely errors extend from consonant to vowel productions to errors in stress, pitch, and voicing (Hull, 2001). Children with bilateral hearing losses are usually described as having speech sound difficulties that are influenced by the amount and quality of acoustic information accessible through their hearing technology and by their listening experiences.

For children with mild to moderate degrees of hearing loss, speech is described as generally intelligible (Eisenberg, 2007). The most common errors involve the production of specific consonants, particularly affricates, fricatives and errors with consonant blends. In this group of children consonant production is generally characterized by deletions and distortions. Vowel productions are generally accurate (Eisenberg, 2007; Elfenbein, Hardin-Jones, & Davis, 1994). Errors are typically described as resembling those of younger children.

In contrast, the speech of children with severe to profound hearing loss has been described as being less intelligible, particularly for those identified late or receive hearing technology at a later age. These children have been described as having difficulties with respiration, phonation, speech rate, consonant production, vowels, suprasegmentals, coarticulatory movements, resonance, and voice quality (e.g., Culbertson, 2007; Ling, 2002). Speech sounds that are particularly difficult include affricates, fricatives, liquids, semivowels, plosives, and, in some cases, nasals (Abraham, 1989). Based on the data obtained from 13 children with severe and profound hearing impairments, Abraham (1989) found that there was a marked difference in the accuracy of production word-initially versus word-finally. All sounds demonstrated a lower percentage of accuracy word-finally. Although the affricates were below 50% accuracy, consonants with even lower percentages of accuracy included [z] and [ð].

Children with hearing impairments have been found to use at least partially rule-governed phonological systems (e.g., Abraham, 1989; Buhler, DeThomasis, Chute, & DeCora, 2007). They use phonological processes similar to those of normally developing young children, although they use these processes more frequently. The overall intelligibility of speech is often reduced, particularly as linguistic complexity increases (Radziewicz & Antonellis, 1997). In a review of several investigations, Flipsen and Parker (2008) identified final consonant deletion, cluster reduction, devoicing of stops, stopping, fronting, liquid simplification, and gliding as the most common developmental processes of children with hearing losses. Among the idiosyncratic processes were initial consonant deletion, glottal stop substitutions, backing, vowel substitution, vowel neutralizations, and diphthong simplification. Final and initial consonant deletions were observed to be very frequent.

In children with cochlear implants, articulatory errors are generally described as being similar to those made by norm hearing children at a younger age. Common phonological processes used by children with cochlear implants have been both developmental and idiosyncratic in nature. They include consonant cluster simplification, stopping, fronting, diphthong simplification, gliding, unstressed syllable deletion, initial consonant deletion, glottal replacement, vowel errors, and assimilation processes (e.g., Buhler et al. 2007; Eriks-Brophy, Gibson, & Tucker, 2013; Flipsen & Parker, 2008).

> Watch this short video of a young girl just getting her first hearing aids. Her reaction is really great.
> youtube.com/watch?v=oyY2JfM1RIM

Clinical Implications: Diagnostics

In addition to audiometric results, the speech-language diagnostician assessing the impact of a client's impaired hearing on the speech sound status needs a host of appraisal data before any diagnostic conclusion can be reached. These include cause, age of onset, and identification of the impairment; its etiology and type; age at which the hearing loss was identified and a hearing device was implemented; and length of previous intervention efforts. Speech intelligibility measures as well as results of formal and informal testing for language skills should also be included in the assessment data. Finally, the client's and caregivers' attitudes toward the disorder and the need for intervention give indications about the degree of motivation and possibly the impact of therapy.

Phonetic and phonological assessments need to be completed for a child with a hearing impairment. Dunn and Newton (1994) outlined the following assessment procedures:

1. *Speech-motor assessment.* This is used to rule out any gross neurological or anatomical limitations that might interfere with speech sound production.
2. *Syllable imitation.* This tests the coordination of the speech mechanism during nonmeaningful speech.
3. *Administration of the Phonetic Level Evaluation (PLE).* This instrument (Ling, 2002) evaluates suprasegmental and segmental skills by imitation of nonsense syllables. The test provides a systematic, comprehensive hierarchy for the assessment of

syllables with varied phonetic contexts. However, the PLE has specific shortcomings (see Dunn & Newton, 1994, pages 130–132) and should not be used as the only evaluative measure for a hearing-impaired child.

4. *Spontaneous speech sample.* Depending on the age and developmental level of a child, this could be either single words or continuous speech. Ideally, the speech sample should include both.

5. *Analysis of the segmental and suprasegmental characteristics of the spontaneous speech sample.* Segmental analysis should include those procedures outlined in this text in Chapter 7 (i.e., consonant and vowel inventory and distribution, syllable shape, and phonological pattern analysis). A suprasegmental analysis determines whether the child uses rate, pauses, stress, and intonational patterns appropriately. This can be done informally with the clinician marking appropriate and inappropriate patterns. Dunn and Newton (1994) suggest a more formal measure developed at the National Technical Institute for the Deaf (Subtelny, 1980). This procedure provides rating scales for a variety of suprasegmental characteristics.

Clinical Implications: Therapeutics

With clients who are hearing impaired, the speech-language clinician's remedial task is mainly directed to improving the client's speech intelligibility. "The term **'speech intelligibility'** may be defined generically as that aspect of oral speech-language output that allows a listener to understand what a speaker is saying" (Carney, 1994, p. 109; emphasis added). Above all, such a task involves, structured work on articulation errors and the selection of a suitable phonetic treatment program. Both of these objectives depend on two prerequisites (Dunn & Newton, 1994):

1. The improvement of the residual hearing by speech signal amplification or cochlear implant and the methodical habituation of its application

2. The maximal use of the level of residual hearing for speech perception through systematic articulatory training.

The first prerequisite presupposes that a client wears an individualized hearing aid at all times and possibly uses auditory trainers during clinical sessions. For a child with a cochlear implant, this means implementing the device and providing training in an intervention program as soon as possible. A primary responsibility of the speech-language clinician called to improve a client's intelligibility level is, therefore, to ensure constant proper amplification, not just during therapy, and to facilitate the client's adjustment to the new hearing situation.

The maximal use of the client's level of residual hearing poses another challenge. Children with hearing impairments miss important information for the recognition of speech signals, which is the main reason for their lack of intelligibility. Essentially, these children produce what they are able to hear, leaving out what they are unable to receive. In directing their attention systematically to specific oral/facial movements accompanying normal suprasegmental and segmental production, their residual hearing can be more effectively used, which in turn, can positively influence intelligibility. In connection with suitable amplification, these efforts should increase speech intelligibility, especially in respect to voice, suprasegmental realization, and vowel production—three especially conspicuous problem areas of children who have hearing impairments.

However, children with hearing impairments also need systematic training on the phonetic as well as the phonological level.

Dunn and Newton (1994) suggest a program that simultaneously teaches phonetic and phonological skills. The training sequence is as follows:

1. *Establish a suprasegmental base.* This is initially achieved through coordination of pitch, duration, and intensity with babbling or vocal play. Once this suprasegmental base is established, it should carry over to the various other stages of treatment. Dunn and Newton state in this context that "clinicians' eagerness to work on consonants before a suprasegmental base is established may result in many of the disordered patterns characteristic of deaf speech" (p. 140).

2. *Teach the segmental speech sounds.* This begins with basic vowel patterns. The patterns are first generated within any context the child can accurately produce, preferably a CV or VC syllable structure. For example, Ling (2002) provides procedures and strategies for achieving a new sound with the population of people who are hearing impaired.

3. *Generalize a stable production by using different phonetic contexts and new syllable types.* Once a production is stable in one basic context, new contexts can be selected. Productions move from various other syllable types to monosyllabic words and, finally, to two-syllable words. With one- and two-syllable words, a child is responsible only for accurate production of the target sound. For example, if the target sound is [b] and the selected word is *boat,* [bo] would be considered an accurate production. Two-syllable words begin with those containing reduplicated syllables such as *bye-bye* or *boo-boo.* In this phase, acceptable speech sound production is applied to meaningful words. In addition, prosodic variation is practiced with these words.

> **CLINICAL EXERCISES**
>
> Which early words could you target that would meet the criteria of numbers 2 and 3 in the Dunn and Newton (1994) guidelines?
>
> How could you establish a suprasegmental base and use these words in therapy?

Motor Speech Disorders: Acquired Apraxia of Speech

Definition and General Features

The general term *apraxia* refers to a disorder in the execution of purposeful movements; reflexive or automatic motor actions remain largely intact. For example, as soon as an otherwise reflexive action is intended—on request, for example, or by one's own volition—gross execution difficulties occur. *Acquired apraxia of speech,* therefore, is the impaired volitional production of articulation and prosody (Ballard, Granier, & Robin, 2000). The primary clinical characteristics considered necessary for the diagnosis of apraxia of speech consists of the following: (1) a slow rate of speech resulting in lengthened sound segments, (2) speech sound errors such as sound distortions or distorted sound substitutions, (3) errors that are relatively consistent in type and location, and (4) disturbed prosody (McNeil, Robin, & Schmidt, 2009). These articulatory and prosodic aberrations do not result from muscle weakness or slowness but from impairment of the central nervous system's programming of oral movements. Apraxia of speech represents an inability to program and sequence articulatory requirements for volitional speech. Thus, **apraxia of speech** is a disorder of expressive communication as a result of brain damage affecting the normal realization of speech sounds, sound sequences, and prosodic features representing speech. Auditory comprehension, in principle, remains intact (Ballard et al., 2000; Duffy, 2005a).

Apraxia of speech is linked to cortical and/or subcortical damage in the language-dominant hemisphere of the brain, but researchers are still uncertain about the specific brain regions involved in apraxia of speech (e.g., Ogar et al., 2006).

Apraxia of speech should be separated from the dysarthrias, another motor speech disorder that affects verbal expression. The following guidelines are given for differentiation between the two (e.g., Shipley & McAfee, 1998):

Apraxia of Speech	Dysarthria
Absence of any muscular weakness, paralytic condition, or discoordination	Presence of muscular weakness; change in muscular tone secondary to neurologic involvement
Speech process of articulation primarily affected	All processes for speech affected: respiration, phonation, resonation, and articulation
Speech errors based on disruption of the central nervous system's programming of oral movements	Speech errors based on disruption of the central and peripheral nervous system's control of muscular movements
Inconsistent articulatory errors	Consistent, predictable articulatory errors

Watch the first few minutes of this individual with apraxia of speech. Note the oral nonverbal apraxic components as the clinician tries to get him to do some nonspeech movements. youtube.com/watch?v=OPjDo03rUd0&list=PLuSyG9vYFwW9Cu2s3tdEZi-5hcz4_LA96

Apraxia of speech differs from the aphasias by the language involvement noted in the aphasias. Apraxia of speech should also be distinguished from **oral (nonverbal) apraxia.** which is a disturbance of planning and executing volitional *nonspeech* movements of oral structures, that is, those movements not representing speech production. For example, a client who is asked to lick her or his lips might blow instead. The same client might be perfectly able to drink some juice, swallow the sip, and lick a drop off her or his lips. On request, though, this person cannot perform the same motor action; attempts probably result in a series of laborious, bizarre trials. As might be expected, clients with apraxia of speech often suffer from oral (nonverbal) apraxia as well.

Articulatory/Phonological Characteristics

The following characteristics of apraxia of speech have been noted (e.g., Croot, 2002; Haley, Ohde, & Wertz, 2000; McNeil et al., 2009):

1. *Effortful, trial-and-error groping of articulatory movements and attempts at self-correction.* This could result in equalization of syllabic stress patterns, slow rate of speech, and other prosodic alterations.
2. *Prosodic disturbances.*
3. *Difficulty initiating utterances.*
4. *Articulatory inconsistency on repeated production of the same utterance.* However, islands of clear, well-articulated speech exist.
5. *Predominance of sound substitution errors.* Additions and prolongations also occur; distortions and omissions are less frequent.
6. *Possible occurrence of sound or syllable transpositions.*
7. *Occasional articulatory errors are complications rather than simplifications.* A consonant cluster could be substituted for a single consonant.
8. *Errors typically related to one another phonetically.* Substitutions, for example, could be related in place or manner of articulation to the intended sound.

9. *More errors on consonants that require more precise articulatory adjustments.* Examples are fricatives and affricates.

10. *Increased number of errors and articulatory struggle as words increase in length.*

11. *Speech comprehension and word recognition abilities often far better than speech production abilities.*

12. *Clients' recognition of their errors.* This could cause numerous retrials or self-correction attempts.

13. *Under otherwise comparable conditions, more sound production errors in stressed than in unstressed syllables.*

> Watch the video of this older woman with apraxia of speech. Which characteristics in the preceding list do you hear? Compare her speech to that of the individual in the previous video. How would you judge her severity? youtube.com/watch?v=dk3oa1cvs04

Clinical Implications: Diagnostics

A diagnosis of apraxia of speech may not have been made before a clinician sees the client. Therefore, the following areas should be included in a thorough evaluation of a client with suspected apraxia of speech (Haynes & Pindzola, 1998):

1. Aphasia test
2. Intelligence, cognitive, and memory tests as needed
3. Apraxia battery
4. Speech-motor mechanism examination
5. Articulation test
6. Spontaneous speech sample

For the purposes at hand, this diagnostic section concentrates on testing procedures that involve only aspects of articulation and phonology—that is, on numbers 3 through 6 of this list of categories.

The speech-motor assessment examines the structure and function of the articulators.

CLINICAL APPLICATION

Formal and Informal Tests for Apraxia of Speech in Adults

Quick Assessment for Apraxia of Speech	Tanner and Culbertson, 1999
The Apraxia Profile Assessment of Apraxia of Speech	Hickman, 1997 Duffy, 2005a
Assessment of Non-Verbal Oral Apraxia	Duffy, 2005b
Test of Oral and Limb Apraxia	Helm-Estabrooks, 1996
Dworkin-Culatta Oral Mechanism Examination	Dworkin and Culatta, 1980
Apraxia Battery for Adults	Dabul, 2000

Some of these tests can be used to evaluate the presence of oral and limb apraxia as well as specific characteristics of apraxia of speech. Others give the clinician information about a client's abilities to sequence words of varying length and complexity.

Although their function is often assessed with one of the apraxia batteries, the oral-mechanism examination can also be used to determine the presence of oral (nonverbal) apraxia. If the structure is intact but commands eliciting nonverbal movements such as "pucker your lips" or "stick out your tongue" result in laborious, bizarre movements, oral apraxia could be suspected.

Both the articulation test and the spontaneous speech sample should answer the following questions:

- *Does the client have difficulty initiating utterances?* Does this difficulty have a pattern? For example, is it better with words or sentences? Does the content of the message play a role?

- *Are there any islands of well-articulated speech?* These are usually automatic-reactive responses such as the days of the week or "I can't say that"; however, are there others?

- *Which sound errors occur?* Evaluate the differences between one-word articulation tests and spontaneous speech. Also note errors that occur as the complexity of the word or utterance increases. Furthermore, register substitutions, additions, prolongations, transpositions, distortions, and omissions.

- *Do sound errors have a pattern?* Errors are typically related to the target sound. A place-manner-voice analysis could demonstrate which patterns are occurring. Observations should include ascertaining difficulties with fricatives, affricates, and consonant clusters, all typical problems for the individual with apraxia of speech.
- *Which prosodic aberrations occur?* Stress realizations (stressed versus unstressed syllables), intonation, rate of speech, and pausing should be observed and analyzed.

Clinical Implications: Therapeutics

In apraxia of speech, the client's ability to program and sequence articulatory requirements for volitional speech is impaired. This impairment ranges from mild to severe; each client demonstrates a different clinical picture. Some could have difficulty only in sequencing certain multisyllabic words or with specific clusters; others could have extreme problems sequencing a simple CV word. Obviously, such varying degrees of impairment influence the selection of therapeutic measures. In addition, certain aspects of motor production affect the error patterns of apraxic speakers (Knock, Ballard, Robin, & Schmidt, 2000; Duffy, 2013; Wambaugh, Martinez, McNeil, & Rogers, 1999). These general guidelines can be used when structuring therapy.

1. *Articulatory accuracy is better for meaningful than for nonmeaningful utterances.* Therefore, avoid nonsense syllables; all treatment stimuli should be meaningful.
2. *Errors increase as words increase in length.* Determine the level at which the client demonstrates accurate production most of the time, and then build on that level. For example, if the assessment reveals that the client can produce CV, CVC, and VC words fairly accurately, start with this level of functioning and slowly build to CVCV structures or "easier" two-syllable words.
3. *Errors increase as the distance between successive points of articulation increases.* Evaluate your word material. Organize it so that this factor is taken into consideration. If you are working on consonant clusters, [st] should be easier than [sk]. If you are structuring words, *toilet* should be easier than *shopping*.
4. *Errors increase on consonants that require more precise articulatory adjustments.* Fricatives, affricates, and consonant clusters are extremely difficult for some clients with apraxia of speech. Begin with other sound classes until more volitional control is achieved.

After an extensive review of the apraxia of speech treatment literature (Wambaugh, Duffy, McNeil, Robin, & Rogers, 2006), the following main categories of treatment for apraxia of speech were noted: (1) articulatory kinematic, (2) rate and/or rhythm, (3) alternative/augmentative communication, and (4) intersystemic facilitation/reorganization. The following is a brief overview of the articulatory kinematic approaches.

1. *Motoric practice.* Stimulation is provided by the clinician, and the client responds with verbal production. Most of these techniques relied on modeling/repetition to elicit productions. A variation was integral stimulation that involved instructing the client to "watch me, listen to me, and say it with me." Repeated practice with limited verbal feedback has been shown to result in improved articulation with persons with chronic apraxia of speech (Wambaugh, Nessler, Cameron, & Mauszycki, 2010).
2. *Use of articulatory placement cues.* This method is used to communicate specific information about sound production. Placement cues have been provided for sounds produced in error and have taken the form of drawings, videotaped models, verbal instructions, and visual modeling. These cues have been used in conjunction with phonetic placement and sound modification techniques.

3. *Use of Prompts for Restructuring Oral Muscular Phonetic Targets (PROMPT, Square, Martin, & Bose, 2001).* This is a technique that provides direct instruction for speech production with a combination of auditory, visual, tactile, and kinesthetic cues that are actively involved in providing sensory input regarding the place of articulatory contact, extent of the jaw opening, and presence and manner of articulation and/ or coarticulation. The cues focus on classes of speech movements and can be applied to isolated sound production gradating to sentence level. This technique has also been utilized with childhood apraxia of speech, children with cerebral palsy, and adults with dysarthria. Because of the relative complexity of the cues provided in the application of PROMPT, therapist training appears to be necessary for correct application. A list of workshops and dates are posted on the PROMPT website.

Motor Speech Disorders: The Dysarthrias

Definition and General Features

The word *articulation* has its origin in the Greek root *arthr-,* referring to the jointed connection between the many different parts of the speaking process. *Dys-arthr-ia,* therefore, literally means "disordered articulation." To be sure, in this context, "articulation" is to be understood in the broadest possible sense, that is, as signifying all articulated movements that result in speech. The technical term *dysarthria,* on the other hand, denotes a rather explicit group of articulation disorders, namely, those caused by neurogenic abnormalities, more specifically by the impairment of a single portion or several portions of the (central and/or peripheral) nervous system that control and coordinate speech. **Dysarthrias** are neuromuscular speech disorders.

Dysarthrias have many different causes. Accident-induced trauma, tumors, cerebrovascular accidents (strokes), congenital conditions, and infectious and degenerative neurogenetic diseases are prominent among them. Each of these events can bring about more or less pronounced paralytic conditions and coordination impairments of the voluntary musculature required for speech production. The result: dysarthrias.

Articulatory/Phonological Characteristics

It is customary to classify the dysarthrias according to the locus of the damage and its neuropathic consequences into five main types:

1. Spastic
2. Ataxic
3. Hypokinetic
4. Hyperkinetic
5. Flaccid

In addition, any simultaneous occurrence of characteristics of several types is categorized as

6. Mixed

Every main type has its cluster of speech impairing phonetic/articulatory production features (Duffy, 2013). They are summarized in Table 11.4

TABLE 11.4 Summary of Features of the Various Types of Dysarthria

Types	Features
Spastic Dysarthria	
(Resulting from upper motor neuron system disorders. Example: pseudobulbar palsy)	
Respiration	Low respiratory frequency with shallow inspiration and lack of expiratory control.
Phonation	Strained, harsh, low-pitch voice; reduced pitch and loudness ranges
Resonation	Hypernasality; nasal air emission
Articulation	Slow, labored, imprecise phoneme realization, especially of consonants.
Ataxic Dysarthria	
(Resulting from cerebellar lesions. Example: cerebellar ataxia)	
Respiration	Shallow inspiration and lack of expiratory control; rapid, irregular, forced breathing patterns
Phonation	Forced, hoarse-breathy, trembling voice; generally reduced (but sometimes excessive) use of pitch and loudness
Resonation	Normal
Articulation	Slow, imprecise phoneme realization, especially of consonants; sound prolongations; irregular pausing between words, syllables, and sounds
Hypokinetic Dysarthria	
(Resulting from disorders of the extrapyramidal system. Example: Parkinsonism)	
Respiration	Frequent respirations with shallow inspiratory phases and lack of expiratory control.
Phonation	Harsh, tremorous voice; reduced pitch and loudness levels
Resonation	Normal
Articulation	Fluctuating imprecise articulation, articulatory bursts, low intelligibility
Hyperkinetic Dysarthria	
(Resulting from disorders of the extrapyramidal system. Examples: athetosis, chorea)	
Respiration	Frequent respirations with shallow inspirations and incomplete expirations; lack of respiratory control
Phonation	Strained, tremorous voice; uncontrolled but generally reduced ranges in the expressive use of pitch and loudness
Resonation	Alternating hypernasality
Articulation	Variable imprecision of sounds, especially consonant, realization
Flaccid Dysarthria	
(Resulting from lower motor neuron system disorders. Example: bulbar palsy)	
Respiration	Shallow, audible inspirations; uneven, incomplete expirations; low respiratory frequency; low expiratory air pressure
Phonation	Breathy, hoarse voice lacking expressive pitch and loudness variation
Resonation	Marked hypernasality with nasal air emission
Articulation	Slow, imprecise phoneme realization, especially of consonants

Source: Summarized from Dworkin (1991); Duffy (2013).

Summaries such as this are helpful, but any division of dysarthric characteristics into just five subtypes suggests more group uniformity than is actually the case. Although some within-group similarities can probably serve as general guidelines, several across-group features overlap considerably. Several of the deficiencies mentioned belong in some measure simply to the clinical picture of most dysarthrias, including the following:

Respiration. Irregular, generally shallow breathing patterns might suddenly become interrupted by some deep breaths, rapid inspiration, incomplete expiration phases, waste of expiratory air during speaking, and lack of respiratory support.

Phonation. Strained voice is characteristic, including deviations from suitable loudness levels (either too loud or too soft) and voice quality (either too harsh or too "breathy," aphonic).

Resonation. Hypernasality and nasal air emission are consequences of incomplete velopharyngeal closure, distorting all speech sounds with the exception of nasals.

Articulation. Labored, indistinct sound articulation, especially of consonants, resulting in distortions or substitutions. Consonant errors might affect whole sound classes; fricatives, for example, might be realized as homorganic stops. Also, second and third elements of consonant clusters might be deleted; rate of speech is usually slower than normal (bradylalia), but bursts of fast speech (tachylalia) might occur as well; qualitative distortions of vowels are also noticeable.

Prosody. Characteristics include a narrow range of intonational configurations ("monopitch") and (often greatly) reduced variety of expressive loudness levels ("monoloudness"). This generally reduced range of prosodic elements is sometimes interrupted by exaggerated stress and intonation patterns (Dworkin, 1991; Patel, 2002).

The physiological basis for all of these characteristics is a striking imbalance in the constant and subtle changes between phases of (relative) muscular tension and relaxation leading to normal speech events. The delicate synergism between the interaction of individual muscles and whole muscle groups to produce speech is in all cases of dysarthria disturbed. Instead, a disproportionate influence of agonistic and antagonistic forces determines dysarthric speech motor activity, distorting its normally smooth flow into effortful, poorly controlled speech production.

Common characteristics such as these exist across and within the main groups of dysarthrias. However, individual clients medically diagnosed with a specific type of dysarthria often show significant deviations from the noted group features. These individual differences are especially important in the assessment and intervention process. The speech-language clinician always needs to find the specific deviations from norm that each individual client displays.

Clinical Implications: Diagnostics

Most clients with dysarthrias are referred to speech-language clinicians by physicians or medical institutions. As a rule, an official diagnosis has already been established, usually down to the subtype the client belongs to medically, for example, spastic dysarthria. What, then, remains for speech-language pathologists to assess and evaluate? Actually, quite a bit.

Even in the appraisal section of the assessment process, speech-language clinicians need to go far beyond the initial (mainly medical) information available. As mentioned earlier, dysarthric subtype characteristics are somewhat vague and indeterminate and, therefore, constitute little more than a point of departure for any appropriate collection of clinical data. They are both helpful and insufficient for clinical purposes. They are helpful because they indicate what to suspect and what to look for. They are insufficient because individual cases more often than not show considerable deviations from average, book-based descriptions. That is why *all* dysarthric symptoms contributing to abnormal voice and speech production need to be appraised as precisely as possible.

CLINICAL APPLICATION

Protocols for the Appraisal of the Speech Characteristics of Clients with Dysarthria

Frenchay Dysarthria Assessment (FDA-2)	Enderby and Palmer, 2008
Dysarthria Examination Battery	Drummond, 1993
Intelligibility Testing in Dysarthria	Kent, Weismer, Kent, and Rosenbek, 1989
Quick Assessment for Dysarthria	Tanner and Culbertson, 1999
Assessments of Intelligibility of Dysarthric Speech	Yorkston and Beukelman, 1981
Robertson Dysarthria Profile	Robertson, 1982

Some of these assessment instruments give profiles for the various diagnostic categories, whereas others provide severity ratings.

One possible aid to precise appraisal is the use of instrumentation. There is certainly no scarcity of instruments available to use to objectify the data. The problem does not lie in a lack of suitable instrumentation but in their proper application to the task at hand. Many clinicians are not trained well enough in instrumentation to feel comfortable with its use or do not have easy access to instrumentation. Another reason for the rare use of instruments in a clinical setting is a time concern: Clinicians feel too pressed for time to engage in the use of instruments to make their appraisal data more objective and verifiable.

A second way to make the appraisal of clients with dysarthrias more comparable, reliable, and precise is the use of a suitable protocol. Such a protocol might look like the one in Appendix 11.1.

After having identified the type and severity of the dysarthric disturbances within the main subsystems contributing to speech, speech/language clinicians are ready to interpret and evaluate them in their totality; that is, they could draw a composite picture of the problem at hand—make a diagnosis in the narrow sense of the term. Diagnoses lead directly into therapy planning and form the very basis for the professional selection of appropriate intervention measures.

Clinical Implications: Therapeutics

The speech-language clinician's main therapeutic goal is the improvement of the client's intelligibility. Because the established deficits are caused by central and/or peripheral nervous system damage, this is done primarily by searching for compensatory measures and training for them. The diagnostic results should provide the necessary information about the type and degree of shortcomings in the various subsystems constituting normal speech production (i.e., respiration, phonation, resonation, and articulation). This information becomes the basis for therapy planning.

Most therapy plans are based on the principle of treating disordered facets of the subsystems contributing to speech thoroughly and methodically (e.g., Dworkin, 1991; McHenry, 2003; Rosenbek & Jones, 2009; Yorkston, 1996). Because speech results from cumulative effects of secondary physiological functions, the primary functions of structures in which speech is rooted must be considered as well. Thus, speech breathing has to evolve out of systematically modified breathing patterns for vital silent breathing; articulatory functions out of natural conditions of lip, tongue, and jaw movements; and the voicing/unvoicing of sound segments and suitable intonation patterning out of previously normalized voice production. In this way, an elaborate system of suitable exercises is created and diligently practiced. If aspects of different subsystems need to be combined—as in the case of respiratory preconditions for specific voice effects such as changes in pitch, loudness, quality, and quantity—matters can quickly become complicated. Superior planning and tenacity as well as flexibility during the implementation of the program are prerequisite ingredients for the successful treatment of practically all clients with dysarthria. A general guideline for this task pertains to the observance of certain sequences. For example, postural adjustments precede every specific measure; respiratory and resonatory dysfunctions must be addressed before phonatory, articulatory, and prosodic ones.

Rosenbek and Jones (2009) summarized the following general treatment goals:

1. *Help the person become a productive patient.* Clinician and client have agreed on the necessity and value of treatment, what is to be accomplished, and the treatment procedures.
2. *Modify abnormalities of posture, tone, and strength.*
3. *Modify respiration.*
4. *Modify phonation.*
5. *Modify resonation.*
6. *Modify articulation.*
7. *Modify prosody.*
8. *If indicated, provide alternative or augmentative modes of communication.*

The ordering of these goals does not imply a certain progression with one exception: The patient must accept an active role in treatment before changes in speech are possible.

Dworkin (1991) provides a procedure based on a specific order of speech subsystems. The first-order subsystems consist of resonation and respiration; the second order is phonation; and the third order consists of articulation and prosody. First-order subsystems are treated first, second-order subsystems next, and third-order subsystems are last in the treatment sequence. Inhibition and facilitation techniques probably need to precede the specific subsystem treatments. Inhibition techniques are implemented for increased tone and any associated weakness and paresis, hyperactive reflexes, hyperkinesia, and hypersensitivity. On the other hand, facilitation techniques are introduced to improve functioning of any of the following abnormal features: decreased tone and associated weakness and paresis, hypoactive reflexes, and hyposensitivity.

Dworkin (1991) provided the following general treatment objectives:

1. Promote adequate orofacial postures.
2. Promote integration of orofacial reflexes.
3. Improve orofacial muscle tone and strength.
4. Improve range, speed, timing, and coordination of orofacial muscle activities.

These general goals must be based on a treatment hierarchy that includes first-, second-, and third-order subsystems. Detailed exercises for each of the subsystems are included in Dworkin (1991).

CLINICAL EXERCISES

According to Dworkin (1991), an ordering of subsystems is worked on in a progressive fashion. The first-order subsystem consists of respiration and phonation.

Explain why these would be first-order subsystems. How do the other subsystems build on these first-order ones?

Based on information in your other textbooks or readings, what are some specific practical techniques you could implement to treat the first-order subsystems?

SUMMARY

Several communication disorders exist with articulatory/phonological deficits as one of their central characteristics. This chapter provided an overview of the most prominent among them. First, the childhood disorders childhood apraxia of speech, cerebral palsy, cleft palate, cognitive impairment, and hearing impairment have been reviewed. Acquired communication disorders with articulatory deficits commonly occurring in adults were then represented by apraxia of speech and the dysarthrias. Each of these disorders has been defined, and general characteristics have been listed. This outline served as a foundation for the subsequent discussion of specific articulatory and phonological problems that are found in these populations. Assessment principles for the respective speech problems noted have been identified followed by selected therapeutic measures for the treatment of individuals within the seven populations.

For each of the disorders mentioned, an impressive list of specialized literature exists. References have been given throughout the chapter to guide interested students and practitioners to more in-depth information. Each disorder represents a complex entity, including many important variables and involving several groups of professionals. This chapter briefly summarized basic considerations of articulatory and phonological features and their clinical intervention.

CASE STUDY

The following results are from the Hodson Assessment of Phonological Patterns (HAPP-3) (Hodson, 2004) for Dillon, age 5;6. Dillon has been diagnosed with childhood apraxia of speech.

1. basket	[bæ.ə]	18. leaf	[jit]
2. boats	[boᵁ]	19. mask	[mæt]
3. candle	[dæ.nə]	20. music box	[mu.ɪt. bɑ]
4. chair	[teᵊ]	21. page	[beˈt]
5. clouds	[daᵁ]	22. plane	[beˈn]
6. cowboy hat	[taᵁ·bə.æt]	23. queen	[din]
7. feather	[bɛ.də]	24. rock	[wɑ]
8. fish	[bɪt]	25. screwdriver	[du.daˈ.ə]
9. flower	[daᵁ.ə]	26. shoe	[du]
10. fork	[fot]	27. slide	[daˈt]
11. glasses	[dæ.ət]	28. smoke	[moᵁt]
12. glove	[dʌb]	29. snake	[deˈt]
13. gum	[dʌm]	30. soap	[doᵁp]
14. hanger	[æn.ə]	31. spoon	[bun]
15. horse	[oᵊt]	32. square	[dɛ.ə]
16. ice cubes	[aˈ.tu]	33. star	[dɑᵊ]
17. jumping	[dʌm]	34. string	[twɪn]

35. swimming	[tɪ.mɪn]		43. crayons	[deˈ.ə]
36. television (TV)	[tɛ.bi]		44. black	[bæt]
37. toothbrush	[tu.bət]		45. green	[din]
38. truck	[tjʌk]		46. yellow	[jɛ.joʊ]
39. vase	[beˈd]		47. three	[ti]
40. watch	[wɑt]		48. thumb	[dʌm]
41. yoyo	[joʊ.joʊ]		49. nose	[noʊd]
42. zip	[jɪp]		50. mouth	[maʊf]

Although Dillon appears to have a fairly complete vowel inventory with the exception of central vowels with r-coloring, his consonant repertoire is extremely limited. There are no fricatives, affricates, lateral, or central approximants represented in this sample. At age 5;6, Dillon was considered highly unintelligible.

THINK CRITICALLY

1. Refer to the case study of Dillon, age 5;6. Which consonants does he have in the prevocalic, intervocalic, and postvocalic positions? Given the fact that most children demonstrate a much larger inventory of consonants in the prevocalic position, what comments could you make about Dillon's inventory?
2. Which syllable shapes are present in the speech sample from Dillon? Do you see any evidence of CC structures?
3. Note the collapse of phonemic contrasts in his speech. Do you see any sound preferences?

TEST YOURSELF

1. Although an exact delineation of symptoms to describe childhood apraxia of speech is controversial, what is considered to be central to the disorder?
   a. oral weakness
   b. sequencing errors
   c. a central nervous system disorder
   d. intellectual impairment
2. Speech-related respiratory, phonatory, articulatory, and prosodic abnormalities, as well as velopharyngeal inadequacies, are primarily associated with
   a. developmental apraxia of speech
   b. hearing losses
   c. cerebral palsy
   d. intellectual disability
3. A management plan for a child with a cleft palate usually involves
   a. long-term care with a team of specialists
   b. short-term care with only a surgeon
   c. long-term care with only a speech-language pathologist
   d. short-term care with a team of specialists
4. Compensatory articulation errors for stop production in children with cleft palate include use of which of the following?
   a. glottal and laryngeal stops
   b. gliding of fricatives
   c. fronting
   d. deaffrication

5. It is estimated that a very large percentage of this group of children has some type of hearing loss.
   a. children with childhood apraxia of speech
   b. children with an intellectual disability
   c. children with a language disorder
   d. all of the above

6. The phonological patterns of children with an intellectual disability can be summarized as
   a. each child has a similar communication difficulty
   b. deletion of consonants is the most frequent error
   c. error patterns are consistent
   d. difficulty is with only r-sounds

7. The degree of speech production difficulty in individuals with a hearing impairment is related to
   a. the type of hearing aid used
   b. the degree of hearing loss
   c. the type of hearing loss
   d. b. and c.

8. Children with a moderate to severe hearing loss need training with which of the following?
   a. suprasegmental aspects of speech
   b. oral-motor movements
   c. velopharyngeal function
   d. swallowing

9. Which of the following is associated with acquired apraxia of speech?
   a. presence of muscular weakness and changes in muscular tone
   b. absence of paralytic conditions
   c. speech errors resulting from the disruption of the central and peripheral nervous systems' muscular movements
   d. consistent, predictable articulatory errors

10. In treating an adult with dysarthria, which of the following is *not* a treatment goal?
    a. modifying respiration
    b. modifying prosodic aspects of speech
    c. modifying the backing of stop consonants
    d. modifying any abnormalities in phonation and resonation

FURTHER READINGS

Duffy, J. R. (2013). *Motor speech disorders: Substrate, differential diagnosis, and management* (3rd ed.). St Louis, MO: Elsevier Mosby.

Falzone, S., Cardamone, J., Karnell, M., & Jones, M. (2006). *The clinician's guide to treating cleft palate speech.* Cambridge, MA: Elsevier.

Hull, R. (2001). *Aural rehabilitation: Serving children and adults.* Clifton Park, NY: Thomson-Delmar Learning.

Velleman, S. (2003). *Childhood apraxia of speech: Resource guide.* Clifton Park, NY: Thomson-Delmar Learning.

Workinger, M. S. (2005). *Cerebral palsy: Resource guide for speech-language pathologists.* Clifton Park, NY: Thomson-Delmar Learning.

APPENDIX 11.1   Protocol for Assessing Respiration, Phonation, Resonation, and Articulation of Dysarthric Speech

1. Rate the degree of normal, near normal, or abnormal behavior on a scale from 1 to 5 by marking the double line at the judged value.

	normal		$\longrightarrow$		abnormal
	1	2	3	4	5

Respiration
Silent breathing --
Speech breathing --
   Inspiration --
   Expiration --
   Breath support --
   Shouting --
   Shortness of breath --

Resonation
Nasality --
Quality of prolonged vowels
(check one) --
   Constant ☐
   Intermittent ☐

Phonation
Voice --
Pitch --
Volume --

Lips
Appearance in resting position --
Lip protrusion --
Movement during speaking --

Jaw
Appearance in resting position --
Movement during speaking --

Tongue
Appearance in resting position --
Protrusion --
Elevating tip of tongue --
Lowering tip of tongue --
Lateral movements --
During speaking --
Strength --

Articulation
Vowels
Quality --
   Duration --
   Consonants --
   Clusters --

Prosody
Stress --
Intonation --
Tempo --
Rhythm --

2. Itemize the most salient characteristic in each of the categories with a rating of 3 or more.

3. Repeat the rating process at least one more time on a different day.

Glossary

acoustic phonenics Study of the transmission properties of speech.

active articulator Parts within the vocal tract that actually move to achieve the articulatory result.

addental [s] A frequent s-sound distortion marked by an articulatory variation in which the tongue approaches the upper incisors, causing the resulting s-sound to lose its regular stridency, giving a "dull" or "flat" sound impression.

affricate Manner of articulation marked by a homorganic release of a stop with the auditory effect of a stop + fricative sequence. Example: [tʃ].

affrication Replacement of fricatives by homorganic affricates. Example: [tʃu] for *shoe*.

age appropriate In accordance with developmental norm values of a given age.

allophones Variations in phoneme realizations that do not change the meaning of a word when they are produced in various contexts.

allophonic variation The phonetic realization of a phoneme; also called *phonetic variation*. *See:* speech sounds.

alveolar Alveolar ridge as place of articulation for consonant production. Example: [t].

alveolarization Change of nonalveolar sounds, mostly interdentals and labio-dentals, into alveolar sounds.

anticipatory assimilation *See:* regressive assimilation.

apical Tip of the tongue as the active articulator for consonant production. Example: [θ].

apico-alveolar Articulated with the apex of the tongue (as active articular) touching or near the alveolar ridge (as passive articulator).

appraisal Collection of data to be interpreted and evaluated in the diagnostic phase.

approximant Speech sounds marked by a much wider passage of air, resulting in a smooth (as opposed to turbulent) airflow for these voiced sounds. Example: [w], [j].

apraxia of speech Disorder of expressive communication as a result of brain damage affecting the normal realization of speech sounds, sound sequences, and prosodic features representing speech.

articulation The totality motor movements involved in production of the actual sounds that comprise speech.

articulation disorder A subcategory of a speech disorder, which is the atypical production of speech sounds characterized by substitutions, omissions, additions, or distortions that may interfere with intelligibility. Articulation-based disorders are phonetic in nature. *See:* phonological disorder.

articulators Anatomical structures used to generate speech sounds: active and passive articulators.

articulatory backing Compensatory measure of children with cleft palate to produce speech sounds more posteriorly in the oral cavity than is normally the case. *See also:* backing.

articulatory phonetics Production features of speech sounds, their categorization, and classification according to specific details of their production.

aspirate Voiceless unlocalized open consonant.

assessment Clinical evaluation of a client's disorder.

assimilation Adaptive articulatory change by which one speech sound becomes similar, sometimes identical, to a neighboring sound segment.

assimilatory process Perfectly natural consequences of normal speech production by which one speech sound becomes similar, sometimes identical, to a neighboring sound. Also called harmony process.

auditory phonetics Study of speech (sound) perception.

augmentative and alternative communication (AAC) Means of compensation for temporary or permanent impairments, activity limitations, and participation restrictions of individuals with severe disorders of speech-language production and/or comprehension, including spoken and written modes of communication

autosegmental phonology One of the nonlinear phonologies proposing that changes within the boundary of a segment could be factored out and put onto another "tier."

avoidance factor The avoidance of words by a child that do not contain sounds within a specific child's inventory.

backing A substitution in which the active and/or passive place of articulation is more posteriorly located than the intended sound.

bifid uvula Uvula that is medially divided into two portions, a split uvula (uvula bifida).

binary system Methodology using a plus (+) and minus (−) system to signal the presence (+) or absence (−) of certain features.

broad transcription Based on the phoneme system of the particular language in which each symbol represents a phoneme.

bunched "r" Referring to the "bunched" corpus of the tongue during an r-sound production.

canonical babbling Term for the reduplicated and nonreduplicated babbling stages.

categorical perception Ability of listeners to perceive speech sounds varied along a continuum according to the phonemic categories of their native language.

centering diphthong A diphthong in which the off-glide, or less prominent element, is the central vowel [ə] or [ɚ]. Examples: *bar* [bɑɚ] or *wear* [wɛɚ].

cerebral palsy (CP) Nonprogressive disorder of motor control caused by damage to the developing brain during pre-, peri-, or early postnatal periods.

checked syllable *See:* closed syllable.

childhood apraxia of speech (CAS) Neurological childhood (pediatric) speech sound disorder in which the precision and consistency of movements underlying speech are impaired in the absence of neuromuscular deficits (e.g., abnormal reflexes, abnormal tone). The main difficulty appears to be the planning and/or programming of spatio-temporal parameters of movement sequences that results in errors in speech sound production and prosody.

citation articulation test Examination of speech sound articulation in selected isolated words.

citing Giving a single-word test response. Example: naming a picture.

clefting Dividing a continuous structure by a cleavage or splitting prominently caused by a failure of the palate to fuse during fetal development.

close Relative nearness of the dorsum of the tongue and the roof of the mouth during vowel production. Example: [u] (when compared to [ʊ]).

closed syllable Checked syllable. A syllable that has a coda. Example: *stop*.

coalescence Merger of neighboring sound segments into a new and different segment.

coarticulation Concept that the articulators are continually moving into position for other segments over a stretch of speech.

coda All sound segments of a syllable following its peak.

code switching Changing back and forth between varieties of dialects, in this case, specifically between African American Vernacular English and General American English; also referred to as *code mixing*.

coding Translating stimuli from one form to another. Example: from auditory to written form or from written to auditory

code mixing In this developmental process, speakers alternate between L1 and L2. This may occur within a phrase or between sentences.

cognate Similarity between two sounds; can refer to similar vowels or consonants that differ only in voicing features. Example: [i] and [ɪ] are i-type vowels, and [p] and [b] are cognates.

communication Sharing information between individuals; any act in which information is given to or received from another person concerning that person's needs, desires, perceptions, knowledge, or affective states.

communication augmentation Addition of any approach designed to support, enhance, or increase the communication of individuals who cannot use speech in all situations.

communication disorder Impairment in the ability to receive, send, process, and comprehend concepts including verbal, nonverbal, and graphic symbol systems.

complete assimilation *See:* total assimilation.

comprehensive evaluation Activities and tests that allows a more detailed and complete collection of data than screenings.

conductive hearing loss Transmission problem affecting the travel of air-conducted sound waves from the external auditory canal to the inner ear.

consonant Speech sound with a significant constriction in the vocal tract, mainly in the oral and pharyngeal cavities, foremost along the oral cavity's sagittal midline.

contact assimilation Adaptive process modifying immediately adjacent sounds; also called *contiguous assimilation.*

contiguous assimilation *See:* contact assimilation.

contoid Nonphonemic consonantlike sound production.

coronal Pertaining to the corona of the tongue (frontal and lateral edges) as the active articulator. Example: [d] is a coronal articulation.

coronal place node Place of articulation of both the tongue tip and the tongue blade segments in feature geometry.

cueing techniques Visual and/or tactile cues used to help a child articulate certain sounds or sound sequences.

culture Way of life developed by a group of individuals to meet psychosocial needs; consists of values, norms, beliefs, attitudes, behavioral styles, and traditions that can impact a dialect.

deaffrication Realization of affricates as homorganic fricatives. Example: [ʃiz] for *cheese.*

deep structure *See:* underlying form

denasalization Replacement of nasals by homorganic stops. Example: [dud] for *noon.*

dental The upper teeth as place of articulation for consonant production. Example: [f] is a dental articulation.

dentalization Nonstandard articulatory variation in the production of nondental consonants: use of the dental place of articulation for a nondental consonant. Example: [s̪] for [s].

derhotacization Loss of r-coloring during the production of [r] and rhotacized central vowels.

derivational morpheme Any grammatically significant addition to a word stem by affixes (prefixes, infixes, suffixes).

developmental apraxia of speech (DAS) *See:* childhood apraxia of speech (CAS).

developmental verbal dyspraxia (DVD) *See:* childhood apraxia of speech (CAS).

diacritics Marks added to sound transcription symbols to give them a particular phonetic value.

diadochokinetic rates Maximum repetitions of the syllables [pʌ], [tʌ], and [kʌ] alone and in various combinations.

diagnosis Result of studying and interpreting of data collected during an appraisal.

dialect Neutral label that refers to any variety of a language that is shared by a group of speakers.

diphthong Gliding monosyllabic speech sound in which a change in quality occurs in its duration.

distinctive features Phonetic constituents that distinguish between phonemes.

distribution of speech sounds Where the norm and aberrant articulations occurred in a word.

dorsal place node In feature geometry, those segments (vowels and consonants) that are articulated with the dorsum of the tongue.

dorsum Surface area of the tongue.

duration symbols Diacritics that mark the length of speech sounds.

dysarthrias Neuromuscular speech disorders.

emerging phonology The time span during childhood in which conventional words begin to appear as a means of communication.

epenthesis Syllable structure process marked by the insertion of a sound segment into a word, primarily (but not always) a schwa insertion between two consonants. Example: [pəliz] for *please*.

ethnic dialects Language variations that are generally related to ethnic background.

ethnicity Commonalities such as religion, nationality, and region that can affect a dialect.

facilitating context Phonetic aspect of neighboring speech sounds able to support sound features to be acquired.

feature geometry Group of nonlinear phonological theories that have adopted the tiered representation of features used in autosegmental phonology; an attempt to explain why some features are affected by assimilation processes (known as *spreading* or *linking* of features), whereas others are affected by neutralization or deletion processes (known as *delinking*).

final consonant deletion A syllable structure process by which a CVC syllable is converted into a CV syllable due to the omission of the final consonant. The omission of a syllable-arresting consonant.

first word An entity of relatively stable phonetic form that is produced consistently by a child in a particular context and that is recognizably related to the adultlike word form of a particular language.

Formal Standard English Language type that applies primarily to written language (and based on it) and the most formal spoken language situations; exemplified in guides of usage or grammar texts.

fortis Production of relatively more articulatory effort among consonant cognates Example: voiceless stop-plosives.

fricative Consonant characterized by an audible friction noise established by forcing expiratory air through a constricted passage in the oral cavity. Example: extensive constriction causes the hissing noise of sibilants, a subcategory of fricatives: [s], [ʃ].

fronting A substitution process marked by more anterior placement of active and passive articulators. Example: t/k substitution.

generative phonology The application of principles of generative (or transformational) grammar to phonology.

glide Manner of articulation; a shift in movement of the articulators from a narrower to a wider consonantal constriction. Example: [w]; also called *semivowel, sonorant.*

gliding Substitution process characterized by the replacement of primarily liquids with glides.

gliding of liquids/fricatives Replacement of liquids or fricatives by glides. Example: [wɛd] for *red.*

glossing Repeating with normal pronunciation what a client has just said for easier identification later.

groping behavior Ongoing series of movements of the articulators in an attempt to find the desired articulatory position.

harmony process *See:* assimilation process.

hearing loss Generic term for any diminished ability in normal sound reception.

holophrastic period Span of time during which a child uses one word to indicate a complete idea.

idiosyncratic (or unusual) error pattern Type of error patterns not (or infrequently) seen in the normal speech development of children.

idiosyncratic processes Phonological patterns found in the speech of individual children with phonemic-based disorders.

independent analysis Assessment that considers only the client's productions without comparing them to the adult norm model.

individual sound approach Traditional or motor method referring to the treatment of individual speech sounds in sequence. *See:* motor approach.

Informal Standard English Based on the assessment by members of the American English-speaking community as they judge the "standardness" of other speakers; relative to a continuum between formal English and vernacular English.

intelligibility Individual's ability to be understood determined by a listener based on how much of an utterance can be recognized.

interdental "s" Frequent s-sound distortion marked by the visibility of the tongue tip between the upper and lower incisors; sounds very much like [θ] and [ð], respectively.

interference Impact of an individual's first language (L1) on English (L2); L2 error results from the direct influence of L1.

intervocalic Referring to consonants or consonant clusters between two vowels, typically at the juncture of two syllables.

inventory of speech sounds List of speech sounds that the client can articulate within normal limits.

item learning Acquisition of word forms as unanalyzed units and as productional wholes.

jargon stage Period characterized by strings of babbled utterances that are modulated primarily by intonation, rhythm, and pausing.

juncture symbols Diacritics that mark juncture phenomena in an utterance. Example: *a + nice man* versus *an + ice man*.

labial Relating to the lips; describes the active articulator as the lower lip or the passive articulator as the upper lip. Example: [m] (bilabial).

labial assimilation Process of changing a nonlabial into a labial sound under the influence of a neighboring labial sound.

labialization Consonant productions with lip rounding. Example: [s^{w}up] for [sup].

labial place node In feature geometry, the place that designates the lip articulation of the rounded vowels and the consonants in General American English.

language Complex and dynamic system of conventional symbols used in various modes for thought and communication.

language disorder Impaired comprehension and/or use of spoken, written, and/or other symbol systems.

laryngeal node In feature geometry, the place that designates the glottal characteristics of the segment.

lateral Description of the manner of articulation in which a midline closure in the oral cavity is accompanied by the lowering of the edges of the tongue which lets the expiratory airstream pass laterally into the cheeks. Example: [l].

lateral "s" Description of the nonstandard s-sound production characterized by (uni- or bilateral) airflow during /s/ realizations.

lax Referring to a lesser degree of muscular activity during vowel production. Example: [ɪ] (when contrasted to [i]).

lenis Comparatively less articulatory effort between consonant cognates. Example: voiced stop-plosives are lenis productions.

limited English proficient Terminology for any individual between the ages of 3 and 21 who is enrolled or preparing to enroll in an elementary or secondary school, who was not born in the United States, or whose native language is a language other than English. Individuals who are Native Americans or Alaska Natives and come from an environment where a language other than English has had a significant impact on the individuals are also included in this definition. The difficulties in speaking, writing, or understanding the English language compromise the individual's ability to successfully achieve in classrooms, where the language of instruction is English or to participate fully in society (PL107-110, The No Child Left Behind Act of 2001).

linear phonologies Phoneme theories characterized by an assumption that all meaning-distinguishing sound segments are serially arranged.

linkage condition Any state or being governing the association of units on different tiers.

lip symbols Diacritics that mark rounding or unrounding of the lips during normally unrounded or rounded consonant realizations. Example: [t^{w}ɪn] = labialized, rounded [t].

liquid Group term for the consonant categories laterals and rhotics.

liquid assimilation Adaptive articulatory influence of a liquid on a neighboring nonliquid sound.

manner of articulation Type of constriction that the active and passive articulators produce for the realization of a particular consonant.

manner of articulation features Term used in generative phonology regarding the way active and passive articulators cooperate to produce sound classes, signaling differences between stops and fricatives, for example.

markedness (of phonemes). Sound that is relatively difficult to produce and less frequent in languages.

mediodorsal Central portion of the tongue as the active articulator for consonant production. Example: [j].

mediopalatal Central portion of the hard palate as the passive articulator for consonant production. Example: [j].

metalinguistic awareness The ability to think about and reflect on the nature of language and how it functions.

metaphonology Conscious awareness of the sounds in a particular language.

metaphon therapy Treatment approach marked by the systematic training of phonological awareness, especially the awareness of sound properties.

metathesis Transposition of sounds in an utterance.

metrical phonology One of the nonlinear theories of phonemes emphasizing stress and using metrical trees that reflect the syntactic structure of an utterance.

micrognathia Condition in which the mandible is unusually small.

minimal pair Set of words that differ in only one phoneme value among their sound constituents. Example: *book* versus *cook*.

minimal pair contrast therapy Treatment that uses pairs of words that differ by one phoneme only.

monophthong Vowel that remains qualitatively the same throughout its entire production; a pure vowel.

morpheme Smallest meaningful unit of a language. Examples: "hits" consists of two morphemes "hit" and "s".

morphology Study of the structure of words.

morphophonemic function Role of phonemes to signal grammatical units. For example, /s/ is a phoneme of the English language as demonstrable by the minimal pair *sick* versus *thick*. However, /s/ also signals plurality, *book* versus *book*s, a morphological function.

morphophonology Study of the different allomorphs of the morpheme and the rules governing their use.

motor approach Procedure that treats individual sounds based on the placement of the articulators for normal speech sound production. *See:* individual sound approach.

motor-based problem Phonetic disorder characterized by misarticulations seen as disruptions at a relatively peripheral level of the articulatory process involving inadequate motor learning.

multilinear phonologies *See:* nonlinear phonologies.

multiple-sound approach Therapy technique in which several error sounds are simultaneously treated.

narrow transcription Recording of sound units with as much production detail as possible; encompasses the use of both the broad classification system noted in the International Phonetic Alphabet and extra symbols that can give a particular phonetic value.

nasal Type of articulation in which consonants are produced with the velum lowered so that the expiratory air can pass freely through the nasal cavity. Example: [m].

nasal assimilation Articulatory adaptation caused by the influence of a nasal on a neighboring non-nasal sound.

nasality symbols Diacritics to mark the passing/nonpassing of expiratory air through the nasal cavity. Only nonnasal sounds can be nasalized, only nasals denasalized.

nasal "s" Irregular s-productions marked by nasal airflow due to incomplete nasal-pharyngeal closure.

natural class Group of phonemes that share one or more features and usually have similar patterns in a language system. *See:* naturalness.

naturalness (of phonemes) Designates (1) the relative simplicity of a sound production and (2) the sound's high frequency of occurrence in languages.

natural phonology Theory that incorporates features of naturalness and was specifically designed to explain the development of a child's phonological system.

natural process Speech sound pattern that is common in the speech development of children across languages.

near-minimal pairs Sets of two words that differ by more than one phoneme; the vowel preceding or following the target sound remains constant in both words.

noncontiguous assimilation *See:* remote assimilation.

nonlinear phonologies Group of theories that regards phoneme segments being governed by more complex linguistic dimensions.

nonphonemic diphthong Vowel that can be realized in its onset only without a change in word meaning. Example: [heɪ] or [he] for *hay*.

nonreduplicated babbling Stage of prelinguistic development that demonstrates variation of both consonants and vowels from syllable to syllable.

obstruents Consonants characterized by a complete or narrow constriction between the articulators hindering the expiratory airstream; includes the stop-plosives, the fricatives, and the affricates.

offglide End portion of a diphthong. Example: [ɪ] in [eɪ].

onglide Beginning portion of a diphthong. Example: [e] in [eɪ].

onset All sound segments of a syllable prior to its peak.

open Referring to the relative open space between the dorsum of the tongue and the roof of the mouth during vowel production. Example: [ʊ] (when contrasted to [u]).

open syllable A syllable that does not contain a coda. Example: *do. See* unchecked syllable.

optimality theory Constraint-based approach, which is one nonlinear (multilinear) theory of phonology.

oral (nonverbal) apraxia Disturbance of the planning and execution of volitional *nonspeech* movements of oral structures.

oral stops Interruptions of articulation by obstruction of the oral cavity but allowances of free airstream passage through the nasal cavity. Example: nasals.

organ of articulation Part in the vocal tract that actually moves to achieve the articulatory result; the active articulator.

palatal Relating to some part of the hard palate as the place of articulation for consonant production.

palatalization Articulatory variation in the production of consonants; use of the palate as place of articulation for nonpalatal consonants.

palatal "s" Irregular s-production characterized by a palatal (rather than alveolar or predorsal)

approximation of the active and passive articulators resulting in an auditory impression approximating a voiceless sh-sound, transcribed as [sʲ].

partial assimilation Adaptive influence of one sound segment on another which results in a higher degree of similarity between the respective sound segments.

passive articulator Area in the vocal tract that is directly involved in the articulation of consonants but is stationary.

peak Most prominent, acoustically intense part of a syllable; usually a vowel.

perceptual constancy Ability to identify the same sound across different speakers, pitches, and other changing environmental conditions.

perseverative assimilation *See:* progressive assimilation.

persisting normal processes Patterns indicating the use of certain phonological processes beyond their typical age limits.

phoneme Smallest linguistic unit that is able, when combined with other such units, to establish word meanings between words.

phonemic awareness An understanding that words are composed of individual sounds.

phonemic diphthong Meaning would change in a particular word if only the vowel onglide was produced. Example: [mas] versus [maᵁs].

phonemic error Replacement of one General American English phoneme with another.

phonemic inventory Repertoire of phonemes used contrastively by an individual.

phonemic problem Misarticulation based on difficulties with the language-specific linguistic function of phonemes.

phonemic transcription Transcription based on the phoneme system of the particular language; each symbol represents a phoneme. *See:* broad transcription.

phonetically consistent form *See:* proto-word, quasi-word, vocable.

phonetic approaches Therapy method that treats each error sound individually, one after the other; also referred to as *traditional-motor approaches.*

phonetic context Segmental, suprasegmental, and phonotactic environment in which a given speech sound occurs.

phonetic inventory Repertoire of speech sounds for a particular client, including all the characteristic production features the client uses.

phonetic placement method Procedure in which a clinician instructs a client how to position the articulators to produce a norm production.

phonetic problem Any misarticulation based on phonetic production difficulties.

phonetics Study of speech emphasizing the description and classification of speech sounds according to their production, transmission, and perceptual features.

phonetic transcription Recording process in which the sound units are written with as much production detail as possible; encompasses the use of both the broad classification system noted in the International Phonetic Alphabet and extra symbols that can be added to give a particular phonetic value; to characterize specific production features. *See:* narrow transcription.

phonetic variability Instability of pronunciations of a child's first 50 words.

phonetic variation Actual realization of a phoneme; also called *allophonic variation.*

phonological awareness The individual's awareness of the sound structure or phonological structure of a spoken word in contrast to written words.

phonological development Acquisition of speech sound form and function in a language system.

phonological disorder/phonemic-based disorder Impaired comprehension and/or use of the sound system of a language and the rules that govern the sound combinations.

phonological idiom Accurate sound productions that are later replaced by inaccurate ones; also called *regression.*

phonological process "Mental operation that applies in speech to substitute for a class of sounds or sound sequences presenting a common difficulty to the speech capacity of the individual" (Stampe, 1979, p. 1).

phonological processing Using sounds of a language to process verbal information in oral or written form that requires working and long-term memory.

phonological rules Notations used to demonstrate the relationship between the underlying (phonological) and the surface (phonetic) forms; in generative

phonological analysis, formalized statements about the patterns of sound substitutions and deletions.

phonology Study of the sound system of a language; examines the sound units of that particular language, how these units are arranged, their systematic organization and rule system.

phonotactics Study of the allowed combinations of phonemes in a particular language.

place node In feature geometry, category that groups together all different places of articulation.

place of articulation The area within the vocal tract that remains motionless during consonant articulation, that is, the passive articulator; the part that the active articulator approaches or contacts directly.

plosive Manner of articulation resulting from a previous complete occlusion at some point in the vocal tract; the sudden release phase of a stop.

postalveolar Posterior portion of the alveolar ridge as place of articulation.

postdorsal Posterior portion of the tongue as active articulator for consonant production. Example: [k].

postpalatal Posterior portion of the hard palate as place of articulation for consonant production.

postvocalic Consonant or consonant cluster following a vowel, typically occurring at the end of a word or utterance.

pragmatics Study of language used to communicate in various social situational contexts, including, among other things, the reasons for talking, conversational skills, and the flexibility to modify speech for different listeners and social situations.

predorsal Anterior portion of the dorsum as active articulator for consonant production. Example: predorsal [z] realization.

predorsal-alveolar Referring to the active articulator (predorsal portion of the tongue) and the passive articulator (alveolar ridge) for the production of speech sounds.

prelinguistic behavior Vocalizations prior to the first actual words.

prepalatal Anterior portion of hard palate as place of articulation for consonant production. Example: [ʒ].

presystematic stage Period in the phonological development of children when contrastive word units (rather than contrastive sounds of phoneme value) are acquired.

prevocalic Consonants or consonant clusters preceding a vowel, typically occurring at the beginning of a word or utterance.

primary functions Life-supporting roles of particular anatomical structures; in this case, the speech mechanism.

progressive assimilation The articulatory influence of a preceding sound on a following sound segment; also called *perseverative assimilation.*

prosodic features Characteristics of large linguistic units, elements that occur across segments, influencing what an individual says.

proto-word Vocalization used consistently by a child in particular contexts but without a recognizable adult model. Also called *vocables, phonetically consistent forms,* and *quasi-words.*

quasi-word *See:* proto-word.

race Biological label defined in terms of observable physical features (such as skin color, hair type and color, head shape and size) and biological characteristics (such as genetic composition).

raised tongue position Tongue location for the production of the vowel in question that is too high.

reduplicated babbling Prelinguistic stage marked by similar strings of consonant–vowel productions.

reduplication Syllable structure process which is a repetition of the first syllable of a word resulting in a syllable that is "simplified." Example: [baba] for *bottle.*

regional dialects Forms of a language corresponding to various geographical locations.

regression *See:* phonological idiom.

regressive assimilation Adaptation of a sound's phonetic production characteristics under the influence of a following consonant. Example: [ɪʃi] for *is she;* also called *anticipatory assimilation.*

remote assimilation Adaptive process modifying a speech sound separated by at least one other segment; also called *noncontiguous assimilation.*

retroflexed Produced with the tip of the tongue "curled back," for example, one form of standard [r] production.

retroflexed "r" Referring to the tip of the tongue curled upward and back during a specific type of [r]-production.

rhotic Relating to the manner of articulation characterized by r-coloring.

rhotic diphthong Vowel in which the offglide is the central vowel with r-coloring [ɚ]. *See also:* centering diphthong.

rhyme Term for the nucleus (vowel) and the coda (the arrest) of a syllable.

rising diphthong During production of these vowels, portions of the tongue move from a lower onglide to a higher offglide position; thus, relative to the palate, the tongue moves in a rising motion.

root node In feature geometry, place that links a segment to the prosodic tiers.

salience factor Child's active selection of words containing sounds that are important or remarkable (salient) to the child in early word production.

screening Activity or test that identifies individuals for further evaluation.

secondary functions Anatomical physiological tasks, including articulation of speech sounds, that occur in addition to the life-supporting ones.

segmental Referring to the discrete, sequentially arranged speech segments to vowels and consonants.

semantics Study of linguistic meaning that includes the meaning of words, phrases, and sentences.

semivowels Sonorants, especially the glides among them, as productionally characterized by an articulatory movement from a sagitally more constricted to a sagitally more open oral cavity.

sensorineural hearing loss Hearing loss that occurs as a consequence of damage to the sensory end organ, the cochlear hair cells, or the auditory nerve.

sequencing errors Disruptions in the production of the correct ordering of speech sounds or syllables.

sibilant Fricative sound characterized by a sharper sound from the presence of high-frequency components. Examples: [s], [ʃ].

silent period Time frame that might occur when English language learners are very quiet, speaking very little as they focus on understanding the new language.

silent posturing Positioning of the articulators for a specific articulation without sound production.

skeletal (or CV) tier Unit of a syllable and its hierarchically related components, onset and rhyme.

social dialects Particular forms of a language that are generally related to socioeconomic status.

sonorant consonants Classes of speech sounds, including the nasals, glides, and liquids produced with a relatively open expiratory passageway.

sonorant Group of vowels and specific consonants that demonstrate increased sonority or more relative loudness in relationship to other sounds with the same length, stress, and pitch.

sonority Sound's loudness relative to that of other sounds with the same length, stress, and pitch.

sound modification method Therapy technique based on deriving the target sound from a phonetically similar sound that a client can accurately produce.

speech Communication or expression of thoughts in spoken words; that is, in oral, verbal communication.

speech disorder Oral, verbal communication that is so deviant from the norm that it is noticeable or interferes with communication.

speech intelligibility "That aspect of oral speech-language output that allows a listener to understand what a speaker is saying" (Carney, 1994, p. 109).

speech sound development The gradual articulatory mastery of speech sound forms in a given language.

speech sound disorder Difficulties making certain sounds that continue past a certain age. ASHA (2014) states that a speech sound disorder includes problems with articulation (making sounds) and phonological processes (sound patterns).

speech sounds Real physical sound entities used in speech; end products of articulatory motor processes.

stimulability testing Examining a client's ability to produce a misarticulated sound in an appropriate manner when "stimulated" by a clinician to do so.

stop Manner of articulation resulting from a complete occlusion at some point in the vocal tract based on the action of an active and a passive articulator; closure preceding the buildup of expiratory airstream pressure. Example: [p].

stopping Substitution process whereby homorganic stops replace a fricative or the omission of the fricative portion of affricates.

stress markers Diacritics that indicate different levels of syllable prominence in an utterance.

strident [s] Irregular s-production named after the auditory impression it creates; that is, a shrill, irritating, often whistle-like sound component.

substitution Replacement of one sound/phoneme with another.

substitution process Describes those sound changes in which one sound or sound class is replaced by another.

suppression Reduction of the use of one or more phonological processes as children move from the innate speech patterns to the adult norm production.

suprasegmental Relating to intonation, stress, juncture, tempo, and rhythm as speech characteristics "added to" speech sound components.

syllabic Relating to a consonant that functions as a syllable nucleus.

syllabification Unit of spoken language that is a division of a (spoken or written) word.

syllable arresting sounds See: coda.

syllable constraint Speech sound restriction or limitation in the production of syllable shapes.

syllable nucleus "Core" of a unit of spoken language carrying its highest intensity and prosodic features, typically a vowel.

syllable releasing sounds See: onset.

syllable shape Structure of the units of spoken language within a word.

syllable shape reduction Diminishment of the shape of a unit of spoken language usually by deleting one of its consonant members.

syllable structure process Sound changes that affect the structure of a unit of spoken language.

syntax Linguistic rules denoting word, phrase, and clause order; sentence organization and the relationship between words, word classes, and other sentence elements.

system Orderly combination of parts forming a complex unity.

systematic sound preference Choice of a single phonetic realization for different phonemes.

system learning Knowledge of phonemic principles that apply to a specific phonological system.

tense Referring to a high degree of muscular activity during vowel production. Example: [i] (when compared to [ɪ]).

tiers Separable and independent levels that represent a sequence of gestures or a unified set of acoustic features.

tone-unit An organizational part imposed on prosodic data.

tongue symbols Diacritics that describe deviations from normal tongue placement for speech sound realizations. Example: [d̪il] = dentalized [d].

tongue thrust Excessive anterior tongue movement during swallowing and a more anterior tongue position during rest.

tongue thrust swallow Excessive anterior tongue movement during swallowing and a more anterior tongue position during rest. *See:* tongue thrust.

total assimilation Influence of a sound segment on another by which all the phonetic properties of the influenced sound are changed; also called *complete assimilation.*

traditional-motor approaches *See:* phonetic approaches.

transfer Incorporation of language features into a nonnative language based on the occurrence of similar features in a native language.

trill Sound produced by the vibratory action of an organ of articulation tapping rapidly against a place of articulation.

unchecked syllable *See:* open syllable.

underlying form Purely theoretical concept that is thought to represent a mental reality behind the way people use language.

unrounding Spreading the lips during sound production. Example: [i] (when compared to [u]).

unstressed syllable deletion A syllable structure process marked by the elimination of the unstressed syllable of a multisyllable word; also called *weak syllable deletion.*

variegated babbling *See:* nonreduplicated babbling.

velar Relating to the soft palate as a passive articulator for consonant production. Example: [g] in [gup].

velar assimilation Adaptation of a nonvelar sound into a velar one under the influence of a neighboring velar sound.

velar harmony Assimilation process (regressive) in which a postdorsal-velar stop-plosive causes a preceding coronal-alveolar stop-plosive to change the position of active and passive articulators. Example: [gɑg] for [dɑg].

velarization A more posterior tongue placement (in the direction of the velum) for palatal sounds.

vernacular dialects Varieties of spoken General American English that are considered outside the continuum of Informal Standard English.

vocable *See:* proto-word.

vocalization (vowelization) Replacement of syllabic liquids and nasals, foremost [l], [r], and [n], by vowels. Example: [lædʊ] for *ladder.*

vocoid Nonphonemic vowel-like sound production.

voice symbols Diacritics that mark the voicing of an unvoiced or the unvoicing of a voiced consonant.

voicing Presence or absence of simultaneous vibration of the vocal cords resulting in voiced or voiceless consonants.

vowel Speech sound formed without significant constriction of the oral and pharyngeal cavities, especially along the sagittal midline of the oral cavity, normally it is the syllable nucleus.

vowelization *See:* vocalization.

weak syllable deletion A syllable structure process marked by the omission of the unstressed syllable of a multisyllable word; also called *unstressed syllable deletion.*

References

Abercrombie, D. (1967). *Elements of general phonetics.* Chicago: Aldine.

Abraham, S. (1989). Using a phonological framework to describe speech errors of orally trained, hearing-impaired school-agers. *Journal of Speech and Hearing Disorders, 54,* 600–609.

Adams, M., Foorman B., Lundberg, I., & Beeler, T. (1997). *Phonemic awareness in young children: A classroom curriculum.* Baltimore: Brookes.

Albery, E., & Russell, J. (1990). Cleft palate and orofacial abnormalities. In P. Grunwell (Ed.), *Developmental speech disorders* (pp. 63–82). New York: Churchill Livingstone.

Almost, D., & Rosenbaum, P. (1998). Effectiveness of speech intervention for phonological disorders: A randomized controlled trial. *Developmental Medicine and Child Neurology, 40,* 319–325.

Altaha, F. (1995). Pronunciation errors made by Saudi University students learning English: Analysis and remedy. *I.T. L.Review of Applied Linguistics,* 109–123.

American Cleft Palate–Craniofacial Association and Cleft Palate Foundation. (1997). *About cleft lip and cleft palate.* Chapel Hill, NC: Author.

American Psychiatric Association. (2000). *Diagnostic and statistical manual of mental disorders* (4th ed.). Arlington, VA: American Psychiatric Publishing.

American Psychiatric Association. (2013). *Diagnostic and statistical manual of mental disorders* (5th ed.). Arlington, VA: American Psychiatric Publishing.

American Speech-Language-Hearing Association Ad Hoc Committee on Communication Processes and Non-speaking Persons. (1980). Nonspeech communication: A position paper. *ASHA, 22,* 267–272.

American Speech-Language-Hearing Association. (1985). Guidelines for identification audiometry. *ASHA, 27,* 49–52.

American Speech-Language-Hearing Association. (1989). Report of the ad hoc committee on labial-lingual posturing function. *ASHA, 31,* 92–94.

American Speech-Language-Hearing Association. (1990). Guidelines for screening for hearing impairments and middle ear disorders. *ASHA, 32* (Suppl. 2), 17–24.

American Speech-Language-Hearing Association. (1991). The role of the speech-language pathologist in management of oral myofunctional disorders. *ASHA, 33* (Suppl. 5), 7.

American Speech-Language-Hearing Association. (1993). *Definitions of communication disorders and variations* [Relevant Paper]. Available from http://www.asha.org/policy

American Speech-Language-Hearing Association. (2005). *Roles and responsibilities of speech-language pathologists with respect to augmentative and alternative communication:* [Position Statement]. Available from www.asha.org/policy

American Speech-Language-Hearing Association. (2007a). *Scope of Practice in Speech-Language Pathology* [Scope of Practice]. www.asha.org/policy

American Speech-Language-Hearing Association. (2007b). *Childhood Apraxia of Speech* [Position Statement]. www.asha.org/policy

American Speech-Language-Hearing Association (2008). *Communication facts: Incidence and prevalence of communication disorders and hearing loss in children-2008 edition.* www.asha.org/research/reports/children.htm.

American Speech-Language-Hearing Association. (2014). *Speech sound disorders: Articulation and phonological processes.* Retrieved from www.asha.org/public/speech/disorders/speechsounddisorders.htm

American Speech-Language-Hearing Association Ad Hoc Committee on Service Delivery in the Schools. (1993). Definitions of communication disorders and variations. *ASHA, 35* (Suppl. 10), 40–41.

American Speech-Language-Hearing Association. Report Ad Hoc Committee on the Feasibility of the Standards of the Clinical Doctorate in Speech-Language Pathology (2013). www.asha.org

American Speech-Language-Hearing Association Audiologic Assessment Panel 1996. (1997). *Guidelines for audiologic screening.* Rockville, MD: Author.

American Speech-Language Hearing Association Committee on Language (1983). *Definition of language. ASHA, 25,* 44.

Anderson, P. (1941). *The relationship of normal and defective articulation of the consonant [s] in various phonetic contexts to auditory discrimination between normal and defective [s] productions among children from kindergarten through fourth grade.* Master's thesis, State University of Iowa, Iowa City.

Andrews, N., & Fey, M. E. (1986). Analysis of the speech of phonologically impaired children in two sampling conditions. *Language, Speech, and Hearing Services in Schools, 17,* 187–198.

Archangeli, D. (1988). Aspects of underspecification theory. *Phonology, 5,* 183–207.

Archangeli, D., & Langendoen, D. (1997). *Optimality theory: An overview.* Oxford: Blackwell.

Archangeli, D., & Pulleyblank, D. (1994). *Grounded phonology.* Cambridge, MA: MIT Press.

Arlt, P. B., & Goodban, M. T. (1976). A comparative study of articulatory acquisition as based on a study of 240 normals, aged three to six. *Language, Speech, and Hearing Services in Schools, 7,* 173–180.

Atkinson-King, K. (1973). Children's acquisition of phonological stress contrasts. *UCLA Working Papers in Phonetics, 25,* 184–191.

Baker, E. (2010). Minimal pair intervention. In A. L. Williams, S. McLeod, & R. J. McCauley (Eds.), *Interventions for speech sound disorders in children* (pp. 41–72). Baltimore: Brookes.

Ball, M. J. (2002). Clinical phonology of vowel disorders. In M. J. Ball & F. E. Gibbon (Eds.), *Vowel disorders* (pp. 187–216). Boston: Butterworth-Heinemann.

Ball, M. J., & Gibbon, F. E. (2002). *Vowel disorders.* Boston: Butterworth-Heinemann.

Ball, M. J., & Kent, R. D. (1997). *The new phonologies: Developments in clinical linguistics.* San Diego, CA: Singular.

Ball, M. J., & Rahilly, J. (1999). *Phonetics: The science of speech.* London: Arnold.

Ballard, K., Granier, J., & Robin, D. (2000). Understanding the nature of apraxia of speech: Theory, analysis, & treatment. *Aphasiology, 14,* 969–995.

Ballard, K. J., Robin, D. A., McCabe, P., & McDonald, J. (2010). A treatment for dysprosody in childhood apraxia of speech. *Journal of Speech, Language, and Hearing Research, 53,* 1227–1245.

Bankson, N. W., & Bernthal, J. E. (1990). *Bankson-Bernthal test of phonology.* Chicago: Riverside Press.

Barlow, J. A. (2001). Case study: Optimality theory and the assessment and treatment of phonological disorders. *Language, Speech, and Hearing Services in Schools, 32,* 242–256.

Barlow, S., & Farley, G. (1989). Neurophysiology of speech. In D. P. Kuehn, M. L. Lemme, & J. M. Baumgartner (Eds.), *Neural bases of speech, hearing, and language* (pp. 146–200). Boston: Little, Brown.

Baudouin de Courtenay, J. (1895). *Versuch einer Theorie phonetischer Alternationen: Ein Capitel aus der Psychophonetik.* Translation in E. Stankiewicz (Ed.), *Selected writings of Baudouin de Courtenay.* Bloomington: Indiana University Press.

Bauer, H. R. (1988). The ethologic model of phonetic development: I. *Clinical Linguistics and Phonetics, 2,* 347–380.

Bauer, H. R., & Robb, M. P. (1989). *Phonetic development between infancy and toddlerhood: The phonetic product estimator.* Paper presented at the national convention of the American Speech-Language-Hearing Association, St. Louis, MO.

Bauman, J. A., & Waengler, H.-H. (1977). Measurements of sound durations in the speech of apraxic adults. *Hamburger Phonetische Beiträge* (Monograph No. 23). Hamburg: H. Buske Verlag.

Bauman-Waengler, J. A. (1991). Phonological processes in three groups of preschool children: A longitudinal study. *Proceedings from the XII International Congress of Phonetic Sciences, Aix-en-Provence, 3,* 354–357.

Bauman-Waengler, J. A. (1993a). *Dialect versus disorder: Articulation errors in African American preschool children.* Presentation at the state convention of the Pennsylvania Speech-Language-Hearing Association, Harrisburg, PA.

Bauman-Waengler, J. A. (1993b). *Language testing of African American children: Assessing assessment instruments.* Seminar presented at the state convention of the Pennsylvania Speech-Language-Hearing Association, Harrisburg, PA.

Bauman-Waengler, J. A. (1994a). Normal phonological development. In R. Lowe (Ed.), *Phonology: Assessment and intervention applications in speech pathology* (pp. 35–72). Baltimore: Williams & Wilkins.

Bauman-Waengler, J. A. (1994b). *Phonetic-phonological features in the speech of African American preschoolers.* Paper presented at the national convention of the American Speech-Language-Hearing Association, New Orleans, LA.

Bauman-Waengler, J. A. (1995). *Articulatory differences between two groups of African American preschoolers.* Paper presented at the national convention of the Canadian Association of Speech-Language Pathologists and Audiologists, Ottawa, Canada.

Bauman-Waengler, J. A. (1996). *Problems in assessing African American children with phonological disorders.* Seminar presented at the national convention of the Black American Speech-Language-Hearing Association, Milwaukee, WI.

Bauman-Waengler, J. A. (2002a). Segmental timing of phonologically disordered children: A developmental perspective. *Beihefte zur Zeitschrift fuer Dialektologie und Linguistik.* Stuttgart, Germany: Steiner Verlag Wiesbaden.

Bauman-Waengler, J. A. (2002b). *Segmental timing of sound errors in the speech of children with phonological disorders.* International Child Phonology Conference, Wichita, KS.

Bauman-Waengler, J. A. (2009). *Introduction to phonetics and phonology: From concepts to transcription.* Boston: Pearson.

Bauman-Waengler, J. A., & Garcia, D. (2011). *Linking Phonology and Language: Approaches, Target Selection and Intervention Ideas.* California Speech-Language-Hearing Association, Monterey, CA.

Bauman-Waengler, J. A., & Garcia, D. (2011). Case 10: Matthew: The changing picture of childhood apraxia of speech—from initial symptoms to diagnostic and therapeutic modifications. In S. S. Chabon & E. R. Cohn (Eds.), *The communication disorders casebook: Learning by example* (pp. 71–81). Boston: Pearson.

Bauman-Waengler, J. A., & Waengler, H.-H. (1988). *Phonological process analysis in three groups of preschool children.* Paper presented at the national convention of the American Speech-Language-Hearing Association, Boston, MA.

Bauman-Waengler, J. A., & Waengler, H.-H. (1990). *Individual variation in phonologically disordered preschoolers: A longitudinal study.* Paper presented at the national convention of the American Speech-Language-Hearing Association, Seattle, WA.

Berko Gleason, J., & Bernstein Ratner, N. (Eds.) (2009). *The development of language* (7th ed.). Boston: Pearson.

Bernhardt, B. (1992). Developmental implications of nonlinear phonological theory. *Clinical Linguistics and Phonetics, 6,* 259–281.

Bernhardt, B. M., Bopp, K. D., Daudlin, B. B., Edwards, S. M., & Daudlin, S. E. (2010). Nonlinear phonological intervention, In A. L. Williams, S. McLeod, & R. J. McCauley (Eds.), *Interventions for speech sound disorders in children* (pp. 315–332). Baltimore: Paul H. Brookes.

Bernhardt, B., & Holdgrafer, G. (2001). Beyond the basics I: The need for strategic sampling for in-depth phonological analysis. *Language, Speech, and Hearing Services in Schools, 32,* 18–27.

Bernhardt, B., & Stemberger, J. P. (1998). *Handbook of phonological development from the perspective of constraint-based nonlinear phonology.* San Diego, CA: Academic Press.

Bernhardt, B., & Stoel-Gammon, C. (1994). Nonlinear phonology: Introduction and clinical application: Tutorial. *Journal of Speech and Hearing Research, 37,* 123–143.

Bernthal, J. E., Bankson, N. W., & Flipsen, P., Jr. (2009). *Articulation and phonological disorders* (6th ed.). Boston: Allyn & Bacon.

Best, C., & McRoberts, G. (2003). Infant perception of non-native consonant contrasts that adults assimilate in different ways. *Language and Speech, 3,* 183–216.

Best, C., McRoberts, G., & Goodell, E. (2001). Discrimination of non-native consonant contrasts varying in perceptual assimilation to the listener's native phonological system. *Journal of the Acoustic Society of America, 109,* 775–794.

Best, S., Bigge, J., & Sirvis, B. (1994). Physical and health impairments. In N. Haring, L. McCormick, & T. Haring (Eds.), *Exceptional children and youth: An introduction to special education* (pp. 300–341). New York: Merrill.

Bird, J., & Bishop, D. V. (1992). Perception and awareness of phonemes in phonologically impaired children. *European Journal of Disorders of Communication, 27,* 289–311.

Bird, J., Bishop, D. V., & Freeman, N. H. (1995). Phonological awareness and literacy development in children with expressive phonological impairments. *Journal of Speech and Hearing Research, 38,* 446–462.

Bishop, D. (1994). Grammatical errors in specific language impairment: Competence or performance limitations. *Applied Psycholinguistics, 15,* 507–550.

Bishop, D., & Adams, C. (1990). A prospective study of the relationship between specific language impairment,

phonological disorders and reading retardation. *Journal of Child Psychology and Psychiatry, 31,* 1027–1050.

Bishop, D., Brown, B., & Robson, J. (1990). The relationship between phoneme discrimination, speech production, and language comprehension in cerebral-palsied individuals. *Journal of Speech and Hearing Research, 33,* 210–219.

Bishop, D., & Robson, J. (1989). Unimpaired short-term memory and rhyme judgment in congenitally speechless individuals: Implications for the notion of "articulatory coding." *Quarterly Journal of Experimental Psychology, 41A,* 123–140.

Blache, S. (1978). *The acquisition of distinctive features.* Baltimore: University Park Press.

Blache, S. (1982). Minimal word-pairs and distinctive feature training. In M. A. Crary & D. Ingram (Eds.), *Phonological intervention: Concepts and procedures* (pp. 61–96). San Diego, CA: College-Hill Press.

Blache, S. (1989). A distinctive feature approach. In N. Creaghead, P. Newman, & W. Secord (Eds.), *Assessment and remediation of articulatory and phonological disorders* (2nd ed., pp. 361–382). New York: Macmillan.

Blachman, B. A. (2000). Phonological awareness. In M. L. Kamil, P. B. Mosenthal, P. D. Pearson, & R. Barr (Eds.), *Handbook of reading research* (pp. 483–502). Mahwah, NJ: Erlbaum.

Bleile, K. (2002). Evaluating articulation and phonological disorders when the clock is running. *American Journal of Speech-Language Pathology, 11,* 243–249.

Blockcolsky, V., Frazer, J., & Frazer, D. (1987). *40,000 selected words.* Tucson, AZ: Communication Skill Builders.

Bloom, L. (1973). *One word at a time: The use of single word utterances before syntax.* The Hague: Mouton.

Bobath, B. (1967). The very early treatment of cerebral palsy. *Developmental Medicine and Childhood Neurology, 9,* 373–390.

Bobath, K., & Bobath, B. (1972). Cerebral palsy, Part II: The neurodevelopmental approach to treatment. In P. H. Pearson & C. E. Williams (Eds.), *Physical therapy services in the developmental disabilities* (pp. 114–185). Springfield, IL: Charles C. Thomas.

Bogliotti, C. (2003). *Relation between categorical perception of speech and reading*

acquisition. Proceedings of the 15th International Congress of Phonetic Sciences, Barcelona, Spain.

Bonvillian, J., Raeburn, V., & Horan, E. (1979). Talking to children—The effect of rate, intonation and length on children's sentence imitation. *Journal of Child Language, 6,* 459–467.

Boone, D. R., & McFarlane, S. C., Von Berg, S. L., & Zraick, R. I. (2013). *The voice and voice therapy.* Boston: Allyn & Bacon.

Botting, N., & Conti-Ramsden, G. (2004). Characteristics of children with specific language impairment. In L. Verhoeven & H. van Balkom (Eds.), *Classification of developmental language disorders: Theoretical issues and clinical implications* (pp. 23–38). London: Lawrence Erlbaum.

Boutsen, F., & Christman, S. (2002). Prosody in apraxia of speech. *Seminars in Speech and Language, 23,* 245–255.

Boysson-Bardies, B., de (2001). *How language comes to children: From birth to two years* (M. DeBevoise, Trans.). Cambridge, MA: NET Press.

Boysson-Bardies, B., de, & Vihman, M. (1991). Adaptation to language. *Language, 67,* 297–339.

Bradley, L., & Bryant, P. (1983). Categorizing sounds and learning to read: A causal connection. *Nature, 301,* 419–421.

Brady, N., Marquis, J., Fleming, K., & McLean, L. (2004). Prelinguistic predictors of language growth in children with developmental disabilities. *Journal of Speech, Language, and Hearing Research, 47,* 663–677.

Bridgeman, E., & Snowling, M. (1988). The perception of phoneme sequence: A comparison of dyspraxic and normal children. *British Journal of Disorders of Communication, 23,* 245–252.

Broen, P. A., & Moller, K. T. (1993). Early phonological development and the child with cleft palate. In K. T. Moller & C. D. Starr (Eds.), *Cleft palate. Interdisciplinary issues and treatment* (pp. 219–249). Austin, TX: PRO-ED.

Bronstein, A. J. (1960). *The pronunciation of American English. An introduction to phonetics.* New York: Appleton-Century-Crofts.

Brown, R. (1973). *A first language: The early stages.* Cambridge, MA: Harvard University Press.

Bruner, J. (1975). The ontogenesis of speech acts. *Journal of Child Language, 2,* 1–19.

Buhler, H., DeThomasis, B., Chute, P., & DeCora, A. (2007). An analysis of phonological process use in young children with cochlear implants. *The Volta Review, 107,* 55–74.

Butcher, A. (1990). The uses and abuses of phonological assessment. *Child Language Teaching and Therapy, 6,* 262–276.

Bzoch, K. (1997). Clinical assessment, evaluation, and management of 11 categorical aspects of cleft palate speech disorders. In K. R. Bzoch (Ed.), *Communication disorders related to cleft lip and palate* (4th ed., pp. 261–311). Austin, TX: PRO-ED.

Camp, B., Burgess, D., Morgan, L., & Zerbe, G. (1987). A longitudinal study of infant vocalizations in the first year. *Journal of Pediatric Psychology, 12,* 321–331.

Carney, A. E. (1994). Understanding speech intelligibility in the hearing impaired. In K. G. Butler (Ed.), *Hearing impairment and language disorders* (pp. 109–121). Gaithersburg, MD: Aspen.

Carney, E. (1979). Inappropriate abstraction in speech assessment procedures. *British Journal of Disorders of Communication, 14,* 123–135.

Carterette, E., & Jones, M. (1974). *Informal speech: Alphabetic and phonemic texts with statistical analyses and tables.* Berkeley: University of California Press.

Carver, C. M. (1987). Dialects. In S. Flexner & L. C. Hauck (Eds.), *The Random House dictionary of the English language* (2nd ed., pp. xxv–xxvi). New York: Random House.

Carvill, S. (2001). Sensory impairment, intellectual disability, and psychiatry. *Journal of Intellectual Disability Research, 45,* 467–483.

Catts, H. (1993). The relationship between speech-language impairments and reading disabilities. *Journal of Speech and Hearing Research, 36,* 948–958.

Catts, H., Fey, M., & Zhang, X. (2001). Estimating the risk of future reading difficulties in kindergarten children: A research-based model and its clinical implementation. *Language, Speech, and Hearing Services in Schools, 32,* 38–50.

Catts, H., & Kamhi, A. (1999). Causes of reading disabilities. In H. Catts & A. Kamhi (Eds.), *Language and reading disabilities* (pp. 95–127). Boston: Allyn & Bacon.

Chan, A., & Li, D. (2000). English and Cantonese phonology in contrast: Explaining Cantonese ESL learners' English pronunciation problems. *Language, Culture, and Curriculum, 13,* 67–85.

Chapman, K. L. (1993). Phonological processes in children with cleft palate. *Cleft Palate-Craniofacial Journal, 30,* 64–71.

Chapman, K. L., & Hardin, M. A. (1992). Phonetic and phonologic skills of two year olds with cleft palate. *Cleft Palate-Craniofacial Journal, 29,* 435–443.

Chapman, K. L., Hardin-Jones, M., & Halter, K. (2003). The relationship between early speech and later speech and language performance for children with cleft lip and palate. *Clinical Linguistics & Phonetics, 17,* 173–197.

Chen, H. P., & Irwin, O. C. (1946). Infant speech: Vowel and consonant types. *Journal of Speech Disorders, 11,* 27–29.

Cheng, L. L. (1994). Asian/Pacific students and the learning of English. In J. Bernthal & N. Bankson (Eds.), *Child phonology: Characteristics, assessment, and intervention with special populations* (pp. 255–274). New York: Thieme.

Chomsky, C. (1971). *Linguistic Development of Children from 6 to 10.* Final Report Project, No. 9A-055, Grant No. Oeg-1-9-090055–0114(010), U.S. Department of Health, Education, and Welfare-Office of Education-Bureau of Research, June 1971.

Chomsky, N. (1957). *Syntactic structures.* The Hague: Mouton.

Chomsky, N., & Halle, M. (1968). *The sound pattern of English.* New York: Harper & Row.

Christensen, M., & Hanson, M. (1981). An investigation of the efficacy of oral myofunctional therapy as a precursor to articulation therapy for pre-first-grade children. *Journal of Speech and Hearing Disorders, 46,* 160–165.

Christian, D., Wolfram, W., & Nube, N. (1988). *Variation and change in geographically isolated communities: Appalachian English and Ozark English.* Tuscaloosa: University of Alabama Press.

Clark, M. C., & Goldstein, B. (1996). *Analysis of vowel error patterns in children with phonological disorders.* Paper presented at the annual convention of the American Speech-Language-Hearing Association, Seattle, WA.

Clarke-Klein, S., & Hodson, B. (1995). A phonologically based analysis of misspellings by third graders with disordered-phonology histories. *Journal of Speech and Hearing Research, 38,* 839–849.

Cohen, L., & Cashon, C. (2003). Infant perception and cognition. In R. Lerner, M. Easterbooks, & J. Mistry (Eds.), *Comprehensive handbook of psychology. Volume 6: Developmental psychology* (pp. 65–90), Hoboken, NJ: John Wiley and Sons.

Cole, R. A., & Perfetti, C. A. (1980). Listening for mispronunciations in a children's story: The use of context by children and adults. *Journal of Verbal Learning and Verbal Behavior, 19,* 297–315.

Compton, A. J. (1976). Generative studies of children's phonological disorders: Clinical ramifications. In D. Morehead & A. Morehead (Eds.), *Normal and deficient child language* (pp. 61–96). Baltimore: University Park Press.

Connolly, J. H. (1986). Intelligibility: A linguistic view. *British Journal of Disorders of Communication, 21,* 371–376.

Conti-Ramsden, G., & Jones, M. (1997). Verb use in specific language impairment. *Journal of Speech and Hearing Research, 40,* 1298–1313.

Coplan, J., & Gleason, J. R. (1988). Unclear speech: Recognition and significance of unintelligible speech in preschool children. *Pediatrics, 82,* 447–452.

Cornwall, A. (1992). The relationship of phonological awareness, rapid naming and verbal memory to severe reading and spelling disability. *Journal of Learning Disabilities, 25,* 532–538.

Crary, M. A. (1983). Phonological process analysis from spontaneous speech: The influence of sample size. *Journal of Communication Disorders, 16,* 133–141.

Crary, M. A. (1993). *Developmental motor speech disorders.* San Diego, CA: Singular.

Croot, K. (2002). Diagnosis of AOS: Definition and criteria. *Seminar in Speech and Language, 23,* 267–280.

Crosbie, S., Holm, A., & Dodd, B. (2005). Intervention for children with severe speech disorder: A comparison of two approaches. *International Journal of Language and Communication Disorders, 40,* 467–491.

Cruttenden, A. (1981). Item-learning and system-learning. *Journal of Psycholinguistic Research, 10,* 79–88.

Cruttenden, A. (1985). Intonation comprehension in 10-year-olds. *Journal of Child Language, 12,* 643–661.

Crystal, D. (1981). *Clinical linguistics.* New York: Springer-Verlag.

Crystal, D. (1986). Prosodic development. In P. Fletcher & M. Garman (Eds.), *Language acquisition* (2nd ed., pp. 174–197). Cambridge: Cambridge University Press.

Crystal, D. (2010). *The Cambridge encyclopedia of language* (3rd ed.). Cambridge: Cambridge University Press.

Culatta, R., Page, J. L., & Wilson, L. (1987). *Speech rates of normally communicative children.* Paper presented at the annual convention of the American Speech-Language-Hearing Association, New Orleans, LA.

Culbertson, D. (2007). Language and speech of the deaf and hard of hearing. In R. Schow and M. Nerbonne (Eds.) *Introduction to audiologic rehabilitation* (5th ed.). (pp. 197–244). Boston, MA: Allyn and Bacon.

Cummings, A. E. (2009). *Brain and behavior in children with phonological delays: Phonological, lexical, and sensory system interaction.* Unpublished doctoral dissertation, University of California, San Diego.

Dabul, B. (2000). *Apraxia battery for adults* (2nd ed.). Tigard, OR: C. C. Publications.

Dalston, R. (1997). The use of nasometry in the assessment and remediation of velopharyngeal inadequacy. In K. R. Bzoch (Ed.), *Communication disorders related to cleft lip and palate* (4th ed., pp. 331–346). Austin, TX: PRO-ED.

Dalston, R., Warren, D., & Dalston, E. (1991). Use of nasometry as a diagnostic tool for identifying patients with velopharyngeal impairment. *Cleft Palate-Craniofacial Journal, 28,* 184–189.

Darley, F. (1991). A philosophy of appraisal and diagnosis. In F. Darley & D. C. Spriestersbach (Eds.), *Diagnostic methods in speech pathology* (2nd ed., pp. 1–23). New York: Harper & Row.

Davis, B. L., Jacks, A., & Marquardt, T. P. (2005). *Vowel patterns in developmental apraxia of speech: Three longitudinal case studies, 19,* 249–274.

Davis, B. L., Jakielski, K., & Marquardt, T. (1998). Developmental apraxia of speech: Determiners of differential diagnosis. *Clinical Linguistics and Phonetics, 12,* 25–45.

Davis, B. L., & MacNeilage, P. F. (1990). Acquisition of correct vowel production: A quantitative case study. *Journal of Speech and Hearing Research, 33,* 16–27.

Dawson, J. I., & Tattersall, P. J. (2001). *Structured photographic articulation test-II.* DeKalb, IL: Janelle Publications.

Dean, E., Howell, J., Hill, A., & Waters, D. (1990). *Metaphon resource pack.* Windsor, UK: NFER Nelson.

DeCasper, A., & Fifer, W. P. (1980). On human bonding: Newborns prefer their mothers' voices. *Science, 208,* 1174–1176.

Delack, J. B., & Fowlow, P. J. (1978). The ontogenesis of differential vocalization: Development of prosodic contrastivity during the first year of life. In N. Waterson & C. Snow (Eds.), *The development of communication* (pp. 93–110). New York: John Wiley.

Delaney, A., & Kent, R. (2004). *Developmental profiles of children diagnosed with apraxia of speech.* Paper presented at the annual meeting of the American Speech-Language-Hearing Association, Philadelphia, PA.

Denes, P. B., & Pinson, E. N. (1973). *The speech chain.* Garden City, NY: Anchor Press.

Dewey, G. (1923). *Relative frequency of English speech sounds.* Cambridge, MA: Harvard University Press.

Dillow, K. A., Dzienkowski, R. C., Smith, K. K., & Yucha, C. B. (1996). Cerebral palsy: A comprehensive review. *The Nurse Practitioner, 21,* 45–61.

Dinnsen, D. A. (1997). Nonsegmental phonologies. In M. J. Ball & R. D. Kent (Eds.), *The new phonologies* (pp. 77–125). San Diego, CA: Singular.

Dinnsen, D. A., & Elbert, M. (1984). On the relationship between phonology and learning. In M. Elbert, D. Dinnsen, & G. Weismer (Eds.), *Phonological theory and the misarticulating child, ASHA Monograph, 22* (pp. 59–68). Rockville, MD: ASHA.

Dodd, B. (1995). *Differential diagnosis and treatment of children with speech disorder.* London: Whurr.

Dodd, B., Crosbie, S., McIntosh, B., Holm, A., Harvey, C., Liddy, M., et al. (2008). The impact of selecting different contrasts in phonological therapy. *International Journal of Speech-Language Pathology, 10,* 334–345.

Dodd, B., Gillon, G., Oerlemans, R., Russell, T., Syrmis, M., & Wilson, H. (1995). Phonological disorder and the acquisition of literacy. In B. Dodd (Ed.), *Differential diagnosis and treatment of children with speech disorder* (pp. 125–146). London: Whurr.

Dodd, B., & Iacano, T. (1989). Phonological disorders in children: Changes in phonological process use during treatment. *British Journal of Disorders of Communication, 24,* 333–351.

Donegan, P. J., & Stampe, D. (1979). The study of natural phonology. In D. A. Dinnsen (Ed.), *Current approaches to phonological theory* (pp. 126–173). Bloomington: Indiana University Press.

Dore, J. (1975). Holophrases, speech acts and language universals. *Journal of Child Language, 3,* 22–39.

Dore, J., Franklin, M. B., Miller, R. T., & Ramer, A. L. (1976). Transitional phenomena in early language acquisition. *Journal of Child Language, 3,* 13–29.

Drummond, S. S. (1993). *Dysarthria examination battery.* Austin, TX: PRO-ED.

Duffy, J. R. (2005a). Assessment of apraxia of speech. *Neuromotor exam form.* Rochester, MN: Mayo Clinic.

Duffy, J. R. (2005b). Assessment of nonverbal oral apraxia. *Neuromotor exam form.* Rochester, MN: Mayo Clinic.

Duffy, J. R. (2013). *Motor speech disorders: Substrate, differential diagnosis, and management* (3rd ed.). St Louis, MO: Elsevier Mosby.

Duncan, L., & Johnston, R. (1999). How does phonological awareness relate to nonword reading amongst poor readers? *Reading and Writing: An Interdisciplinary Journal, 11,* 405–439.

Dunn, C., & Newton, L. (1994). A comprehensive model for speech development in hearing-impaired children. In K. G. Butler (Ed.), *Hearing impairment and language disorders* (pp. 122–143). *Topics in language disorders series.* Gaithersburg, MD: Aspen.

Dunn, L. M., Dunn, L., Whetton, C., & Pintilie, D. (1982). *British picture vocabulary scales.* Windsor: NFER Nelson.

Dworkin, J. P. (1991). *Motor speech disorders: A treatment guide.* St. Louis, MO: Mosby Year Book.

Dworkin, J. P., & Culatta, R. A. (1980). *Dworkin-Culatta oral mechanism examination.* Nicholasville, KY: Edgewood Press.

Dyson, A. T., & Amayreh, M. M. (2007). Chapter 34: Jordanian Arabic speech acquisition. In S. McLeod (Ed.), *The international guide to speech acquisition* (pp. 472–482). Clifton Park, NY: Thomson Delmar Learning.

Edeal, D. M., & Gildersleeve-Neumann, C. E. (2011). The importance of production frequency in therapy for childhood apraxia of speech. *American Journal of Speech-Language Pathology, 20,* 95–110.

Edwards, H. T. (2003). *Applied phonetics: The sounds of American English* (3rd ed.). San Diego, CA: Singular.

Edwards, J., Beckman, M. E., & Munson, B. (2004). The interaction between vocabulary size and phonotactic probability effects on children's production accuracy and fluency in nonword repetition. *Journal of Speech, Language, and Hearing Research, 47,* 421–436.

Edwards, J., Fox, R., & Rogers, C. (2002). Final consonant discrimination in children: Effects of phonological disorder, vocabulary size, and articulatory accuracy. *Journal of Speech, Language, and Hearing Research, 45,* 231–242.

Edwards, M. L. (1992). Clinical forum: Phonological assessment and treatment. In support of phonological processes. *Language, Speech, and Hearing Services in Schools, 23,* 233–240.

Ehren, T. (2010). *What /R/ you doing? Correcting /R/.* American Speech-Language Hearing Association Convention, Philadelphia, PA.

Eisenberg, L. (2007). Current state of knowledge: Speech recognition and production in children with hearing impairment. *Ear and Hearing, 28,* 766–772.

Eisenberg, S. L., & Hitchcock, E. R. (2010). Using standardized tests to inventory consonant and vowel production: A comparison of 11 tests of articulation and phonology. *Language, Speech, and Hearing Services in Schools, 41,* 488-503.

Elbers, L. (1982). Operating principles in repetitive babbling: A cognitive approach. *Cognition, 12,* 45–63.

Elbert, M. (1992). Clinical forum: Phonological assessment and treatment. Consideration of error types: A response to Fey. *Language, Speech, and Hearing Services in Schools, 23,* 241–246.

Elbert, M., Dinnsen, D., & Powell, T. (1984). On the prediction of phonologic generalization learning patterns. *Journal of Speech and Hearing Disorders, 49,* 309–317.

Elbert, M., & Gierut, J. (1986). *Handbook of clinical phonology: Approaches to assessment and treatment.* San Diego, CA: College-Hill Press.

Elfenbein, J., Hardin-Jones, M., & Davis, J. (1994). Oral communication skills of children who are hard of hearing. *Journal of Speech and Hearing Research, 37,* 216–226.

Elliott, L. L. (1979). Performance of children aged 9–17 years on a test of speech intelligibility in noise using sentence material with controlled word predictability. *Journal of the Acoustical Society of America, 66,* 651–653.

Elliott, L. L., Connors, S., Kille, E., Levin, S., Ball, K., & Katz, D. (1979). Children's understanding of monosyllabic nouns in quiet and in noise. *Journal of the Acoustical Society of America, 66,* 12–21.

Enderby, P., & Palmer, R. (2008). *Frenchay dysarthria assessment–2nd edition (FDA-2).* Austin, TX: PRO-ED.

Eriks-Brophy, A., Gibson, S., & Tucker, S.-K. (2013). Articulatory error patterns and phonological process use of preschool children with and without hearing loss. *The Volta Review, 113,* 87–126.

Eyer, J., & Leonard, L. (1994). Learning past tense morphology with specific language impairment: A case study. *Child Language Teaching and Therapy, 10,* 127–138.

Faircloth, S. R., & Faircloth, M. A. (1973). *Phonetic science: A program of instruction.* Englewood Cliffs, NJ: Prentice-Hall.

Farwell, C. B. (1976). Some strategies in the early production of fricatives. *Papers and Reports on Child Language Development, 12,* 97–104.

Fasold, R., & Wolfram, W. (1975). Some linguistic features of Negro dialect. In P. Stoller (Ed.), *Black American English* (pp. 49–87). New York: Deli.

Fasolo, M., Majorano, M., & D'Odorico, L. (2008). Babbling and first words in children with slow expressive development. *Clinical Linguistics and Phonetics, 22,* 83–94.

Ferguson, C. A. (1976). Learning to pronounce: The earliest stages of phonological development in the child. In F. D. Minifie & L. L. Floyd (Eds.), *Communicative and cognitive abilities: Early behavioral assessment* (pp. 273–297). Baltimore: University Park Press.

Ferguson, C. A., & Farwell, C. (1975). Words and sounds in early language acquisition: English initial consonants in the first fifty words. *Language, 51,* 419–439.

Ferguson, C. A., & Garnica, O. (1975). Theories of phonological development. In E. Lenneberg & E. Lenneberg (Eds.), *Foundation of language development* (Vol. 1, pp. 153–180). New York: Academic Press.

Fernald, A., Taeschner, T., Dunn, J., Papousek, M., Boysson-Bardies, B., de, & Fukui, I. (1989). A cross-language study of prosodic modification in mother's and father's speech to preverbal infants. *Journal of Child Language, 16,* 477–503.

Fey, M. E. (1992). Clinical forum: Phonological assessment and treatment. Articulation and phonology: Inextricable constructs in speech pathology. *Language, Speech, and Hearing Services in Schools, 23,* 225–232. (Reprinted from *Human Communication Canada, 1985, 9,* 7–16.)

Firth, J. R. (1948). Sounds and prosodies. *Transactions of the Philological Society.* Oxford: Blackwell.

Fisichelli, R. M. (1950). *An experimental study of the prelinguistic speech development of institutionalized infants.* Unpublished doctoral dissertation, Fordham University.

Fletcher, S. G. (1972). Time-by-count measurement of diadochokinetic syllable rate. *Journal of Speech and Hearing Research, 15,* 763–770.

Fletcher, S. G. (1978). *Time-by-count measurement of diadochokinetic syllable rate.* Austin, TX: PRO-ED.

Fletcher, S. G. (1992). *Articulation. A physiological approach.* San Diego, CA: Singular.

Fletcher, S. G., Casteel, R., & Bradley, D. (1961). Tongue-thrust swallow, speech articulation, and age. *Journal of Speech and Hearing Disorders, 26,* 201–208.

Flipsen, P., Jr., & Parker, R. G. (2008). Phonological patterns in the speech of children with cochlear implants. *Journal of Communication Disorders, 41,* 337–357.

Foster, D., Riley, K., & Parker, F. (1985). Some problems in the clinical application of phonological theory. *Journal of Speech and Hearing Disorders, 50,* 294–297.

Fourcin, A. J. (1978). Acoustic patterns and speech acquisition. In N. Waterson & C. Snow (Eds.), *Development of communication* (pp. 47–72). New York: John Wiley.

Foy, J., & Mann, V. (2012). Speech production deficits in early readers: Predictors of risk. *Reading and Writing, 25,* 799–830.

French, A. (1988). What shall we do with 'medial' sounds? *British Journal of Disorders of Communication, 23,* 41–50.

French, A. (1989). The systematic acquisition of word forms by a child during the first-fifty-word stage. *Journal of Child Language, 16,* 69–90.

Froeschels, E. (1931). *Lehrbuch der Sprachheilkunde* (3rd ed.). Leipzig-Vienna: Deuticke.

Froeschels, E. (1937). Über das Wesen der multiplen Interdentalität. *Acta Otolaryngologica, 25,* 341.

Fudala, J. (2000). *Arizona articulation proficiency scale* (3rd ed.). Los Angeles: Western Psychological Services.

Garnica, O. (1973). The development of phonemic speech perception. In T. Moore (Ed.), *Cognitive development and the acquisition of language* (pp. 215–222). New York: Academic Press.

Garn-Nunn, P., & Lynn, J. (2004). *Calvert's descriptive phonetics* (3rd ed.). New York: Thieme.

Gesell, A., & Thompson, H. (1934). *Infant behavior: Its genesis and growth.* New York: McGraw-Hill.

Gibbon, F. (2002). Personal correspondence.

Gibbon, F., & Wood, S. (2003). Using electropalatography (EPG) to diagnose and treat articulation disorders associated with mild cerebral palsy: A case study. *Clinical Linguistics and Phonetics, 17,* 365–374.

Gierut, J. (1985). *On the relationship between phonological knowledge and generalization learning in misarticulating children.* Bloomington: Indiana University Linguistics Club.

Gierut, J. (1989). Maximal opposition approach to phonological treatment. *Journal of Speech and Hearing Disorders, 54,* 9–19.

Gierut, J. (1990). Differential learning of phonological oppositions. *Journal of Speech and Hearing Research, 33,* 540–549.

Gierut, J. (1991). Homonymy in phonological change. *Clinical Linguistics and Phonetics, 5,* 119–137.

Gierut, J. (1992). The conditions and course of clinically induced phonological change. *Journal of Speech and Hearing Research, 35,* 1049–1063.

Gierut, J. (1998). Treatment efficacy: Functional phonological disorders in children. *Journal of Speech, Language, and Hearing Research, 41,* S85–S100.

Gierut, J. (1999). Syllable onsets: Clusters and adjuncts in acquisition. *Journal of Speech, Language, and Hearing Research, 42,* 708–726.

Gierut J. A. (2001). Complexity in phonological treatment: Clinical factors. *Language, Speech and Hearing Services in Schools, 32,* 229–241.

Gierut, J., Elbert, M., & Dinnsen, D. (1987). A functional analysis of phonological knowledge and generalization learning in misarticulating children. *Journal of Speech and Hearing Research, 30,* 462–479.

Gierut, J., & Hulse, L. E., (2010). Evidence-based practice: A matrix for predicting phonological generalization. *Clinical Linguistics and Phonetics, 24,* 323–334.

Gierut, J. A., & Morrisette, M. L. (2010). Phonological learning and lexicality of treated stimuli, *Clinical Linguistics and Phonetics, 24,* 122–140.

Gierut, J., Morrisette, M. L., Hughes, M. T., & Rowland, S. (1996). Phonological treatment efficacy and developmental norms. *Language, Speech, and Hearing Services in Schools, 27,* 215–230.

Gierut, J., Morrisette, M. L., & Ziemer, S. M. (2010). Nonwords and generalization in children with phonological disorders, *American Journal of Speech-Language Pathology, 19,* 167–177.

Gierut, J., & Neumann, H. (1992). Teaching and learning /θ/: A nonconfound. *Clinical Linguistics and Phonetics, 6,* 191–200.

Gilbert, J. H., & Purves, B. A. (1977). Temporal constraints on consonant clusters in child speech production. *Journal of Child Language, 4,* 417–432.

Gillon, G. (2000). The efficacy of phonological awareness intervention for children with spoken language impairment. *Language, Speech, and Hearing Services in Schools, 31,* 126–141.

Gillon, G. (2002). Follow-up study investigating benefits of phonological awareness intervention for children with spoken language impairment. *International Journal of Language and Communication Disorders, 37,* 381–400.

Gillon, G. (2004). *Phonological awareness: From research to practice.* New York: Guilford.

Gillon, G. (2005). Facilitating phoneme awareness development in 3- and 4-year-old children with speech impairment. *Language, Speech, and Hearing Services in Schools, 36,* 308–324.

Golding-Kushner, K. J. (1995). Treatment of articulation and resonance disorders associated with cleft palate and VPI. In R. J. Shprintzen & J. Bardach (Eds.), *Cleft palate speech management. A multidisciplinary approach* (pp. 327–351). St. Louis, MO: Mosby Year Book.

Goldman, R., & Fristoe, M. (2000). *Goldman-Fristoe test of articulation* (2nd ed.). Circle Pines, MN: American Guidance Service.

Goldsmith, J. A. (1976). *Autosegmental phonology.* Bloomington: Indiana University Linguistics Club.

Goldstein, B. A. (2007). Chapter 33: Spanish-influenced English speech acquisition. In S. McLeod (Ed.), *The international guide to speech acquisition* (pp. 277–287). Clifton Park, NY: Thomson Delmar Learning.

González, G. (1988). Chicano English. In D. Bixler-Marquez & J. Ornstein-Galicia (Eds.), *Chicano speech in the bilingual classroom. Series VI, Vol. 6* (pp. 71–89). New York: Lang.

Gordon-Brannan, M. (1994). Assessing intelligibility: Children's expressive phonologies. In K. Butler & B. Hodson (Eds.), *Topics in Language Disorders, 14,* 17–25.

Gordon-Brannan, M., & Hodson, B. W. (2000). Intelligibility/severity measurements of prekindergarten children's speech. *American Journal of Speech-Language Pathology, 9,* 141–150.

Gordon-Brannan, M., Hodson, B. W., and Wynne, M. K. (1992). Remediating unintelligible utterances of a child with a mild hearing loss. *American Journal of Speech-Language Pathology, 1,* 28–38.

Grames, L. M. (2008). Advancing into the 21st century: Care for individuals with cleft palate or craniofacial differences. *The ASHA Leader.* http://www.asha.org/Publications/leader/2008/f080506a/#1

Greenlee, M. (1974). Interacting processes in the child's acquisition of stop-liquid clusters. *Papers and Reports on Child Language Development* (Stanford University), 7, 85–100.

Grunwell, P. (1975). The phonological analysis of articulation disorders. *British Journal of Disorders of Communication, 10,* 31–42.

Grunwell, P. (1987). *Clinical phonology* (2nd ed.). Baltimore: Williams & Wilkins.

Gutzmann, A. (1895). *Die Gesundheitspflege der Sprache.* Breslau: F. Hirt.

Haelsig, P. C., & Madison, C. L. (1986). A study of phonological processes exhibited by 3-, 4-, and 5-year-old children. *Language, Speech, and Hearing Services in Schools, 17,* 107–114.

Haley, K., Ohde, R., & Wertz, R. (2000). Precision of fricative production in aphasia and apraxia of speech: A perceptual and acoustic study. *Aphasiology, 14,* 619–634.

Hall, M. (1938). Auditory factors in functional articulatory speech defects. *Journal of Experimental Education, 7,* 110–132.

Hall, P. K., Jordan, L. S., & Robin, D. A. (1993). *Developmental apraxia of speech: Theory and clinical practice.* Austin, TX: PRO-ED.

Halle, M. (1962). Phonology in generative grammar. *Word, 18,* 54–72.

Hallé, P. A., Boysson-Bardies, B., de, & Vihman, M. (1991). Beginnings of prosodic organization: Intonation and duration patterns of disyllables produced by Japanese and French infants. *Language and Speech, 34,* 299–318.

Halliday, M. A. (1975). *Learning how to mean: Explorations in the development of language.* New York: Elsevier.

Hanson, M. L. (1988). Orofacial myofunctional therapy: Guidelines for assessment and treatment. *International Journal of Orofacial Myology, 14,* 27–32.

Hanson, M. L., & Barrett, R. H. (1988). *Fundamentals of orofacial myology.* Springfield, IL: Charles C. Thomas.

Hardy, J. C. (1994). Cerebral palsy. In W. A. Secord, G. H. Shames, & E. Wiig (Eds.), *Human communication disorders: An introduction* (4th ed., pp. 562–604). New York: Merrill.

Haskill, A. M., Tyler, A. A., & Tolbert, L. C. (2001). *Months of morphemes: A theme-based cycles approach.* Eau Claire, WI: Thinking Publications.

Haspelmath, M., & Sims, A. D. (2010). *Understanding morphology.* London: Hodder.

Hawkins, S. (1979). Temporal coordination of consonants in the speech of children: Further data. *Journal of Phonetics, 13,* 235–267.

Haynes, W. O., & Pindzola, R. H. (1998). *Diagnosis and evaluation in speech pathology* (5th ed.). Boston: Allyn & Bacon.

Hecht, S., Burgess, S., Torgesen, J., Wagner, R., & Rashotte, C. (2000). Explaining social class differences in growth of reading skills from beginning kindergarten through fourth-grade: The role of phonological awareness, rate of access, and print knowledge. *Journal of Reading and Writing, 12,* 99–128.

Heffner, R-M. S. (1975). *General phonetics.* Madison: University of Wisconsin Press.

Heilmann, J. J., Nockerts, A., & Miller, J. F. (2010). Language sampling: Does the length of the transcript matter? *Language, Speech, and Hearing Services in Schools, 41,* 393–404.

Helm-Estabrooks, N. (1996). *Test of oral and limb apraxia (TOLA).* Chicago: Applied Symbols.

Hesketh, A., Dima, E., & Nelson, V. (2007). Teaching phoneme awareness to preliterate children with speech disorder: A randomized controlled trial. *International Journal of Language and Communication Disorders, 42,* 251–271.

Hickman, L. A., (1997). *The apraxia profile.* San Antonio, TX: Psychological Corporation.

Hidalgo, M. (1987). On the question of "standard" versus "dialect": Implications for teaching Hispanic college students. *Hispanic Journal of Behavioral Sciences, 9,* 375–395.

Hilton, L. (1984). Treatment of deviant phonological systems: Tongue thrust. In W. Perkins (Ed.), *Phonological-*

articulatory disorders (pp. 47–54). New York: Thieme-Stratton.

Himmelmann, N. P. (2000). Tagalog. In G. Booij, C. Lehmann, J. Mugdan, & S. Skopeteas (Eds.), *Morphology: An international handbook on inflection and word formation* (pp. 1473–1490). Berlin: de Gruyter.

Hislop, A., Wigglesworth, J., & Desai, R. (1986). Alveolar development in the human fetus and infant. *Early Human Development, 13,* 1–11.

Hodson, B. W. (1984). Facilitating phonological development in children with severe speech disorders. In H. Winitz (Ed.), *Treating articulation disorders. For clinicians by clinicians* (pp. 75–89). Baltimore: University Park Press.

Hodson, B. W. (1989). Phonological remediation: A cycles approach. In N. A. Creaghead, P. W. Newman, & W. A. Secord (Eds.), *Assessment and remediation of articulatory and phonological disorders* (2nd ed., pp. 323–333). New York: Macmillan.

Hodson, B. W. (1992). Clinical forum: Phonological assessment and treatment, applied phonology: Constructs, contributions, and issues. *Language, Speech, and Hearing Services in Schools, 23,* 247–253.

Hodson, B. W. (1994). Helping individuals become intelligible, literate, and articulate: The role of phonology. *Topics in Language Disorders, 14*(2), 1–16.

Hodson, B. W. (2004). *Hodson assessment of phonological patterns (HAPP-3).* Greenville, SC: Super Duper.

Hodson, B. W. (2007). Identifying phonological patterns and projecting remediation cycles: Expediting intelligibility gains of a 7-year-old Australian child. *Advances in Speech-Language Pathology, 8,* 257–264.

Hodson, B. W., & Paden, E. P. (1981). Phonological processes which characterize unintelligible and intelligible speech in early childhood. *Journal of Speech and Hearing Disorders, 46,* 369–373.

Hodson, B. W., & Paden, E. P. (1983). *Targeting intelligible speech: A phonological approach to remediation.* San Diego, CA: College-Hill Press.

Hodson, B. W., & Paden, E. P. (1991). *Targeting intelligible speech: A phonological approach to remediation* (2nd ed.). San Diego, CA: College-Hill Press.

Hodson, B. W., Scherz, J. A., & Strattman, K. H. (2002). Evaluating communicative abilities of a highly unintelligible preschooler. *American Journal of Speech-Language Pathology, 11,* 236–242.

Hoek, D., Ingram, D., & Gibson, D. (1986). Some possible causes of children's early word extensions. *Journal of Child Language, 13,* 477–494.

Hoffman, P. R., & Norris, J. A. (2010). Dynamic systems and whole language intervention. In A. L. Williams, S. McLeod, R. J. McCauley (Eds.), *Interventions for speech sound disorders in children.* Baltimore: Paul Brookes.

Holmgren, K., Lindblom, B., Aurelius, G., Jalling, B., & Zetterstrom, R. (1986). On the phonetics of infant vocalization. In B. Lindblom & R. Zetterstrom (Eds.), *Precursors of early speech* (pp. 51–63). New York: Stockton Press.

Hornby, P. A., & Hass, W. A. (1970). Use of contrastive stress by preschool children. *Journal of Speech and Hearing Research, 13,* 395–399.

Houston, D. M., & Jusczyk, P. W. (2000). The role of talker-specific information in word segmentation by infants. *Journal of Experimental Psychology, 26,* 1570–1582.

Howell, J., & Dean, E. (1991). *Treating phonological disorders in children: Metaphon-theory to practice.* San Diego, CA: Singular.

Howell, J., & Dean, E. (1994). *Treating phonological disorders in children: Metaphon-theory to practice* (2nd ed.). London: Whurr.

Hsu, H. C., & Fogel, A. (2001). Infant vocal development in a dynamic mother–infant communication system. *Infancy, 2,* 87–109. Available from http://www.nccp.org/publications/pub_948.html

Hull, R. (2001). *Aural rehabilitation: Serving children and adults* (4th ed.). Clifton Park, NY: Thomson-Delmar.

Hurford, D., Darrow, L., Edwards, T., Howerton, C., Mote, C., Schauf, J., et al. (1993). An examination of phonemic processing abilities in children during their first-grade year. *Journal of Learning Disabilities, 26,* 167–177.

Hwa-Froelich, D. A. (2007) Chapter 55: Vietnamese speech acquisition. In S. McLeod (Ed.) *The international guide to speech acquisition* (pp. 580–591). Clifton Park, NY: Thomson Delmar Learning.

Hwa-Froelich, D. A., Hodson, B. H., & Edwards, H. T. (2002). Vietnamese phonology: A tutorial. *American Journal of Speech-Language Pathology, 11,* 264–273.

Ianucci, D., & Dodd, D. (1980). The development of some aspects of quantifier negation. *Papers & Reports on Child Language Development, 19,* 88–94.

Iglesias, A., & Anderson, N. (1995). Dialectal variations. In J. E. Bernthal & N. W. Bankson (Eds.), *Articulation and phonological disorders* (3rd ed., pp. 147–161). Boston: Allyn & Bacon.

Ingram, D. (1974). Phonological rules in young children. *Journal of Child Language 1,* 49–64.

Ingram, D. (1976). *Phonological disability in children.* New York: Elsevier.

Ingram, D. (1989a). *First language acquisition: Method, description, and explanation.* Cambridge: Cambridge University Press.

Ingram, D. (1989b). *Phonological disability in children: Studies in disorders of communication* (2nd ed.). London: Cole & Whurr.

Ingram, D. (2010) The holophrastic stage. In P. C. Hogan (Ed.), *The Cambridge Encyclopedia of the Language Sciences* (pp. 364–366) Cambridge: Cambridge University Press.

Ingram, D., Christensen, L., Veach, S., & Webster, B. (1980). The acquisition of word-initial fricatives and affricates in English by children between 2 and 6 years. In G. H. Yeni-Komshian, J. F. Kavanagh, & C. A. Ferguson (Eds.), *Child phonology: Vol. I. Production* (pp. 169–192). New York: Academic Press.

Ingram, D., & Ingram, K. (2001). A whole-word approach to phonological analysis and intervention. *Language, Speech, and Hearing Services in Schools, 32,* 271–283.

International Phonetic Alphabet Chart (2005). http://www.langsci.ucl.ac.uk/ipa/ipachart.html,.

Irwin, O. C. (1945). Reliability of infant speech sound data. *Journal of Speech Disorders, 10,* 227–235.

Irwin, O. C. (1946). Infant speech: Equations for consonant-vowel ratios. *Journal of Speech Disorders, 11,* 177–180.

Irwin, O. C. (1947a). Infant speech: Consonant sounds according to place of articulation. *Journal of Speech and Hearing Disorders, 12,* 397–401.

Irwin, O. C. (1947b). Infant speech: Consonant sounds according to manner of articulation. *Journal of Speech and Hearing Disorders, 12,* 402–404.

Irwin, O. C. (1948). Infant speech: Development of vowel sounds. *Journal of Speech and Hearing Disorders, 13,* 31–34.

Irwin, O. C. (1951). Infant speech: Consonantal position. *Journal of Speech and Hearing Disorders, 16,* 159–161.

Irwin, O. C., & Chen, H. P. (1946). Infant speech: Vowel and consonant frequency. *Journal of Speech and Hearing Disorders, 11,* 123–125.

Irwin, J. V., & Wong, S. P. (Eds.). (1983). *Phonological development in children 18 to 72 months.* Carbondale: Southern Illinois University Press.

Ivimey, G. P. (1975). The development of English morphology: An acquisition model. *Language and Speech, 18,* 120–144.

Jacobson, J., Boersma, D., Fields, R., & Olson, K. (1983). Paralinguistic features of adult speech to infants and small children. *Child Development, 54,* 436–442.

Jakobson, R. (1949). On the identification of phonemic entities. *Travaux du Cercle Linguistique de Prague, 5,* 205–213.

Jakobson, R. (1962). Zur Struktur des Phonems (pp. 280–310). *Selected Writings I. Vol. 1, Phonological studies.* The Hague: Mouton.

Jakobson, R. (1968). *Child language, aphasia and phonological universals.* The Hague: Mouton. (Original work published 1942)

Jakobson, R., Fant, G., & Halle, M. (1952). *Preliminaries to speech analysis: The distinctive features and their correlates.* Cambridge, MA: MIT Press.

Jakobson, R., & Halle, M. (1956). *Fundamentals of language.* The Hague: Mouton.

Jespersen, O. (1913). *Lehrbuch der Phonetik.* Leipzig: Teubner.

Jones, D. (1938). Concrete and abstract sounds. *Proceedings of the 3rd International Congress of Phonetic Sciences.* Ghent, Belgium.

Jones, D. (1950). *The phoneme: Its nature and use.* Cambridge: Heffer.

Jusczyk, P., & Luce, P. (2002). Speech perception and spoken word recognition: Past and present. *Ear and Hearing, 23,* 2–40.

Justice, L. M., and Redle, E. E. (2014). Communication sciences and disorders: A clinical evidence-based approach (3rd ed.). Boston: Pearson.

Kagan, J. (1971). *Change and continuity in infancy.* New York: John Wiley.

Kamhi, A. G. (1992). Clinical forum: Phonological assessment and treatment. The need for a broad-based model of phonological disorders. *Language, Speech, and Hearing Services in Schools, 23,* 261–268.

Kamhi, A. G., Minor, J. S., & Mauer, D. (1990). Content analysis and intratest performance profiles on the Columbia and the TONI. *Journal of Speech and Hearing Research, 33,* 375–379.

Kantner, C., & West, R. (1960). *Phonetics* (Rev. ed.). New York: Harper & Brothers.

Keating, D., Turrell, G., & Ozanne, A. (2001). Childhood speech disorders: Reported prevalence, comordity, and socioeconomic profile. *Journal of Pediatric and Child Health, 37,* 149–171.

Kent, R. (1982). Contextual facilitation of correct sound production. *Language, Speech, and Hearing Services in Schools, 13,* 66–76.

Kent, R. D. (1997). *The speech sciences.* San Diego, CA: Singular.

Kent, R. D., & Bauer, H. R. (1985). Vocalizations of one-year-olds. *Journal of Child Language, 13,* 491–526.

Kent, R. D., Kent, J. F., & Rosenbeck, J. C. (1987). Maximum performance tests of speech production. *Journal of Speech and Hearing Disorders, 52,* 367–387.

Kent, R. D., Miolo, G., & Bloedel, S. (1994). The intelligibility of children's speech: A review of evaluation procedures. *American Journal of Speech-Language Pathology, 3*(2), 81–95.

Kent, R. D., & Murray, A. D. (1982). Acoustic features of infant vocalic utterances at 3, 6, and 9 months. *Journal of the Acoustical Society of America, 72,* 353–365.

Kent, R. D., & Vorperian, H. K. (2013). Speech impairments in Down Syndrome: A review. *Journal of Speech, Language, Hearing Research, 56,* 178–210.

Kent, R. D., Weismer, G., Kent, J. F., & Rosenbek, J. C. (1989). Toward

phonetic intelligibility testing in dysarthria. *Journal of Speech and Hearing Disorders, 54,* 482–499.

Kercher, M. B., & Bauman-Waengler, J. (1992). *Performances of Black English speaking children on standardized language tests.* Presentation at the national convention of the American Speech-Language-Hearing Association, San Antonio, TX.

Khan, L. (1988). *Vowel remediation: A case study.* Paper presented at the national convention of the American Speech-Language-Hearing Association, Boston, MA.

Khan, L. M. (2002). The sixth view: Assessing preschoolers' articulation and phonology from the trenches. *American Journal of Speech-Language Pathology, 11,* 250–254.

Khan, L., & Lewis, N. (2002). *Khan-Lewis phonological analysis* (2nd ed.). Circle Pines, MN: American Guidance Service.

Kharma, N., & Hajjaj, A. (1989). *Errors in English among Arabic speakers: Analysis and remedy.* London: Longman International Education.

Kim, M., & Pae, S. (2007). Korean speech acquisition. In S. McLeod (Ed.), *The international guide to speech acquisition* (pp. 472–482). Clifton Park, NY: Thomson Delmar Learning.

King, G., & Fletcher, P. (1993). Grammatical problems in school-age children with specific language impairment. *Clinical Linguistics and Phonetics, 7,* 339–352.

Kiparsky, P. (1982). From cyclic phonology to lexical phonology. In H. van der Hulst & H. Smith (Eds.), *The structure of phonological representations* (Vol. II, pp. 131–176). Dordrecht: Foris.

Kiparsky, P., & Menn, L. (1977). On the acquisition of phonology. In J. Macnamara (Ed.), *Language learning and thought* (pp. 47–78). New York: Academic Press.

Kirk, C. (2008). Substitution errors in the production of word-initial and word-final consonant clusters. *Journal of Speech, Language and Hearing Research, 51,* 35–48.

Kisilevsky, B. S., Hains, S. M. J., Jacquet, A.-Y., Grannier-Deferre, C., & Lecanuet, J. P. (2004). Maturation of fetal responses to music. *Developmental Science, 7,* 550–559.

Kitamura, H. (1991). Evidence for cleft palate as a postfusion phenomenon. *Cleft Palate Journal, 28,* 195–211.

Klein, E. S. (1996). *Clinical phonology: Assessment and treatment of articulation disorders in children and adults.* San Diego, CA: Singular.

Klein, H. B., Lederer, S. H., & Cortese, E. E. (1991). Children's knowledge of auditory/articulatory correspondences: Phonologic and metaphonologic. *Journal of Speech and Hearing Research, 34,* 559–564.

Knock, T., Ballard, K., Robin, D., & Schmidt, R. (2000). Influence or order of stimulus presentation on speech motor learning: A principled approach to treatment for apraxia of speech, *Aphasiology, 14,* 653–668.

Kruszewski, N. (1881). *Über Lautabwechslung.* Kasan': Universitätsbuchdruckerei.

Kuhl, P. (2010). Brain mechanisms in early language acquisition. *Neuron, 67,* 713–727.

Kuhl, P., Conboy, B., Padden, D., Nelson, T., & Pruitt, J. (2005). Early speech perception and later language development: Implications for the "critical period." *Language Learning and Development, 1,* 237–264.

Kuhl, P., Stevens, E., Hayashi, A., Deguchi, T., Kiritani, S., & Iverson, P. (2006). Infants show a facilitation effect for native language phonetic perception between 6 and 12 months. *Developmental Science, 9,* F13–F21.

Kumin, L. (1998). Speech and language skills in children with Down syndrome, *Mental Retardation and Developmental Disabilities Research Reviews, 2,* 109–115.

Kumin, L., & Adams, J. (2000). Developmental apraxia of speech and intelligibility in children with Down syndrome. *Down Syndrome Quarterly, 5,* 1–6.

Kussmaul, A. (1885). Die Störungen der Sprache. In H. V. Ziemsson (Ed.), *Handbuch der Speciellen Pathologie und Therapie: Volume 12* (pp. 1–299). Leipzig: F. C. W. Vogel.

Labov, W. (1991). The three dialects of English. In P. Eckert (Ed.), *New ways of analyzing sound change* (pp. 1–44). New York: Academic Press.

Labov, W. (1994). *Principles of linguistic change. Volume 1: Internal factors.* Oxford: Blackwell.

Labov, W. (1996). *The phonological atlas of North America.* Philadelphia: Linguistics Laboratory of the University of Pennsylvania.

Labov, W., Ash, S., & Boberg, C. (2005). *Atlas of North American English.* Berlin: Mouton de Gruyter.

Labov, W., Yaeger, M., & Steiner, R. (1972). *A quantitative study of sound change in progress.* Philadelphia: U.S. Regional Survey.

Ladefoged, P. (1971). *Preliminaries to linguistic phonetics.* Chicago: University of Chicago Press.

Ladefoged, P. & Johnson, K. (2010). *A course in phonetics* (6th ed.). Boston: Thomson Wadsworth.

Ladefoged, P., & Maddieson, I. (1996). *The sounds of the world's languages.* Oxford: Blackwell.

Lahey, M. (1988). *Language disorders and language development.* New York: Macmillan.

Lahey, M., & Bloom, L. (1977). Planning a first lexicon: Which words to teach first. *Journal of Speech and Hearing Disorders, 42,* 340–350.

Lapko, L., & Bankson, N. (1975). Relationship between auditory discrimination, articulation stimulability and consistency of misarticulation. *Perceptual and Motor Skills, 40,* 171–177.

Larrivee, L., & Catts, H. (1999). Early reading achievement in children with expressive phonological disorders. *American Journal of Speech-Language Pathology, 8,* 137–148.

Leafstedt, J., Richards, C., & Gerber, M. (2004). Effectiveness of explicit phonological-awareness instruction for at-risk English learners. *Learning Disabilities Research and Practice, 19,* 252–261.

Lee, H. B. (1999). Korean. In *Handbook of the International Phonetic Association* (pp. 120–122). Cambridge: Cambridge University Press.

Lee, L., Koenigsknecht, R., & Mulhern, S. (1975). *Interactive language development teaching.* Evanston, IL: Northwestern University Press.

Lehiste, I. (1970). *Suprasegmentals.* Cambridge: Massachusetts Institute of Technology.

Leinonen-Davis, E. (1988). Assessing the functional adequacy of children's phonological systems. *Clinical Linguistics and Phonetics, 2,* 257–270.

Leitao, S., Hogben, J., & Fletcher, J. (1997). Phonological processing skills in speech and language impaired children. *European Journal of Disorders of Communication, 32,* 73–93.

Leonard, L. (1988). Lexical development and processing in specific language impairment. In R. Schiefelbusch & L. Lloyd (Eds.), *Language perspectives: Acquisition, retardation, and intervention* (2nd ed., pp. 69–87). Austin, TX: PRO-ED.

Leonard, L. (1994). Some problems facing accounts of morphological deficits in children with specific language impairments. In R. Watkins & M. Rice (Eds.), *Specific language impairments in children* (pp. 91–106). Baltimore: Brookes.

Leonard, L., & McGregor, K. (1991). Unusual phonological patterns and their underlying representations: A case study. *Journal of Child Language, 18,* 261–271.

Leonard, L., McGregor, K., & Allen, G. (1992). Grammatical morphology and speech perception in children with specific language impairment. *Journal of Speech and Hearing Research, 35,* 1076–1085.

Leonard, L., Newhoff, M., & Mesalam, L. (1980). Individual differences in early child phonology. *Applied Psycholinguistics, 1,* 7–30.

Leopold, W. F. (1947). *Speech development of a bilingual child: A linguist's record.* Evanston, IL: Northwestern University Press.

Lepschy, G. C. (1970). *A survey of structural linguistics.* London: Faber and Faber.

Levin, K. (1999). Babbling in infants with cerebral palsy. *Clinical Linguistics and Phonetics, 13,* 249–267.

Lewis, B., Freebairn, L., Hansen, A., Taylor, H., Iyengar, S., & Shriberg, L. (2004). Family pedigrees of children with suspected childhood apraxia of speech. *Journal of Communication Disorders, 37,* 157–175.

Lewis, B., Freebairn, L., & Taylor, H. (2000). Correlates of spelling abilities in children with early speech sound disorders. *Reading and Writing: An Interdisciplinary Journal, 15,* 389–407.

Li, C., & Thompson, S. (1987). Chinese. In B. Comrie (Ed.), *The world's major languages* (pp. 811–833). New York: Oxford University Press.

Liberman, I. Y., & Shankweiler, D. (1985). Phonology and the problems of learning to read and write. *Topical Issues: Remedial and Special Education, 6,* 8–17.

Liberman, M. (1975). *The intonational system of English.* Doctoral dissertation, Massachusetts Institute of Technology, Cambridge, MA.

Liberman, M., & Prince, A. (1977). On stress and linguistic rhythm. *Linguistic Inquiry, 8,* 249–336.

Ling, D. (2002). *Speech and the hearing-impaired child: Theory and practice* (2nd ed.). Washington, DC: Alexander Graham Bell Association for the Deaf.

Lippke, B., Dickey, J., Selmar, J., & Soder, A. L. (1997). *PAT-3: Photo articulation test* (3rd ed.). Austin, TX: PRO-ED.

Lipsitt, L. (1966). Learning processes of human newborns. *Merrill-Palmer Quarterly, 12,* 45–71.

Lipski, J. (2000). The linguistic situation of Central Americans. In S. McKay & S. Wong (Eds.), *New immigrants in the United States* (pp. 189–215). Cambridge: Cambridge University Press.

Local, J. (1983). How many vowels in a vowel? *Journal of Child Language, 10,* 449–453.

Locke, J. L. (1980a). The inference of speech perception in the phonologically disordered child. Part I: A rationale, some criteria, the conventional tests. *Journal of Speech and Hearing Disorders, 45,* 431–434.

Locke, J. L. (1980b). The inference of speech perception in the phonologically disordered child. Part II: Some clinically novel procedures, their use, some findings. *Journal of Speech and Hearing Disorders, 45,* 435–468.

Locke, J. L. (1983). *Phonological acquisition and change.* Orlando, FL. Academic Press.

Locke, J. L. (1990). Structure and stimulation in the ontogeny of spoken language. *Developmental Psychobiology, 23,* 621–643.

Lof, G. L. (2002). Two comments on this assessment series. *American Journal of Speech-Language Pathology, 11,* 255–256.

Long, S. H., & Long, S. T. (1994). Language and children with mental retardation. In V. R. Reed (Ed.), *An introduction to children with language disorders* (2nd ed., pp. 153–191). New York: Merrill.

Lonigan, C., Burgess, S., & Anthony, J. (2000). Development of emergent literacy and early reading skills in preschool children: Evidence from a latent-variable longitudinal study. *Developmental Psychology, 36,* 596–613.

Lonigan, C., Burgess, S., Anthony, J., & Barker, T. (1998). Development of phonological sensitivity in 2- to 5-year-old children. *Journal of Educational Psychology, 90,* 294–311.

Love, R. J. (2000). *Childhood motor speech disability.* (2nd ed.) Boston: Allyn & Bacon.

Lowe, R. J. (1986). *Assessment link between phonology and articulation: ALPHA.* Moline, IL: LinguiSystems.

Lowe, R. J. (1994). *Phonology: Assessment and intervention applications in speech pathology.* Baltimore: Williams & Wilkins.

Lowe, R. J. (1996). *Assessment link between phonology and articulation: ALPHA* (rev. ed.). Mifflinville, PA: Speech and Language Resources.

Lowe, R. J., Knutson, P., & Monson, M. (1985). Incidence of fronting in preschool children. *Language, Speech, and Hearing Services in Schools, 16,* 119–123.

Lowe, R. J., Mount-Weitz, J., & Schmidt, C. (1992). *Activities for the remediation of phonological disorders.* DeKalb, IL: Janelle.

Lund, N. J., & Duchan, J. F. (1993). *Assessing children's language in naturalistic contexts* (3rd ed.). Englewood Cliffs, NJ: Prentice-Hall.

Lundberg, I. (1988). Preschool prevention of reading failure: Does training in phonological awareness work? In R. L. Masland & M. W. Masland (Eds.), *Preschool prevention of reading failure* (pp. 163–176). Parkton, MD: York Press.

Lundberg, I., Olofsson, A., & Wall, S. (1980). Reading and spelling skills in the first school years predicted from phonemic awareness skills in kindergarten. *Scandinavian Journal of Psychology, 21,* 159–173.

Lyytinen, H., Ahonen, T., Eklund, K., Guttorm, T., Laakso, M., Leinonen, S., et al. (2001). Developmental pathways of children with and without familial risk for dyslexia during the first years of life. *Developmental Neuropsychology, 20,* 535–554.

Maas, E., & Farinella, K. A. (2012). Random versus blocked practice in treatment for childhood apraxia of speech. *Journal of Speech, Language, and Hearing Research, 55,* 561–578.

Maassen, B., Groenen, P., & Crul, T. (2003). Auditory and phonetic perception of vowels in children with apraxic speech disorders. *Clinical Linguistics and Phonetics, 17,* 447–467.

Maclean, M., Bryant, P., & Bradley, L. (1987). Rhymes, nursery rhymes and reading in early childhood. *Merrill-Palmer Quarterly, 33,* 255–282.

Magnusson, E. (1991). Metalinguistic awareness in phonologically disordered children. In M. Yavaş (Ed.), *Phonological disorders in children: Theory, research and practice* (pp. 87–120). London: Routledge.

Malabonga, V., & Marinova-Todd, S. (2007). Chapter 38: Filipino speech acquisition. In S. McLeod (Ed.), *The international guide to speech acquisition* (pp. 340–350). Clifton Park, NY: Thomson Delmar Learning.

Malikouti-Drachman, A., & Drachman, G. (1975). The acquisition of stress in Modern Greek. *Salzburger Beiträge zur Linguistik, 2,* 277–289.

Mampe, B., Friederici, A. D., Christophe, A., & Wermke, K. (2009). Newborns' cry melody is shaped by their native language, *Current Biology, 19,* 1994–1997.

Marcos, H. (1987). Communicative function of pitch range and pitch direction in infants. *Journal of Child Language, 14,* 255–268.

Mareschal, D., & French, R. (2000). Mechanisms of categorization in infants. *Infancy, 1,* 59–76.

Marili, J., Andrianopoulos, K., Velleman, M., & Foreman, C. (2004). *Incidence of motor speech impairment in autism and Asperger's disorders.* Paper presented at the annual convention of the American Speech-Language-Hearing Association, Philadelphia, PA.

Marion, M. J., Sussman, H. M., & Marquardt, T. P. (1993). The perception and production of rhyme in normal and developmentally apraxic children. *Journal of Communication Disorders, 26,* 129–160.

Marquardt, T. P., Sussman, H. M., Snow, T., & Jacks, A. (2002). The integrity of the syllable in developmental apraxia of speech. *Journal of Communication Disorders, 35,* 31–49.

Marsh, J. L., & Lehman, J. A. (1988). *Cleft care in 1986: An ACPA survey* [abstract]. American Cleft Palate–Craniofacial Annual Meeting, Williamsburg, VA.

Martinet, A. (1960). *Elements de linguistique général I.* [Elements of general linguistics I]. Paris: Armand Colin.

Masterson, J., Bernhardt, B., & Hofheinz, M. (2005). A comparison of single words and conversational speech in phonological evaluation. *American Journal of Speech-Language Pathology, 14,* 229–241.

Matisoff, J. (1991). Sino-Tibetan linguistics: Present state and future prospects. *Annual Review of Anthropology, 20,* 469–504.

Maye, J., & Gerken, L. (2000). *Learning phonemes without minimal pairs.* Proceedings of the 24th Annual Boston University Conference on Language Development. Somerville, MA: Cascadia Press.

Maye, J., & Weiss, D. (2003). *Statistical cues facilitate infants' discrimination of difficult phonetic contrasts.* Proceedings of the 27th Boston University Conference on Language Development (pp. 508–518). Somerville, MA: Cascadilla Press.

Maye, J., Werker, J., & Gerken, L. (2002). Infant sensitivity to distributional information can affect phonetic discrimination, *Cognition, 82,* B101–B111.

McCabe, P., Rosenthal, J. B., & McLeod, S. (1998). Features of developmental dyspraxia in the general speech impaired population? *Clinical Linguistics and Phonetics, 12,* 105–126.

McCabe, T., Murray, E., Thomas, D., Bejjani, L., & Ballard, K. (2013). *A new evidence-based treatment for childhood apraxia of speech: ReST,* Paper presented at the national convention of the American Speech-Language-Hearing Association, Tampa, FL.

McCarthren, R., Warren, S., & Yoder, P. (1996). Prelinguistic predictors of later language development. In K. Cole, P. Dale, & D. Thal (Eds.), *Assessment of communication and language* (pp. 57–75). Baltimore: Brookes.

McCarthy, J. J., & Prince, A. S. (1995). Faithfulness and reduplicative identity. In *Papers in Optimality Theory: University of Massachusetts Occasional Papers in Linguistics 18* (pp. 249–384). Amherst, MA: Graduate Linguistics Student Association.

McCauley, R.J., & Strand, E.A. (2008). A review of standardized tests of nonverbal oral and speech motor performance in children. *American Journal of Speech-Language Pathology, 17,* 81–91.

McCune, L., & Vihman, M. M. (2001). Early phonetic and lexical development: A productivity approach. *Jour-*

nal of Speech, Language, and Hearing Research, 44, 670–684.

McCurdy, S. (2010). *Hmong learners' deletion and replacement of syllable-final consonants in English.* Unpublished master's thesis, Hamline University, St. Paul, Minnesota.

McDonald, E. T. (1964). *A deep test of articulation—Picture form.* Pittsburgh, PA: Stanwix.

McHenry, M. (2003). The effect of pacing strategies on the variability of speech movement sequences in dysarthria. *Journal of Speech, Language, and Hearing Research, 46,* 702–710.

McLeod, S., van Doorn, J., & Reed, V. (2001). Consonant cluster development in two-year-olds: General trends and individual difference. *Journal of Speech, Language, and Hearing Research, 44,* 1144–1171.

McNeil, M. R., Fossett, T. R., Katz, W. F., Garst, D., Carter, G., Szuminsky, N., & Doyle, P. J. (2007). Effects of on-line kinematic feedback treatment for apraxia of speech. *Brain and Language, 103,* 223–225.

McNeil, M. R., Robin, D. A., & Schmidt, R. A. (2009). Apraxia of speech: Definition, differentiation, and treatment. In M. R. McNeil (Ed.), *Clinical management of sensorimotor speech disorders* (2nd ed.). (pp. 249–268). New York: Thieme.

McNeill, B. C., Gillon, G. T., & Dodd, B. (2009a). Effectiveness of an integrated phonological awareness approach for children with childhood apraxia of speech (CAS). *Child Language Teaching and Therapy, 25,* 341–366.

McNeill, B. C., Gillon, G. T., & Dodd, B. (2009b). A longitudinal case study of the effects of an integrated phonological awareness program for identical twin boys with childhood apraxia of speech (CAS). *International Journal of Speech-Language Pathology, 11,* 482–495.

McReynolds, L. V., & Engmann, D. (1975). Distinctive features analysis of misarticulations. Baltimore: University Park Press.

McReynolds, L. V., Engmann, D., & Dimmitt, K. (1974). Markedness theory and articulation errors. *Journal of Speech and Hearing Disorders, 39,* 93–103.

Mehrabian, A. (1970). Measures of vocabulary and grammatical skills for children up to age six. *Developmental Psychology, 2,* 439–446.

Menn, L. (1971). Phonotactic rules in beginning speech. *Lingua, 26,* 225–251.

Menn, L. (1976). *Pattern, control and contrast in beginning speech: A case study in the development of word form and word function.* Unpublished doctoral dissertation, University of Illinois, Urbana–Champaign.

Menn, L. (1978). *Pattern, control and contrast in beginning speech: A case study in the development of word form and word function.* Bloomington: Indiana University Linguistics Club.

Menn, L., & Velleman, S. (2010). *Framework for decision making in clinical phonology.* Paper presented at the American Speech-Language-Hearing Association, Philadelphia, PA.

Miccio, A. W. (2002). Clinical problem solving: Assessment of phonological disorders. *American Journal of Speech-Language Pathology, 11,* 221–229.

Miccio, A. W., Elbert, M., & Forrest, K. (1999). The relationship between stimulability and phonological acquisition in children with normally developing and disordered phonologies. *American Journal of Speech-Language Pathology, 8,* 347–363.

Migration Policy Institute (2010). State immigration data profiles. Migration Policy Institute tabulations of the U.S. Bureau of the Census' American Community Survey (ACS) and Decennial Census. Washington, D.C.

Miller, J. F. (1988). Facilitating speech and language. In C. Tingey (Ed.), *Down syndrome. A resource book* (pp. 119–133). Boston: College-Hill Press.

Milloy, N., & Morgan-Barry, R. (1990). Developmental neurological disorders. In P. Grunwell (Ed.), *Developmental speech disorders* (pp. 109–132). New York: Churchill Livingstone.

Mines, M., Hanson, B., & Shoup, J. (1978). Frequency of occurrence of phonemes in conversational English language and speech. *Language and Speech, 21,* 221–241.

Mitchell, P. R., & Kent, R. (1990). Phonetic variation in multisyllable babbling. *Journal of Child Language, 17,* 247–265.

Monnin, L., & Huntington, D. (1974). Relationship of articulatory defects to speech-sound identification. *Journal of Speech and Hearing Research, 17,* 352–366.

Monsen, R. B. (1981). A usable test for the speech intelligibility of deaf talkers. *American Annals of the Deaf, 126,* 845–852.

Monsen, R. B., Moog, J. S., & Geers, A. E. (1988). *CID picture SPINE.* St. Louis, MO: Central Institute for the Deaf.

Moran, M. (1993). Final consonant deletion in African American children speaking Black English: A closer look. *Language, Speech, and Hearing Services in the Schools, 24,* 161–166.

Moriarty, B., & Gillon, G. (2006). Phonological awareness intervention for children with childhood apraxia of speech. *International Journal of Language & Communication Disorders, 41,* 713–734.

Morley, M. E., Court, D., & Miller, H. (1954). Delayed speech and developmental aphasia. *British Medical Journal, 2,* 463–467.

Morris, H. L., Spriestersbach, D. C., & Darley, F. L. (1961). An articulation test for assessing competency of velopharyngeal closure. *Journal of Speech and Hearing Research, 4,* 48–55.

Morris, S. R. (2010). Clinical application of the mean babbling level and syllable structure level. *Language, Speech, and Hearing Services in Schools, 41,* 223–230.

Morrisette, M., & Gierut, J. (2002). Lexical organization and phonological change in treatment. *Journal of Speech, Language, and Hearing Research, 45,* 143–159.

Morrison, J., & Shriberg, L. (1992). Articulation testing versus conversational speech sampling. *Journal of Speech and Hearing Research, 35,* 259–273.

Mortensen, D. (2004). *Preliminaries to Mong Leng (Hmong Njua) phonology.* http://ist-socrates.berkeley.edu/~dmort/mong_leng_phonology.pdf

Mortimer, J. (2007). *Effects of speech perception, vocabulary, and articulation skills in morphology and syntax in children with speech sound disorders.* Unpublished doctoral dissertation, McGill University, Montreal, Canada.

Mosher, J. (1929). *The production of correct speech sounds.* Boston: Expression.

Moskowitz, A. (1971). *Acquisition of phonology.* Unpublished doctoral dissertation, University of California, Berkeley.

Munson, B., Edwards, J., & Beckman, M. (2005a). Phonological knowledge in typical and atypical speech-sound development. *Topics in Language Disorders. Clinical Perspectives on Speech Sound Disorders, 25,* 190–206.

Munson, B., Edwards, J., & Beckman, M. E. (2005b). Relationship of non-word repetition accuracy and other measures of linguistic development in children with phonological disorders. *Journal of Speech, Language and Hearing Research, 47,* 61–78.

Murray, E., McCabe, P., & Ballard, K. J. (2014). A systematic review of treatment outcomes for children with childhood apraxia of speech. *American Journal of Speech-Language Pathology, 13,* 1–19.

Myers, F. L., & Myers, R. W. (1983). Perception of stress contrasts in semantic and non-semantic contexts by children. *Journal of Psycholinguistic Research, 12,* 327–338.

Myerson, R. F. (1978). Children's knowledge of selected aspects of sound pattern of English. In R. N. Campbell & P. T. Smith (Eds.), *Recent advances in the psychology of language* (Vol. III4) (pp. 377–402). New York: Plenum Press.

Mysak, E. D. (1959). A servomodel for speech therapy. *Journal of Speech and Hearing Disorders, 24,* 144–149.

Nakazima, S. A. (1962). A comparative study of the speech developments of Japanese and American English in childhood (1): A comparison of the developments of voices at the prelinguistic period. *Studia Phonologica, 2,* 27–46.

Nathani, S., Ertmer, D., & Stark, R. (2006). Assessing vocal development in infants and toddlers. *Clinical Linguistics and Phonetics, 20,* 351–369.

National Center for Children in Poverty: Brief on English language proficiency, family economic security, and child development. (2010). *Mailman School of Public Health.* New York: Columbia University.

National Joint Committee for the Communication Needs of Persons with Severe Disabilities. (2010). *Communication services for individuals with severe disabilities: FAQs and discussion.* American Speech-Language-Hearing Association, Philadelphia, PA.

Nelson, K. (1973). Structure and strategy in learning to talk. *Monographs of the Society of Research in Child Development, 38* (149). Chicago: University of Chicago Press.

Nelson, N. W. (1998). *Childhood language disorders in context: Infancy through adolescence* (2nd ed.). Boston: Allyn & Bacon.

Nemoy, E. M. (1954). *Speech correction through story telling units.* Magnolia, MA: Expression.

Nemoy, E. M., & Davis, S. (1937). *The correction of defective consonant sounds.* Boston: Expression.

Nijland, L., Maassen, B., van der Meulen, S., Gabreëls, F., Kraaimaat, F. W., & Schreuder, R. (2002). Coarticulation patterns in children with developmental apraxia of speech. *Clinical Linguistics and Phonetics, 16,* 461–483.

Nordberg, A., Miniscalco, C., & Lohmander, A. (2014) Consonant production and overall speech characteristics in school-aged children with cerebral palsy and speech impairment. *International Journal of Language & Communication Disorders,16,* 386–395.

Northern, J. L., & Downs, M. P. (2002). *Hearing in children* (3rd ed.). Baltimore: Lippincott, Williams & Wilkins.

Odding, E., Roebroeck, M. E., Stam, H. J. (2006). The epidemiology of cerebral palsy: Incidence, impairments and risk factors. *Disability and Rehabilitation. 28,* 183–191.

Oetting, J., & Horohov, J. (1997). Past tense marking by children with and without specific language impairment. *Journal of Speech and Hearing Research, 40,* 62–74.

Oetting, J., & Rice, M. (1993). Plural acquisition in children with specific language impairment. *Journal of Speech and Hearing Research, 36,* 1236–1248.

Ogar, J., Willock, S., Baldo, J., Wilkins, D., Ludy, C., & Dronkers, N. (2006). Clinical and anatomical correlates of apraxia of speech. *Brain and Language, 97,* 343–350.

O'Grady, W. D., & Archibald, J. (2012). *Contemporary linguistic analysis: An introduction* (7th ed.). Toronto: Pearson Longman.

Oller, D. K. (1980). The emergence of the sounds of speech in infancy. In G. Yeni-Komshian, J. Kavanagh, & C. A. Ferguson (Eds.), *Child phonology: Vol. I. Production* (pp. 93–112). New York: Academic Press.

Oller, D., Eilers, R., Neal, A., & Schwartz, G. (1999). Precursors to speech in infancy: The prediction of speech and language disorders. *Journal of Communication Disorders, 32,* 223–245.

Oller, D. K., Wieman, L. A., Doyle, W. J., & Ross, C. (1976). Infant babbling and speech. *Journal of Child Language, 3,* 1–11.

Olmsted, D. (1971). Out of the mouth of babes: Earliest stages in language learning. The Hague: Mouton.

Osberger, M. J., Robbins, A. M., Todd, S. L., & Riley, A. I. (1994). Speech intelligibility of children with cochlear implants. *The Volta Review, 96,* 169–180.

Otheguy, R., Garcia, O., & Roca, A. (2000). Speaking in Cuban: The language of Cuban Americans. In S. McKay & S. Wong (Eds.), *New immigrants in the United States* (pp. 165–188). Cambridge: Cambridge University Press.

Owens, R. E. (2008). *Language development: An introduction* (7th ed.). Boston: Allyn & Bacon.

Owens, R. E. (2009). Mental retardation/mental disability. In D. K. Bernstein & E. Tiegerman-Farber (Eds.), *Language and communication disorders in children* (6th ed.) (pp. 246–313). Boston: Allyn & Bacon: Pearson.

Paavola, L., Kunnari, S., & Moilanen, I. (2005). Maternal responsiveness and infant intentional communication: Implications for the early communicative and linguistic development. *Child: Care, Health and Development, 31,* 727–735.

Pamplona, M., Ysunza, A., Gonzalez, M., Ramirez, E., & Patino, C. (2000). Linguistic development in cleft palate patients with and without compensatory articulation disorder. *International Journal of Pediatric Otorhinolaryngology, 54,* 81–91.

Panagos, J., & Prelock, P. (1982). Phonological constraints on the sentence production of language disordered children. *Journal of Speech and Hearing Research, 25,* 171–177.

Parker, F., & Riley, K. (2010). *Linguistics for non-linguists: Primer with exercises* (5th ed.). Boston: Allyn & Bacon.

Patel, R. (2002). Prosodic control in severe dysarthria. *Journal of Speech, Language, and Hearing Research, 45,* 858–870.

Paul, R. (1991). Profiles of toddlers with slow expressive language development. *Topics in Language Disorders, 11,* 1–13.

Paul, R. (1993). Patterns of development in late talkers: Preschool years. *Journal of Childhood Communication Disorders, 15,* 7–14.

Paul, R. (2007). *Language disorders from infancy through adolescence: Assessment and intervention.* (3rd ed.) St. Louis, MO: Mosby Year Book.

Paul, R., & Jennings, P. (1992). Phonological behavior in toddlers with slow expressive language development. *Journal of Speech and Hearing Research, 35,* 99–107.

Pena-Brooks, A., & Hegde, M. N. (2000). *Assessment and treatment of articulation and phonological disorders in children.* Austin, TX: PRO-ED.

Pence, K. L., & Justice, L. M. (2008). *Language development from theory to practice.* Upper Saddle River, NJ: Pearson Education.

Penfield, J., & Ornstein-Galacia, J. (1985). *Chicano English: An ethnic dialect.* Philadelphia: John Benjamin.

Perez, E. (1994). Phonological differences among speakers of Spanish-influenced English. In J. Bernthal & N. Bankson (Eds.), *Child phonology: Characteristics, assessment, and intervention with special populations* (pp. 245–254). New York: Thieme.

Pharr, A., Ratner, N., & Rescorla, L. (2000). Syllable structure development of toddlers with expressive specific language impairment. *Applied Psycholinguistics, 21,* 429–449.

Piaget, J. (1952). *The origins of intelligence in children.* New York: International Universities Press.

Pierce, J. E., & Hanna, I. V. (1974). *The development of a phonological system in English speaking American children.* Portland, OR: HaPi Press.

Pike, K. L. (1943). *Phonetics.* Ann Arbor: University of Michigan Press.

Pollock, K. (1991). The identification of vowel errors using traditional articulation or phonological process test stimuli. *Language, Speech, and Hearing Services in Schools, 22,* 39–50.

Pollock, K. E. (2013). Identification of vowel errors: Methodological issues and preliminary data from the Memphis vowel project. In M. J. Ball & F. E. Gibbon (Eds.), *Vowel disorders*

(pp. 83–113). Boston: Butterworth-Heinemann.

Pollock, K. E., & Berni, M. C. (2001). Transcription of vowels. *Topics in Language Disorders, 21,* 22–40.

Pollock, K. E., & Berni, M. C. (2003). Incidence of non-rhotic vowel errors in children: Data from the Memphis Vowel Project. *Clinical Linguistics and Phonetics, 17,* 393–401.

Pollock, K., & Hall, P. K. (1991). An analysis of the vowel misarticulations of five children with developmental apraxia of speech. *Clinical Linguistics and Phonetics, 5,* 207–224.

Pollock, K., & Keiser, N. (1990). An examination of vowel errors in phonologically disordered children. *Clinical Linguistics and Phonetics, 4,* 161–178.

Pollock, K., & Schwartz, R. (1988). Structural aspects of phonological development: Case study of a disordered child. *Language, Speech, and Hearing Services in Schools, 19,* 5–16.

Poole, I. (1934). Genetic development of articulation of consonant sounds in speech. *Elementary English Review, 11,* 159–161.

Powell, T. W., & Elbert, M. (1984). Generalization following the remediation of early- and later-developing consonants clusters. *Journal of Speech and Hearing Disorders, 49,* 211–218.

Powell, T. W., Elbert, M., & Dinnsen, D. A. (1991). Stimulability as a factor in the phonologic generalization of misarticulating preschool children. *Journal of Speech and Hearing Research, 34,* 1318–1328.

Power, T. (2003). Practice for Arabic language backgrounds. http://www.btinternet.com/-ted.power/11 arabic.html

Prather, E. M., Hedrick, D., & Kern, C. (1975). Articulation development in children aged two to four years. *Journal of Speech and Hearing Disorders, 40,* 179–191.

Preisser, D. A., Hodson, B. W., & Paden, E. P. (1988). Developmental phonology: 18–29 months. *Journal of Speech and Hearing Disorders, 53,* 125–130.

Preston, J. L., Hull, M., & Edwards, M. L. (2013). Preschool speech error patterns predict articulation and phonological awareness outcomes in children with histories of speech-sound disorders, *American Journal of Speech-Language Pathology, 22,* 173–184.

Prince, A. S., & Smolensky, P. (1993). Optimality theory: Constraint interaction in generative grammar, *RUCCs Technical Report #2.* New Brunswick, NJ: Rutgers University Center for Cognitive Science.

Pulleyblank, D. (1986). Underspecification and low vowel harmony in Okpe2. *Studies in African Linguistics, 17,* 119–153.

Radziewicz, C., & Antonellis, S. (1997). Considerations and implications for habilitation of hearing impaired children. In D. K. Bernstein & E. Tiegerman (Eds.), *Language and communication disorders in children* (4th ed., pp. 574–603). Boston: Allyn & Bacon.

Ramsdell, H. L., Oller, D. K., Buder, E. H., Ethington, C. A., & Chorna, L. (2012). Identification of prelinguistic phonological categories. *Journal of Speech, Language, Hearing Research, 55,* 1626–1639.

Ratliff, M. (1992). *Meaningful tone: A study of tonal morphology in compounds, form classes, and expressive phrases in White Hmong* (Monograph No. 27, Southeast Asia). De Kalb: Northern Illinois University Center for Southeast Asian Studies.

Reed, V. (2005). *An introduction to children with language disorders* (3rd ed.). Boston: Allyn & Bacon.

Renfrew, C. (1966). Persistence of the open syllable in defective articulation. *Journal of Speech and Hearing Disorders, 31,* 370–373.

Rescorla, L. (1989). The Language Development Survey: A screening tool for delayed language in toddlers. *Journal of Speech and Hearing Disorders, 54,* 587–599.

Rescorla, L., Mirak, J., & Singh, L. (2000). Vocabulary growth in late talkers: Lexical development from 2;0 to 3;0. *Journal of Child Language, 27,* 293–311.

Rescorla, L., & Ratner, N. B. (1996). Phonetic profiles in toddlers with specific expressive language impairment (SLI-E). *Journal of Speech and Hearing Research, 39,* 153–165.

Rescorla, L., & Schwartz, E. (1990). Outcome of toddlers with expressive language delay. *Applied Psycholinguistics, 11,* 393–407.

Reynolds, J. (1990). Abnormal vowel patterns in phonologically disordered children: Some data and a hypothesis. *British Journal of Disorders of Communication, 25,* 115–148.

Reynolds, J. (2013). Recurring patterns and idiosyncratic systems in some English children with vowel disorders. In M. J. Ball & F. E. Gibbon (Eds.), *Handbook of vowels and vowel disorders* (pp. 229–259). East Sussex, UK: Psychological Press.

Rice, M. (1991). Children with specific language impairment: Towards a model of teachability. In N. Krasnegor (Ed.), *Biological and behavioral determinants of language development* (pp. 447–480). Hillsdale, NJ: Lawrence Erlbaum.

Rice, M. (1994). Grammatical categories of children with specific language impairments. In R. Watkins & M. Rice (Eds.), *Specific language impairment in children* (pp. 69–90). Baltimore: Brookes.

Rice, M., & Bode, J. (1993). Gaps in the verb lexicons of children with specific language impairment. *First Language, 13,* 113–131.

Rice, M., & Oetting, J. (1993). Morphological deficits of children with SLI: Evaluation of number marking and agreement. *Journal of Speech and Hearing Research, 36,* 1249–1257.

Rice, M., Wexler, K., & Cleave, P. (1995). Specific language impairment as a period of extended optional infinitive. *Journal of Speech and Hearing Research, 38,* 850–863.

Richardson, U., Leppaenen, P., Leiwo, M., & Lyytinen, H. (2003). Speech perception of infants with high familial risk for dyslexia differ at the age of 6 months. *Developmental Neuropsychology, 23,* 385–397.

Rivera-Gaxiola, M., Silva-Pereyra, J., & Kuhl, P. K. (2005). Brain potentials to native and non-native speech contrasts in 7- and 11-month-old American infants. *Developmental Science, 8,* 162–172.

Robb, M. P., & Saxman, J. H. (1990). Syllable durations of preword and early word vocalizations. *Journal of Speech and Hearing Research, 33,* 583–593.

Roberts, A. (1965). *A statistical linguistic analysis of American English.* The Hague: Mouton.

Roberts, J. E., Burchinal, M., & Footo, M. (1990). Phonological process decline from 2½ to 8 years. *Journal of Communication Disorders, 23,* 205–217.

Roberts, T. (2005). Articulation accuracy and vocabulary size contributions to phonemic awareness and word reading in English language learners. *Journal of Educational Psychology, 97,* 601–616.

Robertson, S. J. (1982). *Robertson dysarthria profile.* San Antonio, TX: Communication Skill Builders.

Roseberry-McKibbon, C. (2007). *Language disorders in children: A multicultural and case perspective.* Boston: Pearson Education.

Roseberry-McKibbon, C., & Brice, A. (2010). *Acquiring English as a second Language: What's "normal," and what's not.* American Speech-Language-Hearing Association http://www.asha.org/public/speech/-development/easl.htm

Rosenbaum, P., Paneth, N., Leviton, A., Goldstein, M., Bax, M., & Jacobsson, B. (2007). A report: The definition and classification of cerebral palsy. *Developmental Medicine & Child Neurology. 109,* 8–14.

Rosenbek, J. C., & Jones, H. N. (2009). Principles of treatment for sensorimotor speech disorders. In M. R. McNeil (Ed.),*Clinical management of sensorimotor speech disorders* (2nd ed.). (pp. 269–288). New York: Thieme.

Rosetti, A. (1959). *Sur la théorie de la syllable.* Gravenhage: Mouton.

Rothgaenger, H. (2003). Analysis of the sounds of the child in the first year of age and a comparison to the language. *Early Human Development, 75,* 55–69.

Ruhlen, M. (1976). *Guide to the languages of the world.* San Diego, CA: Los Amigos Research Associates.

Rvachew, S., & Nowak, M. (2001). The effect of target-selection strategy on phonological learning. *Journal of Speech, Language, and Hearing Research, 44,* 610–623.

Rvachew, S., Rafaat, S., & Martin, M. (1999). Stimulability, speech perception skills, and the treatment of phonological disorders. *American Journal of Speech-Language Pathology, 8,* 33–43.

Ryan, S. (2009). American English pronunciation problems for Filipinos. The Center for Confident American English Communication. Orlando: FL. http://www.confidentvoice.com/blog/american-english-pronunciation-problems-for-filipinos/

Saben, C., & Costello-Ingham, J. (1991). The effects of minimal pairs treatment on the speech-sound production of two children with phonologic disorders. *Journal of Speech and Hearing Research, 34,* 1023–1040.

Sagey, E. (1986). *The representation of features and relations in non-linear phonology.* Unpublished doctoral dissertation, MIT, Cambridge, MA.

Sander, E. K. (1972). When are speech sounds learned? *Journal of Speech and Hearing Disorders, 37,* 55–63.

Sapir, E. (1921). *Language: An introduction to the study of speech.* New York: Harcourt, Brace and World.

Sapir, E. (1925). Sound patterns in language. *Language, 1,* 37–51.

Saussure, F., de (1959). *A course in general linguistics.* (J. Cantineau, Trans.). London: Owen. (Original work published 1916.)

Schmauch, V., Panagos, J., & Klich, R. (1978). Syntax influences the accuracy of consonant production in language-disordered children. *Journal of Communication Disorders, 11,* 315–323.

Schonweiler, R., Schonweiler, B., Schmelzeisen, R., & Ptok, M. (1995). The language and speech skills in 417 children with cleft formations. *Fortschritte in der Kieferorthopädie, 56,* 1–6.

Schwartz, A., & Goldman, R. (1974). Variables influencing performance on speech discrimination tests. *Journal of Speech and Hearing Research, 17,* 25–32.

Schwartz, R. (1992). Nonlinear phonology as a framework for phonological acquisition. In R. Chapman (Ed.), *Processes in language acquisition and disorders* (pp. 108–124). St. Louis, MO: Mosby Year Book.

Schwartz, R., & Leonard, L. B. (1982). Do children pick and choose? An examination of phonological selection and avoidance in early lexical acquisition. *Journal of Child Language, 9,* 319–336.

Scripture, E. W. (1902). *Elements of experimental phonetics.* New York: Charles Scribner's Sons.

Scripture, E. W. (1927). Die Silbigkeit und die Silbe. *Archives für das Studium der neueren Sprachen, CLII,* 74.

Scripture, M., & Jackson, E. (1919). A manual of exercises for the correction of speech disorders. Philadelphia: Davis.

Secord, W. (1981a). *C-PAC: Clinical probes of articulation consistency.* Sedona, AZ: Red Rock Education.

Secord, W. (1981b). *Eliciting sounds: Techniques for clinicians.* San Antonio, TX: Psychological Corporation.

Secord, W. (1989). The traditional approach to treatment. In N. A. Creaghead, P. W. Newman, & W. A. Secord (Eds.), *Assessment and remediation of articulatory and phonological disorders* (2nd ed., pp. 129–158). New York: Macmillan.

Sell, D., Harding, A., & Grunwell, P. (1994). A screening assessment of cleft palate speech (Great Ormond Street Speech Assessment). *European Journal of Disordered Communication, 29,* 1–15.

Seymour, H., Green, L., & Hundley, R. (1991). *Phonological patterns in the conversational speech of African American children.* Paper presented at the national convention of the American Speech-Language-Hearing Association, Atlanta, GA.

Seymour, H., & Miller-Jones, D. (1981). Language and cognitive assessment of Black children. *Speech Language: Advances in Basic Research and Practice, 6,* 203–255.

Share, D., Jorm, A., Maclean, R., & Matthews, R. (1984). Sources of individual differences in reading acquisition. *Journal of Educational Psychology, 76,* 1309–1324.

Shibamoto, J., & Olmsted, D. (1978). Lexical and syllabic patterns in phonological acquisition. *Journal of Child Language, 5,* 417–456.

Shipley, K. G., & McAfee, J. G. (1998). *Assessment in speech-language pathology: A resource manual* (2nd ed.). San Diego, CA: Singular Thomson Learning.

Shprintzen, R. J. (1995). *Cleft palate speech management. A multidisciplinary approach.* St. Louis, MO: Mosby Year Book.

Shriberg, L. D. (1991). Directions for research in developmental phonological disorders. In J. F. Miller (Ed.), *Research on child language disorders: A decade of progress* (pp. 267–276). Austin, TX: PRO-ED.

Shriberg, L. D. (2004). *Diagnostic classification of five subtypes of childhood speech sound disorders (SSD) of currently unknown origin.* Paper presented at the International Association of Logopedics and Phoniatrics, Brisbane, Queensland, Australia.

Shriberg, L. D., Aram, D. M., & Kwiatkowski, J. (1997a). Developmental apraxia of speech: I. Descriptive and theoretical perspectives. *Journal of Speech, Language, and Hearing Research, 40,* 273–285.

Shriberg, L. D., Aram, D. M., & Kwiatkowski, J. (1997b). Developmental apraxia of speech: II. Toward a diagnostic marker. *Journal of Speech, Language, and Hearing Research, 40,* 286–312.

Shriberg, L. D., Aram, D. M., & Kwiatkowski, J. (1997c). Developmental apraxia of speech: III. A subtype marked by inappropriate stress. *Journal of Speech, Language, and Hearing Research, 40,* 313–337.

Shriberg, L. D., Austin, D., Lewis, B., McSweeny, J. L., & Wilson, D. L. (1997). The percentage of consonants correct (PCC) metric: Extensions and reliability data. *Journal of Speech, Language, and Hearing Research, 40,* 708–722.

Shriberg, L. D., & Kent, R. D. (2013). *Clinical phonetics* (4th ed.). Boston: Pearson.

Shriberg, L. D., & Kwiatkowski, J. (1982a). Phonological disorders II: A conceptual framework for management. *Journal of Speech and Hearing Disorders, 47,* 242–256.

Shriberg, L. D., & Kwiatkowski, J. (1982b). Phonological disorders III: A procedure for assessing severity of involvement. *Journal of Speech and Hearing Disorders, 47,* 256–270.

Shriberg, L. D., & Kwiatkowski, J. (1994). Developmental phonological disorders I: A clinical profile. *Journal of Speech and Hearing Research, 37,* 1100–1126.

Shriberg, L. D., Kwiatkowski, J., Best, S., Hengst, J., & Terselic-Weber, B. (1986). Characteristics of children with phonologic disorders of unknown origin. *Journal of Speech and Hearing Disorders, 51,* 140–161.

Shriberg, L. D., Kwiatkowski, J., & Rasmussen, C. (1990). *The prosody-voice screening profile.* Tucson, AZ: Communication Builders.

Shriberg, L. D., & Lof, G. L. (1991). Reliability studies in broad and narrow transcription. *Clinical Linguistics and Phonetics, 5,* 225–179.

Shriberg, L. D., Tomblin, J., & McSweeney, J. (1999). Prevalence of speech delay in 6-year-old children and comorbidity with language impairment. *Journal of Speech, Language, and Hearing Research, 42,* 1461–1481.

Shriberg, L. D., & Widder, C. J. (1990). Speech and prosody characteristics of adults with mental retardation. *Journal of Speech and Hearing Research, 33,* 627–653.

Shvachkin, N. K. (1973). The development of phonemic speech perception in early childhood. In C. A. Ferguson & D. I. Slobin (Eds.), *Studies of child language development* (pp. 91–127). New York: Holt, Rinehart and Winston.

Sievers, E. (1901). *Grundzüge der Phonetik: Zur Einführung in das Studium der indogermanischen Sprachen.* Leipzig: Breitkopf und Hartel.

Singh, S., & Polen, S. (1972). Use of distinctive feature model in speech pathology. *Acta Symbolica, 3,* 17–25.

Skahan, S. M., Watson, M., & Lof, G. L. (2007). Speech-language pathologists' assessment practices for children with suspected speech sound disorders: Results of a national survey. *American Journal of Speech-Language Pathology, 16,* 246–259.

Sloat, C., Taylor, S., & Hoard, J. (1978). *Introduction to phonology.* Englewood Cliffs, NJ: Prentice-Hall.

Small, L. (2012). *Fundamentals of phonetics: A practical guide for students* (3rd ed.). Boston: Pearson.

Smit, A. (1986). Ages of speech sound acquisition: Comparisons and critiques of several normative studies. *Language, Speech, and Hearing Services in Schools, 17,* 175–186.

Smit, A. B. (1993a). Phonologic error distributions in the Iowa-Nebraska Articulation Norms Project: Word-initial consonant clusters. *Journal of Speech and Hearing Research, 36,* 931–947.

Smit, A. B. (1993b). Phonologic error distributions in the Iowa-Nebraska Articulation Norms Project: Consonant singletons. *Journal of Speech and Hearing Research, 36,* 533–547.

Smit, A. B., & Bernthal, J. E. (1983). Voicing contrasts and their phonological implications in the speech of articulation-disordered children. *Journal of Speech and Hearing Research, 26,* 486–500.

Smit, A. B., Hand, L., Freilinger, J., Bernthal, J., & Bird, A. (1990). The Iowa Articulation Norms Project and its Nebraska replication. *Journal of Speech and Hearing Disorders, 55,* 779–798.

Smith, B. L. (1979). A phonetic analysis of consonant devoicing in children's speech. *Journal of Child Language, 6,* 19–28.

Smith, B. L., Brown-Sweeney, S., & Stoel-Gammon, C. (1989). A quantitative analysis of reduplicated and variegated babbling. *First Language, 9,* 175–189.

Smith, N. V. (1973). *The acquisition of phonology: A case study.* Cambridge: Cambridge University Press.

Snow, C., Burns, S., & Griffin, P. (1998). *Preventing reading difficulties in young children.* National Academy of Sciences—National Research Council. Washington, DC: Commission on Behavioral and Social Sciences and Education (BBB21833).

Snow, D. (1998a). Children's imitations of intonation contours: Are rising tones more difficult than falling tones? *Journal of Speech, Language and Hearing Research, 41,* 576–587.

Snow, D. (1998b). A prominence account of syllable reduction in early speech development: The child's prosodic phonology of tiger and giraffe. *Journal of Speech, Language, and Hearing Research, 41,* 1171–1184.

Snow, D. (2000). The emotional basis of linguistic and nonlinguistic intonation: Implications for hemispheric specialization. *Developmental Neuropsychology, 17,* 1–27.

Snowling, M., Bishop, D., & Stothard, S. (2000). Is preschool language impairment a risk factor for dyslexia? *Journal of Child Psychology and Psychiatry, 41,* 587–600.

Snowling, M., Goulandris, N., & Stackhouse, J. (1994). Phonological constraints on learning to read: Evidence from single case studies of reading difficulty. In C. Hulme & M. Snowling (Eds.), *Reading development and dyslexia* (pp. 86–104). London: Whurr.

Square, P., Martin, N., & Bose, A. (2001). The nature and treatment of neuromotor speech disorders in aphasia. In R. Chapey (Ed.), *Language intervention strategies in aphasia and related neurogenic communication disorders* (pp. 847–884). Baltimore: Lippincott, Williams, & Wilkins.

Stackhouse, J. (1982). An investigation of reading and spelling performance in speech disordered children. *British Journal of Disorders of Communication, 17,* 53–60.

Stackhouse, J. (1993). Phonological disorder and lexical development: Two case studies. *Child Language Teaching and Therapy, 9,* 230–241.

Stackhouse, J. (1997). Phonological awareness: Connecting speech and literacy problems. In B. W. Hodson & M. L. Edwards (Eds.), *Perspectives in applied phonology* (pp. 157–196). Gaithersburg, MD: Aspen.

Stampe, D. (1969). The acquisition of phonetic representation. *Proceedings of the Fifth Regional Meeting of the Chicago Linguistic Circle,* 443–454.

Stampe, D. (1972). On the natural history of diphthongs. *Chicago Linguistic Society* (8th Regional Meeting), 578–590.

Stampe, D. (1973). *A dissertation on natural phonology.* Unpublished doctoral dissertation, University of Chicago.

Stampe, D. (1979). *A dissertation on natural phonology.* New York: Garland.

Stanovich, K. (2000). *Progress in understanding reading: Scientific foundations and new frontiers.* New York: Guilford.

Stark, R. (1980). Stages of speech development in the first year of life. In G. Yeni-Komshian, J. Kavanagh, & C. A. Ferguson (Eds.), *Child phonology: Vol. I. Production* (pp. 73–92). New York: Academic Press.

Stark, R. (1986). Prespeech segmental feature development. In P. Fletcher & M. Garman (Eds.), *Language acquisition. Studies in first language development* (pp. 149–173). Cambridge: Cambridge University Press.

Starr, C. D. (1993). Behavioral approaches to treating velopharyngeal closure and nasality. In K. T. Moller & C. D. Starr (Eds.), *Cleft palate: Interdisciplinary issues and treatment* (pp. 337–356). Austin, TX: PRO-ED.

Stathopoulos, E. T., & Sapienza, C. (1993). Respiratory and laryngeal measures of children during vocal intensity variation. *Journal of the Acoustical Society of America, 94,* 2531–2543.

Steriade, D. (1990). *Greek prosodies and the nature of syllabification.* Doctoral dissertation, Massachusetts Institute of Technology. New York: Garland Press.

Stern, D., & Wasserman, G. (1979). *Maternal language to infants.* Paper presented at a meeting of the Society for Research in Child Development.

Stetson, R. H. (1936). The relation of the phoneme and the syllable. *Proceedings of the Second International Congress of Phonetic Sciences,* 245–254.

Stetson, R. H. (1951). *Motor phonetics: A study of speech movements in action.* Amsterdam: North-Holland.

St. Louis, K. O., & Ruscello, D. M. (2000). Oral speech mechanism screening examination (OSMSE) (3rd ed.). Austin, TX: PRO-ED.

Stockman, I. (1996a). Phonological development and disorders in African American children. In A. Kamhi, K. Pollock, & J. Harris (Eds.), *Communication development and disorders in African American children: Research, assessment, and intervention* (pp. 117–154). Baltimore: P. H. Brookes.

Stockman, I. (1996b). The promises and pitfalls of language sample analysis as an assessment tool for linguistic minority children. *Language, Speech, and Hearing Services in Schools, 27,* 355–366.

Stockman, I. (2007). Chapter 23: African American English speech acquisition. In S. McLeod (Ed.), *The international guide to speech acquisition* (pp. 148–160). Clifton Park, NY: Thomson Delmar Learning.

Stockman, I. J., Woods, D. R., & Tishman, A. (1981). Listener agreement on phonetic segments in early infant vocalizations. *Journal of Psycholinguistic Research, 10,* 593–617.

Stoel-Gammon, C. (1985). Phonetic inventories, 15–24 months: A longitudinal study. *Journal of Speech and Hearing Research, 28,* 505–512.

Stoel-Gammon, C. (1987a). Phonological skills of two-year-olds. *Language, Speech, and Hearing Services in Schools, 18,* 323–329.

Stoel-Gammon, C. (1987b). Language production scale. In L. Olswang, C. Stoel-Gammon, T. Coggins, & R. Carpenter (Eds.), *Assessing prelinguistic and early linguistic behaviors in developmentally young children* (pp. 120–150). Seattle, WA: University of Washington Press.

Stoel-Gammon, C. (1998). Phonological development in Down syndrome. *Mental Retardation and Developmental Disabilities Research Reviews, 3,* 300–306.

Stoel-Gammon, C., & Cooper, J. A. (1984). Patterns of early lexical and phonological development. *Journal of Child Language, 11,* 247–271.

Stoel-Gammon, C., & Dunn, C. (1985). Normal and disordered phonology in children. Baltimore: University Park Press.

Stoel-Gammon, C., & Herrington, P. (1990). Vowel systems of normally developing and phonologically disordered children. *Clinical Linguistics and Phonetics, 4,* 145–160.

Stoel-Gammon, C., & Menn, L. (1997). Phonological development: Learning sounds and sound patterns. In J. Berko Gleason (Ed.), *The development of language* (4th ed., pp. 69–121). Boston: Allyn & Bacon.

Stoel-Gammon, C., & Otomo, K. (1986). Babbling development of hearing-impaired and normally hearing subjects. *Journal of Speech and Hearing Disorders, 51,* 33–41.

Storkel, H. (2001). Learning new words: Phonotactic probability in language development. *Journal of Speech, Language, and Hearing Research, 44,* 1321–1337.

Storkel, H. (2003). Learning new words II: Phonotactic probability in verb learning. *Journal of Speech, Language, and Hearing Research, 46,* 1312–1323.

Storkel, H. (2004). The emerging lexicon of children with phonological delays: Phonotactic constraints and probability in acquisition. *Journal of Speech, Language, and Hearing Research, 47,* 1194–1212.

Storkel, H. L., & Rogers, M. A. (2000). The effect of probabilistic phonotactics on lexical acquisition. *Clinical Linguistics and Phonetics, 14,* 407–425.

Strand, E. A., & Debertine, P. (2000). The efficacy of integral stimulation intervention with developmental apraxia of speech. *Journal of Medical Speech-Language Pathology, 8,* 295–300.

Strand, E. A., & McCauley, R. J. (2008). Differential diagnosis of severe speech impairment in young children, The ASHA Leader. www.asha.org/Publications/leader/2008/080812/f080812a.htm

Strand, E. A., & Skinner, A. (1999). Treatment of developmental apraxia of speech: Integral stimulation methods. In. A. J. Caruso & E. A. Strand (Eds.), *Clinical management of motor speech disorders in children* (pp. 109–148). New York: Thieme.

Subtelny, J. D. (1980). *Speech assessment and speech improvement for the hearing impaired.* Washington, DC: Alexander Graham Bell Association for the Deaf.

Swank, L. (1997). Linguistic influences on the emergence of written word

decoding in first grade. *American Journal of Speech-Language Pathology, 6,* 62–66.

Swift, E., & Rosin, P. (1990). A remediation sequence to improve speech intelligibility for students with Down syndrome. *Language, Speech, and Hearing Services in Schools, 21,* 140–146.

Tallal, P., Stark., R. E., Kallman, C., & Mellits, D. (1980). Perceptual constancy for phonemic categories: A developmental study with normal and language-impaired children. *Applied Psycholinguistics, 1,* 49–64.

Tang, G., & Barlow, J. (2006). Characteristics of the sound system of monolingual Vietnamese-speaking children with phonological impairment. *Clinical Linguistics and Phonetics, 8,* 235–255.

Tanner, D., & Culbertson, W. (1999). *Caregiver-administered communication inventory.* Oceanside, CA: Academic Communication Associates.

Taps Richard, J., & Barlow, J. A. (2011). *Phonological assessment and treatment target selection.* Paper presented at the American Speech-Language-Hearing Association, San Diego, CA.

Templin, M. (1957). *Certain language skills in children: Their development and interrelationships* (Institute of Child Welfare, Monograph No. 26). Minneapolis: University of Minnesota Press.

Terrell, S., & Terrell, F. (1993). African American cultures. In D. Battle (Ed.), *Communication disorders in multicultural populations* (pp. 3–37). Boston: Andover Medical.

Thal, D., Oroz, M., & McCaw, V. (1995). Phonological and lexical development in normal and late-talking toddlers, *Applied Psycholinguistics. 16,* 407–424.

Thelwall, R., & Akram Sa'Adeddin, M. (1999). Arabic. In International Phonetic Association, *Handbook of the International Phonetic Association* (pp. 51–54). Cambridge: Cambridge University Press.

Thurlbeck, W. (1982). Postnatal human lung growth, *Thorax, 37,* 465–571.

To, C. K. S., Cheung, P. S. P., & McLeod, S. (2013). A population study of children's acquisition of Hong Kong Cantonese consonants, vowels, and tones. *Journal of Speech, Language, and Hearing Research, 56,* 103–122.

Toppelberg, C., Shapiro, M., & Theodore, M. (2000). Language disorders: A 10-year research update review.

Journal of the American Academy of Child and Adolescent Psychiatry, 39, 143–152.

Torgesen, J. (2000). Individual differences in response to early interventions in reading: The lingering problem of treatment resisters. *Learning Disabilities Research and Practice, 15,* 55–64.

Torgesen, J., Wagner, R., & Rashotte, C. (1994). Longitudinal studies of phonological processing and reading. *Journal of Learning Disabilities, 27,* 276–286.

Torgesen, J., Wagner, R., Rashotte, C., Burgess, S., & Hecht, S. (1997). Contributions of phonological awareness and rapid automatic naming ability to the growth of word-reading skills in second- to fifth-grade children. *Scientific Studies of Reading, 1,* 161–185.

Torgesen, J., Wagner, R., Simmons, K., & Laughon, P. (1990). Identifying phonological coding problems in disabled readers: Naming counting, or span measures? *Learning Disability Quarterly, 13,* 236–243.

Torneus, M. (1984). Phonological awareness and reading: A chicken and egg problem? *Journal of Educational Psychology, 76,* 1346–1358.

Travis, L., & Rasmus, B. (1931). The speech sound discrimination ability of cases with functional disorders of articulation. *Quarterly Journal of Speech, 17,* 217–226.

Trost-Cardamone, J. E. (1990). The development of speech: Assessing cleft palate misarticulations. In D. A. Kernahan & S. W. Rosenstein (Eds.), *Cleft lip and palate: A system of management* (pp. 227–235). Baltimore: Williams & Wilkins.

Trost-Cardamone, J. E., & Bernthal, J. E. (1993). Articulation assessment procedures and treatment decisions. In K. T. Moller & C. D. Starr (Eds.), *Cleft palate. Interdisciplinary issues and treatment* (p. 307 ff.). Austin, TX: PRO-ED.

Trubetzkoy, N. S. (1931). Gedanken über Morphophonologie. *Travaux du Cercle Linguistique de Prague, 4,* 160 ff.

Trubetzkoy, N. S. (1939/1969). *Grundzüge der Phonologie.* Prague: TCLP, 4.

Trubetzkoy, N. S. (1969). *Principles of phonology.* Berkeley: University of California Press. (Original work published 1939)

Tsao, F.-M., Liu, H.-M., & Kuhl, P. (2004). Speech perception in infancy predicts language development in the 2nd year of life: A longitudinal study. *Child Development, 75,* 1067–1084.

Turk, A., Jusczyk, P., & Gerken, L. (1995). Do English-learning infants use syllable weight to determine stress? *Language and Speech, 38,* 143–158.

Tyler, A., & Haskill, A. M. (2011). Morphosyntax intervention. In A. L. Williams, S. McLeod, & R. J. McCauley (Eds.), *Interventions for speech sound disorders in children.* Baltimore: Paul H. Brookes.

Tyler, A., & Langsdale, T. (1996). Consonant–vowel interactions in early phonological development. *First Language, 16,* 159–191.

Tyler, A., & Tolbert, L. (2002). Speech-language assessment in the clinical setting. *American Journal of Speech-Language Pathology, 11,* 215–220.

Tyler, A., Lewis, K. E., Haskill, A. M., & Tolbert, L. C. (2002). Efficacy and cross-domain effects of a morphosyntax and a phonology intervention. *Language, Speech, and Hearing Services in Schools, 33,* 52–66.

Tyler, A., Lewis, K. E., Haskill, A. M., & Tolbert, L. C. (2003). Outcomes of different speech and language goal attack strategies. *Journal of Speech, Language, and Hearing Research, 46,* 1077–1095.

United States Census Bureau. (2010). *Census 2010.* Washington, D.C.: United States Department of Commerce.

United States Census Bureau (2011) *American Community Survey (ACS), Table B05006, Place of Birth for the Foreign-Born Population.* Washington, D.C.: United States Department of Commerce.

United States Census Bureau, *Statistical Abstract of the United States: 2012* (131st Edition) Washington, DC: United States Department of Commerce. http://www.census.gov/compendia/statab/.

United States Department of Education, Office of English Language Acquisition, Language Enhancement, and Academic Achievement for limited English proficient students (June, 2013) The Biennial Evaluation Report to Congress on the Implementation of the Title III State Formula Grant Program for School Years 2008–2010.

Val Barros, A.-M. (2003). *Pronunciation difficulties in the consonant system experienced by Arabic speakers when learning English after the age of puberty.*

Master's thesis, University of West Virginia, Wheeling.

Van Demark, D. R., & Hardin, M. A. (1990). Speech therapy for the child with cleft lip and palate. In J. Bardach & H. L. Morris (Eds.), *Multidisciplinary management of cleft lip and palate.* Philadelphia: W. B. Saunders.

Van Keulen, J. E., Weddington, G. T., & DeBose, C. E. (1998). *Speech, language, learning, and the African American child.* Boston: Allyn & Bacon.

Van Riper, C. (1939a). Ear training in the treatment of articulation disorders. *Journal of Speech Disorders, IV,* 141–142.

Van Riper, C. (1939b). *Speech correction: Principles and methods.* Englewood Cliffs, NJ: Prentice-Hall.

Van Riper, C. (1978). *Speech correction: Principles and methods* (6th ed.). Englewood Cliffs, NJ: Prentice-Hall.

Van Riper, C., & Emerick, L. (1984). *Speech correction: An introduction to speech pathology and audiology* (7th ed.). Englewood Cliffs, NJ: Prentice-Hall.

Van Riper, C., & Irwin, J. (1958). *Voice and articulation.* Englewood Cliffs, NJ: Prentice-Hall.

Velleman, S. (2003). *Childhood apraxia of speech: Resource guide.* Clifton Park, NY: Thomson Delmar Learning.

Velleman, S., & Strand, K. (1994). Developmental verbal dyspraxia. In J. E. Bernthal & N. W. Bankson (Eds.), *Child Phonology: Characteristics, Assessment, and Intervention with Special Populations* (pp. 110–139). New York: Thieme Medical Publishers, Inc.

Velten, H. (1943). The growth of phonemic and lexical patterns in infant language. *Language, 19,* 281–292.

Vihman, M. M. (1992). Early syllables and the construction of phonology. In C. A. Ferguson, L. Menn, & C. Stoel-Gammon (Eds.), *Phonological development: Models, research, implications* (pp. 393–422). Timonium, MD: York Press.

Vihman, M. M. (2004). Early phonological development. In J. E. Bernthal & N. W. Bankson (Eds.), *Articulation and phonological disorders* (5th ed., pp. 63–112). Boston: Allyn & Bacon.

Vihman, M. M., Ferguson, C. A., & Elbert, M. (1986). Phonological development from babbling to speech: Common tendencies and individual differences. *Applied Psycholinguistics, 7,* 3–40.

Vihman, M. M., & Greenlee, M. (1987). Individual differences in phonological development: Ages one through three years. *Journal of Speech and Hearing Research, 30,* 503–521.

Vihman, M. M., Macken, M. A., Miller, R., Simmons, H., & Miller, J. (1985). From babbling to speech: A reassessment of the continuity issue. *Language, 61,* 397–445.

Waengler, H.-H., & Bauman-Waengler, J. A. (1984). *Phonetische Logopädie, Lieferung 2: S-Lautbildungen und ihre Störungen.* Berlin: Marhold Verlag.

Waengler, H.-H., & Bauman-Waengler, J. A. (1989). *Phonological development of normal and speech/language disordered 4-year-olds.* Paper presented at the national convention of the American Speech-Language-Hearing Association, St. Louis, MO.

Wambaugh, J. L., Duffy, J. R., McNeil, M. R., Robin, D. A., & Rogers, M. (2006). Treatment guidelines for acquired apraxia of speech: Treatment descriptions and recommendations. *Journal of Medical Speech-Language Pathology, 14,* 35–97.

Wambaugh, J., Martinez, A., McNeil, M., & Rogers, M. (1999). Sound production treatment for apraxia of speech: Overgeneralization and maintenance effects. *Aphasiology, 13,* 821–837.

Wambaugh, J. L., Nessler, C., Cameron, R., & Mauszycki, S. (2010). *Effects of repeated practice and practice plus pacing control on sound production accuracy in acquired apraxia of speech.* Presentation at the annual Clinical Aphasiology Conference, Isle of Palms, SC.

Ward, I. (1923). *Defects of speech.* New York: E. P. Dutton.

Washington, J. (1998). *African American English research: A review and future directions.* http://www.rcgd.isr.umich.edu/prba/perspectives/spring1998/jwashington.pdf

Washington, J. A., & Craig, H. K. (1994). Dialectal forms during discourse of poor, urban, African American preschoolers. *Journal of Speech and Hearing Research, 37,* 816–823.

Watkins, R., Rice, M., & Moltz, C. (1993). Verb use by language-impaired and normally developing children. *First Language, 13,* 133–143.

Watson, J. (2002). *The phonology and morphology of Arabic.* Oxford: Oxford University Press.

Webb, J. C., & Duckett, B. (1990). *The RULES phonological evaluation.* Vero Beach, FL: The Speech Bin.

Webster, P. E., & Plante, A. S. (1992). Effects of phonological impairment on word, syllable, and phoneme segmentation and reading. *Language, Speech, and Hearing Services in Schools, 23,* 176–182.

Webster, P. E., Plante, A. S., & Couvillion, L. (1997). Phonologic impairment and prereading: Update on a longitudinal study. *Journal of Learning Disabilities, 30,* 365–375.

Webster, R., Majnemer, A., Platt, R., & Shevell, M. (2005). Motor function at school age in children with a preschool diagnosis of developmental language impairment. *Journal of Pediatrics, 146,* 80–85.

Weiner, F. (1979). *Phonological process analysis.* Baltimore: University Park Press.

Weiner, F. (1981). Treatment of phonological disability using the method of meaningful minimal contrast: Two case studies. *Journal of Speech and Hearing Disorders, 46,* 97–103.

Weiner, F., & Bankson, N. (1978). Teaching features. *Language, Speech, and Hearing Services in Schools, 9,* 29–34.

Weinert, H. (1974). *Die Bekämpfung von Sprechfehlern.* Berlin: VEB Verlag Volk und Gesundheit.

Weismer, G. (1984). Acoustic analysis strategies for the refinement of phonological analysis. In M. Elbert, D. Dinnsen, & G. Weismer (Eds.), Phonological theory and the misarticulating child. ASHA Monographs, 22, pp. 30–52. Rockville, MD: ASHA.

Weismer, G. (1997). The role of stress in language processing and intervention. *Topics in language disorders, 17,* 41–52.

Weiss, C. E., & Lillywhite, H. E. (1981). *Communication disorders* (2nd ed.). St. Louis, MO: C. V. Mosby.

Wellman, B. L., Case, I. M., Mengert, I. G., & Bradbury, D. E. (1931). Speech sounds of young children. *University of Iowa Studies in Child Welfare, 5.* Iowa City: University of Iowa Press.

Wells, B., Peppé, S., & Goulandris, N. (2004). Intonation development from five to thirteen. *Journal of Child Language, 31,* 749–778.

Wells, B., Stackhouse, J., & Vance, M. (1996). A specific deficit in onset-rhyme assembly in a 9-year-old child with speech and literacy difficulties. In T. W. Powell (Ed.), *Pathologies of speech and language: Contributions of clinical phonetics and linguistics.* New Orleans, LA: International Clinical Phonetics and Linguistics Association.

Werker, J., & Fennell, C. (2004). Listening to sounds versus listening to words: Early steps in word learning. In D. Hall & S. Waxman (Eds.), *Weaving a lexicon* (pp. 79–110). Cambridge, MA: MIT Press.

Werker, J., & Tees, R. (2005). Speech perception as a window for understanding plasticity and commitment in language systems of the brain. *Developmental Psychobiology, 46,* 233–251.

Wesseling, R., & Reitsma, P. (2000). The transient role of explicit phonological recoding for reading acquisition. *Journal of Reading and Writing, 13,* 313–336.

West, R., & Ansberry, M. (1968). *The rehabilitation of speech* (4th ed.). New York: Harper & Row.

West, R., Kennedy, L., & Carr, A. (1937). *The rehabilitation of speech.* New York: Harpers.

Whalen, D. H., Levitt, A. G., & Wang, Q. (1991). Intonational differences between reduplicative babbling of French- and English-learning infants. *Journal of Child Language, 18,* 501–516.

Whitehill, T., Francis, A., & Ching, C. (2003). Perception of place of articulation by children with cleft palate and posterior placement. *Journal of Speech, Language, and Hearing Research, 46,* 451–461.

Whitehurst, G., Smith, M., Fischel, J., Arnold, D., & Lonigan, C. (1991). The continuity of babble and speech in children with specific expressive language delay. *Journal of Speech and Hearing Research, 34,* 1121–1129.

Wilcox, K., & Morris, S. (1999). *Children's speech intelligibility measure: CSIM Examiner's manual.* Boston: Pearson.

Wilcox, K. A., Schooling, T. L., & Morris, S. R. (1991). *The preschool intelligibility measure (P-SIM).* Paper presented at the annual convention of the American Speech-Language-Hearing Association, Atlanta, GA.

Williams, A. L. (1991). Generalization patterns associated with training least phonological knowledge. *Journal of Speech and Hearing Research, 34,* 722–733.

Williams, A. L. (1992). *Multiple oppositions: An alternative contrastive therapy approach.* Paper presented at the annual convention of the American Speech-Language-Hearing Association, San Antonio, TX.

Williams, A. L. (2000a). Multiple oppositions: Theoretical foundations for an alternative contrastive intervention approach. *American Journal of Speech-Language Pathology, 9,* 282–288.

Williams, A. L. (2000b). Multiple oppositions: Case studies of variables in phonological intervention. *American Journal of Speech-Language Pathology, 9,* 289–299.

Williams, A. L. (2003). *Speech disorders resource guide for preschool children.* Clifton Park, NY: Thomson Delmar Learning.

Williams, A. L., Epperly, R., Rodgers, J. R., & Feltes, L. (1999). *Treatment efficacy in phonological intervention: Clinical case studies.* Poster session presented at the annual convention of the American Speech-Language-Hearing Association, San Francisco, CA.

Williams, G., & McReynolds, L. (1975). The relationship between discrimination and articulation training in children with misarticulations. *Journal of Speech and Hearing Research, 18,* 401–412.

Winitz, H. (1969). *Articulation acquisition and behavior.* New York: Appleton-Century-Crofts.

Winitz, H. (1975). *From syllable to conversation.* Baltimore: University Park Press.

Winitz, H. (1984). Auditory considerations in articulation training. In H. Winitz (Ed.), *Treating articulation disorders: For clinicians by clinicians.* Baltimore: University Park Press.

Winitz, H. (1989). Auditory considerations in treatment. In N. Creaghead, P. Newman, & W. Secord (Eds.), *Assessment and remediation of articulatory and phonological disorders* (2nd ed., pp. 243–264). New York: Macmillan.

Winitz, H., & Irwin, O. C. (1958). Syllabic and phonetic structure of infants' early words. *Journal of Speech and Hearing Research, 1,* 250–256.

Winitz, H., Sanders, R., & Kort, J. (1981). Comprehension and production of the /əz/ plural allomorph. *Journal of Psycholinguistic Research, 10,* 259–271.

Wise, C. M. (1958). *Introduction to phonetics.* Englewood Cliffs, NJ: Prentice-Hall.

Witzel, M. A. (1995). Communicative impairment associated with clefting. In R. J. Schprintzen & J. Bardach (Eds.), *Cleft palate speech management: A multidisciplinary approach.* St. Louis, MO: Mosby.

Wolfram, W. (1986). Language variation in the United States. In O. Taylor (Ed.), *Treatment of communication disorders in culturally and linguistically diverse populations* (pp. 73–116). San Diego, CA: College-Hill Press.

Wolfram, W. (1989). Structural variability in phonological development: Final nasals in vernacular Black English. In R. Fasold & D. Schiffren (Eds.), *Current issues in linguistic theory: Language change and variation* (pp. 301–332). Amsterdam: John Benjamin.

Wolfram, W. (1994). The phonology of a sociocultural variety: The case of African American Vernacular English. In J. Bernthal & N. Bankson (Eds.), *Child phonology: Characteristics, assessment, and intervention with special populations* (pp. 227–244). New York: Thieme.

Wolfram, W., & Schilling-Estes, N. (2006). *American English: Dialects and variation* (2nd ed.). Malden/Oxford: Blackwell.

Wolk, L., & Meisler, A. (1998). Phonological assessment: A systematic comparison of conversation and picture naming. *Journal of Communication Disorders, 31,* 291–313.

WHO, World Health Organization, *Health Topics 2014.* http://www.who.int/topics/disabilities/en/

Wren, Y., Roulstone, S. and Miller, L. L. (2012). Distinguishing groups of children with persistent speech disorder: findings from a prospective population study. *Logopedics, Phoniatrics and Vocology, 37, 1,* 1–10.

Yearbook of immigration statistics. (2003). U.S. Department of Commerce. Springfield, VA: National Technical Information Service.

Yeni-Komshian, G., Flege, J., & Liu, S. (2000). Pronunciation proficiency in the first and second languages of Korean-English bilinguals. Bilingualism: Language. *Cognition, 3,* 131–150.

Yorkston, K. (1996). Treatment efficacy: Dysarthria. *Journal of Speech and Hearing Research, 39,* S42–S57.

Yorkston, K. M., & Beukelman, D. R. (1981). Communication efficiency of dysarthric speakers as measured by sentence intelligibility and speaking rate. *Journal of Speech and Hearing Disorders, 46,* 296–301.

Young, E. H., & Hawk, S. S. (1955). *Motokinesthetic speech training.* Palo Alto, CA: Stanford University Press.

Zeltner, T., Caduff, J., Gehr, P., Pfenninger, J., & Burri, P. (1987). The postnatal growth and development of the human lung I. *Morphometry Respiratory Physiology, 67,* 247–267.

Zemlin, W. R. (1998). *Speech and hearing science: Anatomy and physiology* (4th ed.). Englewood Cliffs, NJ: Prentice-Hall.

Zentella, A. C. (1997). *Growing up bilingual.* Malden, MA: Blackwell.

Zentella, A. (2000). Puerto Ricans in the United States: Confronting the linguistic repercussions of colonialism. In S. McKay & S. Wong (Eds.), *New immigrants in the United States* (pp. 137–164). Cambridge: Cambridge University Press.

Index